CLINICAL
TUBERCULOSIS

CLINICAL TUBERCULOSIS

Edited by

P.D.O. Davies

Consultant Respiratory Physician, Cardiothoracic Centre,
Liverpool NHS Trust, UK

With a Foreword by John Crofton

CHAPMAN & HALL MEDICAL
London · Glasgow · New York · Tokyo · Melbourne · Madras

Published by Chapman & Hall, 2–6 Boundary Row, London SE1 8HN

Chapman & Hall, 2–6 Boundary Row, London SE1 8HN, UK

Blackie Academic & Professional, Wester Cleddens Road, Bishopbriggs, Glasgow G64 2NZ, UK

Chapman & Hall Inc., One Penn Plaza, 41st Floor, New York NY10119, USA

Chapman & Hall Japan, Thomson Publishing Japan, Hirakawacho Nemoto Building, 6F, 1–7–11 Hirakawa-cho, Chiyoda-ku, Tokyo 102, Japan

Chapman & Hall Australia, Thomas Nelson Australia, 102 Dodds Street, South Melbourne, Victoria 3205, Australia

Chapman & Hall India, R. Seshadri, 32 Second Main Road, CIT East, Madras 600 035, India

First edition 1994

© 1994 Chapman & Hall

Typeset in 10/12pt Palatino by Photoprint, 9–11 Alexandra Lane, Torquay
Printed in Great Britain at the University Press, Cambridge

ISBN 0 412 48630 X

∞ Printed on acid-free text paper, manufactured in accordance with ANSI/NISO Z 39.48–1992 (Permanence of Paper).

the stranger, and the fatherless, and the widow, which are within the gates shall come, and shall eat and be satisfied;

Deuteronomy 14:29

This book is dedicated to the disadvantaged of the world, who are at greatest risk from tuberculosis, in the hope that it may help to improve their expectancy of good health.

CONTENTS

CONTRIBUTORS

J. BANKS
Consultant Physician,
Singleton Hospital,
Swansea SA2 8QA,
UK.

S.L. CHAN
Consultant Chest Physician in Charge,
Tuberculosis and Chest Service,
Department of Health,
Kennedy Road,
Hong Kong.

P.D.O. DAVIES
Director,
Tuberculosis Research Unit,
Cardiothoracic Centre,
Liverpool NHS Trust,
Thomas Drive,
Liverpool L14 3PE,
UK.

R.J. DONNELLY
Consultant Surgeon,
Cardiothoracic Centre,
Thomas Drive,
Liverpool L14 3PE,
UK.

S.W. DOOLEY, Jr
Assistant Director for Science Division of
   Tuberculosis Elimination,
Centers for Disease Control and
   Prevention,
1600 Clifton Road, N.E.,
Mailstop E-10,
Atlanta, GA 30333,
USA.

D.A. ENARSON
Scientific Director,
International Union Against Tuberculosis
   and Lung Disease,
68 Blvd Saint-Michel,
Paris 75006,
France.

C.C. EVANS
Consultant Physician,
Royal Liverpool Hospital,
Prescot Street,
Liverpool L7 8XP,
UK.

E. ANNE FANNING
Division of Infectious Diseases,
University of Alberta 8220,
114 Street,
Edmonton,
Alberta T6G 2J3,
Canada.

P. GODFREY-FAUSSETT
Clinical Lecturer, ZAMBART Project,
Department of Clinical Sciences,
London School of Hygiene and Tropical
   Medicine,
London WC1E 7HT,
UK.

PETRA GRAF
Senior Medical Officer,
Tuberculosis and Leprosy Unit,
Dar-es-Salaam,
PO Box 9083,
Tanzania.

J.M. GRANGE
Reader,
Department of Microbiology,
National Heart and Lung Institute,
Royal Brompton Hospital,
Sydney Street,
London SW3 6NP,
UK.

A.D. HARRIES
Professor,
Department of Medicine,
College of Medicine,
Private Bag 360,
Chichiri Blantyre 3,
Malawi,
Central Africa.

M.J. HUMPHRIES
Medical Director,
Roche Asian Research Foundation,
PO Box 98593, Tsimshatsui,
Hong Kong.
Formerly Consultant Physician,
Ruttonjee Sanatorium,
Hong Kong.

P.A. JENKINS
Director,
Mycobacterium Reference Unit,
Public Health Laboratory Service,
University Hospital of Wales,
Heath,
Cardiff CF4 4XW,
UK.

W.K. LAM
Reader in Medicine,
University of Hong Kong;
Physician in Charge,
Cardiorespiratory Section,
University Department of Medicine,
Queen Mary Hospital,
Hong Kong.

A.G. LEITCH
Consultant Physician,
City Hospital,
Greenbank Drive,
Edinburgh EH10 5SB.
Honorary Senior Lecturer,
Department of Medicine,
University of Edinburgh,
UK.

R.J. O'BRIEN
Medical Officer,
Tuberculosis Programme,
Division of Communicable Diseases,
World Health Organization,
1211 Geneva 27,
Switzerland.

S.J. OPPENHEIMER
Professor and Chairman,
Paediatric Department,
Floor 6F,
Clinical Sciences Building,
Prince of Wales Hospital,
Shatin,
Hong Kong.

L.P. ORMEROD
Consultant Physician,
Blackburn Royal Infirmary,
Blackburn,
BB2 3LR,
UK.

H.L. RIEDER
Federal Officer of Public Health,
Division of Epidemiology and Infectious
   Disease,
Hess-Str. 27E,
3097 Liebfeld,
Switzerland;
and
International Union Against Tuberculosis
   and Lung Disease,
68 Blvd Saint-Michel,
Paris 75006,
France.

ANNIK ROUILLON
Executive Director (Emeritus),
International Union Against Tuberculosis
   and Lung Disease,
68 Blvd Saint-Michel,
Paris 75006,
France.

R.J. SHAW
Senior Lecturer and Honorary Consultant,
Chest and Allergy Clinic,
St Mary's Hospital,
London W2 1NY,
UK.

E.A. SHEFFIELD
Senior Lecturer and Honorary Consultant
   Pathologist,
Department of Histopathology,
Bristol Royal Infirmary,
Marlborough Street,
Bristol BS2 8HW,
UK.

PATRICIA M. SIMONE
Medical Officer,
Division of Tuberculosis Elimination,
Centers for Disease Control and
   Prevention,
1600 Clifton Road, N.E.,
Mailstop E-10,
Atlanta, GA 30333,
USA.

P.G. SMITH
Professor of Tropical Epidemiology,
London School of Hygiene and Tropical
   Medicine,
London WC1E 7HT,
UK.

R. TEOH
CNS Department,
Clinical R&D,
Sandoz Pharma,
CH4002 Basle,
Switzerland.

E.G.L. WILKINS
Consultant Physician,
Regional Infectious Diseases Unit,
Monsall Hospital,
Newton Heath,
Manchester M10 8WR,
UK.

CERIDWEN S.D. WILLIAMS
Tuberculosis Health Visitor,
Liverpool and South Sefton Community,
Sefton General Hospital,
Smithdown Road,
Liverpool L15 2HE,
UK.

P.A. WINSTANLEY
Senior Lecturer,
Department of Pharmacology and
   Therapeutics,
University of Liverpool,
Liverpool L69 3BX,
UK.

G.W.K. WONG
Lecturer,
Paediatric Department,
c/o S.J. Oppenheimer,
Floor 6F,
Clinical Sciences Building,
Prince of Wales Hospital,
Shatin,
Hong Kong.

FOREWORD

It is a sad reflection on society's incompetence that, more than thirty years after the methods for cure and prevention were evolved and before the advent of the HIV epidemic, there were already more patients with active tuberculosis in the world than there had been in the 1950s. This was because, over the years, prevalence rates in developing countries had only slightly diminished while, at the same time, their populations had substantially increased. But in recent years there has been an additional and tragic factor. The HIV pandemic has resulted in an explosion of tuberculosis in a number of African countries, adding a grim and tragic dimension to an already challenging problem. Asia and Latin America are similarly threatened.

Even in a number of previously complacent developed countries there has been a reversal of the previously steady downward trend. The causes of this are not always clear. Among these are probably the effect of increasing immigration from high prevalence countries and, at least in some countries such as the USA, the effects of HIV in diminishing resistance to the disease.

Another alarming development is the emergence of multiply-resistant tubercle bacilli. In some countries this is due to previous neglect of the treatment services which resulted in the use of unsatisfactory drug combinations. In others it is due to careless or unscrupulous treatment, either by private medical practitioners or even by those without training in Western medicine. In some places poor quality drugs may be responsible. The potential emergence on a large scale of untreatable tuberculosis, particularly lethal in those infected with HIV, is a nightmare prospect, sadly foreshadowed in certain outbreaks in the USA as described in this book.

On the more optimistic side, there have been considerable advances. In most developed countries, until relatively recently, the classical preventive and therapeutic measures had been effectively applied, with consequent impressive falls in the disease. Unfortunately in some, this had led to complacency with resulting deficiencies in service and consequent resurgence of this disease.

In many developing countries, lack of resource – and often lack of government will – had resulted in failure to develop effective programmes to control the disease. These might exist on paper but were seldom implemented in practice. The British Medical Research Council had pioneered relatively effective and practical therapeutic regimens, but these failed to the systematically applied on a large scale. However, in the last ten years the International Union against Tuberculosis and Lung Disease (IUATLD), under the inspiration and leadership of Karel Styblo and Annik Rouillon, has demonstrated in some of the world's poorest countries that the job could be done. This was achieved through the commitment of the relevant government, the emergence of highly effective local leaders and by applying intensive training and supervision in implementing the National Tuberculosis Control Programme through routine health services. Some external finance was provided through bilateral aid negotiated by IUATLD. Effective control was beginning to be achieved in a number of poor countries when the HIV epidemic struck. In many African countries the burden of tuberculosis has now vastly increased. At the time of writing, this challenge is just being met in the supported countries but we watch with bated breath.

After examining the IUATLD-assisted programmes, the World Bank concluded that these were among the most cost-effective health measures which could be applied worldwide. Consequently the World Health Organization, with World Bank and other support, is now seeking to help countries to implement such programmes along the lines pioneered by IUALTD. Hopefully Asian countries will have their control programmes in place before the HIV epidemic explodes, but time is dangerously short.

This global emergency, now threatening even previously complacent prosperous countries, has resulted in a resurgence of medical interest in tuberculosis. In developed countries many of those made familiar with the clinical aspects during the time when tuberculosis was common have now retired. Peter Davies and his colleagues are therefore to be congratulated on producing a substantial volume which will be of great value to doctors who have had less experience of the disease.

The book is comprehensive and very well referenced. Although particularly valuable to doctors in developed countries, it also addresses the different and difficult problems of developing countries and the complexities of the HIV–tuberculosis interaction.

Everyone concerned with tuberculosis will be grateful for this much needed reference book.

John Crofton

PREFACE

It is 40 years since the last standard textbook on tuberculosis was published in this country[1]. Sir John Crofton and his colleagues have stolen a march on the rest of the world with the publication of their paperback, with the same title as this book, intended for workers in the developing world[2]. With this exception the most recent book on tuberculosis, published in the UK, is not a textbook at all but a potential bestseller written in the style of a thriller[3].

Even without the current increase in cases of tuberculosis, which is occurring in many countries, it would have been time for a new textbook on the subject. However, the increase in cases has sent those working in the field of tuberculosis – clinicians, public health workers, laboratory workers and researchers alike – scurrying to the libraries to look for suitable books only to find the shelves empty.

The reasons for the increase in cases of tuberculosis are still under investigation. HIV-related disease is undoubtedly a major factor in many developing countries and in some developed countries, particularly the USA. However, other factors probably make an appreciable contribution, particularly immigration and an increasing level of social deprivation in some inner city areas of the developed world. Substantial and permanent unemployment is now unfortunately a feature of most national economies. Associated with this is a smaller but tangible population of homeless or temporarily housed, who, because of poor diet and living conditions, are probably contributing to the increase of disease. Whatever the causes of the increase there is now a clear and desparate need for new and authoritative works on tuberculosis.

This book attempts to fill the gap by providing a comprehensive and synoptic account of tuberculosis with up-to-date information on all aspects of the disease. It aims to provide a practical guide on the management of tuberculosis for health workers who may be involved with any aspect of patient management or disease control. It will also provide a source of reference to the doctor in training and interested student. It provides fully referenced chapters on aspects of epidemiology, microbiology, diagnosis and treatment of disease. The more recent problems of tuberculosis are also comprehensively covered, particularly those of disease control and management in immigrants, drug resistance and disease in HIV-infected individuals. Disease prevention and control in both the developed and the developing world is included. A separate section deals with newer methods of diagnosis, such as serological and polymerase chain reaction techniques, not yet available for service work, but which may become standard procedures in the not too distant future.

Each chapter is intended to stand on its own, so that some overlap between chapters is inevitable. Where there is controversy, such as whether prevention of disease in a population is best provided by BCG vaccination or chemotherapy, both sides of the argument are presented. The emergence of HIV-related disease in the developed world has meant that environmental mycobacteria are of increasing importance and so a chapter relevant to this problem is included. The small but important place of animals as a possible vector is also covered. It is perhaps a sad fact but, because of the emergence of multi-drug resistant organisms, surgery once again plays a small but vital role in the treatment of disease. Any coverage of treatment would therefore be incomplete without a section on this aspect.

It is surely a coincidence that the rise of tuberculosis world wide occurred at approximately the same time as the retirement of some of the great names in the research of disease. Within the United Kingdom, Professor Wallace Fox, Professor Denis Mitchison, who are synonymous with short-course chemotherapy, and Dr Ian Sutherland, whose name is inevitably linked with BCG studies, have all retired within the space of a few years. In the international field, Professor Karol Styblo and Doctor Annik Rouillon from the International Union Against Tuberculosis and Lung Disease, have also retired, leaving an enormous gap in expertise and experience to be filled by aspiring newcomers to the scene. To some extent the authorship of this book represents these newly aspiring men and women.

In addition to the retirement of many great names in tuberculosis, the 1980s also saw a dramatic decline in world wide interest and a consequent decrease in funding for tuberculosis research. Some of the resurgence of disease may indeed be due to this neglect, which is only now being corrected. The recent decision of the Chest, Heart and Stroke Association (CHSA) of England to form itself into a purely Stroke Association has resulted in a loss of potential funding of research into tuberculosis in this country. This is particularly sad when it is remembered that the CHSA was originally founded in the last century as the National Association for the Prevention of Tuberculosis. A large proportion of its funds will presumably have been donated specifically towards research into tuberculosis but are now not available for this purpose. Organizations researching specifically into tuberculosis have also seen hard times. The International Union Against Tuberculosis and Lung Disease has seen a number of its national members resign, with consequent loss of funding, and here again the UK contribution, formerly provided by the CHSA, has been lost.

The pressure in academic circles to appoint to research posts, individuals who can attract large grants, has meant, until very recently, a complete absence of appointments in most parts of the world of those interested in tuberculosis research. Researchers in some countries have been lured away from research into tuberculosis by more lucrative research projects available for such diseases as asthma, where pharmaceutical monies are readily available. All this has meant a contraction in the available workforce for research into tuberculosis. Many postgraduate centres specializing in research, teaching and management of respiratory disease now have no research workers or clinicians with a track record in tuberculosis. Indeed it seems to be more by good luck than good management that there is any expertise left in tuberculosis in many developed countries today.

But the greatest tragedy of all, in terms of loss to the world of tuberculosis expertise, has been the closure of the Medical Research Council's Tuberculosis and Chest Diseases Unit, which over several decades has been the driving force behind the development of short-course chemotherapy in the treatment of tuberculosis and its adopted use throughout the world. The closure of this unit and the enforced move of the individuals concerned to other research, is not only a tragic waste, but represents perhaps the greatest blow during the 1980s to the fight against tuberculosis. Even if new drugs are now discovered, which are effective against *M. tuberculosis*, the world has effectively lost its most powerful mechanism to test the efficacy of these drugs in clinical trials. If one wished to find a symbol of the way the developed world has turned its back on the problems of disease in the developing world, which had seen little change in the incidence of disease among its people, then this closure would perhaps be the most poignant.

However, many of the developing nations have not been entirely consistent in their attack on tuberculosis. They too have been distracted by high technology medicine in directions they could ill afford, to the detriment of providing finance for rifampicin-containing short-course chemotherapy in the fight against tuberculosis.

Often it is only the old and poorly serviced hospitals that are available for sufferers from tuberculosis, while the modern, better equipped hospitals are reserved for patients with more 'interesting' conditions. Medical and nursing staff employed to care for tuberculosis patients in these poorer facilities inevitably suffer from low morale and a feeling of being marginalized, just as their patients have been.

It can only be hoped that other organizations may see fit to take up the challenge which the British MRC has chosen to let fall. I hope this book will stimulate individuals and organizations to provide the resources required to help to stamp out this disease which remains the world's commonest cause of morbidity and mortality caused by a single microbe.

In editing this book I am most grateful to many people who have taken the trouble to read and provide constructive comment on manuscripts. Specifically I would like to thank Sir John Crofton and Dr Norman Horne in this respect. I am also very grateful to my secretary Miss Nicola Moon for all the help she has given in the organization of the book and the mountain of secretarial work associated with it.

REFERENCES

1. Keers, R.Y., Ridgen, B.G. and Young, F.H. (1953) *Pulmonary Tuberculosis: a Handbook for Students and Practitioners*, E & S Livingstone, Edinburgh.
2. Crofton, J., Horne, N. and Miller, F. (1992) *Clinical Tuberculosis*. Macmillan, London.
3. Ryan, F. (1992) *Tuberculosis: The Greatest Story Never Told*, Swift, Bromsgrove.

C.C. Evans

Tuberculosis is at least as old as mankind, and the history of the disorder is intertwined inevitably with the history of civilization. Like no other illness, tuberculosis has taken its toll of human life over the millennia, and has spread literally world wide. It is thought to be the oldest of human diseases, which has waxed and waned in its incidence, but has remained a perpetual threat, often in the background without, at least until the present links with AIDS, producing the dramatic epidemics associated with smallpox, plague or cholera. Its worldwide incidence and prevalence has never really been established, but in Europe in the eighteenth century, John Bunyan[1] referred to tuberculosis as the 'Captain of all these Men of Death' and a century later, Oliver Wendell Holmes[2] described tuberculosis as the 'white plague'.

The disease has not only been inseparable from man's progress, but it has been impossible to disentangle the medical issues from the economic and social life of the community. Tuberculosis has been the natural meeting ground for many medical disciplines, including general practitioner, physician, community physician, surgeon, pathologist, microbiologist, radiologist, pharmacologist and medical officer of public health, all of whom with suitable cooperation have been able to benefit both the patient and the community. In the twentieth century, the disease has been the launching pad for the specialties of thoracic medicine and surgery and numerous thoracic societies, and the management

and treatment of the disorder has demonstrated perhaps above all other conditions, the necessity for, and benefits of, clinical trials and structured research.

1.1 ORIGINS OF MYCOBACTERIA

Mycobacteria are believed to be amongst the oldest bacteria on earth, and are ubiquitous in the environment. They are free-living organisms to be found in soil, animal dung, salt and fresh water, mud flats and attached to algae and grasses. They are potentially pathogenic to many animals, including cattle and pigs as well as fish and reptiles.

It has been speculated that cattle were the source of human tuberculosis infection, and that *M. tuberculosis* was a mutant of *M. bovis*, which has a broad host range capable of infecting man and several other species, whereas *M. tuberculosis* is pathogenic only to man and not at all to cattle[3]. Interestingly, cattle first became domesticated in the Neolithic period[4], and studies of human skeletons from that time suggest that Pott's disease, showing collapse and anterior fusion of adjacent mid–thoracic vertebra, represents compelling evidence but not unequivocal proof, of such a hypothesis. The relatively recent finding of acid- and alcohol-fast bacilli in human remains comes from human skeletons in Heidelberg, Germany, dating back to 5000 BC (Fig. 1.1)[5]. Similar proof has been obtained from Egyptian mummies from around 3500 BC[6]. Other examples of prehis-

Clinical Tuberculosis. Edited by P.D.O. Davies. Published in 1994 by Chapman & Hall, London. ISBN 0 412 48630 X

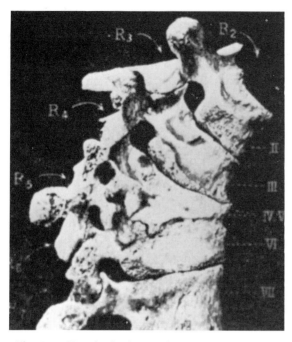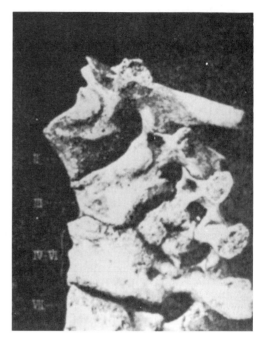

Fig. 1.1   Vertebral column of neolithic skeleton from Heidelberg demonstrating collapse of 4th thoracic vertebra and fusion with 5th. (Reproduced with kind permission from A.S. Lyons and R.J. Petrocelli, *Medicine: An Illustrated History*, Published by N. Abrams, 1987.)

toric skeletal tuberculosis include a Jordanian bronze age skeleton from 3000 BC[7] and a Nesperehan mummy from 1000 BC which revealed not only Pott's disease of the spine, but a psoas abscess[8]. Scandinavian skeletons illustrating Pott's disease have been found in Denmark from about 2000 BC[5] whereas the first UK skeletons are from 200–400 AD[4]. Similar proof of infection has been discovered in Southern Peru from about 700 AD[9], but the first descriptions in North America on skeletal remains were all after Columbus. Similarly, there has been no recorded evidence of tuberculosis in South Africa, Australia or New Zealand prior to colonization.

1.2 TUBERCULOSIS IN ART AND LITERATURE

The Egyptians left many hunchbacks on Dynastic tomb inscriptions of about 3500 BC,

but it cannot be proven whether these are evidence of skeletal tuberculosis or, in view of their abundant presence, mere stylistic art conventions of that culture (Fig. 1.2). It should be noted, however, that the hunchbacks of the early Egyptian Dynastic period are truly angular deformities, whereas the hunchbacked flute players of early prehistoric American art have smooth, rounded deformities, and cannot be accepted as proof of pre-Columbian American tuberculosis (Fig. 1.3)[8].

Early physicians diagnosed disorders on the basis of symptoms and superficial signs, and clearly lacked the precision of diagnosis afforded by modern techniques. Moreover, symptoms of tuberculosis are not always precise, nor confined to a single organ, so that the historian must be aware of the alternative terms used to describe various tuberculous organ disorders and their differential diagnosis that might be attributed to those symptoms and signs (Table 1.1).

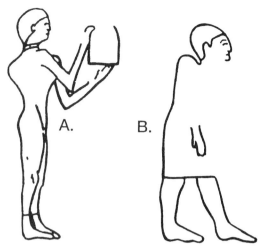

Fig. 1.2 Egyptian tomb inscriptions demonstrating hunchback figures: Dynastic period. (Reproduced with kind permission from D. Morse, D.R. Brothwell and P.J. Ucko, Tuberculosis in Ancient Egypt, *Am. Rev. Respir. Dis.*, 1964,1590, 528)

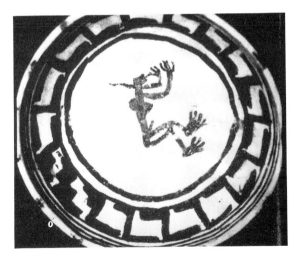

Fig. 1.3 Kokopelli – hunchbacked flute player shown on pottery bowl of Great Pueblo Period 1300 AD. (Reproduced with kind permission from K.F. Wellmann, Kokopelli of Indian Paleology, *J. Am. Med. Assoc.*, 1970, **212**, 1680.)

Egyptian medical papyri refer to cases of cervical lymphadenopathy in the Ebers papyri[10] and tuberculous scrofula might easily be the cause. Chinese writings of 2700 BC describe lung fever and lung cough, which, coupled with the expectoration of blood and sputum and generalized wasting, is strongly suggestive of pulmonary tuberculosis[11]. The Sanskrit writers of 1500 BC were clearly familiar with pulmonary tuberculosis, and the Rig-Veda is an original surviving record. Mesopotamian writings of 675 BC are more suggestive of pulmonary tuberculosis[12] and there are no descriptions to be found in the Old or New Testaments of the Bible.

Greek literature contains numerous references to conditions resembling consumption, including those by Homer (800 BC), Hippocrates (460–377 BC)[12], who probably introduced the term phthisis, Aristotle (384–322 BC), who recognized the contagious nature of the disorder[13], and Plato (430–347 BC), who recommended no treatment because caring for chronic tuberculotic patients was of no advantage to the patient or the state[13]. Galen (131–200 AD), practising in Rome, noticed how contagious phthisis was, and that bronchial obstruction could result in the expectoration of calcified bodies in the sputum[13]. Vegetius (420 AD) remarked that animals were victims of consumption, as well as man. Aretaeus, whose precise dates of living are not known, wrote a classical description of advanced tuberculosis in his book entitled 'On the causes and symptoms of chronic diseases'[14].

The Arabic physicians Rhazes (Al Razi 850–953) and Avicenna (Ibn Sina 980–1037) linked lung cavities with skin ulceration and wrote like the early Greeks, on the benefits to be had of dry air, good food and the potential curability of the disorder. These two Arabic physicians anticipated finding tuberculosis in young people aged 18–30 years with narrow chests and a thin body. At about the same time, Al-Majousi described clubbing of the finger and toe nails[15].

Table 1.1 Historical terms used to describe tuberculosis and other possible causes of that condition

Tuberculosis	Historical synonym	Differential diagnosis
1 Acute progressive	Galloping consumption	Neoplasms and diabetes mellitus
2 Pulmonary	Consumption Phthisis Tabes pulmonali Tissic Hectic fever Gastric fever Asthenia	Bronchial neoplasm Rheumatic and congenital heart disease Pneumonia Lung abscess Empyema
3 Cervical adenopathy	Scrofula Stroma King's Evil	Lymphoma Sarcoidosis Malignancy Syphilis
4 Abdominal	Tabes mesenterica	Colonic neoplasm Crohn's disease Appendix abscess
5 Skin	Lupus vulgaris	CDLE
6 Meningitis	Acute hydrocephalus Infantile encephalitis	Bacterial meningitis Encephalitis
7 Vertebral	Pott's disease	Bacterial spinal abscess Hereditary degenerations

Source: H.M. Coovadia and S.R. Benatar, *A Century of Tuberculosis*, Oxford University Press, 1991, Tables 1.1 and 1.2.

1.3 RENAISSANCE PATHOLOGY

During the Middle Ages, there was no record of the incidence of tuberculosis, although the Montpellier physician Arnold of Villanova (1235–1312) noted that scrofulous patients always had alternative sources of infection within them, and recommended that there was no purpose in operating externally[16]. The healing touch of the monarch was restricted to tuberculosis of the neck glands, and records show that Edward I touched 533 victims in one month, and Philip of Valois (1328–50) put the king's hand on 1500 scrofula cases at a single ceremony[17]. These achievements were insignificant when compared with the 92 102 scrofulous patients on whom Charles II bestowed the royal touch[18].

By 1650, consumption was a leading cause of mortality recorded in London's Bills of Mortality, and there were references in Shakespeare's plays, such as 'the consumptive lover' in *Much Ado About Nothing* and scrofula in *Macbeth*.

Paracelcus (1490–1541) wrote of miners' phthisis[19] and Frascatorius (1483–1553) postulated the existence of imperceptible particles as the cause of the disease some 300 years ahead of the microbiological discovery[17]. By now, pathological dissection was contributing to physicians' understanding of the 'great killer', and Sylvius in Leyden (1614–72) correlated the development of tubercles with various symptoms[20], and at roughly the same time Thomas Willis (1621–75) appreciated that systemic manifestations attributable to consumption must result from internal lung ulceration[21]. Richard Morton (1637–98) described many pathological tuberculous features and gave sound advice about the prevention of phthisis, including the enjoyment of 'an open fresh and kindly air'[22].

Morgagni (1682–1771) believed that there were many potential causes for phthisis[18], but Desault in Bordeaux (1675–1737) believed that the disease was spread by infected sputum[23] – an opinion to be shared by Stark (1741–70)[24].

1.4 FRENCH CLINICAL EXAMINATION

It was Auenbrugger (1722–1809) who originally described the technique of clinical percussion in Austria[25], but it required Corvisart (1775–1821) in Paris to rediscover the technique during the golden age of French medicine[26]. It was he who taught Laennec (1781–1826) who subsequently invented the stethoscope, thereby permitting him to correlate physical findings with pathological dissected states, which had been taught to him by Bayle (1774–1816)[27]. There were opponents to the infective concept of tuberculosis however, and Virchow (1821–1902) asserted in the nineteenth century that phthisis was hereditary[28], whereas Southern Europeans in Italy, Spain and the South of France, centred around Montpellier, came to regard tuberculosis as infectious. Indeed, in the Italian Republic of Lucca in 1699, physicians were instructed to give notice to the Council of the names of patients suspected as suffering from tuberculosis, and Ferdinand VI in Spain introduced tuberculosis notification[29]. In Naples in 1782 it was mandatory to destroy the clothing of a patient dying of tuberculosis, but such foresight into prophylaxis was not sustained, and was lost until Koch's wonderful discoveries in 1882[30].

1.5 BACTERIOLOGY

In Northern Europe, in Britain, France and Germany, the notion existed that tuberculosis was indeed hereditary, and that one inherited the tuberculous diathesis. This so-called eugenic theory was smashed by Villemin (1827–92) who, in 1865, transmitted tuberculosis from man to rabbit by inoculation of tuberculous material, and subsequently from cow to rabbit, when the transmitted disease was much more severe[16].

In Berlin in 1882 Robert Koch (1843–1910) described the tubercle bacillus. Earlier, in his country practice in Wolstein, he had discovered the anthrax bacillus, and laid down his bacteriological postulates. Using aniline dyes and an oil immersion microscope, he was able to identify the tubercle bacillus in every lesion in the human or animal victim, he was able to culture the bacillus outside the body, and when he inoculated the bacillus into an experimental animal, it produced tuberculous lesions. Henceforth, searching for the bacillus in the sputum of suspected cases quickly became standard clinical practice[30].

Koch considered initially that there was no difference between human and bovine tubercle bacilli, but in 1898 Theobald Smith in Harvard showed that there were microscopic, morphological and toxic differences between the various bacilli[31]. In all, five varieties of tubercle bacilli have been distinguished, and these are human, bovine, avian, murine and piscine. The human bacillus is now thought to account for 98% of cases of pulmonary tuberculosis spread by droplet infection by coughing and sneezing, and 70% of non-pulmonary forms. Bovine infection was commonly acquired by drinking infected milk or, rarely, by eating infected beef. Bovine infection is related to the non-pulmonary forms of the condition such as cervical lymphadenopathy, intestinal and abdominal tuberculosis, bone and joint disease, skin infections and tuberculous meningitis, especially seen in children.

1.6 RADIOGRAPHIC DISCOVERY

In 1896 Röntgen (1845–1923) announced the discovery of X-rays, which technique was quickly applied to disorders of the chest and tuberculosis in particular. In time, but sadly not immediately, this advance in diagnostic achievement was to revolutionize the management of tuberculosis.

1.7 PUBLIC ATTITUDES

In the early nineteenth century, during the time of these pivotal pioneering and scientific discoveries, the incidence of tuberculosis was increasing in Europe and the United States, although precise figures are lacking. It has been estimated that 30% of all deaths under 50 years of age in Europe could have been attributed to tuberculosis. Death certification became mandatory in the UK in 1838, although tuberculosis mortality was probably underestimated because of the reluctance of relatives and friends to have the death so registered because of the stigma attached to the disease. Such a stigma reflected the public notion that tuberculosis was an inherited weakness, and as such might interfere with potential marriage and employment of other relatives.

1.8 COLONIZATION

The hereditary theory of tuberculosis historically gained credence because of the apparent increased susceptibility of various ethnic groups consequent upon their first exposure to infected people as a result of colonization, mainly from Europe. The so-called virgin population concept has been seen in the native populations of North America (American Indians)[32], South Africa (Africans)[33], Australia (Aborigines)[34], New Zealand (Maoris)[34] and Papua New Guinea[34], in which the natives developed a higher incidence and more severe form of consumption than the colonizers. Such a concept permitted the colonizers to explain the increased mortality due to tuberculosis in the natives rather than to admit that the changes they had induced in the natives' environment played

any role in the development of the fatal scourge. It was the colonizers who brought the disease to the native population, not only in the nineteenth century, but as early as the Mayflower pilgrims in 1620[32] (Chapter 10, p. 191).

1.9 MIGRATION

European migration in the nineteenth century was also responsible for an increased incidence of tuberculosis. As a result of the Irish potato famine, many Irish immigrants settled in Boston, Massachusetts[35], and Liverpool, England, but smaller epidemics brought about by immigration were described, such as the Outer Hebrideans entering the city of Glasgow. Migration not only occurred for economic reasons, but tuberculous victims were deliberately encouraged to migrate and move to regions where their chances of recovery would be enhanced by allegedly favourable environmental circumstances. Thus, many Europeans with tuberculosis were tempted to travel to the fashionable, sunny, Alpine resorts of Davos and Leysin in Switzerland, Cape Town in South Africa[36], Melbourne in Australia[34], and Colorado in the USA[37].

1.10 SOCIOECONOMIC DEPRIVATION

It is now believed that the common explanation for the increased incidence of tuberculosis both in the colonized and the immigrants is the socioeconomic decline suffered by these groups. Loss of land by natives in colonized countries not only led to overcrowding, but also to loss of valuable food sources. Severe overcrowding during the European industrial revolution in the seventeenth and eighteenth centuries, caused many people to be living in appalling conditions that were dark, damp and congested. Such people were invariably underfed. Whole families lived in rooms no more than 3 m^2 in urban squalor, where they would also be exposed to high doses

Table 1.2 Famous victims of tuberculosis

Henry Purcell	1659–1695	Composer
Voltaire	1694–1778	Philosopher
Sir Walter Scott	1776–1832	Romantic poet and novelist
Niccolo Paganini	1782–1840	Violinist
Percy Bysshe Shelley	1792–1822	Poet
John Keats	1795–1821	Poet
Elizabeth Barrett Browning	1806–1861	Poet
Edgar Allan Poe	1809–1841	Writer
Frederic Chopin	1810–1849	Composer
Charlotte Brontë	1816–1855 ⎫	
Emily Brontë	1818–1848 ⎬	Writers
Anne Brontë	1820–1849 ⎭	
Fyodor Mehailovich Dostoevsky	1821–1881	Writer
Edvard Grieg	1843–1907	Composer
Robert Louis Stevenson	1850–1894	Writer
Anton Chekhov	1860–1904	Playwright
Amadeo Modigliani	1884–1920	Painter
D.H. Lawrence	1885–1930	Writer
Katherine Mansfield	1888–1922	Writer
Joseph Boynton Priestley	1894–1984	Writer
George Orwell	1903–1950	Writer

Source: H.M. Coovadia and S.R. Benatar, A Century of Tuberculosis, Oxford University Press, 1991, Table 1.3.

of infective and infected sputum. In the USA, Trudeau (1848–1915) demonstrated in rabbits the significance of such deprivation. He inoculated ten rabbits with a similar dose of tubercle bacilli setting five free and confining the other five to a damp, sunless existence, and given a poor diet. When those who had been set free were subsequently captured and sacrificed, their bodies showed features of healing from their inoculation, but those confined all died of tuberculosis[38]. A similar intriguing observation linking social deprivation with an increased incidence of tuberculosis was seen in European Jews during the Second World War. Ashkenazim and Sephardim European Jews have been thought traditionally to have a large racial resistance to tuberculosis, but during Jewish persecution, their tuberculosis mortality exceeded that of Gentiles, having hitherto been substantially less[29]. The increase in tuberculosis during the Second World War in Northern Europe has been attributed more to nutritional shortages than overcrowding and housing loss.

1.11 FAMOUS VICTIMS

Many doctors, physicians and pathologists died of tuberculosis, including notably Laennec and Trudeau. Many doctors who survived the disease were to work in sanatoria, and to take up thoracic medicine and surgery as a career. Many famous people suffered and died from tuberculosis, and until this century, the disease was thought to confer a creative energy and skill termed by the Greeks as 'spes phthisica'. No such real association is now thought to exist, and it is not surprising that a disorder accounting for up to one-third of deaths should have affected so many people; millions of less famous people were also victims, but for completeness a list of known creative tuberculotic patients is shown in the Table 1.2.

1.12 CATTLE AS A SOURCE OF INFECTION

At the start of the twentieth century, the elimination of infected milk at source was inaugurated, but not until Koch had acknowledged that there was indeed a difference in the bacilli. Such public health measures were shown to very good effect in the USA from 1917 when there was a dramatic decline in non-pulmonary causes of tuberculosis[35]. In Europe, however, where most forms of the disease were, and are, due to pulmonary tuberculosis, the elimination of infected cattle was not associated with any significant reduction in overall tuberculous mortality.

1.13 MEDICAL MANAGEMENT

Reference has been made already to Hippocratic teaching in which the humoral inbalance of blood, phlegm, yellow bile and black bile required to be corrected for the restoration of health. This was thought to be achieved by venesection or the application of leeches, emetics and aperients, and induction of skin ulceration by blistering agents.

While no fresh air was recommended as a treatment in the Middle Ages, Sydenham extolled the virtues of fresh air taken while riding on horseback or travelling in an open-air carriage. The antiphlogistic therapy of venesection, emetics and purgation continued. All sorts and manners of dietary manipulations were attempted without any proven success. These consisted of the consumption in excess or avoidance of, milk, beef, tea, coffee, cocoa, alcohol and even tobacco: the application locally of ham fat was recommended by some. Laennec surrounded his patients with seaweed from the Brittany coasts. Drugs such as laudanum, digitalis, antimonicals, cod liver oil and astringents were all fashionable at one time or another[16].

1.14 SANATORIA AND NAPT

The sanatorium era lasted almost 100 years. The concept of such an institution was originated by George Bodington of Sutton Coldfield, who, in 1840, with remarkable perspicacity, urged that the tuberculous patient should be in an airy house in the country, which, if on an eminence, so much the better[39]. The neighbourhood should be dry and high, the soil of a light loam, the atmosphere free of damp and fogs, and the cold never too severe to breathe in from the open air. Exercise was encouraged, and the physical well-being sustained with a good diet and generous wine. Bodington's principles of treatment were not favoured in the UK initially however, but were taken up in Germany in particular. The first sanatorium was opened there by Brehmer in Silesia in 1859[40], and this was to be followed by his former patient Dettweiler in Falkenstein. It was here that rest periods in the open air gained popularity, and the Black Forest Institution of Walther at Nordrach became famous[41]. At the same time, sanatoria were being developed in the USA by Trudeau at Lake Saranac and in Denmark at Vejlefjord.

Many British physicians visited Nordrach and set up sanatoria in Wales, England and Scotland, all carrying the Nordrach prefix: Nordrach in Wales, Nordrach upon Mendip, and Nordrach on Dee at Banchory, Scotland[41]. Alexander Spengler founded the famous private sanatorium in Davos in 1866, which was to be the setting for Thomas Mann's novel *The Magic Mountain* ('Der Zauberg') in which he gives an insight into the sanatorium concept where patients become dependent on the protected environment of the mountain and pine forests, and become disabled not only by the disease, but by the cure[42].

Koch's discovery of the tubercle bacillus in 1882 gave fresh impetus to the sanatoria movement. Some cures were achieved, and it became clear that if oxygen was indeed harmful to the tuberculous organism, open-air treatment would have some scientific basis.

In the UK in the second half of the nineteenth century, many consumptive patients were nursed and died in Poor Law Institutions, since there were attempts to keep them out of the voluntary hospitals to protect the beds there for patients suffering from potentially curable diseases. Some of these voluntary hospitals however were specializing as chest hospitals for tuberculosis, such as the Brompton hospital, which opened in London in 1841. In 1898 the National Association for the Prevention of consumption and other forms of Tuberculosis (NAPT) was set up[43]. This was inspired by Sir William Broadbent who informed the Prince of Wales, later King Edward VII, together with Lord Salisbury the Prime Minister, as well as leading physicians that 'this terrible waste of life is preventable', to which his Royal Highness uttered the now famous comment, 'if preventable, why not prevented?'

Nearly 20 years after Koch's discovery, the realization of its importance became apparent, not only to the medical fraternity but to informed members of national associations against tuberculosis. They appreciated not only the scientific achievement of isolating the tubercle bacillus, but also recognized that the former unseen killer was now a visible target against which blows could, and must, be struck. NAPT was part of an international movement already flourishing elsewhere. In the USA, the National Tuberculous Association in 1889 fully realized that tuberculosis was distinctly preventable, that it was not directly inherited, and that it was acquired by direct transmission of the tubercule bacillus in sputum from the sick to the healthy [44]. Such education needed to be made available to the community at large, and similar propaganda was put out by the League against Tuberculosis, which had been inaugurated in France in 1892, its German equivalent established in 1895, and the Dutch association initiated in 1897. The three areas in which NAPT concentrated on prevention were education, the provision of institutional treatment and the elimination of tuberculosis from cattle. NAPT advertised, provided pamphlets and books, and their lecturers travelled all over the country educating people about bad food, bad air and bad drink as well

as overcrowding, overwork and overstrain. It was recognized that there was a higher incidence of tuberculosis in those who were less prosperous, but NAPT did not have the power to improve the lot of city dwellers living in industrialized poverty and squalor. NAPT attempted to educate individuals to be personally responsible for not contracting tuberculosis by improving their lifestyle, but such advice could be neither understood nor taken by poor people. Sanatoria were constructed by public subscription in the UK and were a colossal investment at a time when institutions were an international panacea. They were certainly attractive objects of philanthropy, as the donors could see the results of their charity in a most substantial way.

Patients were admitted to sanatoria for an indefinite period. Discipline was stern, complaints were not tolerated, and the physician superintendent sought a submissive attitude of compliance at his initial interview. The atmosphere in many was like a school, and the attainment of good health was the teaching. Drinking, originally encouraged by Bodington, often resulted in dismissal, but smoking was permitted. Men and women were separated, gathering only for meal times, and the mail was censored in order to avoid mental agitation. Many sanatoria were in the countryside, making access difficult for visitors while at the same time isolating the sputum-positive victims from the community. Most sanatoria faced south, south-east and south-west, with radial pavilions leaving no part in the shade (Fig. 1.4). Design was spartan to resist the notion that luxury led to survival, lest return home might lead to relapse. Sunbathing was encouraged, and ingenious rotating summer houses were installed to maximize sun exposure in the UK (Fig. 1.5). The health-giving properties of the sun were the *raison d'être* for the Swiss clinics of Rollier at Leysin, which specialized in actinotherapy (Fig. 1.6).

The culture in the sanatorium was for a

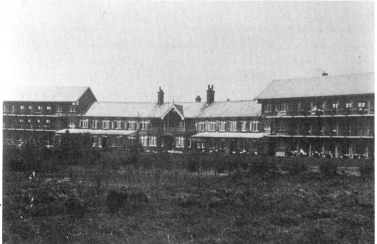

Fig. 1.4 Leasowe Sanatorium, Merseyside, showing south-facing pavillions, all directed towards the sun.

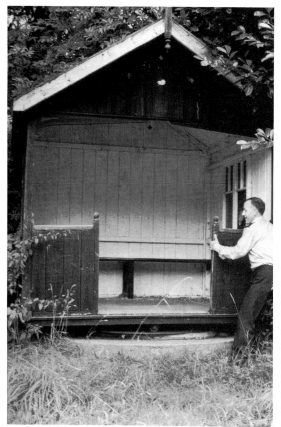

Fig. 1.5 Revolving summer house at Crossley Sanatorium, Cheshire.

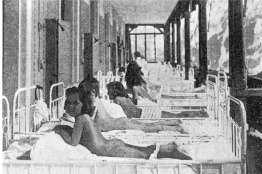

Fig. 1.6 Children taking sunlight on a pavillion ward with the Swiss Alps in the background.

conscientious sustained performance of self-denial, self-restraint and endurance. The medical issues centred around rest, and disease activity was judged by the fever chart. Graded exercises such as receiving the first visitors were only permitted after a fortnight without fever, and washing, feeding and going to the lavatory were then allowed provided that there was no return of fever or haemoptysis. Good food and lots of fresh open air were followed by graded exercises, all carefully supervised with compulsory rest periods every day. With further health improvement and weight gain, patients were encouraged to indulge in gardening, road making, carpentry and poultry keeping, and this formed the basis of the so-called 'pick-axe cure' for consumptives, which was to be the forerunner of the village colonies developed after the First World War in the UK. On discharge, patients were provided with home manuals which contained strict advice as to how to sustain good health[43]. These were to set patterns of public behaviour for years, and indeed generations. Medical follow-up was often carried out in the UK at the dispensaries, and additional drug therapy from a vast pharmacopoeia was tried. These included iron salts, calcium salts, cod liver oil, arsenic, antimony, gold, quinine, salicylates, iodine, creosote, turpentine, carbolic and tuberculin, none of which was demonstrated to be of any practical therapeutic value. Tuberculin, which is a glycerine extract of pure culture of the tubercle bacillus, had been developed by Koch in 1891, and when given subcutaneously in various strengths, showed positive skin reactions in all tuberculous patients. Koch considered that this potential remedy would form an indispensable aid to diagnosis. Unfortunately, tuberculin was introduced internationally prematurely, amid wild enthusiasm and without critical challenge, so that it quickly fell into disrepute as a treatment[45]. It has, of course, remained as a diagnostic tool.

Although sanatorium treatment remained one of the main weapons in the fight against tuberculosis for almost a century, there is no scientifically acceptable evidence that it reduced the toll of the disease. Sanatoria did make some patients feel better, and in others death was delayed. For some, especially children diagnosed as pre-tuberculous but without the disease, sanatorium treatment must have been harmful, as Thomas Mann suspected in *The Magic Mountain*. Comparative results from Saranac, Davos, Brompton and Norway were all similar, demonstrating that about 50% of sputum-positive patients survived for 5 years.

1.15 PUBLIC HEALTH

The International Union against Tuberculosis, with its double-barred cross emblem, was founded in 1902, with offices in Berlin. These were closed down during the First World War but reopened in 1920 in Geneva. The International Union was to encourage a system of tuberculosis control throughout Europe, consisting of notification of all cases, contact tracing and the provision of dedicated dispensaries and institutions, which were usually sanatoria. The prototype for these recommendations had come from Robert Philip in Edinburgh, who founded the Royal Victoria Hospital supported by public subscription; this was to become a model to be emulated world wide for the administrative liasions between the dispensary in the community, the sanatoria and the colonies, the hospital and the Medical Officer of Health, whereby contact tracing and home assessments by Health Visitors were introduced and coordinated[46].

In 1913, national legislation was passed in the UK to verify the notification of all forms of tuberculosis, and this was soon followed by the compulsory isolation of tuberculotics. The 1921 Public Health Tuberculosis Act made local authorities responsible for these aspects of tuberculosis care, and the cost was met from the local rates supplemented by an Exechequer Grant.

1.16 COLLAPSE THERAPY

In addition to first controlling the pulmonary disease by physical rest in the holistic sense in sanatoria, physicians adopted the idea of resting the lung itself by collapsing it with a pneumothorax. James Carson, an Edinburgh graduate, practising in Liverpool, induced artificial pneumothorax in experimental rabbits with beneficial results. When he tried to induce an artificial pneumothorax in man in 1822, in two cases of pulmonary tuberculosis pleural adhesions and loculated empyema prevented a successful outcome[47]. Forlanini 60 years later in Italy induced artificial pneumothorax using nitrogen introduced via a needle with 200 ml instalments on a daily basis[48]. Forlanini's method of repeated small fill-ups was adapted and modified by Murphy in the USA, who gave a 1–3 l large-volume induction of nitrogen under radiographic control[49]. It became apparent that some of Forlanini's patients may have suffered gas embolism, which he termed 'pleural eclampsia' when the needle attached to the nitrogen cylinder was introduced. In Denmark, Christian Saugman added a water manometer to the needle and nitrogen source so that the operator was now able to identify where the tip of the needle was in the pleural space, and thus the safety of the procedure was improved[41]. During the early years of collapse therapy induced by artificial pneumothorax, benefit was thought to accrue only after a long period, but this view was challenged by Ascoli in 1912 who not only obtained effective healing using only a small artificial pneumothorax without significant lung collapse, but he was able to induce bilateral artificial pneumothoraces, further extending the application of the technique to subjects with bilateral pulmonary tuberculosis[50].

It is surprising how few sanatoria were capable of performing radiographs in the UK. In 1914, only 5 of 17 local authority dispensaries and 7 of 96 sanatoria in England and Wales provided facilites for radiography[41]. A notable exception had been Lawson, who installed an X-ray suite in his new sanatorium in Nordrach on Dee in 1900[51]. Morriston Davies had indicated that radiology was of extreme importance in the diagnosis of phthisis, and that it was essential before laying down a rational scheme of treatment[52].

1.17 THORACIC SURGERY

With the wider use of radiology, it was apparent that after induction of the pneu-

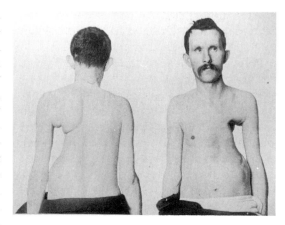

Fig. 1.7   Rib and pulmonary resection. Germany c. 1930.

mothorax, collapse of the diseased part of the lung frequently did not occur due to pleural adhesions. The idea of severing these adhesions was that of Friedrich in 1908, and this was brilliantly developed by Jacaboaeus of Stockholm using a thoracoscope in 1922. This enabled him to dissect and divide the adhesions under direct vision. This technique quickly spread throughout sanatoria in the Western world, and was known as intrapleural pneumonolysis. Impressed with the results of lung collapse achieved by artificial pneumothoraces, surgeons began to deliberately cause lung collapse by other physical methods in which the ribs were removed in part or in whole, and there were some heroic assaults on the thoracic cage and the patient (Fig. 1.7). The early surgical experience of this type caused an unacceptibly high mortality, but thoracoplasty as it was called became modified and refined, being performed in two stages. The first stage involved resection of the paravertebral portions of the lower ribs as proposed by Wilms[53], and this was followed by the second procedure in which the upper ribs were resected as proposed by Sauerbruch[54].

Other forms of surgical collapse therapy, particularly directed to the upper lobe, were invented, and these included extrapleural pneumonolysis, during which various substances were inserted into the extrapleural space in order to maintain lung collapse. In particular, surgeons used abdominal fat and moulded paraffin wax, producing a so-called extrapleural plombage. Collapse of the lung was also achieved by instilling oil rather than air into the pleural space, when an oleothorax was created. These latter procedures were never adopted universally, but phrenic nerve damage causing diaphragmatic paralysis proved very popular. Resection, division and evulsion of the nerve caused permanent injury, but phrenic nerve crush induced a temporary paralysis lasting about 6 months. Phrenic nerve crush was used in conjunction with other simple forms of collapse therapy, but was rarely successful when used on its own. In the 1930s phrenic crush was often used in conjunction with pneumoperitoneum when a 2–3 l insufflation of air was introduced into the peritoneal cavity to elevate both diaphragms and cause some lower lobe collapse.

Thoracic surgical prowess was advancing, and Carl Semb in Oslo combined a modified thoracoplasty with dissection of the apical extrafascial plane, so as to cause collapse of the upper lobe cavity[55]. This issue had been unsuccessfully addressed previously in pulmonary tuberculosis by Monaldi when he introduced the technique of cavity drainage. At the Massachusetts General Hospital, Churchill and Klopstock introduced upper lobectomy[56], and thanks to the further elucidation of bronchopulmonary anatomy by Brock in London, it became possible to perform pulmonary segmentectomy in tuberculous areas[57]. This was usually performed in the apicoposterior segments of the upper lobes and the apical segments of the lower lobes after a technique developed by Chamberlain.

1.18 THORACIC RESEARCH

The scientific role of surgery in pulmonary tuberculosis was considerable, but it is difficult, if not impossible, to estimate its value in reducing mortality and the transmission of the disease. There was neither controlled trial nor rigorous testing of any of the techniques, and such was the faith in collapse therapy and sanatorium treatment that such a trial would have been considered unethical. The close co-operation between physician and surgeon, however, was to strengthen the specialty and led to a much more critical and rational approach to therapy thereafter than in any other branch of medicine. This co-operation led to the inauguration of medical societies composed not only of physicians and surgeons, but of radiologists and pathologists and epidemiologists, and in Britain the current British Thoracic Society and the Society of Thoracic Surgeons of Great Britain and Ireland have in their origins the Society of Medical Superintendents of Tuberculosis Institutions, the joint Tuberculosis Council and the British Tuberculosis Association.

It must be admitted that treatment of pulmonary tuberculosis up to the Second World War was more of an art than a science. The exact size and duration of the artificial pneumothorax was a matter of clinical experience not easily transmitted to others by rational explanation, and other therapeutic or physical manoeuvres were matters of preference and prejudice rather than reason. No major research work was carried out during this time, and monies for any research were directed to NAPT. Nevertheless, the UK figures for tuberculosis mortality from 1850 to 1950 show an astonishing and gratifying reduction, with the notable exceptions of the two great World Wars (Fig. 1.8). It is clear that socioeconomic features as well as medical factors were in operation.

1.19 BCG

In 1924 Calmette, working in the Pasteur Institute in Lille, successfully developed an attenuated strain of tubercle bacillus that was incapable of producing tuberculosis in

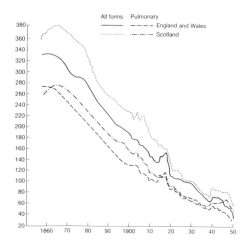

Fig. 1.8 Standardized death rates from tuberculosis per 100 000 population, England and Wales, and Scotland: 1850–1950. (Source: Lynda Bryden, *Below the Magic Mountain*, Clarendon Press, 1988, Fig. 1.)

any laboratory animals[58]. In France, many infants received the oral vaccine of the Bacillus Calmette–Guerin (BCG), but for a variety of reasons, it was not taken up in the rest of Europe. Tragically, in 1930 in Lubeck, Germany, 67 of 249 babies given the vaccine died of acute tuberculosis subsequently shown to be due to the inadvertent administration of virulent tubercle bacilli stored in the same fridge as the BCG[59]. The Scandinavian countries pioneered the use of BCG and administered it intradermally; by 1950 this was being offered throughout Europe in a mass vaccination campaign to all children. From 1954, most health authorities in the UK began voluntary vaccination of 13-year-olds. BCG has never been taken up enthusiastically in the USA. Throughout Europe and the USA, mass miniature radiography was introduced during the Second World War, and this was to play an integral part in identifying unsuspected cases of tuberculosis.

1.20 CHEMOTHERAPY

In 1944 Waksman in the USA discovered streptomycin and found that it was bacteriostatic against *M. tuberculosis*[60]. Clinical trials were set up in the USA and in Britain, where they were supervised by the MRC who set the standard for the scientific assessment of antibiotic efficacy in tuberculosis. Of patients treated with streptomycin, 51% showed radiological improvement of their disease, whereas only 8% of controls did so. Streptomycin was shown to be potentially life-saving in tuberculous meningitis and miliary tuberculosis, but to give rise to adverse effects, most frequently disturbances of balance and hearing. It was appreciated from the onset that resistance to the antibiotic by the tubercle bacillus occurred after 2–3 months continuous therapy, and that special rhythms of treatment or additional therapy would be required to overcome this problem. In fact, this was rapidly realized by Lehmann in Sweden who detected bacteriostatic activity of para-aminosalicylic acid (PAS) against *M. tuberculosis*[61]. The MRC again supervised a trial using streptomycin alone, PAS alone and a combination of both drugs. Unequivocal proof of the action of PAS was established, but a much greater consequence was that combination therapy could be used for prolonged periods without the development of drug resistance[62]. The adverse gastrointestinal effects of high-dose PAS frequently demanded fortitude and endurance by patient and physician, so that the discovery by Robitzek and Selikoff in New York in 1952 of the effectiveness of the relatively inexpensive isonicotinicacid hydrazide (isoniazid) was again welcomed with uncritical enthusiasm[63]. However, the MRC demonstrated that bacterial resistance developed when isoniazid was used singly[64], but in combination with daily streptomycin it was shown to be the most effective remedy available[65]. The use of prolonged combination chemotherapy extended for upwards of 2 years was pioneered in Edinburgh by Crofton and colleagues, and it was possible at long last to envisage cure of pulmonary tuberculosis in all cases[66].

Such chemotherapeutic success challenged the role of traditional management of tuberculosis of bedrest, sanatorium treatment, surgery and rehabilitation, all of which were to become quickly superfluous. Sanatoria have been found a new role as institutions for the elderly, collapse therapy is unnecessary, surgery is hardly ever required unless concurrent lung cancer is suspected, and dispensaries and chest hospitals have been closed down in the Western world. With modern drug therapy, including pyrazinamide introduced in 1954, ethambutol discovered in 1962, and rifampicin discovered in 1969, all that is now necessary is to take the correct drugs in the correct dosage for the correct duration, which nowadays may be as short as 6 months. The tragedy today is that this great potential has not been achieved universally, because tuberculotic patients remain undiscovered, while others remain ill and infectious because money cannot be made available for effective chemotherapy. Most disturbingly, immunosuppression induced by AIDS is permitting a Third World epidemic of proportions akin to those experienced in the sixteenth and seventeenth centuries not with tuberculosis, but with plague, cholera and smallpox.

REFERENCES

1. Bunyan, J. (1905 [1680]) *The Life and Death of Mr Badman* (ed. John Brown), Cambridge.
2. Myers, J.A. (1977) *Captain of All These Men of Death. Tuberculosis Historical Highlights*. Warren H. Green, St Louis.
3. Rich, A.R. (1944) *Pathogenesis of Tuberculosis*, Thomas, Chicago, Ill.
4. Manchester, K. (1984) Tuberculosis and leprosy in antiquity: an interpretation. *Medi. Hist.*, **28**(2), 162–73.
5. Sager, P. Schalimtzek, M. and Moller Christensen, V. (1972) A case of tuberculosis spondylosa in the Danish Neolithic Age. *Dan. Med. Bull.*, **19**(5), 176–80.
6. Zimmermann, M.R. (1979) Pulmonary and osseous tuberculosis in an Egyptian mummy. *Bull. N.Y. Acad. Med.*, **55**(6), 604–8.
7. Ortner, D.J. (1979) Disease and mortality in the early Bronze Age people of Babedh-Dhra, Jordan. *Am. J. Phys. Anthropol.*, **51**(4), 589–97.
8. Morse, D. (1961) Prehistoric tuberculosis in America. *Am. Rev. Respir. Dis.*, **83**, 489–504.
9. Allison, M.J. Mendoza D, and Pezzia, A. (1973) Documentation of a case of tuberculosis in pre-Columbian America. *Am. Rev. Respir. Dis.*, **107**(6), 985–91.
10. Hare, R. (1967) The antiquity of diseases carried by bacteria and viruses: a review of the problem from a bacteriologist's point of view. In *Diseases in Antiquity* (eds D. Brothwell and A.T. Sandison), Charles C. Thomas, Springfield, Ill., ch. 8.
11. Keers, R.Y. (1981) Laennec: his medical history. *Thorax*, **36**(2), 91–4.
12. Morse, D. (1967) Tuberculosis. In *Diseases in Antiquity* (eds D. Brothwell and A.T. Sandison), Charles C. Thomas, Springfield, Ill., ch. 19.
13. Meachen, A. (1978) *A Short History of Tuberculosis*, AMS, New York.
14. Adams, F. (1856) *On the Extant Works of Aretaeus*, Sydenham Society, London.
15. Al-Damluji, S. (1976) *Tuberculosis in Iraq for Medical Students and Practitioners*, William Heinemann, London.
16. Piery M. and Roshem, J. (1931) *Histoire de la tuberculose*, Doin et Cie, Paris, pp. 41–2.
17. Webb, G.B. (1936) *Tuberculosis*, Hoeber, New York.
18. Guthrie, D. (1945) *A History of Medicine*, Thomas Nelson, London, p. 210.
19. Rosen, G. (1943) *History of Miners' Diseases. A Medical and Social Interpretation*, Schuman, New York, pp. 64–7.
20. Flick, L.F. (1925) *Development of Our Knowledge of Tuberculosis*, Flick, Philadelphia, pp. 78–80.
21. Willis, T. (1684) *Practice of Physick*, London, Phar. II, Sect. 1, Ch. VI.
22. Morton, R. (1720) *Phthisiologia*, 2nd edn (trans.), W. and J. Innys, London, p. 74.
23. Desault, P. (1732) *A Treatise on the Venereal Distemper with Dissertation upon Consumption* (trans. J. Andree) London, pp. 272–332.
24. Smyth, J.C. (1788) The Works of the Late William Stark, J. Johnson, London, p. 26.
25. Forbes, J. (1824) On percussion of the chest. A

translation of Auenbrugger's original treatise. *Bull. Hist. Med.* **4**, 373.

26. Beeson, P.B. (1930) Corvisart, his life and works. *Ann. Med. Hist*, **2**, 300.

27. Bayle, G.L. (1810) *Researches on Pulmonary Phthisis*, W. Gapel, Liverpool, p. 2.

28. Virchow, R. (1850) Tuberculosis and its relation to inflammation, scrofulasis and typhoos. In *Collected Essays in Public Health and Epidemiology* (ed. Leland J. Rather). vol. I, Canton, Mass., p. 346.

29. Dubos, R. and Dubos, J. (1953) *The White Plague*, Gollancz, London, pp. 29–30.

30. Koch, R. (1882) 'Die Aetiologie und die Bekampfung der Tuberkulose', lecture delivered to the Physiological Society of Berlin, 24 March 1882 (trans. W. de Rouville), *Medical Classics*, **2** (1938), 853–80.

31. Smith, T. (1898) A comparative study of bovine tubercle bacilli and of tubercle bacille from sputum. *J. Exper. Med.*, **3**, 451.

32. Holmberg, S.D. (1990) The rise of tuberculosis in America before 1820. *Am. Rev. Respir. Dis.*, **142**, 1228–32.

33. Coovadia H.M. and Benatar, S.R. (1991) A *Century of Tuberculosis. South African Perspectives*, Oxford University Press, Cape Town.

34. Proust, A.J. (1991) *History of Tuberculosis in Australia, New Zealand and Papua New Guinea*, Brolga Press, Canberra.

35. Grigg, E.R.N. (1958) The arcana of tuberculosis: Part III. Epidemiologic history of tuberculosis in the United States. *Am. Rev. Tuberc.*, **78**, 426–53.

36. Union of South Africa (1914) *Report of the Tuberculosis Commission*. Cape Times, Cape Town.

37. Rogers, F.B. (1969) The rise and decline of the altitude therapy of tuberculosis. *Bull. Hist. Med.*, **43** (1), 1–16.

38. Trudeau, E.L. (1887) Environment in its relation to the progress of bacterial invasion in tuberculosis. *Am. J. Med. Sci.*, **94**, 118–23.

39. Bodington, G. (1840) *An Essay on the Treatment and Cure of Pulmonary Consumption*, Sinopkin, Marshall, Hamilton and Kent, London.

40. Brehmer, H. (1856) Tuberculosis primis in stadis semper cirabilis. Quoted in A. Latham and A.W. West, The Prize Essay on the Erection of the King Edward VII Sanatorium for consumption (London 1903), p. 5.

41. Keers, R.Y. (1978) *Pulmonary Tuberculosis. A Journey Down the Centuries*, Ballière-Tindall, London.

42. Mann, T. (1928) *The Magic Mountain* (trans. H.T. Lowe-Porter), Martin Secker and Warberg, London.

43. Bryder, L. (1988) *Below the Magic Mountain*, Clarenden Press, Oxford.

44. Knopf, S.A. (1922) *A History of the National Tuberculosis Association*, National Tuberculosis Association, New York, p. 6.

45. Editorial (1890) *Lancet*, p. 1118.

46. Philip, R.W. (1937) *Collected Papers on Tuberculosis*, Oxford University Press, London.

47. Carson, J. (1822) *Essays, Physiological and Practical*, F.B. Wright, Liverpool.

48. Forlanini, C. (1894) Primo tentativi di pneumotorace artificiale della tisi pulmonare. *Gazz. Med. Torino*, **45**, 381.

49. Murphy, J.B. (1898) Surgery of the lung. *J. Am. Med. Assoc.* **31**, 151, 208, 281.

50. Ascoli, M. (1912) Uber den kuntslichen Pneumothorax nach Forlanini. *Dtsch. Med. Wochenschr.*, **38**, 1782.

51. Lawson, D. (1913) X-rays in the diagnosis of lung disease. *Practitioner*, **90**, 53.

52. Davies, H.M. (1924) Surgery in the treatment of pulmonary tuberculosis. *Br. Med. J.*, **2**, 1145.

53. Wilms, M. (1912) Eine neue Methode zur verengerung des thorax bei Lungen tuberkulose. *Munch. Med. Wochenschr.* **58**, 777.

54. Alexander, J. (1937) *The Collapse Therapy of Pulmonary Tuberculosis*, C.C. Thomas, Springfield, Ill.

55. Semb, C. (1935) Thoracoplasty with extrafascial apicolysis. *Acta Chir. Scand.*, **76**, Suppl. 34–7.

56. Churchill, E.D. and Klopstock, R. (1943) Lobectomy for pulmonary tuberculosis. *Ann. Surg.*, **117**, 641.

57. Brock, R.C. (1946) *The Anatomy of the Bronchial Tree*. Oxford University Press, London.

58. Calmette, A. (1923) *Tubercle Bacillus Infection and Tuberculosis in Man and Animals* (trans. W.B. Soper and G.H. Smith), Williams & Wilkins, Baltimore, Md.

59. Calmette, A. (1931) Epilogue de la catastophe de Lubeck. *Presse. Med.* **2**, 17.

60. Schatz, A. and Waksman, S.A. (1944) Effect of streptomycin and other antibiotic substances

upon mycobacterium tuberculosis and related organisms. *Proc. Soc. Exp. Biol. Med.*, **57**, 244.

61. Lehmann, J. (1946) Para aminosalicylic acid in the treatment of tuberculosis. *Lancet*, **1**, 15.

62. Medical Research Council Investigation (1950) Treatment of tuberculosis with streptomycin and para-aminosalicylic acid. *Br. Med. J.*, **2**, 1073.

63. Robitzek, E.H. and Selikoff, I.J. (1952) Hydrazine derivative of isonicotinic acid in the treatment of acute progressive caseous-pneumonic tuberculosis. A preliminary report. *Am. Rev. Tuberc.*, **65**, 402.

64. Medical Research Council Investigation (1952) The treatment of pulmonary tuberculosis with isoniazid. An interim report. *Br. Med. J.*, **2**, 735.

65. Medical Research Council Investigation (1955) Various combinations of isoniazid with streptomycin or with PAS in the treatment of pulmonary tuberculosis. *Br. Med. J.*, **1**, 435.

66. Crofton, J. (1959) Chemotherapy of pulmonary tuberculosis. *Br. Med. J.*, **1**, 1610.

THE EPIDEMIOLOGICAL BASIS OF TUBERCULOSIS CONTROL

2

D.A. Enarson and Annik Rouillon

2.1 THE PROBLEM OF TUBERCULOSIS: EXTENT AND MEASUREMENT

2.1.1 THE EXTENT OF THE PROBLEM

Tuberculosis continues to be a very major problem throughout the world: in the early 1990s as many as 16 million cases of tuberculosis have been reported with, each year, 8 million new cases (one-half of which are infectious) and 3 million deaths due to the disease[1]. These estimates are likely to be high; a more reasonable estimate of the total number of new cases each year is 5.5 million, of which 74% occur in Asia and another 12% in Africa. As many as one billion (one thousand million) people throughout the world may be infected with tuberculosis. Cases of tuberculosis arise either from this large pool of infected people or from those with previous disease, now inactive. The only way to prevent tuberculosis entirely is to stop the transmission of this infection in the community. However, immediate cessation of transmission would be accompanied by only a gradual disappearance, because of disease arising from previously infected individuals who carry a diminishing risk of developing disease throughout their lives.

In spite of the ubiquitous nature of tuberculosis and the 'vicious cycle' that it entails, the bacillus is remarkably inefficient and this inefficiency is the key to its elimination. To become infected requires contact (usually prolonged and intimate contact) with an infectious case[2]. In industrialized countries, the number of contacts per case of infectious tuberculosis appears to be declining; in the middle 1970s, in Canada, the number of contacts per case was seven; at present there are only three contacts per case, only one being under 20 years of age.

2.1.2 MEASURING TUBERCULOSIS IN THE COMMUNITY

When tuberculosis was common and specific treatment was not available, the **mortality rate** was a good indicator of the size of the tuberculosis problem, as there was a fairly constant relationship between incidence and mortality. Rates have been declining ever since the first records were kept. The rate of decline prior to the introduction of chemotherapy was steady at approximately 4% per annum. Around 1945, the rate in industrialized countries plummeted and then began to stabilize again around 1960 following the introduction of streptomycin in 1946, para-aminosalicylic acid (PAS) in 1948 and isoniazid (H) in 1952.

A second measure of tuberculosis in a community is the tuberculin skin test developed by Koch, which indicates the presence of infection with tuberculosis independent of clinical disease. Much of the earliest epidemiological use of this test was in Scandi-

Clinical Tuberculosis. Edited by P.D.O. Davies. Published in 1994 by Chapman & Hall, London. ISBN 0 412 48630 X

navia[3]. Since these early studies, the tuberculin test has been used to determine the prevalence of infection in samples of the general population of many countries. The skin testing of new recruits to the military service of the Netherlands provided the data from which the determination of the **average annual risk of tuberculous infection** was developed[4], although the concept was first described in the study of other infectious diseases (notably smallpox). It indicates the probability of becoming infected within a given year, either estimated from the age-specific prevalence of tuberculin skin sensitivity, or directly measured by repeating the test in the same population at several points in time and calculating the rate of development (incidence) of tuberculin skin sensitivity (indicating infection with tuberculosis). The calculation of the estimate from a single tuberculin survey is based on an algebraic formula $ARI = 1 - (1 - p)^{1/a}$ where ARI is the average annual risk of infection, p is the prevalence of tuberculin sensitivity in the sample and a is the average age of the group tested. This estimation gives the *average* of the experience over the period of time represented by the age (reflecting the average experience at the mid point of the average life span of the tested individuals) and therefore cannot measure short-term changes.

Prevalence rate, from representative samples of the general population, has been determined in some countries, indicating the number of cases of active tuberculosis within the community at a given point in time. The protocol for such work has been developed superbly in Japan and has been undertaken in a number of countries, especially in East Asia. These surveys can identify all infectious sources (the smear-positive cases) at a point in time. Under stable conditions, without intervention, the ratio of prevalence to incidence in a community is 2:1 (that is, the average duration of a case is 2 years). The introduction of specific chemotherapy of tuberculosis has resulted in a disruption of

the ratio of prevalence to incidence, by shortening the duration of cases.

In countries where notification of tuberculosis cases is quite thorough, the incidence of active tuberculosis can be approximated by the **notification rate** of cases, and has been used to monitor the epidemiological situation. This measure requires the supervision and review of all notifications by tuberculosis experts to ensure the validity and completeness of the registration of cases. The incidence of all active cases of tuberculosis is approximately twice that of smear-positive pulmonary cases. An annual risk of infection of 1% is approximately equal to an annual incidence of all active cases of 100 per 100 000[5] where there is no HIV infection; where there is a significant overlap of HIV and tuberculous infection, this ratio is no longer valid.

For purposes of discussion, various 'benchmarks' of tuberculosis (in rates per 100 000 per year) have been proposed as follows[6].

1000   above this rate, tuberculosis can be said to be 'epidemic.'
100   above this rate, groups can be defined as at 'high risk' for tuberculosis.
10   or below this rate, groups can be defined as at 'low risk' for tuberculosis.
1   below this rate, the tuberculosis programmes are entering the elimination phase.
0.1   at this level, tuberculosis can be said to be eliminated.

2.2 THE NATURAL HISTORY OF TUBERCULOSIS

2.2.1 IN THE INDIVIDUAL

In order to be infectious, a patient must have a sufficient concentration of micro-organisms in the sputum to create the floating, infecting dust particles when coughing, sneezing or singing. Tuberculosis patients, to be infectious, must have pulmonary tuberculosis, with the sputum containing acid-fast bacilli visible on direct microscopy[7].

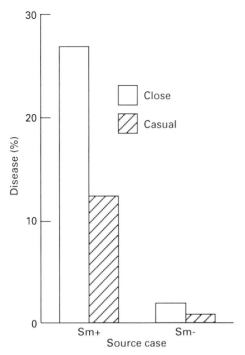

Fig. 2.1 Risk of tuberculous infection due to contact with an active case, by type of case (Sm+, positive on direct smear of sputum microscopy for acid-fast bacilli; Sm−, negative on direct smear but positive on culture for *M. tuberculosis*) and nature of contact (Close, living in the same household as the source case; Casual, acquainted but not living with the source case). (Source: S. Grzybowski *et al.*, *Bull. Int. Union Tuberc.*, 1975, **50**, 90–106.)

The likelihood of infection with tuberculosis, given contact with an infectious case, is a function of the duration and intensity of the contact. Thus, individuals living in the same household (and particularly those sharing the same bedroom) with an infectious case have the greatest risk of becoming infected. The likelihood of infection from casual contact is substantially less (Fig. 2.1). Given contact with an infectious case, on average, approximately one in six persons will become infected. It is much more likely that a contact will remain uninfected than that such a person will become infected after contact with a single infectious case.

Once infected, the likelihood of developing disease is not different, whatever the source. Some studies[2] have suggested that individuals infected by smear-positive source cases are more likely to develop disease. This conclusion is probably incorrect, resulting from the determination of the proportion of infected contacts arising from remote infection based upon population surveys of tuberculin sensitivity which underestimates the prevalence of remote infection among the subset of the population having contact with a case of tuberculosis (and particularly that group whose contact is with a smear-negative, culture-positive case). The likelihood of developing disease is greatest immediately following infection and declines exponentially from that point[8,9]. The incidence of clinically significant disease within the first year after infection is approximately 1.5%. Within the first 5 years after infection (during the steep slope of the decline) the cumulative risk of disease is between 5 and 10% the remainder of the lifetime risk (under stable social and immunological conditions) is probably around 5%. Thus, under usual conditions and on average, the total lifetime cumulative risk of developing disease after becoming infected by contact with an infectious case, is perhaps 15% (about one in six persons). Where repeated contacts with infectious cases are likely, the probability of developing disease may be higher.

Wallgren[10], using the tuberculin skin test to determine the point at which individuals became infected, calculated what he called a 'timetable' of tuberculosis. The type of tuberculosis and the site in the body that was affected bore a striking relationship to the time since the infection occurred. This continues to be true, for example, in Tanzania where the type of tuberculosis varies markedly with age, as Wallgren observed (Fig. 2.2). The first event to occur following infection (within 12 weeks after contact with the infectious case) is the conversion of the tuberculin skin test. In most individuals, systemic response to the infection includes a

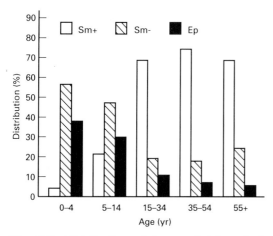

Fig. 2.2 Distribution of types of tuberculosis cases (sm+, positive for acid-fast bacilli on direct smear microscopy of sputum; sm−, negative on direct smear, ep, extrapulmonary) in Kilimanjaro Region, Tanzania in 1989 by age group.

slight rise in temperature, possibly accompanied by flu-like symptoms. Subsequently, the tuberculin skin test demonstrates significant induration for many years, although in some individuals, it may become insignificant or absent in old age[11]. A minority of people who become infected with tuberculosis develop primary disease. Usually, disease is localized in the lung and the regional lymph nodes within the chest, resolving without treatment, leaving a very small calcified scar in the pulmonary parenchyma along with calcification of the hilar lymph node. The appearance of a healed primary complex on chest radiograph has the same significance in terms of probability of subsequent active disease as does a significant tuberculin skin reaction, as both merely reflect previous primary infection. In a small proportion of patients with primary tuberculosis, complications may occur. These include local extension and cavitation (progressive primary tuberculosis), dissemination throughout the body (miliary tuberculosis, often accompanied by tuberculous meningitis), and local complications, the most common of which is obstruction of the right middle lobe bronchus

leading to an obstructive pneumonia with subsequent localized bronchiectasis.

Tuberculous pleurisy occurs, on average, 6 months following primary infection[12]. It is usually a self-limited condition and often resolves spontaneously. In such cases, the likelihood of subsequent relapse (usually in the form of pulmonary tuberculosis) is approximately one in three. A number of hypersensitivity reactions to the tubercle bacillus accompanying primary infection are known to occur, such as dactylitis, erythema nodosum and phlyctenular conjunctivitis. Where tuberculosis is common, tuberculous lymphadenitis (scrofula) is the most common form of extrapulmonary disease. It occurs quite early following infection and is most common in groups in which recent infection with tuberculosis is common (thus young people).

Post-primary pulmonary tuberculosis is the most common form of tuberculosis and occurs most frequently within 5 years of primary infection. Approximately 85% of such cases may be bacteriologically confirmed by sputum culture. Usually more than one-half of these are positive for acid-fast bacilli on direct microscopy of sputum specimens (and are termed smear-positive).

Skeletal tuberculosis may occur at any point in the timetable and has three forms: spondylitis, arthritis and isolated osteomyelitis[13]. Spondylitis most frequently involves the lower intervertebral discs. Tuberculous arthritis most commonly involves the hips, the knees, the shoulders and the elbows, in that order of frequency. A high proportion of patients with tuberculous arthritis have evidence of tuberculosis on the chest radiograph. Abdominal tuberculosis [14,15] occurs in several clinical types. The most common, tuberculous peritonitis, presents with the picture of hepatic failure, abdominal mass or acute abdomen. Ileocecal tuberculosis has all the clinical appearances of Crohn's disease. Anorectal tuberculosis is most frequently a companion of pulmonary tuberculosis and in

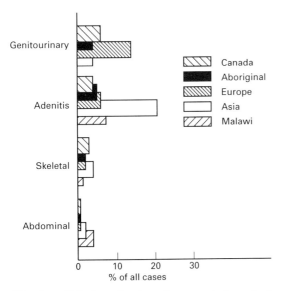

Fig. 2.3   Relation of extrapulmonary tuberculosis to birthplace and ethnic group for cases reported in Canada from 1970 to 1981 (groups Canada, Aboriginal, Europe, Asia) and in Malawi in 1989.

a majority of cases the chest radiograph demonstrates either current or previous disease. The disease presents with non-specific fistula or abscess formation. Mesenteric lymphadenitis usually occurs in young people.

Tuberculosis of the genitourinary system is a late form of the disease, occurring many years after primary infection. For this reason, it preferentially affects individuals after mid life. For reasons that are not clear, it has a predilection for Europeans (Fig. 2.3). It is the most frequent cause of infertility in many developing countries.

Tuberculosis can affect virtually any organ in the body and may present in a large variety of ways; pericarditis, adrenal gland tuberculosis (which may cause Addison's disease), iridocyclitis, mastoid sinus involvement, a space-occupying lesion in the brain, soft-tissue abscess (especially of the breast), and other sites.

2.2.2 IN THE COMMUNITY

When the risk of tuberculous infection is relatively high, the likelihood of first becoming infected is greatest in childhood (before the age of 20 years), and the majority of the population has been infected by that age[11]. Even when the risk is lower and declining, it is likely that the greatest risk of infection is in childhood[16]. If the highest likelihood of developing disease is within the first 5 years after infection, the rate of disease would be greatest between the ages of 20 and 25 years, an observed fact when tuberculosis is common[17–23]. The reason for the higher rates observed in young women, as compared with young men, where tuberculosis is common, is unknown. Where tuberculosis rates are low, if the incidence of disease is calculated only for those who are infected (rather than for the whole community), the peak rates at age 25 in young women are once again observed[24].

A conceptual model of the course of tuberculosis in a human population has been proposed[25 26]. This model indicates that, after introduction of the disease into a group previously without experience of the disease, the incidence of active tuberculosis in the population rapidly rises to a peak. As an increasing proportion of the community becomes infected and their risk of developing disease declines with time, the incidence of disease declines and may stabilize or continue a steady decline[27]. The peak only rarely exceeds 1%[28] and does so only where other factors such as tremendous overcrowding, lack of nutrition or reduced immunity, occur. The rate of decline before the introduction of specific treatment was approximately 4% per annum. With the introduction of chemotherapy, the incidence of active tuberculosis declined much more rapidly (the average annual decline in many industrialized countries has been, until recently, approximately 10%). Recently, however, the rate of decline has either been reduced, or even reversed; the reasons for this development are predictable[25,29].

When tuberculosis is very common, most cases result from recent infection and the disease is most common in young people (especially women). Rates are very high (greater than 100 per 100 000 per annum) and high-risk groups are absent. When tuberculosis is uncommon in the community, very few young people become infected and most cases result from remote infection, the disease affecting predominantly old men. Tuberculosis cases arise from high-risk groups whose risk is determined mainly by the likelihood of having been infected in the past.

The rise in rates immediately following the introduction of tuberculosis into the community, hypothesized by this model, has rarely been observed in human populations. In one example[28], mortality in aboriginal Indians in Canada rose from 1% per annum in 1881 to 9% per annum in 1886 and only slowly declined again to 1% per annum by 1900. Studies of Sudanese recruits to the Egyptian army[30], and Senegalese recruits to the French army in the early 1900s[31], illustrate a similar phenomenon. Young men, who had come from a low prevalence area and who had previously been uninfected, upon moving into a high prevalence area, were exposed to infectious cases, rapidly developed fulminant disease and died at a much higher rate than Europeans.

Detailed information on tuberculosis at the height of its occurrence in the community has been obtained for Inuit (Eskimos) in Canada, Greenland and Alaska[22,23], precisely documented since 1962. In the Northwest Territories of Canada, resident nurses tested and recorded the status of every inhabitant, using the tuberculin skin test, a chest radiograph and bacteriology laboratory. Tuberculosis cases were promptly evacuated to hospitals for prolonged residential treatment. In the early 1960s the incidence of active tuberculosis in the entire community was between 1 and 2% per annum, highest among young people (particularly women); by the 1980s highest rates were much lower and in old men. Between 1964 and 1984, BCG vaccina-tion coverage had increased from less than 50% to over 80% of all children. At the same time the prevalence of previous tuberculosis (fibrotic lesions) in adults had increased from 35% to 42%. During this period, there was an aggressive programme of preventive therapy, which often consisted of 12–18 months of fully supervised, two-drug therapy. By 1984, 43% of those with fibrotic lesions and 34% of those without fibrotic lesions, but who had been infected with tuberculosis, had been treated.

In 1970–1972, the greatest number of cases and highest incidence rate of active tuberculosis was in the group with fibrotic lesions. Lower rates were seen in those who were previously uninfected and in those who had been vaccinated. By 1980–1982, incidence rates in all groups had fallen but the decline was most dramatic in the group with fibrotic lesions; no cases in this group occurred among those who had been previously given preventive chemotherapy.

The level of tuberculosis is very low in some areas. For example, the notification rate of active tuberculosis in Alberta, Canada in 1989, among non-aboriginal Canadian-born persons, was between 1 and 2 per 100 000 with a rate of smear-positive pulmonary tuberculosis near 0.5 per 100 000. Although the transmission of tuberculous infection has virtually ceased, the disease will remain in the community for the lifetime of the last heavily infected cohort and will disappear only when this cohort has completed its life span.

When tuberculosis incidence declines, high-risk groups emerge in the community. These groups, with rates of active tuberculosis at least ten times higher than the national average (with actual rates exceeding 100 per 100 000 per year) have been investigated in the USA[32] and in Canada[33]. In Canada, they included contacts of active cases, with a rate ratio of 62; previous cases, both treated and untreated, 38; silicosis patients, 39; residents of urban slums, 20; Asian-born

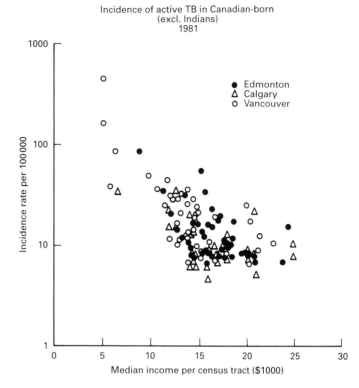

Incidence of active TB in Canadian-born
(excl. Indians)
1981

● Edmonton
△ Calgary
○ Vancouver

Fig. 2.4 Notification rate of active tuberculosis by individual census tract for Edmonton, Calgary and Vancouver, Canada in 1981, related to the median income reported for the census tract.

Canadians, 15, and aboriginal Canadians, 13. Since 1982, a new high-risk group has emerged with the highest relative risk for tuberculosis ever recorded, namely, patients with the acquired immunodeficiency syndrome (AIDS). All high-risk groups together accounted for 80% of all the cases diagnosed at that time: 33% in Asian-born Canadians; 17% in previous cases; 12% in aboriginal Canadians; 8% in contacts; 7% in residents of urban slums and 3% in patients with AIDS.

Urban centres have traditionally experienced higher rates than rural areas[25]. In British Columbia, Canada, from 1970 to 1985[34] notification rates were about twice as high in the large urban centre of Vancouver as compared with the predominantly rural remainder of the province. Although immigrants accounted for some of the difference, when only non-aboriginal Canadian-born persons were considered, the urban/rural

difference remained. To study this further, five separate sections of the city, chosen on the basis of socioeconomic characteristics, were compared; median annual income varied from $6000 to $20 000 per year; rate of unemployment from 18% of employable men to 3%; completion of secondary school education from 59% to 93%. The annual rate of notification of active tuberculosis between 1980 and 1982 also varied across the sections of the city from the lowest socioeconomic level (with an annual notification rate of 242 per 100 000) to the highest level (with a notification rate of 2). A similar relationship was observed for two other Canadian cities, Edmonton and Calgary (Fig. 2.4). The difference in rates typically found between single and married males was entirely due to the concentration of single males in the lowest income census tracts of the city, and, when this was taken into consideration, there were no continuing differences according to marital status. Unemployment was the single most important predictor of level of notification rate in the city. Moreover, in comparing the notification rates with similar reports in poor areas of Buffalo, New York in 1939[35], the rates were quite similar for the two cities, even though there was a much lower likelihood of previous infection with tuberculosis in Vancouver in the later period. These findings indicated that low socioeconomic conditions led to an increase in current transmission of tuberculosis.

Over the two decades since 1970, the proportion of notified cases who had been born outside Canada, rose from 20% of all cases to nearly 50%[36,37], even though some groups had lived in Canada, on average, for more than 40 years, indicating the continuing importance of infection in early life in determining subsequent rates of tuberculosis in low-prevalence countries.

Some investigators[38] have observed that the notification rate of tuberculosis in immigrants is highest in the years immediately following immigration. This higher rate, however, is due to a bias related to incorrect identification of individuals with active tuberculosis as 'immigrants' when, in fact, they were not[36]. Immigrants from high prevalence countries have a higher prevalence of fibrotic lesions than those born in low prevalence countries and those with fibrotic lesions who have never taken chemotherapy have an increased risk of active tuberculosis. A study of immigrants to British Columbia during 1982–1985 from five countries of Asia (Japan, Korea, the Philippines, China and India)[39] found a greater prevalence of fibrotic lesions than in residents of British Columbia (6% compared with 1%). In the years following immigration, a larger number of cases occurred in the group of immigrants who had fibrotic lesions than in those who did not (33 cases compared with 30). In those with fibrotic lesions, the greatest number of the cases were discovered on the initial examin-

ation after entry into Canada, in spite of having been investigated by chest radiograph and bacteriology prior to immigration. Moreover, almost all the cases in those with fibrotic lesions among the immigrants occurred in those who indicated no previous chemotherapy for tuberculosis, with a notification rate for bacillary cases of 1% per annum. As these individuals had been previously identified and were required to have an examination upon arrival, the disease might have been prevented by chemotherapy with isoniazid upon their arrival in the country.

2.3 THE IMPACT OF CHEMOTHERAPY ON TUBERCULOSIS

The principal aim of programmes for control of tuberculosis is to reduce the transmission of tuberculosis and, in this way to eliminate the disease. This is accomplished by the reduction in the number of sources of infection (smear-positive pulmonary cases) by permanently rendering them bacteriologically negative – through treatment or, where no treatment is given, unfortunately only by death of the patient. In evaluating the results of programmes, therefore, it is most important to determine the ability of such programmes to reduce the residual pool of smear-positive cases in the community. The results of treatment programmes under various conditions have been reviewed[40]: when 'no chemotherapy' is given;[41,42] under 'ideal' programme conditions, where chemotherapy is individualized to the patient based upon results of culture and sensitivity of the organism; and under 'mass chemotherapy' conditions prior to the introduction of rifampicin[43,44]. With 'no chemotherapy', one-quarter of the patients die within 2 years and 50% die within 5 years. Another 25% cure themselves (their immunological defence is capable of overcoming the microorganisms within their bodies and render them inactive). Another 25%, however, remain smear-positive sources of infection within the community. Under 'ideal' programmes, 8% of patients die while on treatment, and 84% are cured, leaving 2% smear-positive at the end of treatment (in 6%, results are unknown because they moved or absconded from treatment). With 'mass chemotherapy', the fatality rate is dramatically reduced to only 10%, and the proportion of patients cured is increased to about 60%. This, however, leaves as many as 30% smear-positive or unaccounted for. The irregular treatment of many patients (who leave treatment when feeling better but return when symptoms return) allows them to survive but fails to cure them. Thus, the net effect of such programmes may be to **increase** the number of sources of infection within the community. Under mass treatment conditions what is normally good chemotherapy becomes, in fact, poor chemotherapy. Poor compliance (which is the **normal** state of affairs with patients) is the most important reason. Directly observed chemotherapy is the **only** means to ensure compliance and direct observation of drug-taking **must** be the practice, at a minimum, in that portion of therapy that is most important (the initial intensive phase in smear-positive pulmonary patients).

The second reason is the presence of bacteriological resistance to chemotherapeutic agents. It is very uncommon in countries like Canada[38,45], Algeria[46] or Tanzania[47], where initial resistance to one or more drugs occurs in less than 10% and acquired resistance in more than 35%. In some other countries, however, the problem is very much greater. In Korea, for example, in a national prevalence survey, initial resistance was present in 24% of cases and acquired resistance in 74%[43], in China, the corresponding figures were 27% and 72%[48]. In Korea, 53% and in China, 62% of all cases discovered in the prevalence surveys had previously been treated; these 'residual' cases (representing a failure of the national programme) were drug-resistant sources of

infection in the community. A mathematical model[49] based upon the data derived from the periodic national prevalence surveys of Korea and Taiwan, estimated the relative infectiousness of the two types of cases, new and chronic. A chronic case was estimated to be **more** important as a source of infection in the community (produced more new cases) than a new case.

The introduction of rifampicin-containing regimens of chemotherapy into some national programmes has had a great impact. The most important part of the short-course regimen is the initial intensive phase, continued in smear-positive cases until the sputum smear has become negative (in most cases, after 60 days of treatment). If this period of drug-taking can be assured, overall results can be good enough to have a positive impact on the epidemiological situation through reducing the number of sources of infection in the community, as demonstrated in the National Tuberculosis Programmes (NTP) assisted by the International Union Against Tuberculosis and Lung Disease[50]. In Tanzania, the NTP has been in operation since 1978 (see Chapter 15b). At the outset, the regimen of treatment was 12 months of isoniazid and thioacetazone, supplemented with streptomycin in the first 2 months. Treatment results were poor: less than one-third of patients were cured, one-half of patients abandoned their treatment and one-fifth remained positive. With the same regimen, but improved programme structure, the results were considerably improved, but not yet satisfactory: slightly less than 60% were cured, approximately 30% absconded and 1% remained positive. With the introduction of rifampicin-containing regimens, a further improvement was achieved: nearly 80% were cured, 12% absconded, 6% died and 1% remained positive (results close to those achieved under 'ideal' programmes).

Another example of the impact of rifampicin can be seen by looking at the results of treatment of tuberculosis within the Social Security System[51] in Mexico. This branch of the government is responsible for providing health care for the poorest segment of Mexican society, serving over one-third of the entire population. Rifampicin-containing regimens were introduced into the system in the middle 1980s and gradually replaced 12-month chemotherapy, which was either self-administered or supervised. Results of treatment by cohort analysis for the three types of treatment regimen between 1983 and 1987 indicated successful completion of the regimen in 62% of the self-administered, 68% of the supervised 12-month and 82% of the supervised 6-month treatment groups. The fatality rate was similar in the three groups, at about 5%. The remainder were absconders with highest rates in the self-administered group and lowest in the supervised 6-month group.

Good results with rifampicin-containing regimens are obtained under a precise set of prerequisites[47], including a political commitment to ensure correct operation of the programme (including designated personnel at a central level for supervision, coordination and training and a policy that tuberculosis patients are not discriminated against in obtaining necessary treatment), a regular supply of materials, diagnosis based upon bacteriological examination, correct recording and reporting of diagnosis and treatment results, and direct observation of medication swallowing during the initial, intensive phase. Failure to follow these prerequisites often leads to very poor results, such as those observed in the Harlem district of New York City[52] where the results of treatment are worse than in the poorest developing countries with a consequent and dramatic increase in reported cases (Fig. 2.5), including an alarming increase in the rate of multiple drug resistance.

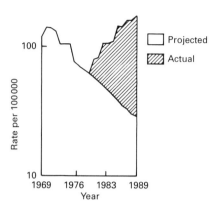

Fig. 2.5 Trend in notification of active tuberculosis in Harlem, New York from 1969 to 1989. (Source: K. Brudney *et al.* (1991) *Am. Rev. Respir. Dis.*, **144**, 745–9.)

2.4 HUMAN IMMUNODEFICIENCY VIRUS (HIV) AND TUBERCULOSIS

Infection with HIV has disrupted the balance that previously existed between the human host and the tubercle bacillus and has thereby increased the rate of development of disease in those who have been infected with tuberculosis. Its action is initially noted in those individuals who are dually infected with both HIV and tuberculosis. Thus, instead of only one in six infected individuals developing tuberculosis during their lifetime, at least one in three who are dually infected can be expected to develop active tuberculosis[53]. The impact of HIV on the tuberculosis situation in the community, however, will be exerted through the increase in the number of infectious cases of tuberculosis in the community caused by HIV infection and the subsequent increase in the rate of transmission within the community.

The impact of HIV on tuberculosis incidence was first noted in the USA[54], where the previous steady decline in tuberculosis incidence was halted and then reversed in the mid 1980s. This effect was, in part, due to the coexistence of the two infections in certain sub populations within the USA, most notably Afro-Americans and the residents of the urban core of the larger cities. Subsequently, the impact has been demonstrated in a number of countries of sub-Saharan Africa. In many countries of Africa, the notification rate of active tuberculosis has been increasing steadily since the beginning of the HIV epidemic[55].

It is possible to identify regions in Africa with an early introduction of HIV and a subsequent high level of the problem and to compare them with regions in which HIV entered later and has not yet reached the same high levels. HIV infection affects groups within any community that are at high risk for the disease and, once these groups become 'saturated' with the infection, the rise in prevalence of cases may stabilize. If this is true, it might be possible that the HIV epidemic, like tuberculosis before it, will reach a peak and then either stabilize or decline following large-scale fatality among the high-risk groups in the community[56]. Infection with both tuberculosis and HIV occurs in young people (between the ages of 15 and 44 years), so that, where tuberculous infection is still common (as in tropical Africa), the two infections exactly coincide and the increase in tuberculosis cases due to HIV is seen in this age range. Where tuberculous infection is now very rare (as in Europe and North America), there is very little overlap between the two infections. Because the mechanism by which HIV first affects the tuberculosis problem in the community is by increasing the likelihood of development of tuberculosis after infection with *M. tuberculosis*, the net impact within different countries may vary considerably. In order to plan for the control of tuberculosis, it is mandatory to determine the level and trend of both HIV and tuberculous infection, and their coincidence, in the community.

Tuberculosis is an early form of opportunistic infection accompanying the immunosuppression resulting from HIV infection[57], as many of the cases of tuberculosis occurring in patients who are diagnosed with AIDS occur prior to any other opportunistic infection. The survival of tuberculosis patients, during the course of treatment, is much better among those who are HIV-negative (about 95%) than among those who are HIV-positive (about 67%). Follow-up of patients in Tanzania who were HIV-positive indicates that 18 months after the beginning of treatment, only 50% remain alive. Of those who survive, however, the response to treatment is not different either between areas with high and low levels of HIV infection, or over time in the regions with a high level of HIV infection. Treatment of infectious cases is as effective in rendering them non-infectious, regardless of HIV infection, and is the most important activity in containing the transmission of tuberculosis caused by the increased number of cases in the community due to HIV infection. Patients who have HIV infection, however, may not tolerate medications as well as those without HIV[58].

It is not possible to know what effect HIV infection will have on tuberculosis in the community. It may have a progressive effect (especially in countries without good treatment programmes) in increasing the number of cases and therefore the transmission of tuberculous infection. On the other hand, it is possible that HIV infection will primarily affect high-risk groups, destroying these groups and then stabilizing within the community, with major impact on the tuberculosis situation only in those high-risk groups in the community. The only effective means of containing the long-term effects of HIV on the tuberculosis situation (the increase in transmission of tuberculous infection) is by means of efficient and extensive programmes of tuberculosis control.

2.5 THE ELIMINATION OF TUBERCULOSIS

There are some very good reasons to support the notion that tuberculosis can be eliminated. The most important reason is the inefficiency of tuberculosis as an infectious disease. Tuberculosis is spread not from an environmental source but from one person (an individual who is sick) to another. Moreover, it is possible to detect such a source by means of sputum microscopy and rapidly to render the patient non-infectious through chemotherapy. Thus it should be possible continuously to reduce the problem of tuberculosis if control measures are applied. Moreover, tuberculosis control activities have what has been termed a 'ratchet' effect, that is, any reduction in the level of the problem, under normal circumstances, can be sustained for some time, even if those activities cease or are interrupted. This is in striking contrast to the situation with such diseases as polio, malaria and tetanus. These arguments make it reasonable to discuss the possibility of elimination of tuberculosis.

On the other hand, with the tools currently available, the elimination of tuberculosis will take place only slowly. This is because the disease, once transmission of tuberculosis infection has ceased, continues to arise for the remainder of the lives of infected individuals (although at an ever-decreasing rate). When transmission is disrupted, there is a 'step-down', a point at which the succeeding birth cohort is very much less likely to be infected. In spite of the cessation of transmission, cases continue to occur unless some form of secondary prevention is applied.

It seems theoretically possible, using the tools that are currently available, to increase the rate of decline of tuberculosis over the 10% seen after the extensive application of effective treatment programmes. This has been demonstrated in the Inuit of the Northwest Territories of Canada among whom the rate was increased to 20% in the 1970s, possibly as a result of extensive use of preventive chemotherapy. The advent of HIV infection threatens this possibility. However, the basis of the fight against tuberculosis (diagnosis and cure of infectious cases) is unchanged. Surprisingly, even in the presence of extensive HIV infection, tubercu-

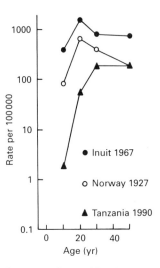

Fig. 2.6 Age-specific notification rate of active, bacillary tuberculosis in males in various groups (Inuit of Canada in 1967, Norway in 1927 and Tanzania in 1990).

losis in Africa today is orders of magnitude less common than it was among the Inuit 30 years ago or even in Europe 70 years ago (Fig. 2.6). Some of the negative thinking concerning the value and effectiveness of contributions to the fight against tuberculosis in Africa[59] (and other developing nations) is clearly not supportable. Nevertheless, the routine application of the types of interventions currently available are fraught with difficulties. It is very hard, among the large number of people infected with tuberculosis, to predict who is at risk of developing disease. The current method of preventive therapy has major limitations, chief of which is the duration of therapy required. Thus, while it is necessary to continue to apply the current tools available, it is important to further refine these tools to improve their administration and performance. With such improvements, it should be possible to hasten the elimination of this disease.

REFERENCES

1. Kochi, A. (1991) The global tuberculosis situation and the new control strategy of the World Health Organization. *Tubercle*, **72**; 1–6.

2. Grzybowski, S. Barnett, G.D. and Styblo, K. (1975) Contacts of cases of active pulmonary tuberculosis. *Bull. Int. Union Tuberc.*, **50**, 90–106.

3. Heimbeck, J. (1936) Tuberculosis in hospital nurses. *Tubercle*, **18**, 97–9.

4. Bleiker, M.A., Griep, W.A. and Beunders, B.J.W. (1964) The decreasing tuberculin index in Dutch recruits. KNCV, The Hague, The Netherlands *Selected Papers*, **8**, 38–49.

5. Murray, C.J.L., Styblo, K. and Rouillon, A. (1990) Tuberculosis in developing countries: burden, intervention and cost. *Bull. Int. Union. Tuberc.*, **65**, 2–20.

6. Clancy, L., Rieder, H.L., Enarson, D.A. and Spinaci, S. (1991) Tuberculosis elimination in the countries of Europe and other industrialized countries. *Eur. Respir.* J. **4**, 1288–95.

7. Loudon, R.G., Williamson, J. and Johnson, J.M. (1958) An analysis of 3485 tuberculosis contacts in the city of Edinburgh during 1954–1955. *Am. Rev. Tuberc.*, **77**, 623–43.

8. Ferebee, S.H. (1970) Controlled chemoprophylaxis trials in tuberculosis: a general review *Adv. Tuberc. Res.*, **17**, 28.

9. Chiba, Y. and Kurihara, T. (1979). Development of pulmonary tuberculosis with special reference to the time interval after tuberculin conversion. *Bull. Int. Union Tuberc.*, **54**, 263–4.

10. Wallgren, A. (1948) The timetable of tuberculosis. *Tubercle* **29**, 245–51.

11. Grzybowski, S. (1965) Ontario studies of tuberculin sensitivity. 1. Tuberculin testing of various populations groups. *Can. Med. Assoc. J.*, **56**, 181–92.

12. Enarson, D.A., Dorken, E. and Grzybowski, S. (1982) Tuberculous pleurisy. *Can. Med. Assoc. J.*, **126**, 493–5.

13. Enarson, D.A., Fujii, M., Nakielna, E.M. and Gtzybowski, S. (1979) Bone and joint tuberculosis: a continuing problem. *Can. Med. Assoc. J.*, **120**, 139–45.

14. Jakubowski, A., Elwood, R.K. and Enarson, D.A., (1987) Active abdominal tuberculosis in Canada 1970–81. *Can. Med. Assoc. J.*, **137**, 897–900.

15. Jakubowski. A., Elwood, R.K. and Enarson, D.A. (1988) Clinical features of abdominal tuberculosis. *J. Infect. Dis.*, **158**, 687–92.

16. Styblo, K., Meijer, J. and Sutherland, I. (1969) The transmission of tubercle bacilli. Its trend in a human population. *Bull. Int. Union. Tuberc.*, **42**, 5–104.

17. Andvoord, K.F. (1930) Der Verlauf der Tuberculose durch Generationen. *Beitr. Klin. Tuberk.* **75**, 552.

18. Frost, W.H. (1939) The age selection of mortality from tuberculosis in successive decades. *Am. J. Hyg.*, **30**, 91–6.

19. Lin, H.T. (1984) *Tuberculosis Problem and its Control in East Asia and South Pacific Area*. Japan Anti-Tuberculosis Association, Tokyo.

20. Gaultung Hansen, O. (1955) *Tuberculosis Mortality and Morbidity and Tuberculin Sensitivity in Norway*. WHO, Geneva, EURO-84/15.

21. Springett, V.H. (1952) An interpretation of statistical trends in tuberculosis. *Lancet*, **i**, 521–5, 575–80.

22. Fellows, D.S. (1934) Mortality in the native races of the Territory of Alaska, with special reference to tuberculosis. *Pub. Health. Rep.*, **49**, 289–99.

23. Grzybowski, S., Styblo, K. and Dorken, E. (1976) Tuberculosis in Eskimos. *Tubercle*, **57** (Suppl. 4).

24. Grzybowski, S. and Allen, E.A. (1964) The challenge of tuberculosis in decline. *Am. Rev. Respir. Dis.*, **90**, 707–20.

25. Grigg, E.R.N. (1958) The arcana of tuberculosis. *Am. Rev. Tuberc.*, **78**, 151–72.

26. Grzybowski, S. and Enarson, D.A. (1985) Tuberculosis, in *Current Pulmonology* (ed. D.H. Simmons), Year Book, Chicago, pp. 73–96.

27. Styblo, K. and Meijer, J. (1978) Recent advances in tuberculosis epidemiology with regard to formulation or re-adjustment of control programmes. *Bull. Int. Union Tuberc.*, **53**, 283–94.

28. Ferguson, R.G. (1955) *Studies in Tuberculosis*, University of Toronto Press, Toronto, pp. 6–9.

29. Rieder, H.L. (1992) Misbehaviour of a dying epidemic: a call for less speculation and better surveillance. *Tubercle Lung Dis.*, **73**, 181–82.

30. Cummins, S.L. (1920) Tuberculosis in primitive tribes and its bearing on tuberculosis of civilized communities. *Int. J. Pub. Health*, **1**, 10–171.

31. Borrel, A. (1920) Pneumonie et tuberculose chez les troupes noires. *Ann. Inst. Pasteur*, **34**, 7–148.

32. Rieder, H.L., Cauthen, G.M., Comstock, G.W. and Snider, D.E. (1989) Epidemiology of tuberculosis in the United States. *Epidemiol. Rev.*, **11**, 79–98.

33. Enarson, D.A., Wade, J.P. and Embree, V.

(1987) Risk of tuberculosis in Canada. *Can J. Pub. Health*, **78**, 305–8.

34. Enarson, D.A. and Dirks, J.M. (1989) The incidence of tuberculosis in a large urban area in Canada. *Am. J. Epidemiol.*, **129**, 1268–76.

35. Terris, M. (1948) Relation of economic status to tuberculosis mortality by age and sex. *Am. J. Pub. Health*, **38**, 1061–70

36. Enarson, D.A., Ashley, M.J., and Grzybowski, S. (1979) Tuberculosis in immigrants to Canada. *Am. Rev. Respir. Dis.*, **119**, 11–18.

37. Enarson, D.A., Sjogren, I. and Grzybowski, S. (1980) Incidence of tuberculosis among Scandinavian immigrants in Canada. *Eur. J. Respir. Dis.*, **61**, 139–42

38. Ashley, M.J., Anderson, T.W. and LeRiche, H. (1974) The influence of immigration on tuberculosis in Ontario. *Am. Rev. Respir. Dis.*, **110**, 137.

39. Wang, J.S., Allen, E.A., Grzybowski, S. and Enarson, D.A. (1991) Tuberculosis in recent Asian immigrants to British Columbia, Canada: 1982–1985. *Tubercle* **72**, 277–83.

40. Grzybowski, S. and Enarson, D.A. (1978) The fate of cases of pulmonary tuberculosis under various treatment programmes. *Bull. Int. Union Tuberc.* **53**, 70–75.

41. Rutledge, C.J.A. and Crouch, J.B. (1919) The ultimate results in 1694 cases of tuberculosis treated at the Modern Woodmen of America Sanatorium. *Am. Rev. Tuberc.* **2**, 755–63.

42. National Tuberculosis Institute (1974) Tuberculosis in a rural population of South India: a 5-year epidemiological study. *Bull. WHO*, **51**, 473–88.

43. Korean National Tuberculosis Association (1975) Report on the Third Tuberculosis Prevalence Survey in Korea, Seoul.

44. Aoki, M. (1984) Comments on the Results of the Sixth Tuberculosis Prevalence Survey in the Taiwan Area. Research Institute of Tuberculosis, Japan Anti-Tuberculosis Association, Tokyo.

45. Wang, J.S., Allen, E.A., Chao, C.W. *et al.* (1989) Tuberculosis in British Columbia among immigrants from five Asian countries. *Tubercle*, **70**, 179–86.

46. Boulahbal, F., Khaled, S. and Tazir, M. (1989) The interest of follow-up of resistance of the tubercle bacillus in the evaluation of a programme. *Bull. Int. Union Tuberc. Lung Dis.* **64**, 23–5.

47. Chonde, T.M. (1989) The role of bacteriological services in the National Tuberculosis and Leprosy Programme in Tanzania. *Bull. Int. Union Tuberc. Lung Dis.*, **64**, 37–9.

48. Nationwide random survey for the epidemiology of pulmonary tuberculosis conducted in 1979 (1981) *Chin. J. Respir. Dis.*, **5**, 67–71.

49. Schulzer M., Enarson D.A., Grzybowski S. *et al.* (1987) An analysis of pulmonary tuberculosis data from Taiwan and Korea. *Int. J. Epidemiol.*, **16**, 584–9.

50. Enarson, D.A. (1991) Principles of IUATLD Collaborative National Tuberculosis Programmes. *Bull. Int. Union Tuberc. Lung Dis.*, **66**, 195–200.

51. Cano Perez, G. (1990) *El programma nacional de la tuberculosis en Mexico*. Secretaria de Salud, Direccion General de Medicina Preventiva, Mexico.

52. Brudney, K. and Dobkin, J. (1991) Resurgent tuberculosis in New York City: Human immunodeficiency virus, homelessness and the decline of tuberculosis control programs. *Am. Rev. Respir. Dis.*, **144**, 745–9.

53. Selwyn, P.A., Haitel, D., Lewis, V.A. *et al.* (1989) A prospective study of the risk of tuberculosis among intravenous drug users with human immunodeficiency virus infection. *N. Engl. J. Med.*, **320**, 345–50.

54. Murray, J. (1989) The white plague; down and out or up and coming? *Am. Rev. Respir. Dis.*, **140**, 1788–95.

55. Slutkin, G., Leowski, J., Mann, J. (1988) The effects of the AIDS epidemic on the tuberculosis problem and tuberculosis programmes. *Bull. Int. Union Tuberc. Lung Dis.*, **63**, 21–4.

56. Styblo, K. and Enarson, D.A. (1991) The impact of infection with human immunodefiency virus on tuberculosis. In *Recent Advances in Respiratory Medicine*, No. 5 (eds D.M. Mitchell), Churchill Livingstone, Edinburgh.

57. Reider, H.L., Cauthen, G.M., Bloch, A.B. *et al.* (1989) Tuberculosis and acquired immunodeficiency syndrom – Florida. *Arch. Intern. Med.*, **149**, 1268–73.

58. Nunn, P., Gathua, S., Brindle, R. *et al.* (1991) Cutaneous hypersensitivity reactions due to thiacetazone in HIV-1 seropositive patients treated for tuberculosis. *Lancet*, **337**, 627–30.

59. Stanford, J.L., Grange, J.M., Pozniak, A. (1991) Is Africa lost? *Lancet*, **338**, 557–8.

THE MICROBIOLOGY OF TUBERCULOSIS

P.A. Jenkins

3.1 INTRODUCTION

The mycobacteria that cause classical tuberculosis are

- *Mycobacterium tuberculosis*
- Asian variant
- African I
- African II
- *Mycobacterium bovis*

M. tuberculosis and *M. bovis* are probably the same species and are more accurately referred to as *M. tuberculosis* var. *hominis* and var. *bovinus* respectively. However it is more convenient to refer to them as above. *M. africanum*[1] and the Asian variants differ from the typical *M. tuberculosis* in minor cultural and biochemical ways only. These distinctions are of purely epidemiological interest and have no bearing on management or prognosis. In the UK, *M. bovis* disease is largely reactivation of infection acquired many years earlier[2]. There is normally little need for contact tracing and patients are rarely smear-positive on direct microscopy. However *M. bovis* is naturally resistant to pyrazinamide and this drug should not be used.

The unique character of the mycobacteria is that they are acid-fast. Once stained by an aniline dye such as carbol fuchsin they resist decolorization with acid and alcohol and are thus termed 'acid- and alcohol-fast bacilli' or AAFB. This is generally shortened to 'acid-fast bacilli' or AFB.

Acid-fastness is thought to be related to the uniquely thick cell wall, which is composed of an interlacing layer of lipids, peptidoglycans and arabinomannans. The aniline dye forms a complex with this layer and is held fast despite the action of the acid–alcohol. This allows the detection of AFB in specimens with a simple staining technique – the Ziehl–Neelsen (ZN) stain, which has been in use for over 60 years.

The uniquely thick cell wall also gives mycobacteria another useful characteristic, which is their resistance to the lethal effects of acids, alkalis and detergents. This is fortunate because most specimens are heavily contaminated with other bacteria, which grow more quickly than mycobacteria and would thus swamp the culture. It is therefore possible to 'treat' the specimen by adding an acid or alkali, thus killing the other bacteria leaving the mycobacteria alive. Ultimately the mycobacteria will also be killed and a balance has to be struck. Ideally between 2% and 3% of cultures should be lost because of contamination, indicating that the treatment procedure is neither too harsh nor too moderate.

The laboratory diagnosis of tuberculosis thus still relies on direct microscopy and culture using techniques devised many years ago. There is no 100% reliable serological test for tuberculosis (Chapter 17a, p. 367 *et seq.*). Many have been tried but all lack specificity

Clinical Tuberculosis. Edited by P.D.O. Davies. Published in 1994 by Chapman & Hall, London. ISBN 0 412 48630 X

and sensitivity. This is due to the ubiquitous nature of mycobacteria. They are widely distributed in the environment and exposure is unavoidable. As a result antibodies develop to the cross-reacting antigens that are present in most mycobacteria and this gives rise to false-positive reactions. On the other hand, individuals respond to different epitopes when infected and the use of a single antigen to detect antibodies gives false-negative results. Finally the widespread use of BCG vaccination may make interpretation difficult (Chapter 15d, p. 345 *et seq.*).

New approaches to the laboratory diagnosis of tuberculosis include the detection of specific substances that can only be present because of the concomitant presence of mycobacteria[3], the detection of mycobacterial antigens by an ELISA technique[4] and the polymerase chain reaction (Chapter 17b). However, microscopy and culture remain the primary methods of laboratory diagnosis and are likely to do so for many years to come.

Accurate and reliable identification and drug sensitivity tests are necessary for the successful treatment of tuberculosis and other mycobacterial diseases. The Public Health Laboratory Service (PHLS) has six laboratories designated as Regional Centres for Tuberculosis Bacteriology. These work in concert with the Mycobacterium Reference Unit to provide a service for England and Wales and currently process over 95% of all requests for identification and sensitivity tests. Standard techniques are used throughout the centres and sensitivity test results are subject to an on-going quality control system.

Most of the mycobacteria that cause disease in man are classed as category 3 pathogens and therefore require specialized handling in designated laboratories. Specimens suspected of containing mycobacteria and cultures thought to be mycobacteria therefore have to be processed in microbiological safety cabinets (class I or II) in a laboratory having a class 3 containment facility. This ensures that any aerosol that

may be produced during the handling of the specimen or culture is unlikely to be a hazard to the laboratory worker[5].

3.2 SPECIMENS

Three specimens of sputum collected on successive days should be provided. Saliva is not adequate. A single specimen of sputum will miss about 25% of microspically positive and about 50% of culture-positive cases. If there is still a problem with diagnosis then an unlimited number of specimens should be sent.

When sputum is not available, for example in children, the gastric contents may be collected. Ideally the patient should cough and swallow for 10 minutes before collection, which should be done early in the morning before food is taken. Laryngeal swabs are less efficient than sputum or gastric contents.

Broncho-alveolar lavage using a fibre-optic bronchoscope provides excellent specimens from specific sites in the lung. However there is an increasing problem of contamination of such specimens because tap water is being used in the machines for rinsing the bronchoscopes instead of sterile distilled water. Unfortunately tap water contains environmental mycobacteria, which lodge in the plastic tubing that connects such machines to the mains supply. *M. chelonei* is the organism most likely to appear as a contaminant and it can be very difficult to eradicate[6]. However any one of the whole range of environmental mycobacteria can cause this problem, ranging from *M. avium* to *M. kansasii*.

Aspirates such as pleural fluids, CSFs etc. should be taken into sterile containers and transported to the laboratory as rapidly as possible. Actual pus is a better specimen than a pus swab but if possible a piece of tissue from the site should be sent. It is often the case that tissue is sent for histology and is placed directly into formalin, thus negating any chance of culture.

Genitourinary tuberculosis is relatively rare

in England and Wales and most laboratories lack the expertise to detect and interpret the significance of AFB in urine. However, when genitourinary tuberculosis is considered a possibility, then 50 ml of early morning urine should be sent on three successive days; 24 h specimens are not recommended.

The examination of faeces used to be rarely necessary. Most cases of tuberculous enteritis have lung lesions and tubercle bacilli in faeces come from swallowed sputum. However, with the advent of the acquired immunodeficiecy syndrome (AIDS) the situation has changed. A significant number of AIDS patients have disseminated disease due to *M. avium* and AFB are often demonstrable in both faeces and biopsies of the intestinal mucosa and can be cultured from these specimens.

3.3 MICROSCOPY

The patient whose sputum is positive on direct microscopy (Plate 1) is most likely to infect his/her close contacts[7]. Such a patient will have at least 5000 organisms/ml of sputum and may have up to ten times that number. Below 5000 organisms/ml it is unlikely that ZN or fluorescence staining will detect AFB. In England and Wales approximately 53% of new cases of pulmonary tuberculosis are positive on direct smear[8].

Direct microscopy of specimens other than sputum is of doubtful utility. Few laboratories have the expertise to interpret ZN-stained smears of urine and most no longer undertake this examination. Very careful scrutiny of smears from aspirates and tissues is necessary to detect the small number that are positive. These are most likely to be biopsy specimens from lymph nodes.

The main role of microscopy is therefore to identify the truly infectious patient so that the chain of infection can be halted by the appropriate treatment of the index patient. It is accepted that 2–3 weeks' chemotherapy with a modern antituberculosis regimen will make most patients non-infectious. Such a regimen will consist of isoniazid, rifampicin and pyrazinamide given for 2 months followed by isoniazid and rifampicin given for an additional 4 months[9] (Chapter 8b, p. 141).

3.4 CULTURE

The definitive diagnosis is the isolation of *M. tuberculosis* in pure culture. However this is only achieved in about 50% of cases and the diagnosis then has to rely on the clinical and/or radiological features, sometimes with histological evidence.

In the UK the most commonly used media for the isolation of tubercle bacilli are Lowenstein–Jensen (LJ) egg medium or Kirchner broth containing an antibiotic mixture. LJ is a simple egg-based medium that may be produced in a buffered form or as an acid egg medium[10]. Two tubes should be used, one containing glycerol and the other sodium pyruvate. Glycerol tends to inhibit the growth of *M. bovis* whereas sodium pyruvate encourages it.

From a sputum specimen positive by direct microscopy, LJ will show growth within 2–3 weeks at 37 °C. The colonies are rough and a beige-to-brown colour and show up well on the green background, which is due to the presence in the medium of the dye malachite green (Plate 2). Smear-negative sputa and specimens from other sites may not give a positive growth until they have been incubated for up to 6 or 8 weeks. Cultures showing no growth are reported negative at this time.

Kirchner being a liquid medium is more difficult to interpret and it is necessary to centrifuge the medium and make a ZN-stained smear of the deposit. If AFB are detected then subcultures are made on LJ but this inevitably entails a delay in reporting.

There are two other methods used in the UK for the culture of mycobacteria. These are the Roche MB check system and the BACTEC

460 radiometric system. Both these rely on the growth of the bacilli in a Middlebrook broth. This is a liquid medium that readily supports the growth of mycobacteria[11]. The Roche MB check system is a biphasic system in which the broth is inoculated with the specimen that has been decontaminated in the usual way. By inverting the system during incubation, this broth culture is flooded over a slope containing, on the one side, Middlebrook 7H-10 agar and, on the other side, a Middlebrook 7H-10 agar containing p-nitro-α-acetylamino-3-hydroxy propiophenone (NAP) and a chocolate agar. Mycobacteria growing in the broth will form visible colonies on the Middlebrook agar. If they do not belong to the tuberculosis complex they will also grow on the Middlebrook agar containing NAP. If they are not myco-bacteria at all they will grow on the chocolate agar[12].

The BACTEC 460 radiometric system also uses a Middlebrook broth but one that incorporates a C^{14}-labelled substrate. During metabolism C^{14}-labelled CO_2 is produced and this is automatically monitored by the machine[11]. Using this system *M. tuberculosis* will grow, on average, 7–10 days more quickly than in the conventional LJ system.

The Middlebrook broth described above will not accommodate blood or bone marrow and is therefore of no use in disseminated disease. There is now available another medium designated Middlebrook 13A, which will take up to 5 ml of blood or a bone marrow. This is not so important from the point of view of classical tuberculosis but is very important in considering the problems of *M. avium* infections in patients with AIDS.

3.5 OTHER METHODS OF DIAGNOSIS

Despite considerable effort there is still no acceptable serological test for tuberculosis (Chapter 17a, p. 367). Such a test would be very useful for smear-negative pulmonary disease, extrapulmonary disease and tuberculosis in children. All the methods that have been tried have lacked specificity and sensitivity due to the diversity of the antigenic determinants of the tubercle bacillus and to exposure to environmental mycobacteria that share antigens with the tubercle bacillus.

ELISA tests have been described for the diagnosis of tuberculosis meningitis[13,14]. However, no ELISA system has yet proved to be acceptable in the UK. A murine monoclonal antibody to the 38 kDa antigen of *M. tuberculosis* has been used in a modified serological competition assay but unfortunately this is not generally available[15]. The application of the polymerase chain reaction for the direct detection of *M. tuberculosis*, while having enormous potential, is not in routine use at present[16–18] (Chapter 17b, p. 381).

Rather than look for antibodies, attempts have been made to detect either antigens themselves or substances specific for myco-bacteria. Rabbit antisera to BCG have been used to detect antigens in CSF[19,20] and gas–liquid chromatography linked with mass spectrometry adapted for selected ion monitoring has been used to detect tuber-culostearic acid (10-methyloctadecanoic acid) in both CSF and sputum[3,21]. Both techniques need further evaluation and the GLC–MS technique requires very expensive equipment.

3.6 IDENTIFICATION OF TUBERCLE BACILLI

It is possible to identify most mycobacteria to the species level with tests based on simple cultural and biochemical properties[22]. It is also possible to identify sub-specific variants by further biochemical tests, by phage-typing or by serotyping but this is of epidemiological value only and has little clinical relevance. It is thus important to identify a strain only as far as is clinically necessary. The recent

Table 3.1 Cultural characters of tubercle bacilli after 2 weeks' incubation

25°C	37°C	45°C	PNB	THIA
−	+	−	−	−

PNB = p-nitro benzoic acid ⎱
THIA = thiacetazone ⎰ incubated at 37°C.

development of DNA fingerprinting using restriction fragment length polymorphism (RFLP) allows a very precise identification of a strain and its possible involvement in an outbreak situation (Chapter 17c, p. 391 *et seq.*).

Tubercle bacilli have a characteristic morphology when a ZN-stained smear is examined by microscopy. However it requires a considerable degree of expertise to interpret this and even then one can be misled. It is therefore necessary to set up a small number of cultural and biochemical tests to confirm the identity of a strain.

A suspension of the strain is inoculated onto LJ slopes for incubation at 25°C, 37°C and 45°C and also on to LJ slopes containing p-nitro-benzoic acid (PNB 500 µ2g/ml) and thiacetazone (10 µg/ml). These are incubated for 2–3 weeks and a tubercle bacillus will show the results illustrated in Table 3.1. Mycobacteria other than tubercle bacilli (MOTT bacilli), also called opportunist or non-tuberculous mycobacteria and even atypical mycobacteria, will show more rapid growth and/or growth at 25°C or 45°C and/or growth on the PNB slope and/or the thiacetazone slope. Some of them will also produce pigment either in the light only (photochromogen) such as *M. kansasii* or in both the light and dark (scotochromogens) such as *M. gordonae* (Chapter 13, p. 265).

Strains belonging to the tuberculosis complex can be divided into a number of variants as described in the introduction. The cultural characteristics for these variants are shown in Table 3.2 but, as said earlier, these are of little clinical importance except in the identification of *M. bovis*, which is naturally resistant to pyrazinamide. The inexpert administration of vaccine strain Bacillus Calmette–Guerin (BCG) can give rise to local abscesses and even regional lymphadenitis and it is not unusual to isolate BCG from such sites (Chapter 14b, p. 297). The characteristics of the strain have been included in Table 3.2 for convenience.

3.7 IDENTIFICATION OF OPPORTUNIST MYCOBACTERIA

The opportunist mycobacteria that most commonly cause pulmonary disease are:

- *M. kansasii*
- *M. avium* ⎫
- *M. intracellulare* ⎬ MAIS complex
- *M. scrofulaceum* ⎭
- *M. malmoense*
- *M. xenopi*

The identification of these organisms is best undertaken by specialist laboratories. The tests described for the identification of *M. tuberculosis* are supplemented by a test for the hydrolysis of Tween 80 and if necessary by thin-layer chromatography of an extract containing the superficial lipids from the cell wall[22,23]. Many species of mycobacteria have lipid patterns that are absolutely characteristic and not shared with other species. Sub-specific variants can also be identified using this technique.

Most if not all species of opportunist mycobacteria are widespread in the environment and they can gain access to specimens. It can therefore be difficult to decide which isolates are clinically significant. Multiple isolates in the absence of any other pathogen and with consistent clinical and/or radiological features will usually indicate significance.

3.8 DRUG RESISTANCE IN TUBERCLE BACILLI

Bacteria change their characters either: (i) in response to a stimulus – that is, by induced

Table 3.2 Variants of the tuberculosis complex

Variant	Oxygen preference[a]	TCH[b]	Nitratase	Pyrazinamide	Cycloserine
M. tuberculosis	A	R	+	S	S
Asian	A	S	+	S	S
African I	M	S	−	S	S
African II	M	S	+	S	S
M. bovis	M	S	−	R	S
BCG	A	S	−	R	R

[a] A, Aerobic; M, microaerophilic; R, resistant; S, sensitive.
[b] Thiophen-2-carboxylic acid hydrazide, 5 mg/l.

adaptation; or (ii) spontaneously (genetically) by mutation. Mutations usually die out but if they have survival value they will multiply more than or instead of the original population of bacilli and will eventually replace it. All populations of tubercle bacilli generate small numbers that are resistant to any particular drug. If the patient is given the drug, a resistant mutant will not be affected and if it is not killed by the body's defences or another drug, it will multiply and replace the sensitive population. When a single drug is given the outcome is finely balanced – the defences may win over the very small initial number of mutants but they may fail. This is why single-drug therapy is often unsuccessful, resulting in drug resistance.

Excluding chemically related drugs, a mutant resistant to one drug is not especially likely to be resistant to a different drug. Thus, if two effective unrelated drugs are given together there is only a small chance of there being any mutant present that is resistant to both drugs at the same time. However, with very severe disease, immunity is low and the bacterial population is very large so doubly-resistant mutants may be present and there can be failure to eliminate them. This is why triple therapy is advisable initially – the chance of a triply-resistant mutant can be ignored. When the bacterial population is reduced (e.g. on conversion to culture-negative) it is safe to drop one of the drugs. Examples of resistant-mutant incidence

are 10^{-6} for rifampicin, 10^{-5} for streptomycin and isoniazid, 10^{-3} for cycloserine and 10^{-2} for pyrazinamide. Therefore the incidence of doubly-resistant mutants would be, for example 10^{-10} for streptomycin plus isoniazid.

3.9 SENSITIVITY TESTS TO TUBERCLE BACILLI

There are opposing views of the need for sensitivity tests. Most would agree that they are helpful in patients who relapse or do not convert and that if the technique is poor then they are not worth the effort. The disagreement arises over the advisability or need for sensitivity tests in new cases and the need to do tests for drugs other than streptomycin, isoniazid, rifampicin and ethambutol.

To plan treatment properly it is necessary to know the incidence of primary resistance in the country as a whole, and to determine this it is necessary to test a good sample of strains not just once but regularly. It seems reasonable therefore to carry out sensitivity tests on new cases if the facilities are available and the technique is adequate. Such tests also provide useful supporting evidence for the identity of the organisms.

There is a further disagreement on how sensitivity tests should be performed. It is simple to determine the minimum inhibitory concentration (MIC) of a drug. A control slope and others containing increasing con-

Table 3.3   Example of a modal resistance control set

		Drug concentrations				
	Control	1	2	4	8	16
Strain A	CG	CG	CG	−	−	−
B	IC	IC	+	−	−	−
C	CG	CG	IC	−	−	−
D	CG	CG	IC	+	−	−
E	IC	IC	−	−	−	−
Mode		CG	IC	−	−	−

CG, confluent growth; IC, innumerable discrete colonies; +, 20–100 colonies; −, less than 20 colonies.

centrations of the drug are inoculated equally and incubated. However, the results differ considerably in different laboratories owing to variations in medium or technique and to some extent at different times in any one laboratory. Even if the MIC is accurate – what does it mean? The MIC can be related to concentrations of drug attainable in the blood or tissues or lesions but these concentrations are not known for all drugs in all situations. Also, in the body the concentrations are always changing – furthermore there are sometimes antagonistic substances present and variations in pH or oxygen tension and other conditions that effect the potency of each drug in an unpredictable way. The MIC is an *in vitro* test under special *in vitro* conditions and there cannot be exact quantitative equivalence (i.e. in μg/ml).

The only valid method of assessing sensitivity tests is to relate the laboratory findings to the results of treatment, initially in animal experiments but then, more importantly, in clinical trials. Such an approach can establish the general outline of sensitivity technique and interpretation but it has only been used in man for a few drugs and then not thoroughly. The chief difficulty is that drugs are not used singly in therapy trials.

The problem has therefore been approached as follows:

1. Establish the behaviour of normal (wild) strains of TB.

2. Determine the response of the patient's strain.
3. Assume that any difference (loss) of sensitivity is harmful.

The normal disc-diffusion methods used to determine the sensitivity of most bacteria are not suitable for mycobacteria. The long incubation period means that plates dry out and the dynamics of the diffusion of the drug into the agar become very complicated. It is necessary therefore to test strains by a titration method. Tubes of medium containing a range of concentrations of the drug (usually doubling) are inoculated and incubated. The results can be expressed in three ways:

1. MIC – the minimal inhibitory concentration.
2. RR – the resistance ratio to a standard strain, usually H37Rv, (i.e. ratio of MICs).
3. MR – modal resistance; this compares the MIC of the test strain with the mode or most common MIC of a group of normal strains.

In the UK the modal resistance method is most commonly used[24]. The mode is determined by testing a large number of strains from new (untreated) cases of tuberculosis. In the example shown in Table 3.3 only five strains are used, but in practice five strains are tested every week, i.e. 260 a year.

3.10 PYRAZINAMIDE

Normal methods cannot be used as the drug is only active in acid medium (pH 5.0 to 5.4) and strains vary in their ability to grow at such low pH levels. It is best to test at three different pH levels, e.g. 5.0, 5.2 and 5.4. Vigorous strains give a true result a pH 5.0, feeble strains at 5.4 and others are intermediate. To reduce the work, each test can be limited to a control and a single drug tube.

3.11 CONCLUSION

The decline in the incidence of tuberculosis has seen a concomitant decline in expertise in general microbiology laboratories. Direct microscopy and culture of specimens is still undertaken in most hospital laboratories but as the number of positives has fallen there is evidence that lack of experience has led to false-positive results being issued. 'Pseudo' outbreaks have aroused unnecessary alarm [25]. False-negative results are much more difficult to identify but it is reasonable to assume that they occur. It is to be hoped that the increased incidence in tuberculosis arising from the problems in the USA and particularly that of multi-drug resistant strains will rekindle interest at all levels in a disease that was well on its way to being eradicated in most developed countries.

REFERENCES

1. Castets, M., Rist, N. and Boisvert, H. (1969) La Variété africaine du bacille tuberculeux humain. *Méd. Afr. Noire*; **16**, 321–2.
2. Hardy, R.M. and Watson, J. (1992) *Mycobacterium bovis* in England and Wales: past present and future. *Epidemiol. Infect.*, **109**, 23–33.
3. French, G.L., Teoh, R., Chan, C.Y. *et al.* (1987) Diagnosis of tuberculous meningitis by detection of tuberculostearic acid in cerebrospinal fluid. *Lancet*, **ii**, 117–19.
4. Watt, G., Zaraspe, G., Bautista, S. and Laughlin, L. (1988) Rapid diagnosis of tuberculous meningitis by using an enzyme-linked immunosorbent assay to detect mycobacterial antigen and antibody in cerebrospinal fluid. *Infect. Dis.*, **158**, 681–6.
5. DHSS (1978) *A Code of Practice for the Prevention of Infection in Clincal Laboratories*, Department of Health and Social Security, HMSO, London.
6. Nye, K., Chadha, D.K., Hodgkin, P. *et al.* (1990) *Mycobacterium chelonei* isolated from broncho-alveolar lavage fluid and its practical implications. *J. Hos. Infect.*, **16**, 257–61.
7. British Thoracic and Tuberculosis Association (1978) A study of standardized contact procedure in tuberculosis. *Tubercle*, **59**, 245–59.
8. Medical Research Council Cardiothoracic Epidemiology Group (1992) National Survey of notification of tuberculosis in England and Wales. *Thorax*, **47**, 770–5.
9. British Thoracic Society (1984) A controlled trial of 6 months chemotherapy in pulmonary tuberculosis. Final report: Results during the 36 months after the end of chemotherapy and beyond. *Br. J. Dis. Chest*, **78**, 330–6.
10. Zaher, F. and Marks, J. (1977) Methods and medium for the culture of tubercle bacilli. *Tubercle*, **58**, 143–5.
11. Middlebrook, G., Reggiardo, A. and Tigertt, W.D. (1977) Automatable radiometric detection of growth of *Mycobacterium tuberculosis* in selective media. *Am. Rev. Respir. Dis.* **115**, 1066–9.
12. Damato, R S., Isenberg, H.D., Hochstein, L. *et al.* (1991) Evaluation of the Roche Septi Check AFB system for the recovery of mycobacteria. *J. Clin. Microbiol*, **29**, 2906–8.
13. Grange, J.M., Gibson, J., Nassau, E. and Kardijito, T. (1980) Enzyme-linked immunosorbent assay (ELISA): a study of antibodies to *Mycobacterium tuberculosis* in the IgG, IgA and IgM classes in tuberculosis and sarcoidosis. *Tubercle*, **61**, 145–52.
14. Sada, E.D., Ferguson, L.E. and Daniel, T.M. (1990) An ELISA for the serodiagnosis of tuberculosis using a 30 000 Da native antigen of *Mycobacterium tuberculosis*. *J. Infect. Dis.*, **162**, 928–31.
15. Wilkins, E.G.L. and Ivanyi, J. (1990) Potential value of serology for diagnosis of extra pulmonary tuberculosis. *Lancet*, **336**, 641–4.
16. Brisson-Noel, A., Gicquel, B., Lecossier D *et al.* (1989) Rapid diagnosis of tuberculosis by amplification of mycobacterial DNA in clinical samples. *Lancet*, **ii**, 1069–71.
17. Sjobring, U., Meckleburg, M., Bengard, A.A.

and Miorner, H. (1990) Polymerase chain reaction for detection of *Mycobacterium tuberculosis*. *J. Clin. Microbiol.*, **28**, 2200–4.

18. Shankar, P., Manjunath, N., Mohan, K.K. *et al.* (1991) Rapid diagnosis of tuberculosis meningitis by polymerase chain reaction. *Lancet*, **337**, 5–7.

19. Sada, E., Ruiz-Palacios, G.M., Lopez-Vidal, Y. and de Leon, S. (1983) Detection of mycobacterial antigens in cerebrospinal fluid of patients with tuberculous meningitis by enzyme-linked immunosorbent assay. *Lancet*, **ii**, 651–2.

20. Radhakrishan, V.V., Sehgal, S. and Mathai, A. (1990) Correlation between culture of *Mycobacterium tuberculosis* and detection of mycobacterial antigens in cerebrospinal fluid of patients with tuberculous meningitis. *J. Med. Microbiol.*, **33**, 223–6.

21. Oldham, G., Larsson, L. and Mardh, P. (1979) Demonstration of tuberculostearic acid in sputum from patients with pulmonary tuberculosis by selected ion monitoring. *J. Clin. Invest.*, **63**, 813–19.

22. Marks, J. (1976) A system for the examination of tubercle bacilli and other mycobacteria. *Tubercle*, **57**, 207–52.

23. Marks, J. and Jenkins, P.A (1971) Thin layer chromatography of mycobacterial lipids as an aid to classification: technical improvements: *Mycobacterium avium, M. intracellulare* (Battey bacilli). *Tubercle*, **52**, 219–25.

24. Marks, J. (1961) The design of sensitivity tests of tubercle bacilli. *Tubercle*, **42**, 314–16.

25. Davies, P.D.O. Williams, C.S.D., Shears, P. *et al.* (1992) Pseudo-outbreak of tuberculosis in a paediatric oncology ward [Abstract]. *Thorax*, **47**, 220 P.

THE PATHOLOGY OF TUBERCULOSIS 4

E.A. Sheffield

4.1 THE MORPHOLOGY OF GRANULOMATA

The histological features of tuberculosis are characteristic and similar in all sites of infection. The hallmark of active infection is the necrotizing epithelioid cell granuloma. It is also important to point out that tuberculous granulomata are identical morphologically and immunologically to granulomata due to other infectious causes such as histoplasmosis and blastomycosis[1]. Before describing the pathology of tuberculosis, some general points will be covered.

The predominant cells in all granulomata, whether organized into epithelioid cell foci or not, are non-lymphoid mononuclear cells[2,3]. This diverse group, known as the reticulo-endothelial or mononuclear phagocyte system[4], includes blood monocytes, tissue macrophages (or histiocytes), and organ-specific forms such as the Kupffer cells of the liver. In epithelioid cell granulomata they are represented by macrophages, epithelioid cells and giant cells of predominantly Langerhans type[2,5,6]. The nuclei of these giant cells are arranged in an arc around central granular cytoplasm. Tuberculous granulomas typically show necrosis; as described later this is due to the inherent toxicity of the bacilli and the release of cytokines such as tumour necrosis factor and interleukin-1[7].

Mononuclear phagocytes arise from immature bone marrow precursors, circulate briefly as monocytes and then populate the tissues as macrophages. They are capable of rapid differentiation and activation. Mackaness[8] used the term 'activation' to describe increased activity against ingested pathogens; such macrophages can be recognized functionally[9] and morphologically[10].

An epithelioid cell granuloma consists of a collection of partly or highly specialized mononuclear phagocytes in response to a persistent inflammatory agent. Epithelioid cells appear large with abundant eosinophilic cytoplasm and show indistinct cell boundaries[11]. Enzyme histochemistry and immunochemistry support the concept that the cell population of a granuloma is mixed, with different activities of cells in varying regions of the granuloma.

Inclusions, such as asteroid or Schaumann bodies, may be found in the giant cells in long-standing granulomatous inflammation. Asteroid bodies are also seen in giant cells and are formed from a radial arrangement of cytoskeletal elements. Schaumann bodies are laminated calcified bodies 10–100 μm in diameter found within epithelioid cells and giant cells. They may lie free in areas of fibrosis and indicate previous granulomatous inflammation. They show a central crystalline core containing iron and calcium. They are probably of lysosomal origin[12]. They have been reported as occurring in up to 6% of tuberculous granulomata.

On electron microscopy, macrophages have a deeply indented nucleus with fairly dense chromatin. A nucleolus may be prominent. Mitochondria are relatively numerous.

Clinical Tuberculosis. Edited by P.D.O. Davies. Published in 1994 by Chapman & Hall, London. ISBN 0 412 48630 X

Strands of rough endoplasmic reticulum and lysosomes lie in the cytoplasm. Variable numbers of microfilaments and microtubules are also present throughout the cytoplasm.

The most striking feature is the presence of large numbers of cytoplasmic vacuoles[13,14]. These inclusions are circular or elongated and measure 0.05–0.25 μm in diameter. Some are electron dense and resemble lysosomes. The majority, however, contain fluffy material that appears homogenous. This latter type of vacuole appears to be unique to epithelioid cells[15,16]. Fragments of micro-organisms may be seen within these vacuoles[17]. Epithelioid cells show prominent rough endoplasmic reticulum and Golgi lamellae, therefore suggesting that in epithelioid cell granulomas macrophages change from a predominantly phagocytic to a secretory role[18,19]. Well-developed epithelioid cells show numerous cytoplasmic projections, which frequently interdigitate and occasionally form junctions[19,20]. This feature accounts for the indistinct and cytoplasmic boundaries of epithelioid cells seen on light microscopy.

The intercellular junctions that form between epithelioid cells resemble desmosomes. Subplasmalemmal densities present on the opposing cells closely relate to a plaque of electron-dense extracellular material. Immature cells in granulomata generally lack such membrane interconnecting elements. Isolated subplasmalemmal linear densities of the type seen in relation to intercellular junctions in granulomas are frequently seen in cells of the mononuclear-phagocyte system[21]. The large number of junctions between epithelioid cells suggests cell-to-cell communication is prominent. Adhesion molecules are associated with these junction complexes. Cell adhesion due to these molecules has been localized by immunocytochemistry, in particular integrin VLA-3[22]. This integrin is strongly associated with intercellular contact sites. Subplasmalemmal densities are associated with areas of the cell membrane where cytoskeletal filaments relate to the extracellular matrix[23].

4.2 THE IMMUNOLOGY OF GRANULOMATA

The immunological response to tuberculosis is almost entirely cell-mediated, the epithelioid cell being the effector cell. Macrophages in association with a delayed hypersensitivity reaction show increased phagocytic and intracellular killing ability[24]. There is substantial evidence that the mononuclear and epithelioid cells seen within granulomata are derived from the bone marrow via the circulation. Cells of the mononuclear phagocytic system from different anatomical sites show marked functional and phenotypic differences[25]. This heterogeneity may reflect either the influence of environmental factors stimulating circulating monocytes to differentiate in a particular way, or the existence of different macrophage subsets[26]. Different subsets of macrophages are seen in B and T cell-dependent areas of peripheral human lymphoid tissues[27]. Further evidence that epithelioid cells are derived from monocytes is provided by the retention of the monocyte–macrophage marker RFD-2 by epithelioid cells throughout granulomata[28]. Epithelioid cells also show the macrophage marker OKMI[29,30]. However, mononuclear phagocytes in the centre and periphery of granulomata differ in their immunological phenotype[31]. Activated macrophages and epithelioid cells within the centre of granulomata strongly express HLA-DR and show marked acid phosphatase activity. In the periphery of granulomata there is an additional population of non-lymphoid HLA-DR positive cells, which show only a small degree of acid phosphatase activity. These cells appear to function as antigen-presenting cells[32]. Epithelioid giant cells also strongly express HLA-DR, and may also function as antigen-presenting cells[30].

4.2.1 THE ROLE OF T CELLS

The feature that distinguishes hypersensitivity granulomata from non-specific foreign-body type granulomata is the presence of lymphocytes (Plate 3). In hypersensitivity type epithelioid cell granulomata, lymphocytes are seen in close association with the activated macrophage–monocyte cells. These T cell–macrophage interactions are important in the immunology of tuberculosis[33]. The majority of lymphocytes seen in epithelioid cell granulomata are T cells[34]. These cells show features of activation[35]. A higher proportion of CD4 helper cells are present in the centre of granulomata than at the periphery[36]. CD8 suppressor and B cells tend to be associated with epithelioid cells at the periphery, particularly in tuberculosis[37], where occasionally they form a mantle separating the granuloma from the surrounding tissue[30]. Paradoxically, some CD4 helper cells can show suppressor functional activity. These features support the concept that a function of a granuloma is the formation of an isolated microenvironment[38] with immunoregulation occurring at the periphery. Some workers have emphasized the role of T lymphocytes in granulomatous inflammation, hypothesizing that these cells may initiate epithelioid cell granulomata[39,40]. In tuberculous granulomata, T lymphocytes produce interferon-1[41]. There are reports, however, of epithelioid cell granulomata being induced in the absence of T cell function[42]. The importance of cytokine activity in granulomata is shown by the suppressive role of corticosteroids. The macrophages in granulomata show decreased activation and number in the presence of steroids in experimental situations. There is also decreased tissue necrosis, with steroids showing an anti-inflammatory effect[43]. The release from granulomata of cytokines such as tumour necrosis factor and gamma interferon may be responsible for systemic effects such as fever in tuberculous infection[44].

Studies have shown that there is T cell receptor gene restriction in individuals with tuberculosis[45]. It is of interest that gamma-delta T cells are increased in the peripheral blood; this is a feature seen in mycobacterial infections[46]. Gamma-delta lymphocytes react to mycobacterial antigens[47]. They appear not to be increased in number in the granulomata themselves[48]. Some mononuclear cells in granulomata stain for S100 antigen, a marker of certain members of the mononuclear macrophage system, in particular Langerhans cells and so-called T-zone histiocytes. These are believed to function as antigen-presenting cells. Epithelioid cells and the monocytes in granulomata strongly express leucocyte function associated antigen-1 (LFA-1) and its ligand intercellular adhesion molecule-1 (ICAM-1). This supports the view that the monocyte-macrophage cells in granulomata are involved in antigen presentation.

The concept of high- and low-turnover granulomas was introduced by Spector [49–51]. 'High' turnover granulomata are dependent on continued recruitment from the bone marrow. Most foreign-body type granulomata are of 'low'-turnover type. These differ in being very long lived with a low level of monocyte recruitment and minimal fibrosis. The lack of fibrosis in foreign-body granulomata may be due to the low level of macrophage turnover with subsequent small amounts of free lysosomal enzymes and other fibrogenic substances[52]. In the case of high-turnover granulomata it appears that activated macrophages stimulate the proliferation of fibroblasts[53]. For example, by secreting fibronectin, activated macrophages attract fibroblasts and by secreting a growth factor the absolute number of fibroblasts is increased[54]. Granulomas have therefore been classified by the presence or absence of an associated immunological response[55]. They fall into two main groups: immunological or hypersensitive type[56] and the non-immunological foreign-body type.

4.3 THE PATHOLOGY OF TUBERCULOSIS

Tuberculosis can cause lesions in any tissue or organ of the body, but most frequently involves the lung. In view of this, the following account will focus mainly on this organ. Other organ sytems will be then be described.

4.3.1 PULMONARY TUBERCULOSIS

(a) Primary tuberculosis

The pathology of tuberculosis takes into account the inherent virulence of the organism, the immunity of the person infected, the development of hypersensitivity and the formation of epithelioid cell granulomata. Primary tuberculosis is the first infection of an unsensitized host. Tubercle bacilli usually enter the lung via the airways, and when in small groups of one to three can reach the alveolar spaces[57] in droplets smaller than 5 μm in diameter. The very early cellular reaction in tuberculosis is not known, but it is probable that neutrophils are responsible for phagocytosis initially, and macrophages are recruited later. They are then phagocytosed and the majority of the organisms will be killed. This has been termed stage I of the disease[57,58]. However, a proportion of the bacilli will survive and replicate within the macrophages and cause cell death (stage II). Further monocytes are recruited from the circulation and transform into macrophages, but unless they are activated they are inefficient at destroying the tubercle bacilli. Chemotactic factors such as complement component C5a and various cytokines such as monocytic chemotactic protein 1 (MCP-1) recruit macrophages[59]. Acid-fast bacilli are easily seen at this stage. Tubercle bacilli are transported via lymphatics to regional lymph nodes, in which epithelioid cell granulomata develop. Granulomata develop typical central necrosis as delayed hypersensitivity to the bacilli develops (stage III). This takes about 2–4 weeks, as measured by the tuberculin test. The necrosis in the granulomata is most probably due to local toxic lysosomal or cytokine effect rather than ischaemia. Tuberculous bacilli are also directly cytotoxic. The epithelioid cells that result are much more efficient at killing the intracellular bacilli. The majority of the bacilli are now extracellular and have a reduced ability to multiply and are more difficult to find at microscopy. A spectrum of reactivity to the tubercle bacilli appears to exist[60]. There may be a florid granulomatous reaction with few identifiable bacilli comparable with tuberculous leprosy. The other end of the spectrum is the presence of quiescent macrophages with abundant necrosis and large numbers of bacilli[60–62] (Plate 4).

This initial focus of caseous bronchopneumonia together with the lymphadenopathy is known as a Ghon complex. This type of infection is seen mainly in early childhood in endemic areas with a maximum incidence at 1–3 years[63]. The lymph nodes on the same side as the Ghon focus form a mass usually larger than the Ghon focus. Histologically there is marked fibrinous exudate and numerous acid-fast bacilli surrounded by granulation tissue. Connective tissue stains will show that initially the underlying lung architecture is preserved. Features correspond to the grey hepatization phase of lobar pneumonia. Infection may be centred on blood vessels[64]. The primary pulmonary focus is usually unilateral and found in a subpleural position above or below the lobar fissure between the upper and lower lobes, or less commonly the basal part of the lower lobes. Grossly it appears as a yellow-white area of softening 10–20 mm in diameter surrounded by a grey capsule. The soft area represents the 'caseous' necrosis. There may be an associated pleural effusion.

Similar primary complexes occur in organs infected by less frequent routes of infection, such as the gastrointestinal tract, oropharyngeal lymphoid tissue and the skin. Regional lymph nodes are involved by lymphatic transport of bacilli from the initial site of infection.

From the lymphatics, the bacilli enter veins and spread to other parts of the body, including the lungs, the brain, kidney and bone. If bacilli enter a pulmonary artery, spread to other parts of the lung will result. The systemic haematogenous stage is frequently marked by acid-fast bacilli in the urine. Despite this wide distribution, in the majority of cases the infection is controlled and lesions resolve without clinical features. Areas of infection smaller than a millimetre in size resolve with no fibrosis. Larger areas of infection, greater than 5 mm across show fibrosis and dystrophic calcification and occasionally ossification. They have the appearance of friable white material surrounded by a grey capsule with fibrosis in the adjacent lung. These larger lesions appear to be a source of reactivation. Hilar lymph nodes typically show dense hyaline fibrosis. In the infant, however, there may be uncontrolled proliferation of the tubercle bacilli; the Ghon focus may penetrate a blood vessel or bronchus to cause bronchopneumonia and other satellite lesions or 'miliary' disseminated disease such as meningitis, or renal disease. Infected organs show numerous small, white nodules resembling millet seed. Oesophageal perforation has also been rarely described [65].

Congenital tuberculosis is rare and generally lethal. Infection appears to be by a haematogenous route or from aspiration of infected amniotic fluid[66].

(b) Secondary tuberculosis

After resolution of the primary infection, small numbers of bacilli survive within the scarred foci for many years. The majority of infections, at least 90%, do not progress any further. Reactivation of the disease (post-primary or secondary tuberculosis) occurs when host resistance is impaired. This may be due to immunosuppression from any cause, including malnutrition, alcoholism, malignant disease, silicosis, diabetes[67] and acquired immune deficiency syndrome (AIDS). Post-primary pulmonary tuberculosis may also be the result of further infection from an exogenous source. This disease is mainly a disease of the elderly[68], who were infected at a young age when tuberculosis was more common. It is usually seen in the apical or posterior segments of the upper lobes (Simon's foci) 10–20 mm from the pleura and apical segments of the lower lobes. Clinically the disease presents as an acute necrotizing pneumonia (Plate 5). Hilar lymphadenopathy is not a prominent feature. In view of the sensitivity of the host there is a very florid response to the bacilli, with marked caseous and liquefactive necrosis. The liquefaction and cavitation is due to the hydrolysis of protein, lipid and nucleic acids by the enzyme products of large numbers of macrophages recruited in view of the hypersensitivity of the host[69]. The organisms are able to multiply extracellularly in large numbers. This is stage IV of the disease as described by Lurie. The lesion often ruptures into a bronchus and may result in progressive pulmonary tuberculosis localized to one area of the lung. Endobronchial and endotracheal infection may result. Large numbers of bacilli are usually present in the sputum. There may be a dominant florid hypersensitivity reaction to this liquefied material in the distal lung, particularly in children. Diffuse bronchopneumonia can occur. A tuberculous empyema may result if the secondary lesion ruptures into the pleural cavity. Organisms may be coughed up and infect the larynx or be swallowed and infect the lymphoid tissue of the gastrointestinal tract. Other paths of spread within the lung are via arteries, with miliary spread to all parts of the lung, or via a pulmonary vein with dissemination to all areas of the body. Common sites of spread are the bone marrow, eye, lymph nodes, liver, spleen, kidneys, adrenal, prostate, seminal vesicles, uterine tubes, endometrium and the meninges. The eye is another important site of involvement. The disease may then progress in any one of these organs to dominate the clinical picture. Common sites of isolated infection are cervical lymph nodes (scrofula), meninges, kidney, adrenals, bones, uterine tubes and the epididymis. Diagnosis of such extrapulmonary sites often requires biopsy [70].

In renal disease, infection of the renal pelvis and the bladder may result. Tuberculosis of the uterine tubes may spread to the endometrium and the adjacent pelvic structures. In infection of the spine (Pott's disease), the disease may spread along the psoas fascia along a tract opening in the groin. Chronic tuberculous infection is a well-known cause of reactive systemic amyloid (secondary, AA type).

In severely immunosuppressed individuals, particularly in AIDS, in view of the reduced T lymphocyte population there is almost a total absence of granulomata and large numbers of mycobacteria proliferate uncontrolled within macrophages. Rarely patients show loss of skin sensitivity and loss of cell-mediated immunity to the mycobacteria[71].

Another rare form of disseminated spread of infection is cryptic disseminated tuberculosis. This occurs in immunodeficient individuals and the elderly. Very small lesions are present with large numbers of bacilli[72]. The cause of such reduced response to the infection is not known but may be due to abnormal expression of HLA-DR gene products[73].

Secondary lesions are associated with a great deal of lung destruction. Much of the destruction may be due to overproduction of cytokines such as tumour necrosis factor[74].

The liquified cavity becomes surrounded by dense fibrous tissue. It is lined by caseous material with soft nodules and may contain remnants of pulmonary vessels. Cavities usually measure from 3–10 cm across. If they are developing they have thin walls; more chronic cavities are surrounded by fibrosis. Pulmonary artery aneurysm[75] and bronchopleural fistula[76] are complications that may result. A late problem with a chronic cavity is colonization by a fungus such as aspergillus with the development of a mycetoma.

4.4 SYSTEMIC INVOLVEMENT IN TUBERCULOSIS

The more common sites of involvement are described.

4.4.1 LYMPH NODES

Lymph nodes may become an isolated site of disease in secondary tuberculosis; involvement of cervical nodes is termed 'scrofula'. A sinus may develop, connecting with the skin. Cervical lymphadenopathy may occur in primary tuberculosis where the site of infection is the oropharynx, including the tonsil. The nodes may become adherent and form a multinodular mass that may imitate metastatic carcinoma.

Lymph nodes infected with tuberculosis may enlarge when antituberculosis chemotherapy is started. It is suggested that the breakdown of degenerating bacilli stimulates cell-mediated immunity[77].

4.4.2 SKIN

Primary tuberculosis of the skin is very rare and is usually the result of direct inoculation. The lesion develops within 2–4 weeks after the inoculation. The earliest response is a neutrophilic reaction with necrosis and ulceration. Macrophages are recruited and necrotizing epithelioid cell granulomata develop.

Miliary tuberculosis of the skin can occur in primary pulmonary tuberculosis and is characterized by numerous micro-abscesses surrounded by macrophages containing acid-fast bacilli.

Involvement of the skin in secondary tuberculosis is manifested by lupus vulgaris. These chronic lesions are found on the head and neck as red-brown patches with nodules. Well-formed epithelioid cell granulomata with Langerhans giant cells are seen histologically, although necrosis is minimal. Acid-fast bacilli are rarely seen.

Occasionally disseminated skin lesions are seen in active tuberculous infection. They show well-formed granulomata without acid-fast baciili. Regression occurs on treatment and they probably represent a local response to fragments of tuberculous antigenic material[78]. They are known as tuberculids (papulonecrotic, lichen scrofulosorum and erythema induratum). Necrosis and vasculitis may be seen.

4.4.3 CENTRAL NERVOUS SYSTEM

Tuberculous meningitis may occur after the escape into the subarachnoid space of bacilli from a focus of infection in the meninges or cortex. There is a diffuse meningitis with severe inflammation and fibrin exudation and eventual fibrosis. Nerves and blood vessels may be compromised; obliterative endarteritis develops. A rare form of tuberculosis in an epidural site may result from spread of tuberculous infection from the middle ear. Subdural tuberculosis manifests as large confluent plaques of exudate.

Tuberculomas are localized space-occupying masses within the brain tissue with central necrosis and surrounding granulomatous inflammation. In adults they are supratentorial while in children they tend to occur in the posterior fossa. Old lesions may calcify. In only half the cases is there a previous history of tuberculosis[79].

A hypersensitivity phenomenon manifesting as acute haemorrhagic leucoencephalopathy may occur in tuberculous patients. This may also be associated with upper respiratory tract infections due to organisms other than tuberculosis and in septicaemia. There is diffuse oedema, focal demyelination and a perivascular macrophage reaction. Spinal cord involvement has been described[80].

4.4.4 FEMALE GENITAL TRACT

(a) Uterine tubes and ovary

Primary tuberculosis is rare; secondary infection is almost always by the haematogenous route. The uterine tubes are the most common site of infection. Although a pulmonary lesion may not be evident, involvement of the peritoneum or kidneys may be present. Lymphatic spread from primary intestinal infection may occur or there may be direct spread from the bladder or gastrointestinal tract.

As the disease becomes chronic, there is thickening and nodularity of the tube. Dense fibrous adhesions between the ovary and tube develop, and the fimbriae and ostium may obliterate. The ovary can be involved by direct spread from the uterine tube, but this is less common than tube involvement itself[81]. It is rare to see necrotizing granulomata within the ovarian stroma. The uterine tube can dilate and form a hydrosalpinx. Mucosal granulomata are seen, which extend into the muscle wall and to the serosa. They can become confluent and cause obstruction. The granulomata ulcerate and infectious material is released into the tube lumen. Tubal obstruction is almost always the end result of this process[82]. Calcification is common in old lesions.

(b) Endometrium

Involvement of the endometrium follows infection of the uterine tubes. The resulting granulomatous inflammation may be focal and poorly formed in view of the monthly shedding of the endometrium. The inflammation can, however, be diffuse with numerous necrotizing granulomata. The only manifestation of the disease may be a chronic endometritis with plasma cells. The inflammation is normally superficial: deep granulomatous inflammation is rare[83]. Reactive changes may be seen in the adjacent endometrial glands. Placental tuberculous infection is rare[84]. Infection of the cervix and vulva may follow tuberculous endometritis. Tuberculous cervicitis may resemble carcinoma macroscopically.

4.4.5 KIDNEY AND MALE GENITAL TRACT

Tuberculosis of the kidney results from secondary spread from a pulmonary site and it may be either unilateral or bilateral. The resulting necrotizing granulomata involve the cortex and medulla and eventually rupture into the renal pelvis.

Tuberculous cystitis, epididymitis and orchitis may result from this. Tuberculous epidiymitis may also originate from the prostate. In haematogenous spread, the head of the epididymis is most frequently involved, the vas being spared. In spread from the prostate, both the vas and tail are involved. Testicular involvement may simulate a neoplasm.

4.4.6 BONE AND JOINT

Tuberculosis at these sites is normally secondary by the haematogenous spread from the lung. The most common site involved is the spine, in the area of the tenth thoracic vertebra, although any bone may be involved. There is bone destruction with replacement by caseous inflammation. A paravertebral abscess may result. Spinal cord compression is a recognized complication. The infection can track along anatomical planes to discharge a distance from the involved bone.

Poncet's disease may occur in association with tuberculosis. Hypertrophic osteoarthropathy may also occur where pulmonary disease is long-standing or extensive. Organisms are not found at the involved sites and the conditions probably have an immunological basis. Tuberculous arthritis may originate in the synovium itself or develop from direct spread from tuberculous arthritis. The knee and hip joints are the most commonly involved sites. The end result is joint restriction or ankylosis.

4.4.7 GASTROINTESTINAL

As with the lung, tuberculosis can be divided into primary and secondary types. Tuberculosis can affect any part of the gastrointestinal tract, but it is most commonly found in the terminal ileum and ileocaecal region. It is rare to see tuberculosis in the colon and rectum. Acute obstruction and perforation are frequent complications. The differential diagnosis of tuberculosis always includes Crohn's disease. Tuberculosis can cause single or multiple strictures with mucosal ulceration. The ulcers tend to be annular in distribution, the base being raised. The submucosa is characteristically obliterated in tuberculosis, with severe associated fibrosis. This fibrosis results in hypertrophic or ulceroconstrictive forms of the disease. Fissures and fistulae are rare. Granulomata are well formed, found in Peyer's patches and lymphoid follicles, and almost always are found in regional lymph nodes. Enterocolitis may result from acute infection and perforation with the development of peritonitis, and ascites may occur. In peritonitis the surface is studded with myriads of tubercles, which can fuse to form caseous masses. Involvement of the greater omentum predominates.

Anorectal tuberculosis is common in areas with a high incidence of pulmonary and intestinal tuberculosis[85]. One clinical type is in patients presenting with active tuberculosis with anal ulceration in which acid-fast bacilli are numerous. The second clinical type is more chronic with marked fibrosis and fistulae in which bacilli are sparse; differentiation from Crohn's disease is difficult.

Gastric tuberculosis is almost always secondary and presents with chronic ulceration associated with destruction but minimal fibrosis. A tuberculous mass may develop at the pylorus. Regional lymph nodes are normally involved[86].

4.4.8 CARDIOVASCULAR

Tuberculous pericarditis is associated with generalized infection; myocarditis is less frequent. Constrictive pericarditis with heart failure may result. Although involvement of small vessels is common in tuberculosis, large vessel involvement is rare. The aorta is most commonly involved.

4.4.9 ENDOCRINE

The adrenal is the most frequently involved endocrine gland and tuberculosis is a typical cause of Addison's disease. In extensive multi-system disease, the adrenals are spared. In contrast to this, when the adrenals are involved and destroyed by necrotizing granulomatous inflammation, extra-adrenal tuberculosis is rare[87]. Involvement of the pituitary, in particular the hypophysis, follows pulmonary infection.

REFERENCES

1. Collins, F.M. (1982) The immunology of tuberculosis. *Am. Rev. Respir. Dis.*, **125** (3):, 42–9.
2. Adams, D.O. (1976) The granulomatous inflammatory response. A review. *Am. J. Pathol.*, **84**, 164–91.
3. Williams, G.T. and Jones Williams, W. (1983) Granulomatous inflammation – a review. *J. Clin Pathol.*, **36**, 723–33.
4. van Furth, R., Langevoort, M.L. and Schaberg, A. (1975) Mononuclear phagocytes in human pathology – proposal for an approach to improved classification. In *Mononuclear Phagocytes in Immunity, Infection and Pathology* (ed. R. van Furth), Blackwell Scientific, London, pp. 1–15.
5. Dannenberg, A.M. (1975) Macrophages in inflammation and infection. *N. Engl. J. Med.*, **298**, 489–93.
6. Spector, W.G and Mariano, M. (1975) Macrophage behaviour in experimental granulomas. In *Mononuclear Phagocytes in Immunity, Infection and Pathology* (ed. R. van Furth), Blackwell Scientific, London, pp. 927–38.
7. Rook, G.A.W., Taverne, J., Leveton, C. and Steele, J. (1987) The role of gamma interferon, vitamin D3 metabolites and tumour necrosis factor in the pathogenesis of tuberculosis. *Immunology*, **62**, 229–34.
8. Mackaness, G.B. (1971) Delayed hypersensitivity and the mechanisms of cellular resistance to infection. In *Progress in Immunology* (ed. B. Amos), Elsevier, New York, pp. 413–24.
9. Rhodes, J.M. and Bennedsen, J. (1979) Activation of macrophages assessed by *in-vivo* and *in-vitro* tests. *Adv. Exp. Med. Biol*, **121**, 203–9.
10. van der Rhee, H.J., van der Burgh-de-Winter, C.P.M. and Daems W.T. (1979) The differentiation of monocytes into macrophages, epithelioid cells and multinucleate giant cells in subcutaneous granuloma. 1. Fine structure. *Cell Tissue*, **197**, 355–78.
11. Kitaichi, M. (1986) Pathology of pulmonary sarcoidosis. *Clin. Dermatol.*, **4**, 108–15.
12. Jones Williams, W. and Williams, D. (1968) The properties and development of conchoidal bodies in sarcoid and sarcoid-like granulomas. *J. Pathol. Bacteriol.*, **96**, 491–4.
13. Jones Williams, W., Erasmus, D.A., James, E.M. Valerie and Davis, T. (1970) The fine structure of sarcoid and tuberculous granulomas. *Postgrad. Med. J.*, **46**, 496–500.
14. Jones Williams, W., Erasmus, D.A., Jenkins, E.M., James, E.M. Valerie and Davis, T. (1971). A comparative study of the ultrastructure and histochemistry of sarcoid and tuberculous granulomas. In *Proceedings of the 5th International Conference on Sarcoidosis* (eds L. Lovinski and F. Macholda), University of Karlova, Prague, pp. 115–20.
15. Carr, I. and Norris, P. (1977) The fine structure of human macrophage granules in sarcoidosis. *J. Pathol.*, **12**, 229–33.
16. Judd, P.A., Finnegan, P. and Curran, R.C. (1975) Pulmonary sarcoidosis: a clinicopathological study. *J. Pathol.*, **115**, 191–8.
17. Narayanan, R.B., Badenoch-Jones, P. and Turk, J.L. (1981) Experimental mycobacterial granulomas in guinea pig lymph nodes:

ultrastructural observations. *J. Pathol.*, **134**, 253–65.

18. James, E.M. Valerie and Jones Williams, W. (1974) Fine structure and histochemistry of epithelioid cells in sarcoidosis. *Thorax* **29**, 115–20.

19. Fuse, Y., Imazeki, N., Asakawa, M. *et al.* (1980) Ultrastructural study of sarcoid granulomas – lymphocyte alterations within sarcoid granulomas. In *Proceedings of the 8th International Conference on Sarcoidosis*, Cardiff (eds W. Jones Williams and B.H. Davies), Alpha Omega Press, pp. 19–22.

20. Beaumont, D., Soler, P., Leguern, G. and Basset, F. (1981) Mise en evidence de complexes jonctionnels entre cellules d'origine monocytaire des granulomes sarcoidiens. (Evidence of junctional complexes of monocytic origin in sarcoid granulomas). *Pathol. Biol. (Paris)*, **29**, 229–32.

21. Kawanami, O., Ferrans, V.J., Crystal, R.G. (1980) Subplasmalemmal linear densities in cells of the mononuclear phagocyte system in the lung. *Am. J. Pathol.* **100**, 131–50.

22. Burridge, K., Fath, K., Kelly, T. *et al.* (1988) Focal adhesions: Transmembrane junctions between the extracellular matrix and the cytoskeleton. *Ann. Rev. Cell Biol.*, **4**, 487–525.

23. Kaufmann, R., Frosch, D., Westphal, C. *et al.* (1989) Integrin VLA-3: Ultrastructural localization at cell–cell contact sites of human cell cultures. *J. Cell Biol.*, **109**, 1807–15.

24. Mariano, M., Mikitin, T. and Malucelli, B.E. (1977) Phagocytic potential of macrophages from within delayed hypersensitivity-mediated granulomata. *J. Pathol.*, **123**, 27–33.

25. Baroni, C.D., Vitolo, D., Remotti, D. *et al.* (1987) Immunohistochemical heterogeneity of macrophage subpopulations in human lymphoid tissues. *Histopathology*, **11**, 1029–42.

26. Wood, G.S., Turner, R.R., Shiurba, R.A. *et al.* (1985). Human dendritic cells and macrophages. *In-situ* immunophenotypic definition of subsets that exhibit specific morphologic and microenvironmental characteristics. *Am. J. Pathol.*, **119**, 73–82.

27. Fossum, S. and Ford, W.L. (1985) The organisation of cell populations within lymph nodes: their origin, life history and functional relationships. *Histopathology*, **9**, 469–99.

28. Poulter, L.W. (1983) Antigen presenting cells *in-situ*: their identification and involvement in immunopathology. *Clin. Exp. Immunol.*, **53**, 520–3.

29. Bjerke, J.R., Matre, R. and Nilsen, R. (1983) Characterisation of mononuclear cells in sarcoid skin lesions using monoclonal antibodies. *Acta Pathol. Immunol. Scand. Sect. C*, **91**, 233–6.

30. van der Oord, J.J., de Wolf-Peeters, C., Facchetti, F. and Desmet, V.J. (1984) Cellular composition of hypersensitivity-type granuloma. Immunohistochemical analysis of tuberculous and sarcoidal lymphadenitis. *Hum. Pathol.*, **15**, 559–65.

31. Munro, C.S., Campbell, D.A., Collings, L.A. and Poulter, L.W. (1987) Monoclonal antibodies distinguish macrophages and epithelioid cells in sarcoidosis and leprosy. *Clin. Exp. Immunol.*, **68**, 282–7.

32. Poulter, L.W., Campbell, D.A., Munro, C.S. and Janossy, G. (1986) Discrimination of human macrophages and dendritic cells using monoclonal antibodies. *Scand. J. Immunol.*, **24**, 351–7.

33. Kaufmann, S.H. and Flesch, I.E. (1988) The role of T cell-macrophage interactions in tuberculosis. *Springer Semin. Immunopathol.*, **10**, 337–58.

34. Ridley, H., Turk, J.C. and Badenoch-Jones, P. (1978) Cellular responses in leprosy and related diseases with particular reference to cells of the mononuclear phagocyte series. In *Proceedings of the 8th International Conference on Sarcoidosis*, Cardiff (eds W. Jones Williams and B. H. Davies), Alpha Omega Press, pp. 743–5.

35. Popp, W., Zwick, H., Wanke, T. *et al.* (1992) Nucleolar silver staining patterns of lymphocytes in sarcoidosis. *Path of Res. Pract.*, **188**, 131–4.

36. Modlin, R.L., Hofmann, F.M., Schama, O.P. *et al.* (1984) Demonstration *in-situ* of subsets of T-lymphocytes in sarcoidosis. *Am J Dermatopathol.*, **6**, 423–7.

37. van den Oord, J.J., de Wolf-Peeters, C., Fachetti F. and Desmet, V.J. (1984) Cellular composition of hypersensitivity-type granulomas: immunohistochemical analysis of tuberculous and sarcoidal lymphadenitis. *Hum. Pathol.*, **15**, 559–65.

38. Buckley, P.J., Smith, M.R., Braverman, M.F. and Dickson, S.A. (1987) Human spleen contains phenotypic subsets of macrophages and dendritic cells that occupy discrete microanatomic locations. *Am. J. Pathol.*, **128**, 505–20.

39. Hunninghake, G.W. and Crystal, R.G. (1981) Pulmonary sarcoidosis. A disorder mediated by excess helper T-lymphocyte activity at sites of disease activity. *N. Eng. J. Med.*, **305**, 420–34.

40. Thomas, P.D. and Hunninghake, G.W. (1987) Current concepts of the pathogenesis of sarcoidosis. *Am Rev. Respir. Dis.*, **135**, 747–60.

41. Fujiwara, H., Kleinhenz, M.E., Wallis, R.S. and Eliner, J.J. (1986) Increased interleukin-1 production and monocyte suppressor cell activity associated with human tuberculosis. *Am. Rev. Respir. Dis.*, **133**, 73–7.

42. Tanaka, A., Emori, K., Nagao, S. *et al.* (1982) Epithelioid granuloma formation requiring no T-cell function. *Am. J. Pathol.*, **106**, 165–70.

43. McCue, R.E., Dannenberg, A.M. Jr, Higuchi, S. and Sugimoto, M. (1978) The effect of cortisone on the accumulation, activation, and necrosis of macrophages in tuberculous lesions. *Inflammation*, **3**, 159–76.

44. Barnes, P.F., Fong, S.J., Brennan, P.J. *et al.* (1990) Local production of tumour necrosis factor and IFN-gamma in tuberculous pleuritis. *J. Immunol.*, **145**, 149–54.

45. Grunewald, J., Janson, C.H., Eklund, A., *et al.* (1992) Restricted V alpha 2.3 gene usage by CD4+ T lymphocytes in bronchoalveolar lavage fluid from sarcoidosis patients correlates with HLA-DR3. *Eur. J. Immunol.*, **22**, 129–35.

46. Holroyd, K.J., Tamura, N., Banks, T. *et al.* (1990) Limited diversity of gamma delta T-cell antigen receptor junctional region sequences in individuals with sarcoidosis compared to broad diversity in normal subjects. *Trans. Assoc. Am. Phys.*, **103**, 102–11.

47. Ohmen, J.D., Barnes, P.F., Uyemura, K. *et al.* (1991) The T cell receptors of human gamma delta T cells reactive to *Mycobacterium tuberculosis* are encoded by specific V genes but diverse V-J junctions. *J. Immunol.*, **147**, 3353–59.

48. Tazi, A., Fajac, I., Soler, P. *et al.* (1991) Gamma/delta T-lymphocytes are not increased in number in granulomatous lesions of patients with tuberculosis or sarcoidosis. *Am. Rev. Respir. Dis.*, **144**, 1373–5.

49. Spector, W.G. and Lykke, A.W.J. (1966) The cellular evolution of inflammatory granulomata. *J. Pathol. Bacteriol.*, **92**, 163–77.

50. Ryan, G.B. and Spector, W.G. (1969) Natural selection of long-lived macrophages in experimental granulomata. *J. Pathol.*, **99**, 139–45.

51. Spector, W.G. and Ryan, G.B. (1969) New evidence for the existence of long lived macrophages. *Nature*, **221**, 860–2.

52. Bowers, R.R., Stapleton, M.E. and Lew, P.D. (1983) An ultrastructural study of the macrophages of the carrageenan-induced granuloma in the rat lung. *J. Pathol.*, **140**, 29–40.

53. Spector, W.G. (1976) Epithelioid cells, giant cells and sarcoidosis. *Ann. NY Acad. Sci.*, **278**, 3–6.

54. Bitterman, P.B., Adelberg, S. and Crystal, R.G. (1983) Mechanisms of pulmonary fibrosis. Spontaneous release of the macrophage-derived growth factor in the interstitial lung disorders. *J. Clin. Invest.*, **72**, 1801–13.

55. Warren, K.S., Domingo, E.O. and Cowan, R.B.T. (1967) Granuloma formation around schistosome eggs as a manifestation of delayed hypersensitivity. *Am. J. Pathol.*, **51**, 735–56.

56. Epstein, W.L. (1967) Granulomatous hypersensitivity. *Progr. Allergy*, **11**, 36–88.

57. Lurie, M.B. (1964) *Resistance to Tuberculosis: Experimental Studies in Native and Acquired Defense Mechanisms*, Harvard University Press, Cambridge, Mass.

58. Dannenburg, A.M. (1991) Review. Delayed-type hypersensitivity and cell-mediated immunity in the pathogenesis of tuberculosis. *Immunol. Today*, **12**, 228–33.

59. Leonard, E.J. and Yoshimura, T. (1990) Human monocyte chemoattrant protein-1 (MCP-1). *Immunol. Today*, **11**, 97–101.

60. Lenzini, L., Rottoli, P. and Rottoli, L. (1977) The spectrum of human tuberculosis. *Clin. Exp. Immunol.*, **27**, 230–7.

61. Ridley, D.S. and Ridley, M.J. (1987) Rationale for the histological spectrum of tuberculosis. A basis for classification. *Pathology*, **19**, 186–92.

62. Ridley, M.J. and Ridley, D.S. (1986) Histochemical demonstration of mycobacterial antigen-specific antibody and complement in the lesions of tuberculosis. *Histochem. J.*, **18**, 551–6.

63. Auerbach, O. (1959) The natural history of the tuberculous pulmonary lesion. *Med. Clin. North. Am.*, **43**, 239–51.

64. Ojeda, V.J. and Joske, R.A. (1986) Angiocentric pulmonary granulomas in tuberculosis. *Pathol. Res. Pract.* **181**, 344–88.

65. Auerbach, O. and Dail, D.H. (1988) Mycobacterial infections. In *Pulmonary Pathology*

(eds H.D. Dail and S.P. Hammar), Springer Verlag, New York, pp. 173–88.

66. Snider, D.E. and Bloch, A.B. (1984) Congenital tuberculosis. *Tubercle*, **65**, 81–2.

67. Stead, W.W. (1967) Pathogenesis of a first episode of chronic pulmonary tuberculosis in man: recrudescence of residuals of the primary infection or exogenous reinfection? *Am. Rev. Respir. Dis.*, **95**, 729–45.

68. Slavin, R.E., Walsh, T.J. and Pollack, A.D. (1980) Late generalised tuberculosis. A clinical pathologic analysis and comparison of 100 cases in the pre-antibiotic and antibiotic eras. *Medicine*, **59**, 352–66.

69. Dannenberg, A.M. (1982) Pathogenesis of pulmonary tuberculosis. *Am. Rev. Respir. Dis.*, **125** (3), 25–9.

70. Banner, A.S. (1979) Tuberculosis. Clinical aspects and diagnosis. *Arch. Intern. Med.*, **139**, 1387–90.

71. Howard, W.L., Klopfenstein, M.D., Steininger, W.J. and Woodruf, C.E. (1970) The loss of tuberculin hypersensitivity in patients with active pulmonary tuberculosis. *Chest*, **57**, 530–4.

72. Proudfoot, A.T. (1971) Cryptic disseminated tuberculosis. *Br. J. Hosp. Med.*, **5**, 773–80.

73. Ellner, J.J. (1986) Immune dysregulation in human tuberculosis. *J. Lab. Clin. Med.*, **108**, 142–9.

74. Kindler, V. and Sappino, A.P. (1991) The beneficial effects of localised tumour necrosis factor production in BCG infection. *Behring Inst. Mitt.*, **88**, 120–4.

75. Auerbach, O. (1939) Pathology and pathogenesis of pulmonary arterial aneurysm in tuberculous cavities. *Am. Rev. Tuberc.*, **29**, 99–115.

76. Donath, J. and Khan, F.A. (1984) Tuberculous and post-tuberculous bronchopleural fistula: Ten year clinical experience. *Chest*, **86**, 697–703.

77. Lucas, S.B. (1988) Histopathology of leprosy and tuberculosis – an overview. *Br. Med. Bull.* **44**, 584–99.

78. Morrison, J.G.L. and Fourie, E.D. (1974) The papulonecrotic tuberculide from Arthus reaction to lupus vulgaris. *Br. J. Dermatol.*, **91**, 263–70.

79. DeAngelis, L.M. (1981) Intracranial tuberculoma: case report and review of the literature. *Neurology*, **31**, 1133–6.

80. Dastur, D.K. (1986) The pathology and pathogenesis of tuberculous encephalopathy and myeloradiculopathy: a comparison with allergic encephalomyelitis. *Childs Nerv. Syst.*, **2**, 13–19.

81. Ylinen, O. (1961) Genital tuberculosis in women. Clinical experience with 348 proved cases. *Acta Obstet. Gynecol. Scand.*, **40** (Suppl 2), 1–213.

82. Haines, M. (1958) Tuberculous salpingitis as seen by the pathologist and the surgeon. *Am. J. Obstet. Gynecol.*, **75**, 472–81.

83. Nogales-Ortiz, F., Taranco, I. and Nogales, F.F. Jr. (1979) The pathology of female genital tuberculosis. A 31 year study of 1436 cases. *Obstet. Gynecol.*, **53**, 422–8.

84. Warthin, A.S. (1907) Tuberculosis of the placenta: a histological study with especial reference to the nature of the earliest lesions produced by the tubercle bacillus. *J. Infect. Dis.* **4**, 347–68.

85. Logan, V. St C.D. (1969) Anorectal tuberculosis. *Proc. R. Soc. Med.*, **62**, 1227–30.

86. Morson, B.C. and Dawson, I.M.P. (1990) *Gastrointestinal Pathology*, 3rd edn, Blackwell Scientific, London, pp. 110–11.

87. Sloper, J.C. (1955) Pathology of adrenals, thymus and certain other endocrine glands in Addison's disease: analysis of 37 necropsies. *Proc. R. Soc. Med.*, **48**, 625–8.

THE IMMUNOPHYSIOLOGY AND IMMUNOPATHOLOGY OF TUBERCULOSIS

5

J.M. Grange

The course, characteristics and outcome of tuberculosis vary enormously from patient to patient. Almost without exception, these variations are attributable to the immune responses of the host rather than to differences in the virulence of the causative organism. The mechanism of virulence of the tubercle bacillus remains shrouded in mystery but it has been apparent for almost a century that it does not owe its virulence to the synthesis of toxic substances but to its ability to survive the host's various immune defence mechanisms. More recently, it has become clear that virtually all the clinical and pathological manifestations of tuberculosis, as well as the infectivity of some patients, are the result of inappropriate, tissue-damaging immune reactions. Thus, in tuberculosis, the host's immune response is a two-edged sword – mediating protective responses but also facilitating progression of the disease in the patient and in the community.

The characteristic lesion of tuberculosis, and indeed of most chronic infections, is the granuloma (Plate 6). This consists of a compact aggregate, many layers thick, of macrophages in an activated form around the pathogen and a peripheral zone containing lymphocytes responsible for macrophage activation. The closely interdigitated macro-phages bear a resemblance to epithelial cells and are therefore termed 'epithelioid cells'. Some of the macrophages fuse to form multinucleate giant cells (Langerhans cells) which, though not unique to tuberculosis, strongly support the histological diagnosis.

5.1 THE NATURAL HISTORY OF TUBERCULOSIS

Despite the enormous variation in the clinical features of tuberculosis, the disease nevertheless tends to follow a common pattern or 'timetable' of events (Table 5.1)[1]. Most cases of human tuberculosis are the result of inhalation of small, moist, expectorated droplets containing tubercle bacilli. These lodge in the alveoli or terminal air passages of the lung and establish a local focus of disease termed the Ghon focus. Bacilli are transported to the lymph nodes at the hilum of the lung where additional foci of disease develop. The Ghon focus together with the hilar lymphadenopathy is termed the primary complex (of Ranke). Bacilli disseminate further by the lymphatic and blood streams and lodge in many organs of the body. Thus, primary tuberculosis is a systemic infection. Primary complexes may also be acquired by ingesting tubercle bacilli, usually *M. bovis* in milk, in which case the implantation focus

Clinical Tuberculosis. Edited by P.D.O. Davies. Published in 1994 by Chapman & Hall, London. ISBN 0 412 48630 X

Table 5.1   The 'timetable of tuberculosis'

Stage	Duration	Principal features
1	3–8 weeks	Development of primary complex. Conversion to tuberculin positivity
2	3 months	Serious forms of tuberculosis due to haematogenous dissemination: miliary and meningeal disease
3	3–4 months	Tuberculous pleurisy due to haematogenous spread or direct spread from enlarging primary lesion
4	Up to 3 years	Resolution of primary complex. Appearance of more slowly developing extrapulmonary lesions: bone and joint and renal tuberculosis

Adapted from A. Wallgren, *Tubercle*, 1948, **29**, 245–51.

will be in the tonsil or intestinal wall and the lymphatic lesion will be in the cervical or mesenteric nodes. A minority of primary lesions follow traumatic inoculation, most typically as an occupational hazard of anatomists and pathologists – the lesion being termed 'prosector's wart'[2].

In most cases, the host's immune defences overcome the primary infection, which often passes unnoticed. In the minority of cases, the Ghon focus may enlarge progressively and possibly rupture into the pleural cavity, causing pleurisy. The hilar lymph node enlargement may be sufficient to compress a bronchus, causing collapse of a lobe of the lung, or it may erode into the pericardial space, causing tuberculous pericarditis. Alternatively, one of the foci of infection in more distant organs may progress, leading to the serious non-pulmonary sequelae of primary tuberculosis including bone and joint, renal and meningeal disease.

Healed primary complexes may remain dormant; in about 10% of infected persons, reactivation eventually occurs, resulting in post-primary tuberculosis. Exogenous re-infection may, of course, also cause this form of tuberculosis.

For reasons that are not known, post-primary tuberculosis of whatever origin tends to occur in the upper parts of the lung. The necrotic element in the post-primary lesion is much more evident than in primary disease, resulting in very large lesions, which often rupture and discharge their necrotic contents into the bronchi, thereby forming pulmonary cavities (Fig. 5.1). Unlike primary disease, the regional lymph nodes are rarely involved and associated disease in other organs is uncommon. Post-primary tuberculosis is therefore more localized and contained than the primary form of the disease. On the other hand, secondary lesions may develop in the same and opposite lung and the larynx due to spread of bacilli through the bronchi and trachea. Bacilli may be swallowed and cause secondary indurated lesions in the alimentary tract. This spread of disease is, however, quite distinct from the haematogenous spread in primary tuberculosis.

The cavity formation and containment of disease in post-primary tuberculosis is the result of active immune responses. Old patients and those whose immunity is suppressed by, for example, AIDS, renal failure and post-transplant immunosuppressive therapy, tend to develop spreading pulmonary lesions with little or no cavity formation and widespread haematogenous dissemination of the disease.

5.2 HOST RESPONSES IN EARLY INFECTION

Little is known of the events occurring in the first few days after primary infection of human beings by the tubercle bacillus: our

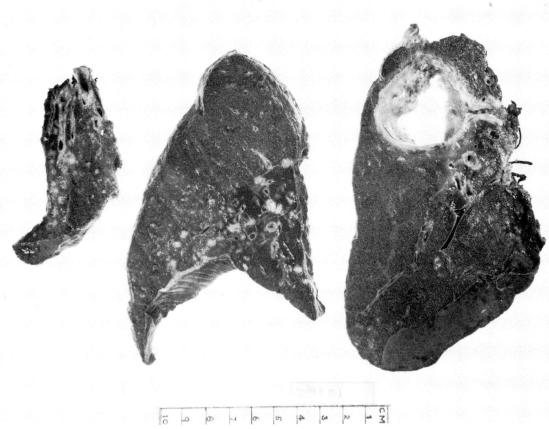

Fig. 5.1 Post-primary tuberculosis showing a cavity and secondary lesions resulting from bronchial spread of bacilli.

knowledge of these events comes mostly from studies on the rabbit[3]. An inflammatory reaction develops at the site of implantation and initially consists of an accumulation of blood-derived white cells, principally polymorphonuclear leucocytes. Subsequently, macrophages infiltrate the lesion leading first to a mixed appearance of acute pyogenic and chronic granulomatous inflammation and eventually to a distinct epithelioid cell granuloma. The early inflammation and granuloma formation is induced non-specifically by various components of the mycobacterial cell wall and probably

inhibits the spread of the infection. There is also evidence that a population of T cells known as gamma-delta T cells is able to respond non-specifically to a limited range of bacterial components and cause macrophage aggregation and activation before the specific immune responses have developed[4].

The non-specific protective reactions in the early stages of the infection are unable to prevent dissemination of the bacilli by the lymphatic system to the regional lymph nodes, resulting in formation of the primary complex, or further dissemination by the blood stream to more distant organs.

5.3 INDUCTION OF IMMUNE RESPONSIVENESS IN TUBERCULOSIS

Antigens of *M. tuberculosis* are taken up and processed by the antigen-presenting cells and presented in close association with products of the major histocompatibility complex (MHC) genes to antigen-specific T cells. There are two classes of MHC gene products and these determine the subsets of T cells to which the antigen is presented. The T cells that induce and help immune functions (CD4$^+$ T cells) recognize antigens in association with the Class II MHC antigens, coded for by the HLA-D genes, while T cells with suppressor and cytotoxic functions (CD8$^+$) recognize antigen in association with Class I MHC antigens, coded for by the HLA-A and -B genes.

The 'repertoire' of antigens that may be presented on the surface of the antigen-presenting cell is affected by genetically determined factors and varies from one person to another. This genetic polymorphism affecting antigen recognition is thought to be an evolutionary mechanism to ensure that no single pathogen can eliminate an entire mammalian species[5].

After binding to the antigen/MHC complex, the antigen-specific T cells undergo activation and clonal expansion and then participate in the wide range of possible immune reactions. Thus T cells responsible for the induction and suppression of protective immunity, delayed hypersensitivity, cytolysis and antibody production as well as memory cells, with varying kinetics of appearance and disappearance, are produced in response to challenges by *M. tuberculosis* [6]. Although clones of T cells capable of recognizing mycobacterial antigens have been produced *in vitro*, it has not been easy to relate the subset of T cells to the type of immune response, whether protective or tissue-damaging, that they facilitate. This may be easier in the future as there is now evidence that the CD4$^+$ and CD8$^+$ cells may be further divided into distinct functional subclusters. In the mouse, helper T cells are divisible into two such subclusters, one of which (T$_H$1) secretes interleukin 2 and gamma interferon and helps cell-mediated immunity reactions and the other (T$_H$2) secretes interleukins 4 and 5 and helps antibody production[7]. Human helper T cells appear to be divisible into analogous subclusters[8].

5.4 GENETIC CONTROL OF IMMUNE RESPONSES IN TUBERCULOSIS

The existence of genes that determine resistance to tuberculosis has long been suspected. In the mouse, a *bcg* gene confers resistance to early stages of infection by BCG and other intracellular pathogens[9], apparently by affecting the innate ability of the macrophages to inhibit or kill the pathogens. There is suggestive evidence for a similar gene determining disease susceptibility in man.

There have been many unsuccessful attempts to find linkages between susceptibility to tuberculosis and the class I HLA genes (HLA-A and -B). Studies on class II (HLA-D) genes have been more promising and have revealed that the HLA-DR2 gene appears to predispose to the development of tuberculosis, particularly radiologically advanced, smear-positive disease[10–12]. The HLA-DR2 specificity may affect antigen recognition as persons of this genotype have higher levels of antibody to epitopes on a 38 kilodalton protein unique to *M. tuberculosis* than those lacking this genotype[10].

It has been suggested that the class II genes may determine the functional type of T cell (e.g. T$_H$1 or T$_H$2) to which mycobacterial antigen is presented. On the other hand, the lack of a very close linkage between tuberculosis and HLA has led to the concept that the selection of the type of immune response by mycobacteria is a multifactorial event based not only on specific antigen recognition but also on more primitive systems that recognize a range of common bacterial components[8]. A predetermined tendency to an induction of predominantly T_H1- or T_H2-mediated responses to mycobacterial antigens in man is suggested by a study of healthy hospital workers exposed to tuberculosis patients. Some of these workers reacted strongly to PPD and had low levels of antibody to *M. tuberculosis* (suggesting a T_H1 response) while others reacted poorly to PPD but had higher antibody levels (suggesting a T_H2 response)[13].

Class II genes also affect reactivity to skin testing with tuberculin. Thus, skin testing with a range of mycobacterial sensitins revealed that persons lacking the HLA-DR3 gene tend to respond poorly to all sensitins, while those of HLA-DR4 phenotype respond relatively strongly to species-specific antigens of *M. tuberculosis*[14].

5.5 PROTECTIVE IMMUNITY AND THE ROLE OF THE MACROPHAGE

In the classical theory of cell-mediated immunity to mycobacteria and other intracellular pathogens, antigens of the pathogens are specifically recognized by helper T cells, which then activate macrophages non-specifically so that they are then able to destroy a wide range of intracellular pathogens[15]. The experiments that led to this theory were conducted principally with mice. Problems have been encountered with this theory in respect to human tuberculosis as this differs considerably from the disease in the mouse. Thus the latter is more resistant than human beings to tuberculosis and the disease is principally an intracellular one. Furthermore, although activated mouse macrophages undoubtedly kill tubercle bacilli, attempts to demonstrate such killing by human macrophages have, with few exceptions, been unsuccessful[16]. Mouse macrophages may owe their greater mycobactericidal powers to their ability to generate toxic nitrogen metabolites, i.e. nitric oxide and nitrogen dioxide. Activated human macrophages, unlike those of the mouse, are able to utilize vitamin D to induce further activation and, as outlined below, this phenomenon may account for further differences between immune responses in mice and man.

While the isolated human macrophage may be of limited effectiveness against tubercle bacilli, collectively they may form a powerful defence mechanism in the form of the granuloma. Being metabolically very active, the macrophages consume oxygen diffusing into the granuloma so that the interior region becomes anoxic and necrotic – a process termed caseation on account of the cheese-like appearance of the necrotic material. The acidic and anoxic conditions within the granuloma inhibit the growth of mycobacteria and may be bactericidal. This, together with bacterial inhibition by the activated macrophages, leads to quiescence. The granuloma becomes dormant and is entombed in fibrous scar tissue, which may become calcified. Unfortunately, a few mycobacteria may remain viable within these biological sarcophagi and re-emerge as the cause of disease years or decades later.

5.6 MYCOBACTERIAL PERSISTENCE

The nature of the mycobacteria that persist for many years within the tissues is one of the mysteries of mycobacteriology[17]. It has been shown that mycobacteria may remain viable for long periods without replication under anaerobic conditions[18]. This could explain dormancy, but several authors have advanced more elaborate theories, including the existence of cell-wall-free forms or microspores (Much's granules)[17,19]. Host immunity certainly plays a part in maintaining dormancy as reactivation is often associated with a weakening of immune defences. This suggests that persisting bacilli are not truly dormant but undergo replication, perhaps intermittently and slowly, at a rate that is matched by their destruction by immune or other mechanisms. Overt disease would then develop if the rate of host-mediated bacterial destruction failed to keep up with the replication rate. This possibility is suggested by the fact that a 6–12 month course of isoniazid, a drug that is reported to kill only those tubercle bacilli that are actively replicating, eliminates these persistors in a high proportion of infected people.

5.7 POST-PRIMARY TUBERCULOSIS

This form of tuberculosis usually occurs in the upper part of the lung. The immunological reaction with granuloma formation is initially similar to that seen in primary disease but tissue necrosis is much more evident, resulting in very large caseous lesions termed tuberculomas. Proteases released by activated macrophages cause softening or liquefaction of the caseous material. The acidic and anoxic conditions within the lesion, together with free fatty acids in the softened caseous material, do not favour mycobacterial growth and relatively few acid-fast bacilli are present. Many lesions eventually erode into bronchi and their softened contents are discharged, resulting in the formation of cavities. The environment of the cavity wall is quite different from that of the solid tuberculoma. Air enriched with carbon dioxide, the ideal atmosphere for cultivation of tubercle bacilli, enters the cavity and neutralizes the previously acidic conditions. As a result, there is a massive increase in the numbers of acid-fast bacilli in the cavity wall and many gain access to the sputum, rendering the patient infectious. Bacilli are also able to spread to other parts of the lung through the bronchial tree and to set up additional foci of disease. In the days before effective chemotherapy, surgical procedures designed to obliterate pulmonary cavities appeared to limit the progression of the disease and to encourage resolution.

It is generally assumed that cavity forma-tion and the other manifestations of post-primary tuberculosis are a consequence of the necrotizing reaction known as delayed hypersensitivity. Although obviously causing extensive tissue damage, this reactivity may have some protective value. Thus, in contrast to primary tuberculosis, bacilli rarely spread from the site of disease via the lymphatic or blood streams. (As mentioned earlier, they may spread to other parts of the lung through the bronchial tree.) Also, the tissue destruction may lead to massive fibrosis and scarring that, in turn, may wall off the active lesions, leading to quiescence. In the pre-chemotherapeutic era, spontaneous resolution occurred in about one-fifth of patients with cavitary post-primary tuberculosis[20]. In the chemotherapeutic era, such excessive scarring may be distinctly disadvantageous by favouring bacillary dormancy and inhibiting the diffusion of antituberculosis agents into the lesion[21].

To understand the immunological phenomena responsible for the extensive tissue necrosis and other characteristics of post-primary tuberculosis it is necessary to look back to the studies of Robert Koch, who discovered the tubercle bacillus in 1882.

5.8 THE KOCH PHENOMENON AND DELAYED HYPERSENSITIVITY

In 1891 Koch described the series of studies that had, in the previous year, led him to claim that he had discovered a cure for tuberculosis[22]. During these studies, he inoculated guinea-pigs with cultures of virulent tubercle bacilli by intradermal injection and observed the development of disease (Fig. 5.2). After 10–14 days, a small nodule developed at the inoculation site. This subsequently ulcerated and remained open until the animal died. The regional lymph nodes were grossly involved about 1 month later, after which the disease spread to many organs and the animal died between 3 and 4 months after inoculation. It was found,

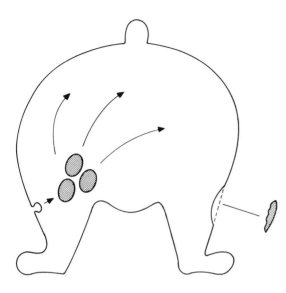

Fig. 5.2 A diagrammatic representation of the Koch phenomenon in the guinea-pig. The first challenge (left side) leads to an ulcer at the inoculation site and enlarged draining lymph nodes (primary complex) and further haematogenous dissemination. Subsequent challenge (right side) leads to a flat ulcer with sloughing off of the bacilli-laden dermis and no involvement of the draining lymph nodes.

however, that if infected guinea-pigs were re-inoculated at another site 4–6 weeks after the initial inoculation, the ensuing reaction was quite different. Within a day or two, an area of skin 0.5 to 1 cm across at the inoculation site became darkened and, after a further few days, it became necrotic and sloughed off, leaving a shallow ulcer that rapidly healed. Regional lymph nodes were not involved and it appeared that the second infection had been successfully eliminated. Koch then found that an identical reaction occurred after injection of killed tubercle bacilli and also of a filter-sterilized broth culture of the bacilli concentrated by evaporation. Koch named this preparation Old Tuberculin and administered it to tuberculosis patients by subcutaneous injection in the belief that it would induce a systemic protec-

tive reaction. This, unfortunately, did not occur: the remedy was ineffective for pulmonary disease and a few patients died of 'tuberculin shock' but some patients with long-standing skin tuberculosis made dramatic recoveries. These findings suggested that the necrotic 'Koch phenomenon' was protective when the disease was confined to the skin and could be sloughed off but was ineffective in those cases in which the disease involved internal organs.

Tissue damage may be an unavoidable consequence of a protective immune reaction. Nevertheless, some tissue-damaging immune processes appear to confer no benefit to the host and are referred to as hypersensitivity reactions. Four types were defined by Gell and Coombs – the first three are relatively rapid in onset and are the result of various forms of antigen-antibody reactions[23]. Type IV reactions, of which the Koch phenomenon is the classical example, appears to be mediated by cells rather than antibody and is of more delayed onset than the former three. Thus it is usually termed delayed type hypersensitivity (DTH).

5.9 THE TUBERCULIN REACTION

Although abandoned as a therapeutic agent, Koch's Old Tuberculin was used as a skin-testing reagent by the Austrian physician Clemens von Pirquet. On the basis of extensive clinical and post-mortem studies, von Pirquet established that reactivity to tuberculin indicated that the person had previously been infected by the tubercle bacillus[24]. The procedure for skin testing has been somewhat modified over the ensuing decades. In the original test, a drop of Old Tuberculin was placed on the skin, which was scratched through the drop, but reagents are now administered by intradermal injection (Mantoux method) or by multiple pronged devices (Heaf and tine tests). Old Tuberculin has been replaced by Purified Protein Derivative (PPD), the reagents are now standardized and their strength is expressed in International Units (previously termed Tuberculin Units). Nevertheless, the principle of the test remains unchanged and, in countries where tuberculin reactivity has not been artificially induced by BCG vaccination, provides a useful indication of the extent of transmission of tuberculosis in the community[25].

Histological examination of biopsies of the tuberculin reaction reveals a dense infiltration of blood-derived white cells around the capillaries, hair follicles and sweat glands[26,27]. Some of the mononuclear cells (macrophages and lymphocytes) migrate from these inflammatory foci into the intervening dermis, especially into the subepidermal region. This migration is, at least in part, in response to specific mycobacterial antigens as more migration occurs in reactions to tuberculin than to leprosin in tuberculosis patients and *vice versa* in leprosy patients. There is no correlation between the number of cells in the test site, estimated as the percentage of the dermis occupied by the perivascular and periappendicular inflammatory foci, and the presence or extent of clinically evident swelling and induration. Indeed, subjects who are clinically tuberculin-negative may have an intense cellular infiltrate in the dermis. Thus, although the reaction is cell-mediated, it is not a direct consequence of the bulk of the cellular infiltrate.

The greatly increased cellularity of the dermis at the tuberculin test site leads to increased oxygen consumption and a compensatory increase in blood flow, accounting for the zone of erythema that surrounds the area of induration. Blood flow measurements have, however, revealed that in many tuberculin reactions, notably the larger and more obviously indurated ones, there is a central slowing of the blood flow[28]. This results in tissue anoxia, acidosis and, in a few reactions, overt tissue necrosis. The mechanism of this central relative slowing of blood flow is unknown but it is likely that it is related to the mechanisms, discussed below, that are responsible for the tissue necrosis and pulmonary cavity formation in postprimary tuberculosis.

Each mycobacterial species contains antigens unique to that species and also those that are common to all mycobacteria. As both groups of antigens may elicit tuberculin reactions, exposure to other mycobacterial species in the environment may induce crossreactive responses on skin testing with tuberculin. In some countries or regions, crossreactions are clearly differentiated by their size from genuine responses to tuberculin but in others the distinction between genuine and cross-reactions is not clear. For this reason, the diameter of a tuberculin reaction considered as being diagnostically significant varies from region to region. In veterinary practice, simultaneous testing of cattle with reagents prepared from *M. bovis* and from a common environmental mycobacterium (*M. avium*) is used to distinguish specific reactivity from cross-reactivity but this technique is rarely used in human studies.

Skin testing studies with reagents prepared from filter-sterilized ultrasonicates of many mycobacterial species (new tuberculins) have revealed three categories of reactor[29,30]. Persons in Category 1 fail to react to any reagent, even if they have been infected by *M. tuberculosis* or have received BCG vaccine. This non-reactivity appears to have a genetic basis (p. 59). Category 2 responders react to any mycobacterial species, even if it is not present in the environment, indicating that these persons respond to common mycobacterial antigens. Category 3 responders only react to certain mycobacteria, indicating that they recognize species-specific, but not common, mycobacterial antigens. While most healthy people are Category 2 responders, those with overt tuberculosis or other mycobacterial disease are mostly Category 3 responders, suggesting that they have lost the ability to recognize the common mycobacterial antigens, which may include protective epitopes. The significance of this finding to the development of effective immunotherapy is discussed in section 5.14 on p. 66.

5.10 PROTECTIVE IMMUNITY AND DELAYED HYPERSENSITIVITY

The relation between protective and non-protective immune reactions in tuberculosis, and the relation of both to tuberculin reactivity, has been the topic of considerable debate and confusion for many decades[31]. Much of the confusion is due to nomenclature, as both types of reaction have been grouped under the umbrella title of 'cell-mediated immunity' (CMI).

During his pioneering studies on tuberculin testing, von Pirquet observed that patients with very advanced tuberculosis were often tuberculin-negative[32]. He thus concluded that a positive tuberculin reaction was a correlate of protective immunity. This idea has been challenged on many occasions and there is still controversy as to whether protective immune responses and necrotic DTH reactions are quite distinct or whether they are manifestations of the same response, but differing in intensity. This controversy has been extensively reviewed[31,33–35] but, although several questions remain unanswered, modern immunological and molecular biological approaches are close to permitting a resolution of the issue.

5.11 THE NATURE AND MECHANISM OF DELAYED HYPERSENSITIVITY

Following their activation and clonal expansion, helper T cells secrete gamma interferon (IFN-g) and other cytokines that activate the macrophages (Fig. 5.3). *In vitro* studies show that IFN-g *per se* does not increase the resistance of human macrophages to *M. tuberculosis* but that it has another important effect. It induces a 1-hydroxylase in human macrophages, which converts the inactive 25-OH vitamin D3 to the active 1,25 $(OH)_2$ vitamin D3 (calcitriol)[36]. This increases the ability of the macrophages to inhibit the intracellular replication of *M. tuberculosis* but it also sensitizes them to the triggering of the release of tumour necrosis factor (TNF) and other cytokines[16]. One potent trigger of TNF release from such sensitized macrophages is *M. tuberculosis* and the active substance is a cell wall component termed lipoarabinomannan B (LAM)[37].

Under normal circumstances, TNF plays a protective role in infections by rapidly activating phagocytic cells and contributing to the process of granuloma formation. By contrast, excessive release as occurs, for example, in Gram-negative septicaemia, causes the toxic shock syndrome. TNF is also termed cachectin and is said to be responsible for the severe wasting (consumption, phthisis or cachexia) seen in advanced untreated tuberculosis. TNF is, however, undetectable in sera from tuberculosis patients without such advanced disease and, indeed, these patients have a circulating inhibitor of the toxic effects of TNF. The question has thus been raised as to whether the relatively low levels of TNF released from tuberculosis granulomata are protective or lead to necrosis.

Rook and his colleagues have shown that infection of cell lines by *M. tuberculosis*, or indeed the mere addition of crude culture supernatants of this bacillus, greatly enhances the susceptibility of the cells to killing by TNF[16,38]. *In vivo*, injection of tuberculin followed 24 h later by an injection, at the same site, of a minute amount of TNF leads to a necrotic reaction. This sensitization appears to be T cell-dependent.

Thus the sequence of events in a necrotic tuberculin reaction or tuberculous lesion could be as follows. Mycobacterial antigen is recognized by T cells, which then release gamma interferon and other cytokines that activate macrophages and induce the 1-hydroxylase enzyme, which, by generating

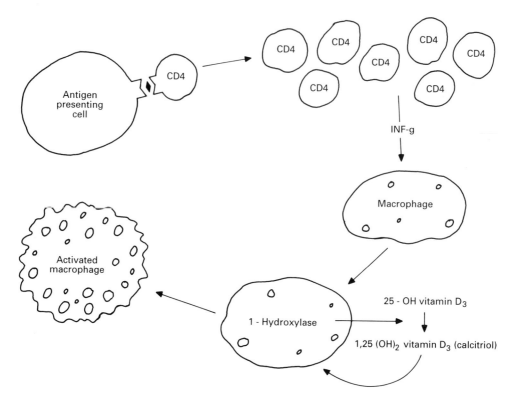

Fig. 5.3 The pathway of macrophage activation. Mycobacterial antigen is presented by the antigen presenting cell to an inducer T cell (CD4+). This undergoes clonal expansion and the resulting cell population secretes gamma interferon and other cytokines that activate the macrophage. Induction of a 1-hydroxylase enables the macrophage to convert inactive 25-OH vitamin D_3 to the active 1,25 $(OH)_2$ vitamin D_3, resulting in further activation.

calcitriol, primes these cells for TNF release. Other T cell products sensitize cells at the site to the toxic effects of TNF. Mycobacterial components, notably LAM, then trigger TNF release from the primed macrophages and this kills the sensitized cells in the neighbourhood (Fig. 5.4). (In this context it is noteworthy that sarcoid granulomata produce large quantities of 1,25 $(OH)_2$ vitamin D3, enough indeed to induce hypercalcaemia, but necrosis of the lesions is very uncommon, presumably as there is no LAM or other TNF releasing factor of bacterial origin.)

At first view, it might seem that this explanation of necrosis occurring in tuberculosis would imply that all reactions, whether lesions or tuberculin test sites, would be necrotic and counter-protective. Non-necrotic reactions may be explained by postulating that, while T cell products may sensitize cells to the toxic effects of TNF, this is the property of a particular subset of T cells. Antigen recognition by other subsets might have the opposite effect. Although the mechanism is unknown, there is very strong evidence that the immune system may make a 'decision' between a necrotic and non-necrotic response to infection by *M. tuberculosis* and that an inappropriate decision may be reversed by an appropriate immunotherapeutic intervention.

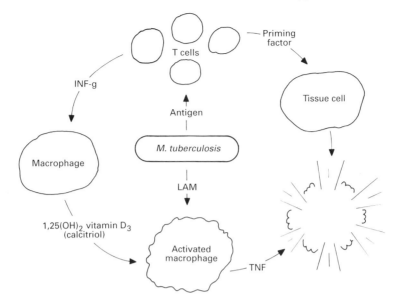

Fig. 5.4 The role of tumour necrosis factor (TNF). Macrophages are primed to release TNF and T cell factors either protect from, or enhance susceptibility of cells to killing by TNF. Mycobacterial lipoarabinomannan B (LAM) triggers the release of TNF from macrophages. (Adapted from G.A.W. Rook and R. Al Attiyah, *Tubercle*, 1991, **72**, 13–20.)

5.12 'SPECTRUM' OF IMMUNE REACTIVITY IN TUBERCULOSIS

Attempts have been made to classify cases of tuberculosis according to a 'spectrum' of immune reactivity similar to that evident in leprosy. There are, however, fundamental differences between the two diseases that render such a comparison difficult[39]. In leprosy, there is a hyper–reactive (tuberculoid) form with extensive granuloma formation but very few bacilli and an anergic (lepromatous) form in which there are huge numbers of bacilli and a very specific suppression or absence of cellular immune responses to the leprosy bacillus and various borderline forms in which the immune responsiveness is unstable and liable to cause severe reactions. The nearest equivalent in tuberculosis to tuberculoid leprosy is lupus vulgaris, a very chronic cutaneous form of tuberculosis in which there are well-organized, non-necrotic epithelioid cell granulomata and very few bacilli.

There is no real form of tuberculosis equivalent to anergic lepromatous leprosy. Although disseminated, multibacillary tuberculosis may occur, this is usually a consequence of generalized immunosuppression rather than the specific failure to recognize antigens of the pathogen. Also, *M. tuberculosis* is much more toxic and rapidly growing than *M. leprae* so that, unless treated, disseminated tuberculosis rapidly progresses to a fatal outcome.

Ridley and Ridley thus described a three-group 'spectrum' of tuberculosis, with group 1 corresponding to chronic cutaneous disease and group 3 to disseminated disease in immunosuppressed persons. Most cases of tuberculosis are of the localized pulmonary and non-pulmonary types and belong to group 2[40].

5.13 IMMUNOSUPPRESSION AND TUBERCULOSIS

It has long been known that suppression of immune reactivity may lead to endogenous reactivation of tuberculosis and this fact has been particularly evident since the advent of the HIV pandemic[41]. Persons dually infected by HIV and *M. tuberculosis* have a much greater chance of developing reactivation tuberculosis than those only infected by the latter, i.e. an increase in the annual reactivation rate from 1% to 10%. Tuberculosis in HIV-positive patients differs from that in non-immunocompromised patients in that the disease is much less contained and cavity formation is less apparent. Thus, the disease may present as a spreading pulmonary lesion with rather non-specific radiological features or as disseminated disease. This emphasizes that both cavity formation and the 'walling-off' process seen in post-primary disease have an immunological basis.

Not only does HIV infection predispose to tuberculosis, the latter may adversely affect the progress of the former. Tuberculosis, even if effectively treated, often leads to a rapid progression of HIV infection to AIDS. This appears to be due to tumour necrosis factor, which induces the production of a nuclear factor, which in turn activates the transcription of the DNA provirus of the HIV leading to viral replication[42].

Tuberculosis itself may induce a degree of immunosuppression, which reverts to normal after successful therapy of the disease. Various defects in immune function have been described in tuberculosis and, in particular, HIV–negative patients with active disease may show a CD4+ T cell lymphopenia[43].

Relatively high numbers of CD8 cells were found in broncho-alveolar lavage (BAL) fluid from patients with miliary tuberculosis. The time taken for the radiographs to clear on therapy was related to the number of these cells, suggesting that they had an adverse effect on protective immunity. The number of lymphocytes in BAL fluid was much higher after 8 weeks of therapy and there was a distinct shift from CD8+ to CD4+ dominance [44].

5.14 VACCINATION AND IMMUNOTHERAPY

Bacille Calmette-Guerin (BCG) was produced from a tubercle bacillus of bovine origin by repeated subculture on potato-bile medium. This approach to vaccine development was based on the finding that children who developed, and recovered from, tuberculous cervical lymphadenopathy (scrofula) as a result of consuming milk contaminated with *M. bovis* appeared to be protected against the more serious pulmonary forms of tuberculosis later in life (Marfan's law)[45]. In accord with this theory, BCG was initially given as an oral suspension to infants although, for reasons of safety and standardization, it is now given by intradermal injection. The mode of action of BCG is unknown. It is particularly effective in preventing the serious non-pulmonary forms of primary tuberculosis such as meningitis. Thus its principal effect may be to prevent dissemination of bacilli from the primary infection.

BCG protects, to some extent, against leprosy[46] and against lymphadenitis due to environmental mycobacteria in children[47], indicating that some, or all, of the determinants of protection are to be found among the antigens common to all mycobacteria.

The efficacy of BCG varies greatly from region to region (see Fig. 14b.1, p. 299). In regions where the vaccine is relatively ineffective, greater protection is obtained by vaccinating children shortly after birth[48]. Various explanations have been given for the regional variation: one of the more plausible ones is that immunity to mycobacterial disease may be conferred by exposure to environmental mycobacteria and that subsequent BCG vaccination cannot add substantially to the level of protection. Alternatively, some species or populations of environmental mycobacteria may induce inappropriate tissue-damaging responses that BCG cannot counteract or may even boost[49]. In this respect, tuberculin reactions may be divided into non-necrotic 'Listeria-type' and necrotic 'Koch-type' responses by careful clinical inspection[50] and detection of central slowing of the blood flow by laser Doppler velicometry[51].

There is therefore abundant evidence that, depending on various factors, immune responses may confer protection or cause excessive tissue damage and permit bacillary replication in the cavity wall. Any means of switching from the latter to the former would be of great therapeutic benefit. Skin testing with mixtures of sensitins prepared from various mycobacteria showed that necrotic Koch-type reactions are converted to non-necrotic reactions by the inclusion of antigens of the non-pathogenic, rapidly growing species such as *M. vaccae*[52]. Subsequent extensive studies revealed that an injection of 10^9 killed *M. vaccae* has a systemic effect in replacing Koch-type reactivity with a protective response[21]. It also restores immune recognition of the common mycobacterial antigens, which, as described above, is absent in patients with active mycobacterial disease. The precise mode of action of *M. vaccae* has not been determined but clinical studies indicate that it is a valuable adjunct to short-course chemotherapy, possibly permitting the duration of therapy to be reduced from 5 months or more to 2 months or less[53].

5.15 OTHER IMMUNOLOGICAL PHENOMENA IN TUBERCULOSIS

Attention has focused recently on the possibility that immunity to mycobacteria may, to some extent, involve lysis of cells harbouring mycobacteria, a process that would also contribute to the immunopathological features of the tissue reactions. Such cell killing may be due to antigen-specific cytotoxic (CD8$^+$) T cells as, in the mouse, these have been shown to confer resistance to infection by *M. tuberculosis* by *in vivo* depletion and adoptive transfer studies[54]. As yet, however, there is no evidence for

the involvement of cytotoxic CD8$^+$ cells in human tuberculosis[44]. In addition, natural killer (NK) and CD4$^-$ CD8$^-$ T cells have been implicated in non-specific intracellular killing of mycobacteria, as well as killing of infected macrophages[55]. Large numbers of cytolytic gamma-delta T cells have been found in the necrotic lesions of tuberculous lymphadenitis[56], although their precise role in such lesions is not clear.

There have been extensive studies on antibody assay in tuberculosis in the hope of developing a serological test for this disease. Unfortunately no test has proved sensitive or specific enough to justify its introduction into routine diagnostic services[57]. Serological studies have been used to relate immune responses to various mycobacterial epitopes to susceptibility to tuberculosis in the hope of delineating those antigens that confer protective immunity. Thus, for example, healthy subjects exposed to open tuberculosis have high levels of antibody to a 14 kDa protein of *M. tuberculosis* while those with progressive tuberculosis have low levels of that antibody[58] (Chapter 17a, p. 369).

A characteristic of tuberculosis is an increase in the proportion of a form of immunoglobulin in the IgG class that lacks a terminal galactose from a sugar component of this macromolecule. Raised levels of this so-called 'agalactosyl IgG' also occur in other diseases, including rheumatoid arthritis (RA) and Crohn's disease, which are characterized by tissue damage due to cytokines released by T cells and an acute-phase protein response[16]. A tenuous connection between tuberculosis and RA has emerged from studies on the so-called heat-shock proteins (HSP). These form a class of structurally highly conserved proteins found in all living creatures and are also termed 'chaperone' or 'nurse-maid' proteins as they assist in the folding and assembly of other protein macromolecules. It has been shown that T cells from patients with RA react to mycobacterial HSPs and to the human homologues and that adjuvant arthritis in rats is adoptively transferable by T cell clones reacting to a 65 kDa mycobacterial HSP[59]. Clearly, tuberculosis is not a regular cause of RA (although a very few patients develop an arthritis-like condition termed Poncet's disease), but mycobacteria could, by antigen mimicry, be one of the triggers for the onset of RA. Whether or not this proves to be the case, mycobacteria may, by antigen mimicry, induce autoimmune phenomena that contribute to tissue damage in both tuberculosis and leprosy[60].

A further factor suggesting a link between the immunopathology of tuberculosis and of RA is the finding that the HLA-DR4 phenotype, which is known to predispose to RA, is associated with large dermal reactions to specific antigens of *M. tuberculosis* but not to those of other mycobacteria[14].

5.16 CONCLUSIONS

Immune reactions in tuberculosis are complex and, depending on various genetic and environmental factors, result in either protective immunity or excessive tissue damage. Tuberculosis passes through two stages – primary and post-primary. In the former, bacilli disseminate to regional lymph nodes and to more distant sites. Nevertheless, most primary lesions resolve although a few bacilli may persist within healed lesions and subsequently reactivate. Post-primary disease is characterized by excessive tissue necrosis, which, though having some protective effect by walling off the active lesions, generates cavities that favour massive bacillary multiplication, rendering the patient infectious, and dissemination of disease throughout the lung by bronchial spread. This necrotic hypersensitivity is analogous to the Koch phenomenon in the guinea-pig.

There is evidence that necrotizing immune responses are the result of the sensitization of tissues by T cell-derived factors to killing by tumour necrosis factor (TNF) released by macrophages primed for such release by endogenously generated calcitriol. The TNF release is triggered by mycobacterial cell wall components, especially lipoarabinomannan. In protective immune responses, however, TNF has a more beneficial effect by activating macrophages and facilitating granuloma formation. The factors determining the nature of the response are poorly understood. The immunopathological response is characterized by elevated levels of an abnormal immunoglobulin (agalactosyl IgG), suggesting immune dysregulation. In addition, patients with active tuberculosis often fail to react in skin testing to shared mycobacterial antigens.

Both the protective immune responses and the necrotic hypersensitivity responses responsible for walling off the infection are suppressed in HIV positive and other immunocompromised tuberculosis patients so that progressive disseminated disease is commonly seen. The immune response in tuberculosis activates the HIV so that tuberculosis predisposes to the rapid onset of AIDS.

The mode of action of BCG is not understood. Its efficacy varies enormously from region to region but, in all regions, it is most effective when given neonatally. Thus extrinsic factors, probably exposure to environmental mycobacteria, may induce inappropriate immune reactions that administration of BCG cannot override. There is, however, strong evidence that the administration of killed cells of a rapidly growing mycobacterium, *M. vaccae*, which is rich in shared mycobacterial antigens, replaces a necrotic Koch-type response by a non-necrotic protective one. Such immunomodulation may be the key to future prevention and treatment of tuberculosis.

REFERENCES

1. Wallgren A. (1948) The 'time-table' of tuberculosis. *Tubercle*, **29**, 245–51.
2. Grange J.M., Noble, W.C., Yates, M.D. and Collins, C.H. (1988) Inoculation mycobacterioses. *Clin. Exp. Dermatol.*, **13**, 211–20.

3. Medlar, E.M. (1955) The behaviour of pulmonary tuberculosis. A pathological study. *Am. Rev. Tuberc.*, **71** (Part 2, Suppl.), 1–244.

4. Inoue, T., Yoshikai, Y., Matsuzaki, G., and Nomoto, K. (1991). Early appearing g/d-bearing T cells during infection with Calmette Guerin bacillus. *J. Immunol.*, **146**, 2754–62.

5. de Vries, R.R.P. (1991) An immunogenetic view of delayed type hypersensitivity. *Tubercle*, **72**, 161–7.

6. Orme, I.M. (1987) The kinetics of emergence and loss of mediator T lymphocytes acquired in response to infection with *Mycobacterium tuberculosis*. J. Immunol., **138**, 293–8.

7. Mossman, T.R. and Moore, K.W. (1991) The role of Il-10 in crossregulation of T_H1 and T_H2 responses. In *Immunoparasitology Today* (eds C. Ash and R.B. Gallagher), Elsevier, New York A49–A53.

8. Rook, G.A.W. (1991) Mobilising the appropriate T cell subset: the immune response as taxonomist? *Tubercle*, **72**, 253–4.

9. Schurr, E., Malo, D., Radzioch, D. *et al.* (1991) Genetic control of innate resistance to mycobacterial infections. *Immunol. Today*, **12**, A42-A45.

10. Bothamley, G.H., Beck, J.S., Geziena, M. *et al.* (1989) Association of tuberculosis and *M. tuberculosis*-specific antibody levels with HLA. *J. Infect. Dis.*, **159**, 549–55.

11. Brahmajothi, V., Pitchappan, R.M., Kakkanaiah, V.N. *et al.* (1991) Association of pulmonary tuberculosis and HLA in South India. *Tubercle*, **72**, 123–32.

12. Khomenko, A.G., Litvinov, V.I., Chukanova, V.P. and Pospelov, L.E. (1990) Tuberculosis in patients with various HLA phenotypes. *Tubercle*, **71**, 187–92.

13. Pitchappan, R.M., Brahmajothi, V., Rajaram, K. *et al.* (1991) Spectrum of immune reactivity to mycobacterial (BCG) antigens in healthy hospital contacts in South India. *Tubercle*, **72**, 133–9.

14. Ottenhoff, T.H.M., Torres, P., de las Aguas, J.T. *et al.* (1986) Evidence for an HLA-DR4-associated immune response gene for *Mycobacterium tuberculosis*. Lancet, **2**, 310–12.

15. Mackaness, G.B. (1967) The immunology of antituberculous immunity. *Am. Rev. Respir. Dis.*, **97**, 337–44.

16. Rook, G.A.W. and Al Attiyah, R. (1991) Cytokines and the Koch phenomenon. *Tubercle*, **72**, 13–20.

17. Grange, J.M. (1992) The mystery of the mycobacterial persistor. *Tubercle Lung Dis.*, **73**, 249–51.

18. Wayne, L.G. and Lin, K-Y. (1982) Glyoxylate metabolism and adaptation of *Mycobacterium tuberculosis* to survival under anaerobic conditions. *Infect. Immun.*, **37**, 1042–9.

19. Stanford, J.L. (1987) Much's granules revisited. *Tubercle*, **68**, 241–2.

20. Springett, V.H. (1971) Ten year results during the introduction of chemotherapy for tuberculosis. *Tubercle*, **52**, 73–87.

21. Stanford, J.L. (1991) Koch's phenomenon: can it be corrected? *Tubercle*, **72**, 241–9.

22. Koch, R. (1891) Weitere Mitteilungen uber ein Heilmittel gegen Tuberculose. *Dtsch. Med. Wochenschr.*, **171**, 101–2.

23. Coombs, R.R.A. and Gell, P.G.H. (1975) Classification of allergic reactions responsible for hypersensitivity and disease. In *Clinical Aspects of Immunology*, 3rd edn, (eds P.G.H. Gell and R.R.A. Coombs), Blackwell, Oxford, pp. 761–81.

24. von Pirquet, C. (1909) Demonstration zur Tuberculindiagnose durch Hautimpfung. *Berl. Klin. Wochenschr.*, **481**, 699.

25. Styblo, K. (1980) Recent advances in epidemiological research in tuberculosis. *Adv. Tuber. Res.*, **201**, 1–63.

26. Beck, J.S., Morley, S.M., Gibbs, J.H., *et al.* (1986) The cellular responses of tuberculosis and leprosy patients and of healthy controls in skin tests to new tuberculin and healthy subjects. *Clin. Exp. Immunol.*, **64**, 484–94.

27. Beck, J.S. (1991) Skin changes in the tuberculin test. *Tubercle*, **72**, 81–7.

28. Beck, J.S., Gibbs, J.H., Potts, R.C. *et al.* (1989) The relation between cutaneous blood flow and cell content in the tuberculin reaction. *Scand. J. Immunol.*, **291**, 33–9.

29. Stanford, J.L., Nye, P.M., Rook, G.A.W., *et al.* (1981) A preliminary investigation of the responsiveness or otherwise of patients and staff of a leprosy hospital to groups of shared or specific antigens of mycobacteria. *Lepr. Rev.*, **52**, 321–7.

30. Kardjito, T., Beck, J.S., Grange, J.M. and Stanford, J.L. (1986) A comparison of the responsiveness to four new tuberculins among Indonesian patients with pulmonary tuberculosis and healthy subjects. *Eur. J. Respir. Dis.*, **69**, 142–5.

31. Bothamley, G.H. and Grange, J.M. (1991) The

Koch phenomenon and delayed hypersensitivity: 1891–1991. *Tubercle*, **72**, 7–11.

32. von Pirquet, C. (1908) Verlauf der tuberculosen Allergie bei einen Falle von Masern und Miliartuberkulose. *Wein. Klin. Wochenschr.*, **21**, 861–5.

33. Youmans, G.P. (1975) Relation between delayed hypersensitivity and immunity in tuberculosis. *Am. Rev. Respir. Dis.*, **111**, 109–18.

34. Lefford, M.J. (1975) Delayed hypersensitivity and immunity in tuberculosis. *Am. Rev. Respir. Dis.*, **111**, 243–46.

35. Salvin, S.B. and Neta, R. (1975) A possible relation between delayed hypersensitivity and cell-mediated immunity. *Am. Rev. Respir. Dis.*, **111**, 373–77.

36. Rook, G.A.W. (1988) The role of vitamin D in tuberculosis. *Am. Rev. Respir. Dis.* **138**, 768–70.

37. Moreno, C., Taverne, J., Mehlert, A. *et al.* (1989) Lipoarabinomannan from *Mycobacterium tuberculosis* induces the production of tumour necrosis factor from human and murine macrophages. *Clin. Exp. Immunol.*, **76**, 240–45.

38. Al-Attiyah, R.J. (1991) The regulation of necrosis in mycobacterial lesions. Doctor of Philosophy Thesis, University of London.

39. Skinsnes, O.K. (1968) Comparative pathogenesis of mycobacterioses. *Ann. NY Acad. Sci.*, **154**, 19–31.

40. Ridley, D.S. and Ridley, M.J. (1987) Rationale for the histological spectrum of tuberculosis. A basis for classification. *Pathology*, **19**, 186–92.

41. Festenstein, F. and Grange, J.M. (1991) Tuberculosis and the acquired immune deficiency syndrome. *J. Appl. Bacteriol.*, **71**, 19–30.

42. Osborn, L., Kunkel, S. and Nabel, G.J. (1989) Tumour necrosis factor and interleukin 1 stimulate the human immunodeficiency virus enhancer by activation of the nuclear factor kappa B. *Proc. Natl Acad. Sci. USA*, **86**, 2236–40.

43. Beck, J.S., Potts, R.C., Kardjito T. and Grange, J.M. (1985) T4 lymphopenia in patients with active pulmonary tuberculosis. *Clin. Exp. Immunol.*, **60**, 49–54.

44. Ainslie, G.M., Solomon, J.A. and Bateman, E.D. (1992) Lymphocyte and lymphocyte subset numbers in blood and in bronchoalveolar lavage and pleural fluid in various forms of human pulmonary tuberculosis at presentation and during recovery. *Thorax*, **47**, 513–18.

45. Savage, W.G. (1929) *The Prevention of Human Tuberculosis of Bovine Origin*, Macmillan, London.

46. Brown, J.A.K., Stone, M.M. and Sutherland, I. (1966) BCG vaccination of children against leprosy in Uganda. *B. Med. J.*, **1**, 7–14.

47. Romanus V. (1988) Swedish experiences 12 years after the cessation of general BCG vaccination of new borns in 1975. *Bull. Union Int. Tuberc. Lung Dis.*, **63**(4), 34–8.

48. Tripathy, S.P. (1987) Fifteen year follow-up of the Indian BCG prevention trial. *Proceedings of the 24th International Union Against Tuberculosis Conference on Tuberculosis and Respiratory Diseases*, Singapore, Professional Postgraduate Services, pp. 69–72.

49. Stanford, J.L., Shield, M.J. and Rook, G.A.W. (1981) How environmental mycobacteria may predetermine the protective efficacy of BCG. *Tubercle*, **62**, 55–62.

50. Stanford, J.L. and Lema, E. (1983) The use of a sonicate preparation of *Mycobacterium tuberculosis* (new tuberculin) in the assessment of BCG vaccination. *Tubercle*, **64**, 275–82.

51. Potts, R.C., Beck, J.S., Gibbs, J.H. *et al.* (1992) Measurements of blood flow and histometry of the cellular infiltrate in tuberculin skin test responses of the Koch-type and Listeria-type in pulmonary tuberculosis patients and apparently healthy controls. *Int. J. Exp. Pathol.*, **73**, 565–72.

52. Nye, P.M., Price, J.E., Revankar, C.R. *et al.* (1983) The demonstration of two types of suppressor mechanism in leprosy patients and their contacts by quadruple skin-testing with mycobacterial reagent mixtures. *Lepr. Rev.*, **54**, 9–18.

53. Stanford, J.L., Grange, J.M. and Pozniak, A. (1991) Is Africa Lost? *Lancet*, **338**, 557–8.

54. Muller, I., Cobbold, S.P., Waldmann, H. and Kaufmann, S.H.E. (1987) Impaired resistance against *Mycobacterium tuberculosis* infection after selective *in vitro* depletion of L3T4⁻ and Lyt2⁺ T cells. *Infect. Immun.*, **55**, 2037–41.

55. Restrepo, L.M., Barrera, L.F. and Garcia, L.F. (1990) Natural killer cell activity in patients with pulmonary tuberculosis and in healthy controls. *Tubercle*, **71**, 95–102.

56. Modlin, R.L., Pirmez, C. Hofman, F.M. *et al.*, (1989) Lymphocytes bearing antigen-specific gd T-cell receptors accumulate in human infectious disease lesions. *Nature*, **339**, 544–8.

57. Grange, J.M. and Laszlo, A. (1990) Serodiag-

nostic tests for tuberculosis: a need for assessment of their predictive accuracy and acceptability. *Bull. WHO*, **681**, 571–6.

58. Bothamley, G.H., Beck, J.S., Potts, R.C. *et al.*, (1992) Specificity of antibodies and tuberculin response following occupational exposure to tuberculosis. *J. Infect. Dis.*, **166**, 182–6.

59. Rook, G.A.W. (1988) Rheumatoid arthritis, mycobacterial antigens and agalactosyl IgG. *Scand. J. Immunol.*, **28**, 487–93.

60. Das, P.K. and Grange, J.M. (1993) Mycobacteria in relation to tissue immune response and pathogenesis. *Rev. Med. Microbiol.*, **4**, 15–23.

RESPIRATORY TUBERCULOSIS

L.P. Ormerod

6.1 PRIMARY TUBERCULOSIS

6.1.1 CLINICAL FEATURES

The majority of primary infections are asymptomatic, the only evidence being the development of a positive tuberculin test. Symptoms are often mild and non-specific and cannot be differentiated from other childhood illnesses. Clinical signs are unusual and are limited to signs of collapse such as bronchial breathing or localized wheeze caused by compression or occlusion of a bronchus by enlarged lymph glands. Cough is also uncommon unless bronchial compression is present.

6.1.2 DIAGNOSIS

The diagnosis depends on demonstrating tuberculin conversion, which becomes positive 3–6 weeks after initial infection and which may be accompanied by radiographic changes. The peripheral lung lesion (Ghon focus) may be visible, accompanied by ipsilateral hilar lymphadenopathy (Fig. 6.1). Visible radiographic abnormality varies with ethnic group. In some, such as those of Indian subcontinent (ISC) ethnic origin, marked hilar or paratracheal lymphadenophaty may be the only feature. After some 12 months the Ghon focus or regional nodes may calcify. In the presence of radiographic changes tubercle bacilli can sometimes be cultured from gastric washings.

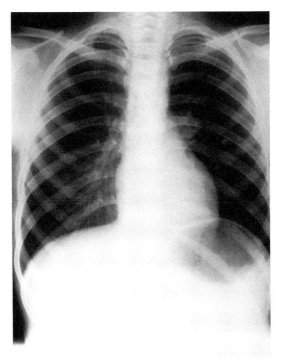

Fig. 6.1 Primary tuberculosis. Left-sided primary complex with calcifying Ghon focus in the mid zone. Mother sputum smear-positive.

6.1.3 COMPLICATIONS

(a) Pneumonitis/collapse (so-called epituberculosis)

Regional lymphadenopathy can compress or occlude a segmental or lobar bronchus lead-

Clinical Tuberculosis. Edited by P.D.O. Davies. Published in 1994 by Chapman & Hall, London. ISBN 0 412 48630 X

ing to dense shadowing. This can result from extrinsic pressure, bronchostenosis or discharge of caseous material into the affected lobe or segment. Local physical signs are often present in such cases (see Fig. 11.1, p. 213).

(b) Obstructive emphysema

Occasionally the obstructing lymph node or caseous stenosis sets up a ball-valve effect with so-called 'obstructive emphysema' of the lobe. This is not true emphysema but an overdistension of the lobe involved. It is best seen on a radiograph taken in expiration, when overdistension of the lung will be apparent, often with some degree of mediastinal displacement to the contralateral side.

(c) Bronchiectasis

Involvement of a lobar or segmental bronchus by primary tuberculosis can lead to the development of bronchiectasis in the distal lung[1]. The middle lobe may be particularly prone to this complication because the orifice is surrounded by glands[2]. This may lead to persistent symptoms and be the only evidence of previous primary tuberculosis (Fig. 11.1, p. 213).

(d) Pleural effusion

The primary infection can be accompanied by a small ipsilateral pleural effusion. This is usually small and transient.

(e) Associated hypersensitivity phenomena

Erythema nodosum

Erythema nodosum is a dermal lesion caused by perivascular inflammation of arteries and veins, but can also involve fat and connective tissues. It is attributed to a response to high circulating levels of immune complexes, but is not specific to tuberculosis. When due to tuberculosis, it usually occurs within 3–8

weeks of infection[3]. In developed countries erythema nodosum is now rarely caused by tuberculosis; sarcoidosis, streptococcal infection and inflammatory bowel disease being much more common causes. In developing countries it is much more likely to be due to tuberculosis, but the association with leprosy should be borne in mind.

Phylectenular conjunctivitis

Phylectenular conjunctivitis is associated with tuberculin hypersensitivity. It is rare in developed countries, but is still seen in the Third World[4], usually in children within 12 months of primary infection. The usual appearance is of small grey or yellow nodules in the conjunctiva near the limbus with dilated vessels radiating outwards, giving symptoms of irritation, pain, lacrymation and photophobia in one or both eyes[5]. The lesions can appear and disappear spontaneously. The lesions may resolve on anti-tuberculosis drugs alone, but local treatment with atropine drops to dilate the pupil or hydrocortisone drops to reduce inflammation may be required.

6.2 MILIARY TUBERCULOSIS

6.2.1 PATHOGENESIS

Miliary tuberculosis occurs when tubercle bacilli are spread acutely through the blood stream. In high prevalence areas the majority of cases follow shortly after primary infection. In low prevalence areas the majority of cases occur in the elderly, representing reactivation. Bacilli spreading into vessel walls may reach the intima and discharge into the blood stream causing spread to other parts of the body. The lung is always involved, but other organs variably so. Miliary tuberculosis derives its name from the small, seed-like macroscopic appearance of the lesions (Latin *milia* = seed), which can be seen on chest radiography as discrete diffuse lesions.

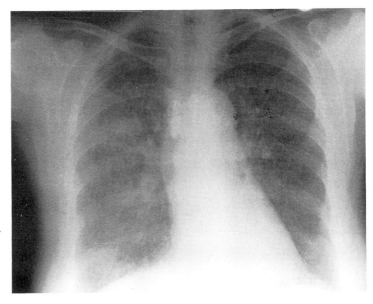

Fig. 6.2 Miliary tuberculosis. Radiograph of a 74-year-old patient with miliary tuberculosis. Calcified paratracheal glands show this to be reactivated infection. Diagnosis confirmed by CSF microscopy.

Microscopically the miliary lesions consist of Langerhans giant cells, epithelioid cells and lymphocytes, containing acid-fast bacilli, and sometimes central caseation. In the elderly or in immunosuppressed patients non-reactive pathological appearances are described with necrotic lesions containing no specific tuberculous features, but with many acid-fast bacilli. The diagnosis is usually made at post-mortem examination[6].

Symptoms the onset of which are usually insidious[7], include anorexia, malaise, fever and weight loss, which occur in 'acute' and cryptic forms.

6.2.2 ACUTE MILIARY TUBERCULOSIS

In addition to general symptoms, headache from co-existent tuberculous meningitis frequently occurs and should alert the clinician to perform a lumbar puncture. Cough, dyspnoea and haemoptysis are less common symptoms. Physical signs may be few. The chest almost invariably sounds clear to auscultation. Enlargement of the liver, spleen or lymph nodes may be found in a small number of cases[8]. Involvement of the serosal surfaces can lead to the development of small pericardial or pleural effusions or a mild ascites. On examination of the fundus it is important to seek the presence of choroidal tubercles, which are commoner in children. The lesions are usually few and appear as small slightly raised yellowish plaques, which may flatten and become white as the illness progresses. Skin lesions may also occur in the form of papules, macules or purpuric lesions. These probably represent local vasculitic lesions caused by reaction to mycobacterial antigen.

The typical radiograph (Fig. 6.2) shows an even distribution of uniform-sized lesions throughout all zones of the lung. The size of the lesions is usually 1–2 mm but occasionally large lesions are seen. There may be evidence of a primary complex or a previous tuberculous lesion to suggest reactivation. Small bilateral pleural effusions may also be present. An unusual variation with reticular shadowing due to lymphatic involvement has been described[9].

Table 6.1 Comparison of characteristic and cryptic miliary TB

Feature	Cryptic	Characteristic
Age	Majority over 60 years	Majority under 40 years
TB history or contact	Up to 25%	Up to 33%
Malaise/weight loss	75%	75%
Fever	90%	75%
Choroidal tubercles	Absent	Up to 20%
Meningitis	Rare unless terminal	Up to 20%
Lymphadenopathy	Absent	Up to 20%
Miliary shadowing on radiograph	Rare	Usual except in early stages
Tuberculin test	Usually negative	Usually positive
Pancytopenia/leukaemoid reaction	Common	Rare
Bacteriological confirmation	Urine; sputum	Sputum; urine
	Bone marrow	CSF
Biopsy evidence	Liver up to 75%	Seldom required
	Bone marrow	
	Lymph node	

6.2.3 CHRONIC 'CRYPTIC' MILIARY TUBERCULOSIS

As tuberculosis declines in incidence in developed countries, a form of miliary tuberculosis without typical radiographic shadowing, so-called 'cryptic' miliary tuberculosis, has been seen more frequently. This is usually found in patients over the age of 60[10], but may be seen in young patients in some immigrant groups. The symptoms are usually insidious with weight loss, lethargy and intermittent fever[11]. Physical signs such as choroidal tubercles or meningitis are usually absent. Mild hepato-splenomegaly may be present, but no other physical signs are usually found. A high index of suspicion is required to make the diagnosis, and most patients are diagnosed at post-mortem[12]. The main differential diagnosis is disseminated carcinoma. Table 6.1 compares various features of the acute and chronic forms.

6.2.4 DIAGNOSIS

The characteristic form of miliary disease is usually easy to diagnose because of the typical radiographic appearances, which are only absent in the early stages. The tuberculin test is usually positive, and bacteriological confirmation may be obtained from sputum, urine or CSF cultures. The diagnosis of cryptic miliary tuberculosis depends on clinical suspicion leading to specific tests and/or response to a trial of antituberculosis drugs. In the cryptic form, blood dyscrasias are not uncommon. Pancytopenia[13,14], leukaemoid reactions[15,16] and other granulocyte abnormalities[17] have all been described. Bone marrow aspiration may yield both granulomata on microscopy and acid-fast bacilli on culture, and should be considered particularly in the presence of blood dyscrasias. Liver biopsy has the highest yield of granulomata which have been reported in up to 75% of cases. In cases where the patient is unwilling to have the appropriate tests, or where the facilities for them do not exist, a clinical trial of antituberculosis drugs should be given. The fever usually responds within 7–10 days and clinical improvement takes place in 4–6 weeks.

6.2.5 COMPLICATIONS

(a) Meningitis

TB meningitis may complicate miliary tuberculosis, and is a manifestation of acute

Plate 1   (Chapter 3) **Ziehl-Neelsen stained smear of sputum showing acid-fast bacilli.** ($\times$ 500; oil immersion.)

Plate 2   (Chapter 3) **Colonies of** *M. tuberculosis* **growing on Lowenstein–Jensen medium.**

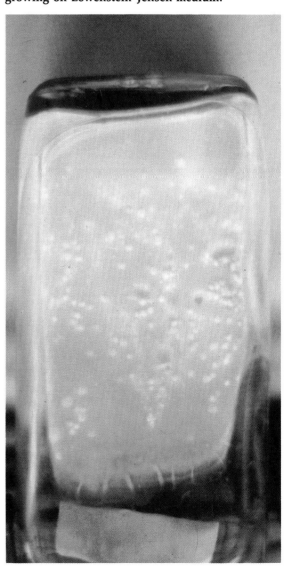

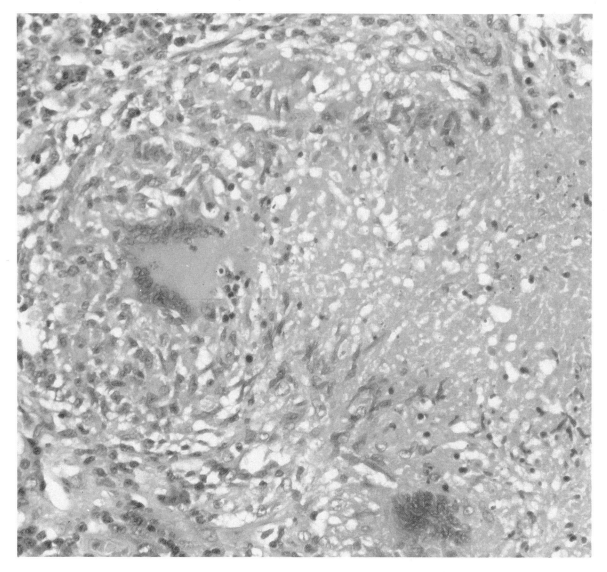

Plate 3 (Chapter 4) **A caseating granuloma showing epithelioid cells and lymphocytes.** A giant cell is present centre left.

Plate 4 (Chapter 4) **Macroscopic section showing tuberculoma in an upper lobe.**

Plate 5 (Chapter 4) **Macroscopic section showing caseating pneumonia in a lower lobe.**

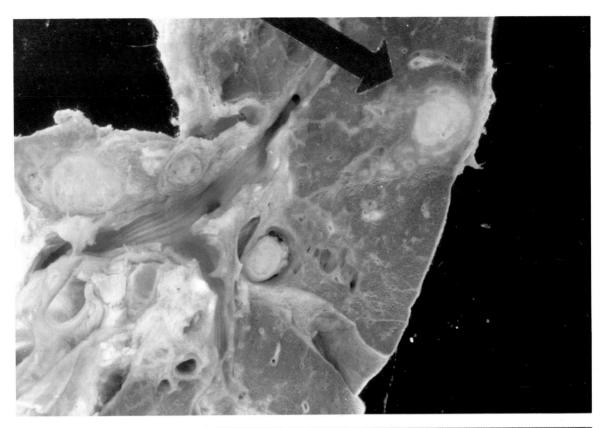

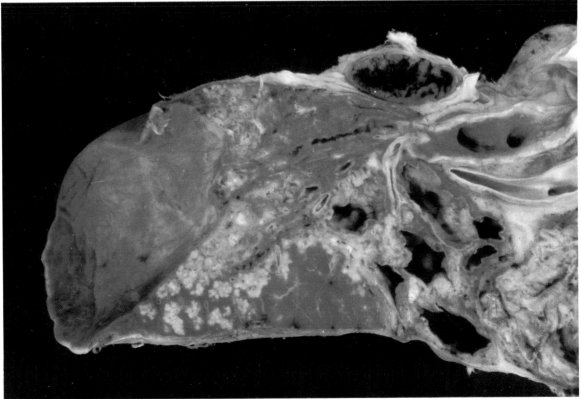

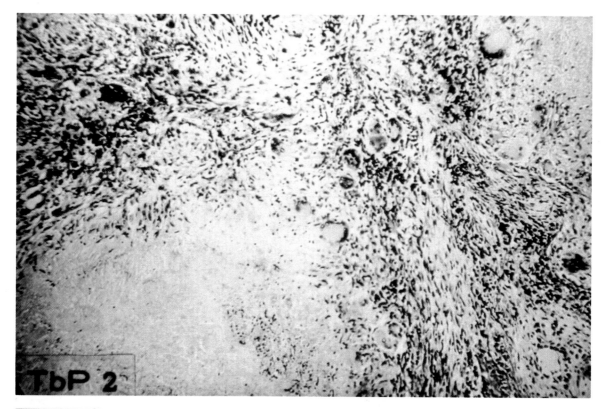

Plate 6 (Chapter 5) **A tuberculous granuloma showing epithelioid cells, giant cells and central caseous necrosis.**

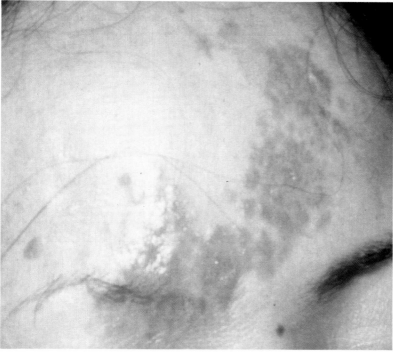

Plate 7 (Chapter 7) **Cutaneous tuberculosis (lupus vulgaris).**

haematogenous spread. It occurs overtly in up to 20% of cases. Lumbar puncture should be performed if there is any suggestion of meningeal irritation or headache. A positive microscopy for acid-fast bacilli in the CSF may be the most rapid way of confirming the clinical diagnosis of miliary tuberculosis.

(b) Adult respiratory distress syndrome (ARDS)

Occasionally disseminated tuberculosis presents as ARDS[18]. In these cases breathlessness due to the ARDS may predominate, and the characteristic chest radiograph appearances may be obscured by diffuse confluent or ground-glass shadowing[19,20].

6.3 POST-PRIMARY TUBERCULOSIS

Post-primary pulmonary tuberculosis is much the commonest type of tuberculosis, and is important not only because of clinical disease, but because patients with this disease are the source of continuing infection in the community. Post-primary tuberculosis can arise by one of the following mechanisms.

(a) Direct progression of primary disease

If the local immune response at the primary site does not arrest the infection, the disease can progress to caseation and cavitation. Alternatively a pleural effusion or empyema may result. Infection may also spread to distant sites by the haematogenous route. Whether this occurs in an individual varies with the infecting dose of bacilli, the immune response, the presence of other diseases and the presence of previous BCG vaccination.

(b) Reactivation of quiescent primary disease

Local immune responses usually contain the primary infection within the lung, which is then said to be 'arrested'. The site of the primary infection may be visible on chest

radiography and may calcify at a later stage, but there is often no radiographic evidence of prior infection; a positive tuberculin skin test being the only evidence. Although the disease is 'arrested', tubercle bacilli may remain dormant and sequestered in pulmonary macrophages or in scar tissue where they may remain viable for many years[21]. If the effectiveness of local defences or general immunity falls due to age, intercurrent illness, immunosuppression from drugs[22] or HIV infection, the dormant bacilli may become active and clinical disease develops. This is thought to be the main mechanism of development of tuberculosis in the middle-aged or elderly, and particularly in the homeless[23].

(c) Haematogenous spread to the lung

Bacilli may sometimes be disseminated from a primary complex, via the blood stream, to the lungs. Symmetrical upper zone mottling is thought to result but this is unproven.

(d) Exogenous reinfection

Reinfection by inhaled tubercle bacilli is thought to be uncommon as it is likely to be prevented by immunity derived from the primary infection. This again is difficult to prove as the majority of tubercle bacilli, whether endogenous or exogenous, are fully sensitive to drugs. This mechanism can be shown to have occurred on the rare occasions when individuals, who once had tuberculosis with fully sensitive organisms, have a second episode with organisms resistant to drugs they have never received[24]. In the future the occurrence of exogenous reinfection may be proved by DNA fingerprinting if cultures from the original and recurrent infections are available. This is only likely to occur in areas of high prevalence.

6.3.1 CLINICAL

(a) Symptoms

The symptoms of respiratory tuberculosis may be non-specific and constitutional or

Table 6.2 Presentations of respiratory tuberculosis

Common	Less common
Asymptomatic pick-up on radiography	Chest wall pain
Persistent cough	Hyponatraemia
Malaise/weight loss	ARDS
Non-resolving pneumonia	
Haemoptysis	

specific and respiratory. General symptoms include tiredness, a feeling of malaise, or anorexia. Weight loss occurs as disease progresses, and may be accompanied by sweating associated with fever, particularly at night. Amenorrhoea may occur in females if weight loss is significant. Cough is the commonest respiratory symptom, the sputum being mucoid or purulent and may be accompanied by haemoptysis. This is usually light with blood-stained sputum or small amounts of blood. Occasionally it can be severe, with several hundred millilitres due to rupture of a bronchial artery into a cavity. Chest pain is rare but may be dull and poorly localized or localized and pleuritic in nature. As lung damage (or pleural effusion) progresses, breathlessness of effort may develop which is related to the extent of disease, and possibly associated anaemia. The development of symptoms is usually insidious over a period of weeks to months, but a presentation with a relatively short history of cough, fever and dyspnoea simulating pneumonia is recognized. A list of presentation symptoms is given in Table 6.2.

(b) Signs

The signs of respiratory tuberculosis can be non-specific or respiratory. General signs include pallor due to anaemia, fever or evidence of weight loss. Clubbing may occur in extensive or long-standing disease[25]. If the lung involvement is only mild or moderate there may be no clinical signs. Upper zone crackles may be heard, or there may be signs of consolidation. Localized wheeze may be present because of bronchial narrowing, but 'amphoric' breathing is rarely heard. In chronic tuberculosis the trachea may be deviated towards the side of greatest lung destruction. Examination may provide evidence of extrapulmonary tuberculosis, such as cervical lymphadenopathy. The co-existence of respiratory and non-respiratory tuberculosis occurs in up to 10% of cases in some countries, particularly in immigrants of ISC ethnic origin[26,27]. The usual combination is of intrathoracic and cervical lymphadenopathy[28]. In HIV infected patients the proportion presenting with two or more sites is higher.

6.3.2 RADIOGRAPHIC CHANGES

(a) Radiographic spectrum (Figs 6.3–6.8)

No radiographic pattern is absolutely diagnostic of tuberculosis, but some patterns are highly suggestive though capable of being mimicked by other diseases. The distribution of shadowing in parenchymal post-primary disease shows a strong tendency for the upper lobes, with a predilection for the posterior segments. Disease in the lower lobes tends to be in the apical segment [29,30]. Bilateral disease, especially in the upper zones, is common, the shadowing being a patchy or nodular infiltration initially. As the infiltration becomes more confluent, cavitation develops. Loss of volume and fibrosis leads to elevation of the hilae, with tracheal or mediastinal deviation if the disease is predominantly unilateral. Calcification develops in the later stages of arrested or treated disease. A normal chest radiograph can occur even in the presence of a positive sputum smear or culture. This is because endobronchial disease either from an ulcerated area in a bronchus, or a gland eroding into a major bronchus may discharge caseous material into an airway[31].

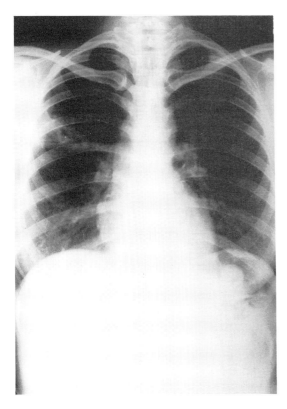

Fig. 6.3 Pulmonary tuberculosis. Early infiltration of right upper zone.

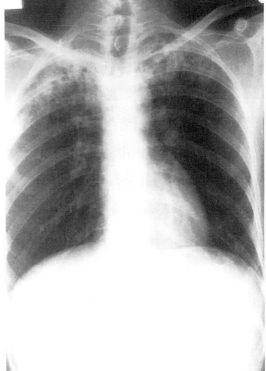

Fig. 6.4 Pulmonary tuberculosis. Infiltration of both upper zones. Bronchoscopy washings are positive on microscopy.

(b) Differential diagnosis

The main differential diagnoses are listed in Table 6.3. The distribution of radiographic shadowing is often a useful guide to diagnosis with upper zone predilection and bilateral involvement being features in favour of tuberculosis.

Segmental or lobar pneumonic shadowing, particularly in the upper zones, can mimic tuberculosis. Symptoms of bacterial or viral pneumonia are usually more profound and of a shorter duration than in tuberculosis. If bacterial pneumonia is suspected, antibiotics should be given. Failure of the chest radiograph to improve in 3 weeks should lead to the consideration of tuberculosis and examination of the sputum for acid-fast bacilli if this has not already been undertaken.

In older patients, carcinoma of the bronchus can mimic tuberculosis, particularly squamous cell carcinoma, which also has a tendency to cavitate. Bronchoscopy may be needed to exclude carcinoma, and washings should routinely be taken in upper zone lesions where there is no endobronchial abnormality for staining for acid-fast bacilli and for cytological examination. Sometimes carcinoma and tuberculosis can co-exist, the carcinoma being the cause of reduced immunity, allowing reactivation of latent infection. Where isolated pulmonary lesions are present, the presence of calcification or satellite lesions on tomography or CT scan favours tuberculosis. Fine-needle biopsy[32,33] or transbronchial lung biopsy may be required

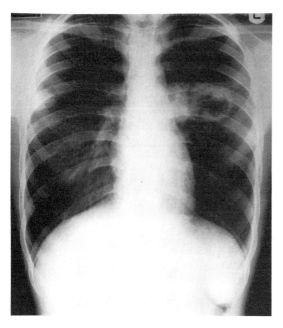

Fig. 6.5 Pulmonary tuberculosis. Cavitation involving left mid zone (apical segment of left lower lobe).

to provide a diagnosis, if sputum is negative on smear. Occasionally thoracotomy is required to establish the diagnosis (Chapter 8c, p. 157)

Other cavitating lesions such as lung abscess or pulmonary infarction may give rise to diagnostic difficulty. Acute lung abscess or cavitating pneumonia due to either *Klebsiella pneumoniae* or *Staphyloccus pyogenes* is usually easy to differentiate because of the acute systemic illness and the isolation of the appropriate organism from blood and/or sputum. Less acute lung abscesses such as those following aspiration cause more difficulty, with a longer history and more insidious onset, which can mimic tuberculosis. Cavitory tuberculosis is typically sputum microscopy-positive. If three negative smears are obtained the diagnosis of tuberculosis is less likely. Pulmonary emboli cause infarction, which may cavitate and in the upper zones can sometimes mimic tuberculosis.

Here the radiograph usually shows rapid changes, which help differentiate the two conditions. Ultrasonography or contrast studies may be helpful and show underlying venous thrombosis. Clinical features such as nasal or renal involvement are common in vasculitic causes of cavitation such as Wegener's granulomatosis. Upper zone fibrosis and loss of volume can arise in the later stages of extrinsic allergic alveolitis, allergic bronchopulmonary aspergillosis and sarcoidosis. The presence of calcification suggests tuberculosis. Specific immunological tests are available for allergic alveolitis and aspergillosis, and in sarcoidosis the tuberculin test is negative or only weakly positive.

(c) 'Activity' of disease

The presence of radiographic shadowing is not necessarily a guide to disease activity. Shadowing from arrested disease is quite common, particularly in older patients. The inactivity of a lesion is shown by negative sputum cultures and failure of a particular radiographic lesion to change with time or treatment. Activity of disease is better judged by sputum examination and the eliciting of associated clinical features.

A positive sputum culture is an absolute indication of activity and hence for treatment. The presence of weight loss, haemoptysis or fever suggest activity and the need for sputum examination. Extensive and softly edged shadowing on radiography shadowing that is increasing on serial films, or the presence of cavitation without a prior history of effective treatment, favour activity and the need for sputum examination. An individual with radiographic shadowing, which is static and shown to be inactive by sputum tests, is at substantially greater risk of reactivation than a tuberculin-positive person with a normal radiograph[34,35]. Treatment of such lesions with isoniazid had been shown to reduce reactivation rate[36], but serial radiographs are not economic or helpful as most

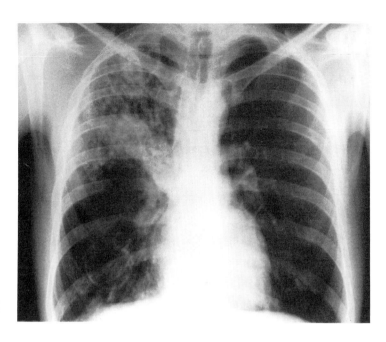

Fig. 6.6 Pulmonary tuberculosis. Cavitation involving right upper and mid zones.

reactivations occur between follow-up intervals[37]. The decision as to whether or not to give chemoprophylaxis in an individual case will depend on local incidence, resources and the balance between possible adverse effects and the elimination of the risk of reactivation.

(d) Altered pattern of disease

In the substantial majority of cases of post-primary tuberculosis the lung is involved with most patients being sputum smear-positive or smear-negative culture-positive. The pattern is altered in two circumstances: some immigrant groups and HIV-positive patients. Immigrants of Indian Subcontinent ethnic origin presenting with tuberculosis in developed countries have lower smear and culture positivity rates, a greater incidence of isolated mediastinal lymphadenopathy or pleural effusion, and smear- and culture-negative parenchymal disease[28]. The reasons for these differences are not clear, but co-existent HIV infection is not implicated (Chapter 10, p. 202).

In other parts of the world, particularly Africa, HIV infection is associated with re-duced smear-positivity rates and cavitation, less frequent presentation with characteristic radiographic appearances, increased disseminated disease, mediastinal and peripheral lymphadenopathy, pleural effusion and extrapulmonary disease. This altered pattern has been reported in Zaire[38], Zambia[39] and in sub-Saharan Africa in general[40], in the USA in Haitians[41] and other groups [42], and in Europe[43]. The reduced proportion of smear-positive cases and typical radiographic changes has important implications for developing countries, by making the diagnosis harder to confirm with limited health resources (Chapter 12b, p. 241).

6.3.3 OTHER INVESTIGATIONS

(a) Sputum bacteriology

Microscopy of sputum for acid-fast bacilli is the only test that may be available for diagnosis in developing countries. A positive smear for acid-fast bacilli by the Ziehl–Nielsen technique makes a diagnosis of tuberculosis highly probable as the proportion of non-tuberculous mycobacteria causing

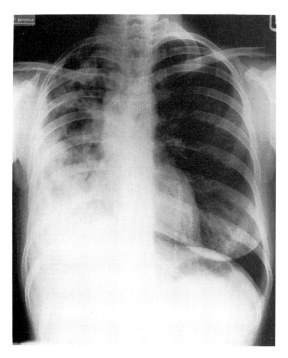

Fig. 6.7 Pulmonary tuberculosis. Cavitation involving entire right lung, with additional pleural shadowing.

pulmonary disease is very low in both the developed world and developing countries. In developed countries the Ziehl–Nielsen technique has been replaced largely with rhodamine-auramine staining, which fluoresces under ultra-violet light and has a greater sensitivity. Ideally the diagnosis should be confirmed by culture, which also allows drug-sensitivity testing.

Often pulmonary tuberculosis is suspected but not confirmed by sputum microscopy. Fibre-optic bronchoscopy if available may enable a rapid diagnosis to be made from bronchial brushings and washings[44–47], and is particularly useful in non-sputum producers[48]. Bronchoalveolar lavage combined with bronchoscopy may give a useful yield[49], and has been shown to be better than gastric washings[50]. Transbronchial

lung biopsy in addition to washings may increase the yield[51]. Care must be taken with sterilization of the bronchoscope, as inadequate sterilization can allow transmission of tuberculosis[52]. In areas of high TB prevalence it may be worthwhile routinely sending cultures from patients undergoing bronchoscopy at the time of examination[53]. Yields of up to 14% in patients with negative pre-bronchoscopy sputum smears and no clinical suspicion of tuberculosis have been reported[54]. Although invasive methods of diagnosis are very safe, occasional worsening of radiographic appearances after bronchoscopy has been described[55]. Where bronchoscopy is not available, gastric washings may be used. This method has a low sensitivity but a high specificity[56]. Laryngeal swabs may also be useful for obtaining specimens for microbiology. Where facilities permit, induced sputum using nebulized hypertonic saline can provide specimens.

(b) Other tests

Elevation of the ESR, the presence of normochromic normocytic anaemia, elevation of gammaglobulin, and reduced serum sodium can all occur in pulmonary tuberculosis and are related to disease severity[57–58] but are non-specific. The tuberculin test is a poor indicator of clinical disease in asymptomatic adults, because it can be depressed by extensive tuberculosis. Conversely there is poor correlation between a strongly positive tuberculin test and the presence of clinical tuberculosis, particularly in individuals over the age of 35 years. The possible usefulness of serodiagnostic tests and polymerase chain reaction in the diagnosis of TB are covered in later chapters (Chapters 17a, 17b).

6.3.4 COMPLICATIONS

(a) Early

Pleurisy

Pleurisy may accompany the lung infiltration and be accompanied by a rub.

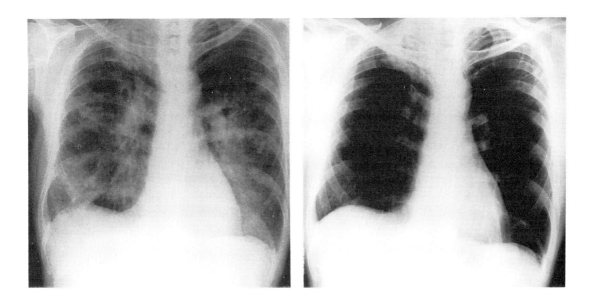

Fig. 6.8 Tuberculous bronchopneumonia. Widespread shadowing from material aspirated from reactivated right apical lesion. Sputum smear-positive. Radiographs at presentation (a) and after 2 months' therapy (including steroids) (b).

Table 6.3 Main differential diagnoses on radiography

Pattern	Alternative diagnosis
Unilateral infiltration	Carcinoma lung; pneumonia
Bilateral infiltration	Sarcoidosis (histoplasmosis; coccidiomycosis[a])
Bilateral upper-zone fibrosis	Extrinsic allergic alveolitis
	Sarcoidosis
	Allergic bronchopulmonary aspergillosis
Solitary cavitated lesion	Carcinoma lung
	Lung abscess
	Klebsiella pneumonia
	Rheumatoid nodule
	Pulmonary infarction
Bilateral cavitation	Staphylococcal pneumonia
	Wegener's granulomatosis
	Progressive massive fibrosis
Mediastinal lymphadenopathy	See p. 85

[a] To be considered in some geographical areas, e.g. North and South America and parts of Africa.

Pleural effusion

This is discussed on p. 86.

Empyema

A pleural effusion can become purulent developing into an empyema with many acid-fast bacilli spreading into the fluid from exudative lung lesions. The cytology of the fluid can be polymorphonuclear but is more often lymphocytic. Acid-fast bacilli may be seen on microscopy. Rarely an acute pyo-pneumothorax can occur if a cavitating lesion ruptures into the pleural cavity.

Laryngitis

In extensive smear-positive tuberculosis, tuberculous laryngitis may occur, presenting with painful hoarseness. This usually responds rapidly to antituberculosis chemotherapy. Continuing hoarseness after a few weeks of drug treatment should raise the possibility of laryngeal carcinoma being present.

Spread to other organs

Sputum containing bacilli may be swallowed and cause disease in the alimentary tract, particularly in the small intestine.

Poncet's arthropathy

Poncet[59] described a fleeting polyarthritis associated with tuberculosis, not due to direct involvement, but as an immunological reaction to tuberculoprotein. It is seen occasionally[60] but usually resolves within 8 weeks on antituberculosis treatment. The diagnosis is one of exclusion, other causes of inflammatory polyarthritis not being found, together with the resolution on specific anti-tuberculosis therapy.

Death

Despite effective drug treatment, even in the developed world tuberculosis still has an appreciable mortality. Studies in the UK[61] showed that in a series of 1312 adults with pulmonary disease, 163 (12%) died before completion of treatment, half due directly to tuberculosis and half in which tuberculosis was a contibuting factor. A further 51 died before the diagnosis was made. The radiographic extent of disease before treatment, age, extent of cavitation and smear positivity, but not sex or ethnic group, were shown to be independent factors in mortality[61]. A later study[62] showed a 12.9% case fatality rate, with a death rate ten times greater than age-matched controls. The cause of death can be difficult to pinpoint[63] but may be due to subclinical adrenal insufficiency.

(b) Late complications

Airflow obstruction

Damage to the bronchi from endobronchial fibrosis, causes airflow obstruction[64,65]. The proportion of patients with airflow obstruction after treatment depends on their age, sex and ethnic group. Smoking, increasing age and increasing extent of disease are all factors associated with airflow obstruction[64]. The presence of one factor doubles the proportion with airflow obstruction, and two factors quadruples the proportion. Co-existent chronic cough with some sputum simulating chronic bronchitis can also occur[65].

Severe lung damage

Cor pulmonale can occur as a late consequence of pulmonary damage following extensive fibrosis with airflow obstruction[64,65]. The left lung appears more prone to extensive damage than the right[66]. Respiratory failure secondary to severe restrictive disease is still occasionally seen following calcified empyema, the so-called 'lung en curaisse', or following previous thoracoplasty due to a severe restrictive defect[67,68].

Aspergilloma

The colonization of chronic healed cavities by the spores of *Aspergillus fumigatus* is well documented[69]. These usually cause few symptoms but haemoptysis, which can be recurrent and minor, or massive, can occur. Some conservatively managed cases progress to respiratory failure and death[70]. In patients with unilateral disease and well-preserved lung function, resection has good results[71,72] (Chapter 8c, p. 157). In patients unfit for surgery, other treatment options to reduce or stop haemoptysis have been tried with some success, including selective bronchial artery embolism[73], intracavitatory treatments[74] and radiotherapy[75].

Amyloid

This is now a rare complication but has been observed in chronic empyema and following chronic aspergilloma. Proteinuria sufficient to cause nephrotic syndrome is the usual clinical presentation. The presence of amyloid deposits in the rectal mucosa, liver or kidney on biopsy confirm the diagnosis.

Carcinoma of the lung

Since tuberculosis and carcinoma are both common in smokers, and can occur simultaneously, it is difficult to separate any discrete risk from tuberculosis. Anecdotal reports of scar carcinomas have not been borne out in detailed epidemiological surveys[76].

Adult respiratory distress syndrome (ARDS)

ARDS has been described in the presence of cavitatory tuberculosis[77] as well as with miliary tuberculosis (section 6.2.5).

6.4 MEDIASTINAL GLANDS

6.4.1 CLINICAL

Mediastinal (paratracheal or hilar) lymphadenopathy accompanies primary infection in children and some young adults. It may be the only radiographic feature, with the Ghon focus often being undetectable (Fig. 6.9). The lymphadenopathy is usually unilateral[78,79] but can be bilateral[80,81]. Symptoms may be absent or non-specific with fever, dry cough, poorly localized chest discomfort and mild weight loss. In primary tuberculosis (p. 73) significant compression or direct involvement of the airway is common in children, but is much less common in adults because of the greater calibre of the major bronchi. Erosion into the oesophagus may also occur[82]. Hilar lymphadenopathy is a very uncommon manifestation of tuberculosis in young White adults, but is common in Asian immigrants to developed countries[26–28;83] and accounts for up to 15% of disease in the 15–34 year age group. It is sometimes associated with cervical lymphadenopathy[27,28]. Until recently, isolated mediastinal lymphadenopathy was unusual in Africans, but is being seen more often as a result of reactivated disease in HIV-positive individuals, particularly as CD4 counts fall[40,42]. A similar increase in mediastinal lymphadenopathy associated with HIV infection has been seen in minority ethnic groups such as Haitians in the USA[41].

6.4.2 DIFFERENTIAL DIAGNOSIS AND INVESTIGATION

The differential diagnosis is largely between lymphoma and sarcoidosis. Since the lymphadenopathy in tuberculosis is related to primary or immediate post-primary infection, the skin tuberculin test is usually strongly positive. The tuberculin response is reduced or negative in lymphoma or sarcoidosis, although the clinical usefulness of the tuberculin test is reduced in areas of high HIV seroprevalence because of a false-negative or weak response caused by a reduced CD4 lymphocyte count. A negative tuberculin test in an HIV-negative patient virtually excludes tuberculosis as a cause of lymphadenopathy.

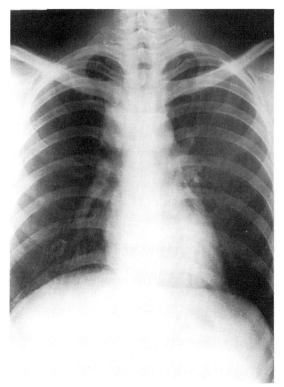

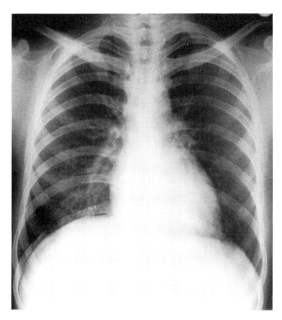

Fig. 6.9 Mediastinal glands. Right paratracheal glands in a 24-year-old Asian male; (a) before and (b) after treatment.

In tuberculosis there may be evidence of lung disease in addition to lymphademopathy. This tends to be unilateral, or asymmetrical if bilateral. Lymphadenopathy in sarcoidosis is usually bilateral and symmetrical, asymptomatic and associated with erythema nodosum. In the presence of a negative tuberculin test, these features are sufficient to make a clinical diagnosis of sarcoidosis. In the absence of erythema nodosum, a positive Kveim test may avoid the need for invasive biopsy. Very bulky mediastinal lymphadenopathy is likely to be due to lymphoma.

Where appropriate, tissue diagnosis by mediastinoscopy, or biopsy of associated cervical lymphadenopathy, should be performed. In a White patient with no history of contact with tuberculosis and a negative tuberculin test, an alternative diagnosis should be sought. In persons with a greater chance of tuberculosis, such as Asian immigrants or in high-prevalence areas, clinical management with a trial of antituberculosis drugs may be appropriate. Pyrazinamide-containing regimens result in a significant reduction in node size by 2 months[84], whereas with non-pyrazinamide-containing regimens the response takes longer. In persons with a high probability of tuberculosis, drug treatment for 3 months, with pyrazinamide in the initial 2 months, can be given. Mediastinoscopy can be reserved for those who show no radiographic response to such treatment[85]. In some ethnic groups such as Chinese, in whom tuberculous lymphadenopathy is uncommon, bronchascopically confirmed endobronchial disease has been described in some patients[86].

6.5 PLEURAL EFFUSION

6.5.1 DIFFERENTIAL DIAGNOSIS (Fig. 6.10)

The presence of a pleural effusion only on a chest radiograph does not differentiate tuberculosis from other causes. If the radiograph shows mediastinal lymphadenopathy or lung

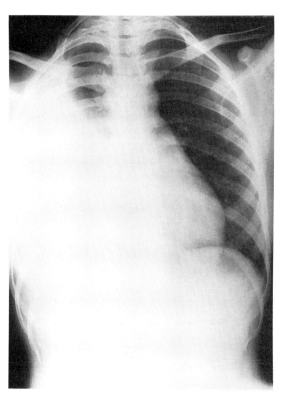

Fig. 6.10 Pleural effusion. Large right pleural effusion in a 20-year-old Asian girl. Pleural biopsy showed multiple granulomata.

infiltration in addition, tuberculosis is more likely to be present. A history of contact with tuberculosis within the previous 12 months increases the likelihood of disease as most pleural effusions occur within 6 months of contact[3].

6.5.2 DIAGNOSIS

The pleural fluid caused by tuberculosis is usually a straw-coloured exudate but may be bloodstained. The protein content is usually above 30 gm/l, and the glucose reduced. The cytology of the fluid shows plentiful lymphocytes for which there is some evidence of preferential sequestration in the fluid[87].

Because of the difficulty of confirming the diagnosis by pleural fluid culture, the use of immunological tests has been investigated (Chapter 17a, p. 367). Polymerase chain reaction has been shown to be superior to culture[88], and detection of mycobacterial antigen by ELISA has a high sensitivity and specificity[89] (Chapter 17b, p. 381). The usefulness may depend on the antigen used as a high level of false-positive results using anti-BCG antibody is reported[90]. The gold standard for confirmation of tuberculosis in pleural fluid must remain positive culture, which occurs in up to 50% of cases. The speed of obtaining a positive culture may be improved in the future by bedside inoculation into a BACTEC system[91] (p. 36). A raised level of adenosine deaminase in the pleural fluid was initially thought to be specific[92], but studies have shown an appreciable overlap with other causes of pleural effusion[91].

Granulomata with caseation and Langerhans giant cells are found on biopsy in 30–70% of cases. Because the distribution of granulomata is not uniform, multiple biopsies[93] increase the diagnostic yield. Where available, thoracoscopy can be used to give a visually guided biopsy to increase the chances of a positive result.

REFERENCES

1. Thompson, B.C. (1950) Bronchiectasis in primary tuberculous lesions associated with segmental collapse. *Lancet*, **i**, 386–8.
2. Brock, R.C. (1950) Post-tuberculous bronchostenosis and the middle lobe syndrome. *Thorax*, **5**, 5–39.
3. Wallgren, A. (1948) The timetable of tuberculosis. *Tubercle*, **29**, 245–51.
4. Aderele, W.I. (1979) Pulmonary tuberculosis in childhood: analysis of 263 cases seen at Ibadan, Nigeria. *Trop. Geograph. Med.*, **31**, 41–51.
5. Miller, F.J.W. (1982) *Tuberculosis in Children: Evolution, Epidemiology, Treatment, Prevention*, Churchill Livingstone, Edinburgh.
6. Bobrowitz, I.D. (1982) Active tuberculosis

undiagnosed until autopsy. *Am. J. Med.*, **72**, 650–8.

7. Monie, R.D.H., Hunter, A.M., Rocchiccioli, K.M.S. *et al.* (1983) Retrospective survey of the management of miliary tuberculosis in South and West Wales 1976–8. *Thorax*, **38**, 369–72.

8. Sahn, S.A. and Neff, T.A. (1974) Miliary tuberculosis. *Am. J. Med.*, **56**, 495–505.

9. Price, M. (1968) Lymphangitis reticularis tuberculosa. *Tubercle*, **49**, 377–84.

10. Proudfoot, A.T., Akhtar, A.J., Douglas, A.C. *et al.* (1969) Miliary tuberculosis in adults. *Br. Med. J.*, **ii**, 273–7.

11. Proudfoot, A.T. (1971) Cryptic disseminated tuberculosis. *Br. J. Hosp. Med.*, **5**, 773–80.

12. Grieco, M.H. and Chmel, H. (1974) Acute disseminated tuberculosis as a diagnostic problem. *Am. Rev. Respir. Dis.*, **109**, 554–60.

13. Medd, W.E. and Hayhoe, F.G.J. (1955) Tuberculous miliary necrosis with pancytopenia. *Q. J. Med.*, **24**, 351–64.

14. Cooper, W. (1959) Pancytopenia associated with disseminated tuberculosis. *Ann. Intern. Med.*, **50**, 1497–501.

15. Hughes, J.T., Johnstone, R.M., Scott, A.C. *et al.* (1959) Leukaemoid reactions in disseminated tuberculosis. *J. Clin. Pathol.*, **12**, 307–11.

16. Twomey, J.J., Leavell, B.S. (1965) Leukaemoid reactions to tuberculosis. *Arch. Intern. Med.*, **116**, 21–8.

17. Oswald, N.C. (1963) Acute tuberculosis and granulocytic disorders. *Br. Med. J.*, **ii**, 1489–96.

18. So, S.Y. and Yu, D. (1981) The adult respiratory distress syndrome associated with miliary tuberculosis. *Tubercle*, **62**, 49–53.

19. Heap, M.J., Bion, J.F., and Hunter, K.R. (1989) Miliary tuberculosis and the adult respiratory distress syndrome. *Respir. Med.*, **83**, 153–6.

20. Dyer, R.A., Chappell, W.A. and Potgeiter, P.D. (1985) Adult respiratory distress syndrome associated with miliary tuberculosis. *Crit. Care Med.*, **13**, 12–15.

21. Blacklock, J.W.S. (1932) Tuberculous disease in children: its pathology and bacteriology. *Medical Research Council. Special Report Series*, No. 172, HMSO, London.

22. Friedman, L.N., Sullivan, G.M., Bevilaqua, R.P. *et al.* (1987) Tuberculosis screening in alcoholics and drug addicts. *Am. Rev. Respir. Dis.*, **136**, 1188–92.

23. Patel, K.R. (1985) Pulmonary tuberculosis in residents of lodging houses, night shelters and common hostels in Glasgow: a five year prospective survey. *Br. J. Dis. Chest.*, **79**, 60–6.

24. Ormerod, L.P. and Skinner, C. (1980) Reinfection tuberculosis: two cases in the family of a patient with drug resistant disease. *Thorax*, **35**, 56–9.

25. Reeve, P.A. Harries, A.D., Nkhoma, W.A. *et al.* (1987) Clubbing in African patients with pulmonary tuberculosis. *Thorax*, **42**, 986–7.

26. Medical Research Council Tuberculosis and Chest Diseases Unit (1980) National survey of tuberculosis notifications in England and Wales 1978/9. *Br. Med. J.*, **281**, 895–8.

27. Medical Research Council Tuberculosis and Chest Diseases Unit (1985) National survey of tuberculosis notifications in England and Wales 1983. *Br. Med. J.*, **291**, 658–61.

28. Medical Research Council Tuberculosis and Chest Diseases Unit (1987) National survey of tuberculosis notifications in England and Wales 1983; characteristics of disease. *Tubercle*, **68**, 19–32.

29. Chang, S.C., Lee, P.Y., Perng, R.P. (1987) Lower lung field tuberculosis. *Chest*, **91**, 230–2.

30. Farman, D.P. and Speir, W.A. (1986) Initial roentgenographic manifestations of bacteriologically proven *M. tuberculosis*: typical or atypical. *Chest*, **89**, 75–7.

31. Ip, M.S.M., Yo, S.Y., Lam, W.K. *et al.* (1986) Endobronchial tuberculosis revisited. *Chest*, **89**, 727–30.

32. Gomes, I., Trindade, E., Vidal, O. *et al.* (1991) Diagnosis of sputum smear-negative forms of pulmonary tuberculosis by transthoracic fine needle aspiration. *Tubercle*, **72**, 210–13.

33. Robicheaux, G. Moinuddin, S.M. and Lee, L.H. (1985) The role of aspiration biopsy cytology in the diagnosis of pulmonary tuberculosis. *Am. J. Clin. Pathol.*, **83**, 719–22.

34. Grzybowski, S., Ashley, M.J. and Pinkus, G.J. (1976) Chemoprophylaxis in inactive tuberculosis: long term evaluation of a Canadian trial. *Canad. Med. J.*, **114**, 607–11.

35. Gryzbowski, S., Fishaut, H., Rowe, J. *et al.* (1971) Tuberculosis among patients with various radiologic abnormalities followed by the chest service. *Am. Rev. Respir. Dis.*, **104**, 605–8.

36. International Union against Tuberculosis Committee on Prophylaxis (1982) Efficacy of various durations of isoniazid preventive therapy for tuberculosis: 5 years of follow-up in the IUAT trial. *Bull. WHO*, **60**, 555–64.

37. Pearce, S. and Horne, N.W. (1974) Follow-up

of patients with pulmonary tuberculosis adequately treated with chemotherapy. Is it really necessary? *Lancet*, **ii**, 641–3.

38. Coleblunders, R.L., Ryder, R.W., Nzilambi, N. *et al.* (1989) HIV infection in patients with tuberculosis in Kinshasa: Zaire. *Am. Rev. Respir. Dis.*, **139**, 1082–5.

39. Elliott, A.M., Luo, N. and Tembo, G. (1990) Impact of HIV on tuberculosis in Zambia: a cross sectional study. *Br. Med. J.*, **301**, 412–15.

40. Harries, A.D. (1990) Tuberculosis and HIV infection in developing countries. *Lancet*, **335**, 387–90.

41. Pitchenik, A.E. and Rubinson, H.A. (1985) The radiographic appearance of tuberculosis in patients with the acquired immunodeficiency syndrome (AIDS) and pre-AIDS. *Am. Rev. Respir. Dis.*, **131**, 393–6.

42. Modilevsky, T., Sattler, F.R. and Barnes, P.F. (1989) Mycobacterial disease in patients with HIV infection. *Arch. Intern. Med.*, **149**, 2201–5.

43. Soriano, E., Mallolas, J., Gatell, J.M. *et al.* (1988) Characteristics of tuberculosis in HIV-infected patients: a case-control study. *AIDS*, **2**, 429–32.

44. Danek, S.J. and Bower, J.S. (1979) Diagnosis of pulmonary tuberculosis by flexible fibreoptic bronchoscopy. *Am. Rev. Respir. Dis.*, **119**, 677–9.

45. Willcox, P.A., Benatar, S.R. and Potgeiter, P.D. (1982) Use of the flexible fibreoptic bronchoscope in the diagnosis of sputum negative pulmonary tuberculosis. *Thorax*, **37**, 598–601.

46. Funahashi, A., Lohaus, G.H., Politis, J. *et al.* (1983) Role of fibreoptic bronchoscopy in the diagnosis of mycobacterial diseases. *Thorax*, **38**, 267–70.

47. Chawla, R., Pant, K., Jaggi, O.P. *et al.* (1988) fibreoptic bronchoscopy in smear-negative pulmonary tuberculosis. *Eur. Respir. J.*, **1**, 804–6.

48. Al-Kassimi, F.A., Azhar, M., Al-Hajed, S. *et al.* (1991) Diagnostic role of fibreoptic bronchoscopy in tuberculosis in the presence of typical X-ray pictures and adequate sputum. *Tubercle*, **72**, 145–8.

49. De Gracia, J., Currull, V., Vidal, R. *et al.* (1988) Diagnostic value of bronchoalveolar lavage in suspected pulmonary tuberculosis. *Chest*, **93**, 329–2.

50. Norrman, E., Keistinen, T., Uddenfeldt, M. *et al.* (1988) Bronchoalveolar lavage is better than gastric lavage in the diagnosis of pulmonary tuberculosis. *Scand. J. Infect. Dis.*, **20**, 77–80.

51. Wallace, J.M., Deutsch, A.L., Harrell, J.M. *et al.* (1981) Bronchoscopy and transbronchial biopsy in the evaluation of patients with suspected acute tuberculosis. *Am. J. Med.*, **70**, 1189–94.

52. Nelson, K.E., Larson, P.A., Schraufnagel, D.E. *et al.* (1983) Transmission of tuberculosis by flexible fiberbronchoscopes. *Am. Rev. Respir. Dis.*, **127**, 97–100.

53. Ip, M., Chau, P.Y., So, S.Y. *et al.* (1989) The value of routine bronchial aspirate culture at fibreoptic bronchoscopy for the diagnosis of tuberculosis. *Tubercle*, **70**, 281–5.

54. Sarkar, S.K., Sharma, T.N., Purohit, S.D. *et al.* (1982) The diagnostic value of routine culture of bronchial washings in tuberculosis. *Br.J. Dis. Chest*, **76**, 358–60.

55. Rimmer, J., Gibson, P. and Bryant, D.H. (1988) Extension of pulmonary tuberculosis after fibreoptic bronchoscopy. *Tubercle*, **69**, 57–61.

56. Berean, K. and Roberts, F.J. (1988) The reliability of acid fast stained smears of gastric aspirate specimens. *Tubercle*, **69**, 205–8.

57. Morris, C.D.W. (1989) The radiography, haematology and biochemistry of pulmonary tuberculosis in the aged. *Quart. J. Med.*, **71**, 529–35.

58. Morris, C.D.W., Bird, A.R. and Nell, H. (1989) Haematological and biochemical changes in severe pulmonary tuberculosis. *Quart. J. Med.*, **73**, 1151–9.

59. Poncet, A. (1897) De la polyarthrite tuberculeuse deformant ou pseudo-rheumatism chronic tuberculeux. *Congr. Franç. Chir.*, **1**, 732–6.

60. Wilkinson, A.G. and Roy, S. (1984) Two cases of Poncets disease. *Tubercle*, **65**, 301–8.

61. Humphries, M.J., Byfield, S.P., Darbyshire, J.H. *et al.* (1984) Deaths occurring in newly notified patients with pulmonary tuberculosis in England and Wales. *Br. J. Dis. Chest*, **78**, 149–58.

62. Cullinan, P. and Meredith, S.K. (1991) Deaths in adults with notified pulmonary tuberculosis 1983–5. *Thorax*, **46**, 347–50.

63. Ellis, M.E., Webb, A.K. (1983) Cause of death in patients admitted to hospital for pulmonary tuberculosis. *Lancet*, **i**, 665–7.

64. Snider, G.L., Doctor, L., Demas, T.A. *et al.* (1971) Obstructive airway disease in patients

with treated pulmonary tuberculosis. *Am. Rev. Respir. Dis.*, **103**, 625–40.

65. Biruth, G., Caro, J., Malmberg, R. *et al.* (1966) Airways obstruction in pulmonary tuberculosis. *Scand. J. Respir. Dis.*, **47**, 27–36.

66. Ashour, M., Pandya, L., Mezragji, A. *et al.* (1990) Unilateral post-tuberculous lung destruction: the left bronchus syndrome. *Thorax*, **45**, 210–12.

67. Sawicka, E.H., Branthwaite, M.A., Spencer, G.T. (1983) Respiratory failure after thoracoplasty: treatment by intermittent negative pressure ventilation. *Thorax*, **38**, 433–5.

68. Phillips, M.S., Kinnear, W.J.M. and Schneerson, J.M. (1987) Late sequelae of pulmonary tuberculosis treated by thoracoplasty. *Thorax*, **42**, 445–51.

69. Research Committee of the British Thoracic and Tuberculosis Association (1970) Aspergillomas and residual tuberculous cavity. The result of a resurvey. *Tubercle*, **51**, 227–45.

70. Butz, R.O., Zvetina, J.R. and Leininger, B.J. (1985) Ten year experience with mycetomas in patients with pulmonary tuberculosis. *Chest*, **87**, 356–8.

71. Al-Majed, S., Ashour, M., Al-Kassimi, F.A. *et al.* (1990) Management of post-tuberculous complex aspergilloma of the lung: role of surgical resection. *Thorax*, **45**, 846–9.

72. Jewkes, J., Kay, P.H., Paneth, M. *et al.* (1983) Pulmonary aspergilloma: analysis of prognosis in relationship to haemoptysis and survey of treatment. *Thorax*, **38**, 572–8.

73. Remy, J., Arnaud, A., Fardou, H. *et al.* (1977) Treatment of haemoptysis by embolisation of bronchial arteries. *Radiology*, **122**, 33–7.

74. Shapiro, M.J., Albelda, S.M., Maycock, R.L. *et al.* (1988) Severe haemoptysis associated with pulmonary aspergilloma – percutaneous intracavitatory treatment. *Chest*, **94**, 1225–31.

75. Schneerson, J.M., Emerson, P.A. and Phillips, R.H. (1980) Radiotherapy for massive haemoptysis for an aspergilloma. *Thorax*, **35**, 953–4.

76. Sternitz, R. (1965) Pulmonary tuberculosis and carcinoma of the lung: a survey from two population-based disease registers. *Am. Rev. Respir. Dis.*, **92**, 758–66.

77. Dyer, R.A. and Potgeiter, P.D. (1984) The adult respiratory distress syndrome and bronchogenic pulmonary tuberculosis. *Thorax*, **39**, 383–7.

78. Miller, W.T. and Macgregor, R.R. (1978) Tuberculosis: frequency of unusual radiographic findings. *Am. J. Radiol.*, **130**, 867–75.

79. Hadlock, F.P., Park, S.K., Awe, R.J. *et al.* (1980) Unusual radiographic findings in adult pulmonary tuberculosis. *Am. J. Radiol.*, **134**, 1015–18.

80. Sakowitz, A.J. and Sakowitz, B.H. (1979) Bilateral hilar lymphadenopathy: an uncommon manifestation of adult tuberculosis. *Chest*, **71**, 421–3.

81. Dhand, S., Fisher, M. and Fewell, J.W. (1979) Intrathoracic tuberculous lymphadenopathy in adults. *J. Am. Med. Assoc.*, **241**, 505–7.

82. Bloomberg, T.J. and Dow, C.J. (1980) Contemporary mediastinal tuberculosis. *Thorax*, **35**, 392–6.

83. Enarson, D., Ashley, M.J. and Grzybowski, S. (1979) Tuberculosis in immigrants to Canada. *Am. Rev. Respir. Dis.*, 119, 11–18.

84. Ormerod, L.P. (1988) A retrospective comparison of two drug regimens RHE2/RH10 and RHZ2/RH10 in the treatment of tuberculous mediastinal lymphadenopathy. *Br. J. Dis. Chest*, **82**, 274–81.

85. Farrow, P.R., Jones, D.A., Stanley, P.J. *et al.* (1985) Thoracic lymphadenopathy in Asians resident in the United Kingdom: role of mediastinoscopy in initial diagnosis. *Thorax*, **40**, 121–4.

86. Chang, S., Lee, P. and Perng, R. (1988) Clinical role of bronchoscopy in adults with intrathoracic tuberculous lymphadenopathy. *Chest*, **93**, 314–17.

87. Rossi, G.A., Balbi, B. and Manca, F. (1987) Tuberculous pleural effusions. *Am. Rev. Respir. Dis.*, **138**, 575–9.

88. Manjunath, N., Shankar, P., Rajan, L. *et al.* (1991) Evaluation of a polymerase chain reaction for the diagnosis of tuberculosis. *Tubercle*, **72**, 21–7.

89. Ramkisson, A., Coovadia, Y.M. and Coovadia, H.M. (1988) A competition ELISA for the detection of mycobacterial antigen in tuberculous exudates. *Tubercle*, **69**, 209–12.

90. Dhand, R., Ganguly, N.K., Vaishnavi, C. *et al.* (1988) False-positive reactions with enzyme-linked immunosorbent assay of *M. tuberculosis* fluid antigens in pleural fluid. *J. Med. Microbiol.*, **26**, 241–3.

91. Maartens, G. and Bateman, E.D. (1991) Tuber-

culous pleural effusions: increased culture yield with bedside inoculation of pleural fluid and poor diagnostic yield. *Thorax*, **46**, 96–9.

92. Ocana, I., Martinez-Vazquez, J.M., Segura, R.M. *et al.* (1983) Adenosine deaminase in pleural fluid: test for diagnosis of tuberculous pleural effusion. *Chest*, **84**, 51–3.

93. Mungall, I.P.F., Cowen, P.N., Cooke, N.T. *et al.* (1980) Multiple pleural biopsy with the Abrams needle. *Thorax*, **35**, 600–2.

M.J. Humphries, W.K. Lam and R. Teoh

7.1 INTRODUCTION

Tuberculosis can affect any organ in the body and although the most common presentation is pulmonary, extrapulmonary disease is also an important manifestation. Non-respiratory presentations may be atypical or relatively insidious and tuberculosis may not be considered initially in the differential diagnosis. This is an important phenomenon as the dangers of delayed diagnosis may be crippling or even life-threatening, particularly in spinal, meningeal, pericardial or abdominal tuberculosis.

In a survey of notifications of tuberculosis in England and Wales conducted by the Medical Research Council (MRC) in 1983[1], the disease was classified as respiratory only in 68%, non-respiratory in 25% and both in 7%. Hence, 32% of newly notified patients with tuberculosis presented with extrapulmonary manifestations. For White patients in the survey, the figures were 78%, 18% and 4% respectively, while for patients of Indian subcontinent (ISC) ethnic origin, the figures were 54%, 34% and 12%. Hence 46% of newly diagnosed patients with tuberculosis of ISC origin in England and Wales had non-respiratory manifestations.

In 1983 the overall notification rate for non-respiratory disease was 51 times as high for the ISC (81 per 100 000) as for the White group (1.6 per 100 000). The difference in rates varied considerably for different lesions, being 72 times as high for lymph node disease but only ten times as high for genitourinary disease (Table 7.1).

In a more recent survey[2] of 2163 previously untreated patients notified in 1988, 698 (32%) had non-respiratory disease, of whom 395 (57%) were of ISC ethnic origin. For both the White and ISC groups, lymph node tuberculosis was the most common manifestation, accounting for 52% of non-respiratory disease in the ISC group and 37% in the White patients; abdominal disease was more than twice as common (14% versus 6%) (Table 7.2). By contrast, genitourinary tuberculosis was much more common in the White group (28% versus 4%).

The other sites were equally involved in the two ethnic groups; the pattern of the other ethnic origins followed that of the ISC group. (See also Table 10.1, p. 196.)

In the USA the proportion of all reported cases of extrapulmonary tuberculosis has risen from 8% in 1964 to 15% in 1981 and 17.5% in 1986[3,4]. The same trends have been observed in Hong Kong, where the total tuberculosis notification rates have decreased from 404 (per 100 000) in 1960 to 254 in 1970 and 112 in 1990. The proportion of non-respiratory cases, however, has increased from 1.2% in 1967 to 6.6% in 1990[5].

Patients infected with HIV have a higher risk of developing tuberculosis of all forms, particularly extrapulmonary manifestations, which may occur in up to 70% of all HIV-infected individuals who develop tuberculosis[6]. Furthermore HIV-infected persons

Clinical Tuberculosis. Edited by P.D.O. Davies. Published in 1994 by Chapman & Hall, London. ISBN 0 412 48630 X

Table 7.1   Sites of non-respiratory disease for all newly notified previously untreated patients in a 6-month period[a]

Site	Ethnic group							
	White			ISC			All ethnic groups	
	No.	%	Annual rate per 100 000	No.	%	Annual rate per 100 000	No.	%
Lymph nodes[b]	136	37	0.6	268	53	43	454	47
cervical	112			247			404	
other	26			28			60	
Bone or joint	40	11	0.2	99	20	16	150	15
spine	18			39			60	
hip	5			3			10	
knee	2			9			12	
elbow	3			6			10	
ankle	1			6			9	
wrist	5			2			7	
other	12			46			61	
Genitourinary tract	98	27	0.4	24	5	4	134	14
kidney and urinary tract	54			7			69	
female genital	20			9			30	
male genital	20			3			25	
unspecified	9			6			16	
Abdominal	38	10	0.2	64	13	10	121	12
Central nervous system	27	7	0.1	25	5	4	61	6
meningitis	27			21			55	
other	2			7			11	
Miliary	23	6	0.1	18	4	3	46	5
Abscesses	7	2	0.03	17	3	3	24	2
Pericardium	7	2	0.03	5	1	0.8	14	1
Cutaneous	8	2	0.04	4	1	0.6	12	1
All other sites	22	6	0.1	18	4	3	45	5
Total number of patients in the 6 months	359[c]	100	1.6	503[c]	100	81	970[c]	100

[a] Data taken from the Medical Research Council Survey of 1983, with estimated annual notification rates per 100 000 population for the main sites for England only in 1983. The annual notification rates were estimated using populations derived from the 1983 Labour Force Survey (Office of Population Censuses and Surveys, unpublished data).
[b] Excluding intrathoracic nodes
[c] 82 patients (including 32 White, 40 ISC) had disease involving more than one site.

who develop tuberculosis are relatively more likely to develop rapidly progressive disease[7] and certain extrapulmonary sites such as lymph nodes and meninges are more frequently affected in HIV-infected individuals compared with those not infected[8].

Hence the recognition and diagnosis of extrapulmonary lesions are likely to assume a greater importance in the foreseeable future.

7.2 LYMPH NODE TUBERCULOSIS

7.2.1 EPIDEMIOLOGY AND PATHOGENESIS

Lymph node tuberculosis, occurring predominantly in the cervical region, is the most common manifestation of non-respiratory tuberculosis worldwide. In the USA it accounted for about 30% of cases of extrapulmonary tuberculosis in 1986[9]. In England

Table 7.2 Non-respiratory disease sites by ethnic origin[a]

Disease site/lesion	White		ISC		Other	
	No.	%	No.	%	No.	%
Lymph node	86	37	205	52	38	54
Bone and joint	31	13	51	13	5	7
Genitourinary tract	65	28	16	4	3	4
Abdomen	14	6	57	14	13	19
Central nervous system	10	4	21	5	5	7
Miliary	19	8	27	7	5	7
Abscess	10	4	14	4	3	4
Other	18	8	32	8	4	6
Total patients[b]	233	100	395	100	70	100

[a] Data taken from the Medical Research Council Survey of 1988.
[b] Some patients had lesions at more than one site.

and Wales, it is most commonly seen in immigrants from Africa and the Indian subcontinent, and comprises more than one-half of the non-respiratory cases seen in these groups[1,10]. In Hong Kong, it accounts for 45% of cases of extrapulmonary tuberculosis[5].

Formerly, lymph node tuberculosis was often caused by *M. bovis*, but now *M. tuberculosis* is the commonest isolate[10–12]. Environmental mycobacteria such as *M. scrofulaceum* and *M. avium–intracellulare* are occasionally isolated, particularly in cervical lymph node tuberculosis in young children [12].

Lymph node tuberculosis occurs either as a result of primary infection, as reactivation of previously contained foci, or by extension from a contiguous focus. In a prospective study searching for associated mycobacterial infection of the upper aerodigestive tract in 75 patients with cervical tuberculous lymphadenitis[13], 25 patients (39%) had radiographic evidence of active or healed pulmonary tuberculosis, with two patients showing *M. tuberculosis* in sputum culture, and five patients (6%) had tuberculous nasopharyngitis. Mycobacterial infection of other parts of the upper aerodigestive tract was not found. In primary infection, most commonly

acquired by airborne infection, a non-specific inflammatory reaction occurs as soon as the mycobacteria reach the alveoli, and phagocytosis and intracellular replication take place. A bacteraemia is thought to occur with dissemination throughout the body. Lymphatic involvement is thought by most to be an integral part of the tuberculous infection with generalized lymphatic and haematogenous spread rather than a localized disease process. The vast majority of the primary lesions heal, and reactivation as a result of decreased body defence due to various causes is the mechanism by which tuberculosis in the adult usually develops, whether it is in the lung or in lymph nodes or other extrapulmonary sites.

Supraclavicular lymph node tuberculosis is usually caused by lymphatic spread from mediastinal disease[11].

7.2.2 CLINICAL FEATURES

In populations with high rates of tuberculosis, tuberculous lymphadenitis has its greatest incidence in early childhood, but would occur in later adulthood in populations with low incidence. In the USA and the UK, the highest incidence of tuberculous lymphadenitis occurs between 25 and 50

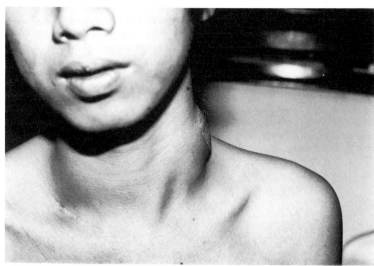

Fig. 7.1 Cervical lymph node with abscess formation.

years of age[12, 14, 15], while in Hong Kong it is between 20 and 40 years of age with a male to female ratio of about 1:1.3.

Cervical nodal involvement (scrofula) is commonest, and accounts for about 70% of all lymph node tuberculosis cases[16]. It may be associated with tuberculosis in the lungs or elsewhere in about 40–50% of the cases. The lymph node swelling is usually of insidious onset and is painless, although it may be tender early in the infection when it is enlarging more rapidly. Initially, the lymph nodes are discrete and firm, but later they become matted together and fluctuant (Fig. 7.1). The overlying skin may break down with formation of abscesses and chronic discharging sinuses, which heal with scarring.

Between one-third to two-thirds of patients have constitutional symptoms, with fever, night sweats, weight loss and malaise. Tuberculous lymphadenitis in an immunosuppressed patient may be acute and resemble an acute pyogenic bacterial infection[17].

Hilar and paratracheal lymph node enlargement is often seen in post-primary tuberculosis in some Asian and African ethnic groups. Mediastinal abscesses may occur with involvement of trachea, bronchi and superior vena cava, which might require urgent surgical intervention. Oesophageal symptoms are uncommon although dysphagia secondary to an adjacent tuberculous mediastinal lymph node has been reported[18,19]. Rarely, acute polyarthritis may be the presenting feature[20].

7.2.3 DIAGNOSIS

The age, ethnic group and typical clinical features of a patient may suggest the diagnosis of lymph node tuberculosis, so may a positive chest radiograph (hilar or mediastinal lymphadenopathy, calcified granuloma, pulmonary infiltrates or pleural thickening, in about 40–50%) and a positive tuberculin skin reaction (present in 90% or more of the cases). A definite diagnosis, however, requires demonstration of *M. tuberculosis* in the pus from draining sinuses or smear, culture and histology of lymph nodes. Acid-fast bacilli can be demonstrated in 25–50% of lymph node biopsy smears[21]. The isolation rate on culture from biopsy or pus aspirated is about 60–70%[10,21]. This relatively low isolation rate probably reflects a very small population of organisms within the lymph nodes, which become enlarged as a result of a hypersensitivity response to tuberculoprotein. Histologically, tuberculous lymphadenitis may show mild reactive hyperplasia or granuloma, usually with caseation and necrosis. Fine-needle aspiration cytology (FNAC), by showing granulomatous changes, can also establish the diagnosis in 71–83% of cases[16,22–25] and the combined use of a tuberculin skin test and FNAC can diagnose 90% of the cases[23]. The specificity of FNAC was 93% in one study[24]. Thus, FNAC is a sensitive, specific and cost-effective way to diagnose tuberculous cervical lymphadenopathy and is recommended.

For mediastinal lymph node tuberculosis, which is commonly associated with pulmonary disease, sputum may show acid-fast bacilli even if pulmonary infiltrates are not apparent. A study of CT scanning of the thorax[26] has shown special characteristics of the tuberculous mediastinal lymph nodes, i.e. preponderance of involvement of the right paratracheal and tracheobronchial nodes, and with contrast medium, nodes larger than 2 cm in diameter invariably showed central areas of relatively low density and peripheral rim enhancement. Some smaller nodes did not show low-density areas, but showed varying degree of homogeneous enhancement instead. Although metastatic nodes can be of low density, this study suggests that in the setting of mediastinal lymphadenopathy in a young adult, the CT findings described above are characteristic enough to support a diagnosis of tuberculosis. The diagnosis can be confirmed by lymph node smear, culture and biopsy obtained by mediastinoscopy, although in the setting of the typical ethnic group, radiographic and clinical features and a strongly positive tuberculin test, the diagnosis is so likely that biopsy confirmation is usually not needed. It should be noted that mediastinoscopy may produce considerable morbidity (e.g. haemorrhage, chronic tuberculosis sinus in the mediastinoscopy tract)[27]. More recently, mediastinal mycobacterial lymphadenopathy

has been diagnosed successfully in a patient with AIDS by transbronchial needle aspiration[28], which, on microscopy, revealed respiratory mucosa with lymphocytes and on smear was positive for numerous acid-fast bacilli. (See also Chapter 6, p. 85.)

The main clinical differential diagnoses include lymphoma, carcinomatous metastasis and sarcoidosis, and the main histological differential diagnosis of granuloma (especially if non-caseating) includes sarcoidosis, brucellosis, fungal infections, syphilis and berylliosis.

7.2.4 TREATMENT

Modern antituberculosis chemotherapy has become the cornerstone of therapy for lymph node tuberculosis. An 18-month regimen of isoniazid (H) plus rifampicin (R) or ethambutol (E), both supplemented by streptomycin (S) for the first 2 months, was found to be effective by a British Thoracic Association study in 1979[29]. More recently, a controlled trial by the British Thoracic Society Research Committee[15,30] has shown equal efficacy of 9- versus 18-month chemotherapy regimens (isoniazid plus rifampicin for 9 or 18 months, supplemented initially by ethambutol for 8 weeks). There was no clinical or microbiological relapse at 5 years and cosmetic results were good in both groups. The 9-month regimen (isoniazid 300 mg daily, plus rifampicin 450 mg daily for patients weighing less than 50 kg and 600 mg daily for those weighing more than 50 kg, supplemented by ethambutol 15–25 mg per kg body weight in the first 8 weeks) is therefore recommended as effective therapy for superficial lymph node tuberculosis.

Pyrazinamide (Z) has been shown to have an important place in the initial 2 months of treatment of pulmonary tuberculosis (see also Chapter 8b, p. 144). Its role in lymph node tuberculosis has been studied by a retrospective radiographic comparison of two regimens (2HRE/10HR versus 2HRZ/10HR) in the treatment of tuberculous mediastinal lymphadenitis[31]. It was found that the pyrazinamide group responded more rapidly at 2, 5 and 7 months compared with the ethambutol group. Thus, it may be possible to reduce the total duration of treatment to 6 months if pyrazinamide is given for the first 2 months instead of ethambutol. In one retrospective study, McCarthy and Rudd[32] reported successful treatment in 40 out of 41 patients treated with 6 months' chemotherapy, including initial 2 months of pyrazinamide (2HRZ/4HR). A recent Indian study in children[33] used three times weekly supervised isoniazid, rifampicin, pyrazinamide and streptomycin for 2 months followed by twice-weekly streptomycin/isoniazid for 4 months, on an outpatient basis, and showed a 97% cure rate at the end of 3 years' follow-up. It is notable that despite severe and multiple site lymph node involvement in many of these patients, clinical response to treatment was rapid, and 81% of these lesions disappeared within 1 month of start of treatment. Currently, the British Thoracic Society[34,35] is undertaking a trial in 199 patients to test whether a 6-month regimen using pyrazinamide would enable the duration of treatment for lymph node tuberculosis to be reduced from 9 months (2HRE/7HR versus 2HRZ/7HR versus 2HRZ/4HR). A preliminary report[35] showed that there was little difference between the regimens in speed of resolution of nodes, or in the percentage with residual nodes at the end of treatment. Aspiration after commencing chemotherapy was, however, required in seven patients on ethambutol compared with one patient on pyrazinamide, a difference that was significant ($P=0.005$). This is probably the result of a more powerful, bactericidal action of pyrazinamide compared with ethambutol. This study is being followed up to 30 months from commencement of treatment to determine relapse rates, and the results are awaited with interest.

Lymph nodes may increase in size and new nodes may appear both during and after chemotherapy without indicating a failure of treatment or relapse[15,33]. In the British study[15], existing lymph nodes increased in size in 12% of patients and fresh lymph nodes appeared in another 12% within the first 8 months of chemotherapy. At the end of chemotherapy, residual nodes were palpable in 9% of the patients, and new nodes appeared in 11%. The incidence of these events was similar in both the 9- and 18-month chemotherapy groups, and showed no further changes at 5-year follow-up[30]. These nodes were sterile on culture, and their enlargement or new appearance may be due to hypersensitivity to tuberculoprotein released from disrupted macrophages[10,15] and did not indicate an unfavourable outcome.

With the advent of modern, effective antituberculosis chemotherapy, routine surgical excision or therapeutic aspiration of enlarged cervical lymph nodes would be unnecessary[16], and indeed has been shown to confer no advantage[15,30]. Even for the nodes that enlarge after chemotherapy, operation is not necessarily indicated, as the enlargement is usually transient. Surgery would be reserved for diagnostic biopsy and the unusual situation of persistent discharging abscess or sinuses, or mediastinal abscesses involving the trachea, bronchi or superior vena cava. Total surgical excision would be preferable to simple incision and drainage for cervical abscesses or sinuses[36], and is certainly the procedure of choice for mediastinal abscesses.

7.3 ORTHOPAEDIC TUBERCULOSIS

7.3.1 TUBERCULOSIS OF THE SPINE

(a) Epidemiology

Tuberculosis of the spine is the commonest manifestation of orthopaedic tuberculosis[37]. The condition is a rare form of extrapulmonary tuberculosis but is an important illness as crippling deformities may result. In many technically advanced countries, tuberculosis of the spine is rarely seen, indeed the diagnosis may be over-looked[38], but it may be seen more commonly in immigrant populations. For example, the notification rate for orthopaedic tuberculosis in England and Wales in 1983 was 0.2 per 100 000 for White patients but was 16 per 100 000 in patients of ISC ethnic origin[1]. In Hong Kong, it was 0.6 per 100 000 population in 1990[5]. In many developing nations, orthopaedic tuberculosis is a significant cause of crippling deformities.

7.3.2 CLINICAL FEATURES

The most common presentation of tuberculosis of the spine is of back pain of variable duration. Most patients have had symptoms for some months, occasionally even years. In one report including six patients with spinal tuberculosis the duration of symptoms before diagnosis ranged from 4 months to 4 years[39]. Rarely there may be radicular pain, which may be referred to the loin or abdomen and may be mistaken for an abdominal condition[40]. There may be lower limb symptoms or sphincter disturbance due to cord compression by associated abscess formation.

Examination may reveal local tenderness or muscular spasm and mild kyphosis. In more advanced cases there may be gross kyphosis at presentation. If there is associated psoas abscess formation, a fluctuant mass may appear in the groin. Large psoas abscesses may occasionally be palpated abdominally.

7.3.3. DIAGNOSIS

Tuberculous infections of the spine often start as a discitis of the intervertebral disc and then spread along the anterior and longitudinal ligaments to involve the adjacent vertebral bodies. Hence on plain radiography

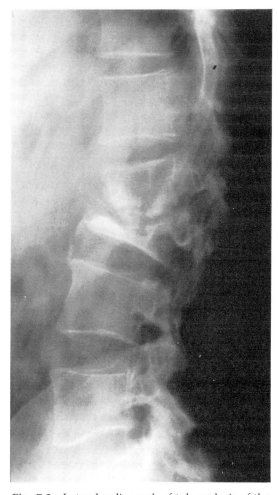

Fig. 7.2 Lateral radiograph of tuberculosis of the spine showing collapse of the L2 and L3 vertebrae and the intervertebral disc. (Courtesy of Professor Alan Scher, University of Stellenbosch, South Africa.)

films of the spine the anterior edges of the superior and inferior borders of adjacent vertebral bodies are often eroded with narrowing of the disc space (Fig. 7.2). There is progressive destruction of the vertebral bodies with loss of height and subsequent kyphosis. Occasionally more than one disc space may be involved, and lesions may 'skip', with healthy vertebrae in between. The lower thoracic, lumbar, and lumbosacral

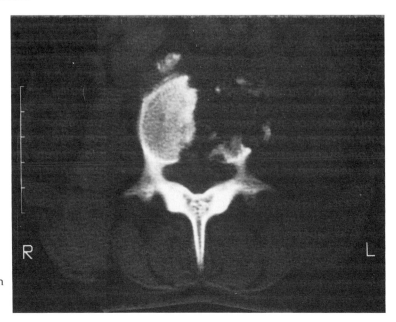

Fig. 7.3 Computerized tomographic (CT) scan of tuberculosis of the spine with destruction of the vertebral body.

vertebrae are the sites most commonly involved. Infections of the cervical vertebrae are relatively rare. Paravertebral abscess formation is a common complication of spinal tuberculosis.

Computerized tomographic (CT) scanning is valuable in demonstrating and assessing the extent of tuberculous skeletal involvement[41–3], and the CT scan may be abnormal before changes appear on plain radiography films[42]. In tuberculosis of the spine, it may clearly demonstrate the extent of the spinal destruction (Fig. 7.3). Paravertebral and psoas abscess formation may be seen in some patients. Magnetic resonance imaging may also be helpful in delineating tuberculous spinal lesions[44,45], T2-weighted images may be helpful in those lesions with associated epidural sepsis and inflammation[45]. Multiple views including both coronal and sagittal cuts can define the lesions completely[46].

In a patient with evidence of pulmonary tuberculosis and a suggestive spinal lesion, it is often unnecessary to confirm the diagnosis by invasive investigations of the spinal site.

The differential diagnosis includes other pyogenic spinal infections and malignancy . Malignant spinal metastases tend to erode the pedicles and spinal bodies and leave the disc intact, in contrast to tuberculous infections, which erode the disc early in the disease process. However, diagnostic confusion may occur[38]. The onset of pyogenic infection is often more acute and the pain may be more severe. Invasive procedures either by needle biopsy or by open exploration may be undertaken to establish a firm diagnosis, and it is important that all specimens are collected not only for histology, but also for culture for both pyogenic organisms and for *M. tuberculosis*. The yield for cultures of *M. tuberculosis* may be increased by the use of special media, including the selective Kirchner medium[47]. Where there is doubt every effort should be made to obtain sufficient tissue to make an accurate diagnosis.

7.3.4 TREATMENT (see also Chapter 8b, p. 141)

A number of studies conducted over a 20-year period by the British Medical Research

Council have provided very valuable conclusions in the treatment of tuberculosis of the spine. In these studies, patients who had received previous treatment for 12 months or more, or those with paralysis who could not walk unaided were excluded.

In the earliest studies that involved centres in Hong Kong, Korea and Rhodesia, chemotherapy with isoniazid and PAS for 18 months was found to be highly effective, with over 80% of patients achieving favourable status by 3 years. Further, there was no additional benefit derived from 6 months' bed rest, a plaster jacket, debridement operations, or the addition of streptomycin for 3 months[48–51].

Although the results were very good at 3 years, patients in Hong Kong who underwent resection of the spinal focus and bone grafting with anterior spinal fusion (the so-called 'Hong Kong Operation'), achieved more rapid bony fusion and less residual spinal deformity[52]. However, the procedure requires considerable surgical, anaesthetic and nursing expertise. As a result of these studies, the MRC recommended ambulatory chemotherapy as the treatment of choice for tuberculosis of the spine[53].

In recent years the evolution of short-course chemotherapy for the treatment of pulmonary tuberculosis stimulated research into shorter regimens for treatment of tuberculosis of the spine, based on isoniazid and rifampicin. Results from Hong Kong, Korea and India demonstrated that short-course regimens of isoniazid plus rifampicin for 6 or 9 months were highly effective in the treatment of tuberculosis of the spine[54]. Further, the results were as good as 18-month standard regimens with isoniazid and PAS. Regimens consisting of 9 months of either isoniazid plus PAS or isoniazid plus ethambutol were found to have less favourable results and cannot be recommended[55]. In Hong Kong, a comparison of patients who underwent the 'Hong Kong Operation' and those who were treated with ambulatory chemotherapy alone, showed that the operation conferred no added benefit[54]. In conclusion, ambulatory short-course chemotherapy has been proven to be highly effective in the treatment of tuberculosis of the spine, and for the great majority of the patients operative procedures are unnecessary. However, patients who develop acute cord compression may require early surgical intervention. This should only be undertaken by someone well experienced in the technique of spinal decompression.

Although the spine is the most commonly involved orthopaedic site, tuberculosis can affect any bone or joint in the body and should be suspected in any patient with an unusual orthopaedic or articular lesion, which may be single[56] or multiple [57]. Unusually, there may be disseminated lesions throughout the skeleton whose bizarre or cystic nature may mimic the picture of metastatic carcinoma[58,59]. Non-tuberculous arthropathies have also been described in patients with pulmonary tuberculosis, including hypertrophic pulmonary osteoarthropathy[60]; and so-named Poncet's disease[61], a sterile, mono- or polyarthritis affecting large joints. However, these manifestations are very rare.

7.3.5 MANAGEMENT OF DISEASE AT OTHER ORTHOPAEDIC SITES

Most tuberculous bone or joint lesions will respond to short-course chemotherapy comprising 2 months of isoniazid, rifampicin and pyrazinamide, followed by 4 months of isoniazid and rifampicin.

Surgical intervention is not normally required but may be necessary early in the disease process, either to obtain material for diagnosis, or to relieve pressure and allow drainage from an abscess. Surgery may rarely be necessary once chemotherapy has been completed in order to relieve pain and gain stability by arthrodesis of an unstable joint. Replacement of a hip or knee joint, destroyed by tuberculosis, has been attempted. A further course of chemotherapy is sometimes given following such operative intervention.

7.4 TUBERCULOUS MENINGITIS

7.4.1 INTRODUCTION

Tuberculous meningitis (TMB) is a life-threatening form of tuberculosis and the commonest form of central nervous system (CNS) tuberculosis. The condition is a serious cause of morbidity and mortality in developing countries and has emerged as a serious complication in patients with AIDS and its related complex[62,63]. In one review, CNS involvement by tuberculosis developed at a rate of more than 2000 per 100 000 in HIV-infected individuals[64]. The importance of TB meningitis is disproportionate to its rarity, as patients often spend many months in hospital and there is a real risk of irreversible neurological damage, which may require institutional care. Hence the early recognition and prompt treatment of TB meningitis are important clinical considerations.

While treatment of pulmonary tuberculosis is based on numerous well-conducted, clinical trials[65], no substantial controlled studies have been conducted in TB meningitis. Treatment is largely empirical: larger doses of antituberculosis agents are prescribed in the hope of overcoming the blood-brain barrier, and the optimum duration of treatment is unknown. Although this situation is unsatisfactory, it is possible to suggest appropriate guidelines for treatment based on relatively recent data on the penetration of antituberculosis drugs into the cerebrospinal fluid (CSF). The overall management of a patient with TB meningitis involves properly supervised antituberculosis chemotherapy, judicious use of corticosteroids and careful surveillance of clinical progress. Computerized tomographic scanning and prompt neurosurgical consultation are also important features of management.

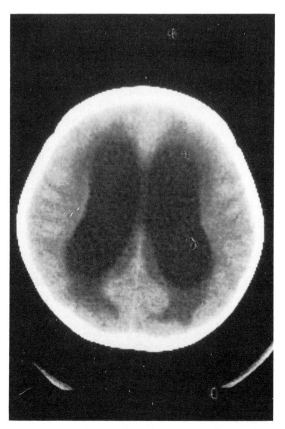

Fig. 7.4 Marked hydrocephalus and periventricular oedema in a patient with tuberculous meningitis.

7.4.2 PATHOGENESIS AND PATHOLOGY

When *M. tuberculosis* infects the meninges, there is nearly always a focus elsewhere. Tubercle bacilli usually gain access to the CSF via small subpial tuberculomata; direct spread from blood is unlikely[66].

Macroscopically, the meninges appear opaque and give the brain a greyish gelatinous appearance. If exudate around the medulla is exuberant, the exit foramina may be obstructed resulting in hydrocephalus (Fig. 7.4). The meningeal changes may extend to the spinal roots, thus explaining the common finding of depressed or absent deep tendon reflexes in the limbs. Focal neurological signs

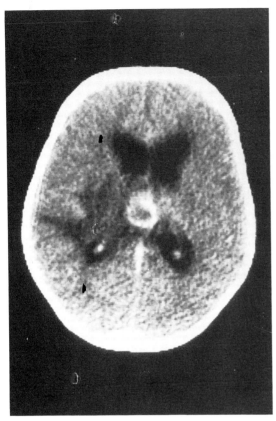

Fig. 7.5 Intracranial tuberculoma with associated cerebral oedema.

may be caused by tuberculomata (Fig. 7.5) but more commonly result from vascular occlusion, particularly at the base of the brain. This explains the common clinical finding of pyramidal tract and basal ganglia signs.

7.4.3 CLINICAL FINDINGS

The prodromal symptoms of malaise, anorexia, headache, nausea, and vomiting may last 2–8 weeks. These are non-specific and diagnosis may be difficult, particularly when there is no evidence of tuberculosis in the lungs or elsewhere. Children feed poorly, become irritable or drowsy or may present with behavioural changes.

As an assessment of severity of disease and a guide to prognosis, it is useful to stage patients clinically at the time of diagnosis, based on the British Medical Research Council classification[67]. In stage I (early disease), consciousness is undisturbed and no focal neurological signs are present. In stage II (medium severity), consciousness is disturbed but the patient is not comatose or delirious; focal neurological signs and cranial nerve palsies may be present. In the most advanced disease, stage III, patients are stuporose or in coma with or without focal neurological signs.

Once meningeal symptoms are evident, there is invariably a low-grade fever, which is rarely above 39°C. Infants become irritable or somnolent with neck retraction and tense fontanelles. In older patients, the neck is usually only moderately stiff and rarely as rigid as in bacterial meningitis.

Cranial nerve palsies develop in up to one-third of patients. Papilloedema is common and may be found in the absence of hydrocephalus or raised intracranial pressure, usually without visual impairment. When visual impairment develops, tuberculoma compressing the optic nerve or ethambutol toxicity should be excluded. Oculomotor nerve palsies (IIIrd and VIth) are common, whereas VIIth and VIIIth nerve palsies are seen less frequently. The pupils may be large and slowly reactive to light, even in the absence of other signs of a IIIrd nerve palsy. Rarely, internuclear ophthalmoplegia and horizontal gaze pareses may develop. This indicates intrinsic brain stem dysfunction and a poor prognosis, possibly because adjacent vital structures are involved[68]. In contrast, oculomotor nerve pareses do not imply a poor prognosis. The finding of choroid tubercles on fundoscopic examination is very helpful but they may resemble cytoid bodies seen in systemic lupus erythematosus.

The most common findings are mono-, hemi-, or paraparesis and less frequently mild dysphasia. Cerebellar signs, extrapyramidal and hypothalamic disturbances may also occur.

Involuntary movements are more commonly seen in children and may present early in the disease and usually subside after 6 weeks. A fine resting tremor, dystonic posturing of the limbs and chorea have all been described. Persistent involuntary movements after recovery from TB meningitis may occur in children[69] and the resultant dystonia and or choreoathetosis can be most disabling.

Epileptic seizures may present at any stage. They are more frequent in children than adults and are usually the direct effect of meningeal inflammation on the cerebral cortex. When increasing drowsiness or seizures develop during treatment, it is mandatory to ascertain the exact cause as cerebral oedema, obstructive hydrocephalus, expanding intracranial tuberculomata and hyponatraemia due to inappropriate antidiuretic hormone secretion must all be considered and managed appropriately.

Children with TB meningitis may develop the rare but therapeutically important entity, tuberculous encephalopathy. This presents as increasing drowsiness, decerebrate spasm and coma, or involuntary movements and seizures. Its recognition is important, because of the excellent response to corticosteroids[70].

While the brunt of TB meningitis falls on the basal meninges and cerebrum, the spinal meninges are also frequently affected. Indeed, depressed or absent deep tendon reflexes are a frequent finding, though this is not generally accompanied by other motor or sensory problems. In contrast, TB meningitis can on occasion, directly involve the spinal meninges – so-called spinal TB meningitis[71]. This manifests as sciatica or root pain with flaccid or spastic limbs, and the early loss of control of bladder and anal sphincters. Full recovery of movement and sphincter control is rare.

Clinical deterioration may develop 2–18 months after the start of chemotherapy and may be due to enlargement of previously clinically silent intracranial tuberculomata[72,73]. These tuberculomata may present with symptoms of raised intracranial pressure, epilepsy, or neurological deficit. Such events may appear alarming but perseverence with the therapeutic regimen is usually required. The addition of steroids may be beneficial.

7.4.4 PROGNOSIS

The change in therapy over the years has not been reflected by an improved prognosis. Despite advances in the treatment of tubercolosis, the most important prognostic factors are still the stage of disease when treatment is started, and the patient's age[74].

Children under 3 years have a significantly worse prognosis and this factor is independent of stage. In our series of 199 children, nearly all those presenting in stage I (mild), made a complete recovery (96%); complete recovery occurred in 78% of children with stage II. In contrast, only 21% presenting with the most severe disease, stage III, made a full recovery. Multivariate analysis of patient characteristics and chemotherapy regimens revealed that only two statistically significant independent variables predicted prognosis: these being (a) stage at presentation and (b) the age. The introduction of rifampicin and pyrazinamide did not appear to influence the outcome[75]. This further emphasizes the importance of early diagnosis and treatment of TB meningitis.

TB meningitis occasionally develops during pregnancy, when the prognosis is said to be poor. The reason for this is unclear. It is possible that pregnancy alters the patient's response to the tubercle bacillus, yet pregnancy *per se* was not associated with relapse in 215 cases of treated pulmonary TB[76]. Adults over the age of 65 years generally have a poorer prognosis than those below this age.

Infection with HIV does not appear to alter the clinical manifestations or prognosis of TB meningitis, except that patients with CD4 counts less than $0.2 \times 10^9/l$ have a significantly reduced survival[8].

7.4.5 DIAGNOSIS

Routine blood tests are not particularly helpful nor is the tuberculin test. A chest radiograph is often very helpful as pulmonary TB may be apparent in up to one-half of patients[75]. But when radiological evidence of active tuberculosis is missing, the diagnosis rests almost entirely on the CSF examination as the finding of an entirely normal CSF is exceedingly rare. Lumbar puncture is safe in this chronic meningitis and can be carried out even in patients with papilloedema. When the diagnosis remains in doubt after the first CSF sample, serial CSF examinations may be helpful. The glucose and cellular changes in partially treated bacterial meningitis generally return to normal in weeks, whereas the changes in TB meningitis are more persistent.

The CSF opening pressure is usually elevated, even up to 600 mmH$_2$O.

An elevated CSF cell count is invariable, however the rise is moderate compared with bacterial meningitis and is usually under 500/mm^3[75]. Characteristically, lymphocytes predominate in the CSF: however, polymorphonuclear leucocytes may predominate early in the infection particularly during the first 10 days[77]. In our series, 17% of patients had a predominance of polymorphonuclear leucocytes in the first CSF specimen; lymphocytes predominate thereafter[75,78]. The CSF is usually clear and only rarely turbid; the CSF protein is almost invariably raised, in our series the mean was 2.58 g/l and was elevated in 96% of patients. The glucose concentration in CSF is usually low, the mean value in our series was 1.76 mmol. More pertinent perhaps is that the glucose level may be within the normal range.

The identification of acid-fast bacilli in CSF is diagnostic. Although stating the obvious, an assiduous and careful examination for acid-fast bacilli in CSF is crucial. Success rates can be improved if large volumes of CSF (8–10 ml) are examined. The first CSF specimen is the most likely one to be culture-positive[79], but all subsequent samples should be sent for microscopic examination and culture.

When repeated CSF smear examinations are negative, samples of sputum, early morning urine and gastric aspirate should be sent for culture, even in the absence of clinical or radiological evidence of disseminated disease, as miliary tuberculosis may present with an apparently normal chest radiograph[80].

As the direct smear examination of CSF for acid-fast bacilli is usually negative in TB meningitis, and cultures take many weeks, a rapid confirmatory laboratory test would be a considerable advantage. Various methods have been employed[81–84] to detect antigen from, and antibody to, *M. tuberculosis* in the CSF but regrettably none is at present commercially available. Polymerase chain reaction techniques appear very promising as a rapid diagnostic tool[84], however this method is likely to be relatively expensive (Chapter 17b, p. 381).

7.4.6 MEDICAL TREATMENT

Sucessful treatment of TB meningitis depends to a great degree on the levels in the CSF achieved by antituberculosis drugs. However, reliable data concerning the penetration of antituberculosis drugs into the CSF were limited until relatively recently.

Antituberculosis chemotherapy should be started as soon as the diagnosis is suspected, which is often before confirmatory evidence is available. Both the choice of drugs and the duration of therapy have to be considered [85]. Our regimen, used in Hong Kong, is based on quadruple therapy of daily intramuscular streptomycin, oral isoniazid, rifampicin and pyrazinamide. These drugs are employed because they form the most bactericidal combination, with pyrazinamide and isoniazid making the largest contribution (see also Chapter 8b, p. 144).

In general, larger doses are prescribed to overcome the blood–brain barrier, but with the recent publication of additional data on CSF pharmacokinetics, lower doses have been used. Isoniazid is given at a dose of 10 mg/kg with a maximum dose of 600 mg per day, but half this amount may well be adequate[86,87]. Rifampicin 10 mg/kg is normally given, but it is uncertain whether effective CSF concentrations are achieved [88]. Adequate CSF concentrations of pyrazinamide are reported with 30–40 mg/kg[89]; we now prescribe 35 mg/kg daily for adults and children. Streptomycin (20 mg/kg) with a maximum dose of 1 g per day, is given for the first 2–3 months of treatment, on the assumption that this is when the meninges are inflamed and CSF penetration is likely to be optimal.

The total duration of treatment for TB meningitis is not based on any firm data and the advice from various authors differs considerably. We recommend that the duration of treatment be adjusted to take into account the important prognostic factor of the clinical stage of disease when treatment is started. Those presenting with stage I (mild) and II (medium) disease may be safely treated for 9–12 months, although 6 months may be adequate[90,91]. Patients presenting with stage III (severe) disease are treated for at least 12 months. Those with intracranial tuberculoma should probably be treated for at least 18–24 months. However, there are no conclusive data supporting our recommendations. Certainly there is no evidence that the longer treatments given to patients with stage III disease are required or improve prognosis.

In pregnant women, normal doses of isoniazid, rifampicin and pyrazinamide may be safely prescribed without untoward tera-

togenic effects. Streptomycin should not be used[91] and ethionamide avoided.

7.4.7 THE ROLE OF CORTICOSTEROIDS

The role of corticosteroids in treatment has long been a source of debate and controversy. Although there is some agreement on their use under certain specific clinical situations, considerable disagreement exists on their 'routine' administration in TB meningitis.

Based on our own experience and review of the literature[92,93], we recommend adding corticosteroids to antituberculosis chemotherapy for all patients with stage II (medium) or III (severe) disease.

Other indications for the use of corticosteroids include tuberculous encephalopathy in children[71]. Steroids can result in rapid improvement and make the child manageable without recourse to major tranquilizers. The occasional adult may also develop encephalopathic features without frank disturbance of consciousness or focal signs: the irritability and photophobia normally also respond to steroids.

A controversial indication for steroids is TB meningitis complicated by spinal arachnoiditis (with or without spinal block). Like others, we prescribe steroids in this situation but the evidence that this improves the outcome is uncertain.

7.4.8 SURGICAL TREATMENT

The most important role of surgery is the prompt drainage of obstructive hydrocephalus. The combination of deterioration in the conscious level plus suspicion of an enlarging hydrocephalus should be treated urgently; surgical drainage should not be delayed by attempts to control the hydrocephalus with steroids. The theoretical risk of spreading the tubercle bacilli from the CSF to other organs via the shunt is not a reasonable justification for delay in operation.

Occasionally surgical decompression of an intracranial tuberculoma in patients with TB meningitis is indicated by its location. Excision or debulking is indicated when the anterior optic pathways are compressed with resultant visual impairment[94] or when the brain stem is compressed by a cerebellar tuberculoma or abscess formation[95].

7.5 ABDOMINAL TUBERCULOSIS

7.5.1 EPIDEMIOLOGY

Abdominal tuberculosis is a relatively rare condition in many technically advanced countries, being largely confined to immigrant groups where the rates for tuberculosis are very much higher than the indigenous population[96–98]. In a survey of notifications of tuberculosis in England and Wales in 1983, the notification rates for abdominal tuberculosis were 50 times higher in patients of Indian subcontinent ethnic origin, compared with White patients[1]. In many developing nations, abdominal tuberculosis is still seen commonly. For example in one series of patients reported from Nigeria, tuberculosis accounted for 25% of all patients with ascites[99] and 42% in one further series of patients in Lesotho[100].

With the widespread pasteurization of milk in technically advanced countries, *M. bovis* is no longer a significant source of abdominal tuberculosis. The most frequently isolated mycobacterium is *M. tuberculosis*. In patients with advanced HIV infection, both *M. tuberculosis* or *M. avium-intracellulare* may occur either as an isolated infection or as part of disseminated disease. Intra-abdominal adenopathy, particularly of the peri-pancreatic and mesenteric compartments, are predominant features[101].

7.5.2 CLINICAL FEATURES

Tuberculosis can infect any part of the gut from the mouth and gums to the anus. Upper gastrointestinal involvement is relatively rare. In a series of 500 patients with abdominal tuberculosis who underwent surgery, lesions of the upper gastrointestinal tract were found in only 2.8% of patients[102].

Tuberculous lesions in the oesophagus may present as dysphagia and on endoscopy the lesion may resemble an ulcerating tumour[103,104]. However most tuberculous lesions of the upper gastrointestinal tract present either as gastrointestinal bleeding or as an acute abdomen. The lesions may perforate and at laparotomy there may be associated mesenteric lymphadenopathy[105]. The diagnosis is usually made on histology of an endoscopic or laparotomy specimen and is often an unexpected finding. Ileo-caecal tuberculosis is a relatively common form of tuberculous enteritis and accounts for between 24 and 85%[106–108] of all tuberculous lesions of the gut. The colon is occasionally involved and may present with massive gastrointestinal bleeding[109]. Granulomatous lesions of the anus are a rare manifestation of the disease.

The symptoms of abdominal tuberculosis are often non-specific and insidious in onset, although occasionally the presentation is one of acute abdominal pain. In one series the most common symptoms were fever (72%), anorexia (58%), chronic abdominal pain (36%) and nausea and vomiting (22%). Acute abdominal pain (22%), diarrhoea (17%) and constipation (14%) were also described[110]. In addition, pulmonary tuberculosis was present in 36% of patients while for 14% the condition was asymptomatic, being discovered at diagnostic laparotomy. In one other series 67% of patients noticed abdominal swelling[108].

On examination there are no pathognomonic physical findings of abdominal tuberculosis[111]. The classical 'doughy' consistency of the abdomen on palpation has been rarely described with conviction in recent series. Indeed in one small series of 11 patients none was reported to have a 'doughy' abdomen[112]. Most patients will be febrile[113] and approximately half the patients have abdominal distension or ascites whereas abdominal tenderness and hepatomegaly are less common. Examination may reveal a mass in the right iliac fossa in patients with ileo-caecal tuberculosis, indeed abdominal masses may be palpated in any part of the abdomen due to matted loops of bowel.

Subacute or sometimes total intestinal obstruction may occur[114], with the symptoms of vomiting and the presence of a distended tympanic abdomen on physical examination, with or without the presence of an abdominal mass. Perforation of bowel or fistula formation may also occur and are associated with a relatively poorer prognosis[110]. Rarely, the presentation may be one of acute appendicitis.

In one large series of 182 patients, 80 (48%) had either strictures of the ileum, jejunum or a hyperplastic ileo-caecal lesion[115].

Disseminated infection of the peritoneal cavity (tuberculous peritonitis) usually presents with ascites as a prominent feature, with the accompanying symptoms of fever, abdominal distension and weight loss with or without chronic abdominal pain. Peritonitis has been reported as being less common than intestinal tuberculosis in one large study. Bhansali[116] reported 300 patients with abdominal tuberculosis, at operation 196 were found to have intestinal tuberculosis and in the other 104 patients the peritoneum and lymph nodes were affected.

7.5.3 PATHOLOGY

Tuberculous peritonitis may result from ingestion, local extension from the gut into lymphatics, or from haematogenous spread. Tuberculous salpingitis may spread to cause generalized peritonitis[117].

In the peritoneal cavity there is frequently ascites and white tubercles scattered throughout the omentum, bowel wall and other organs. The mesentery is usually thickened and oedematous and there may be collections of pus or caseous masses. Signs of perforation, obstruction or fistula formation may be apparent.

Tuberculous involvement of the bowel is most commonly seen at the ileo-caecal junction. The terminal ileum is thickened and the whole circumference of the bowel is usually involved.

On macroscopic examination the bowel may be indistinguishable from Crohn's disease and strictures may mimic those observed in lymphoma or ischaemia[107]. Adjacent lymph nodes may be enlarged and be either firm or fleshy in character, occasionally there may be abscess formation within the nodes, or even calcification.

Other organs in the abdominal cavity may be affected, particularly the liver.

Tuberculosis of the liver is rare but may have a variety of presenting features similar to other more common conditions. There may be a diffuse infiltration with tubercles giving a miliary appearance[118,119]. There is also a macronodular form, which may mimic hepatocellular carcinoma, including the presence of marked hypervascularity on angiography[120]. Portal hypertension[121] and bleeding gastric varices have been reported in association with the nodular form of hepatic tuberculosis[122].

Abscesses may develop that may be solitary, mimicking the ultrasonographic and computerized tomographic appearances of a pyogenic or amoebic abscess[123,124]. Alternatively there may be tuberculous micro-abscesses throughout the liver[125]. Occasionally, tuberculous masses (pseudo-tumours) may occur[126]. Clearly, liver biopsy is diagnostic, and hepatic involvement may also be discovered at laparotomy. Tuberculosis of the pancreas[127,128], spleen and gallbladder have also been reported.

Histological features of abdominal tuberculosis are those of caseating granulomata with Langerhans giant cells often associated with a lymphocytic infiltrate. Acid-fast bacilli may be demonstrated on Ziehl–Neelsen staining, either in the bowel wall, mesentery, lymph nodes or the gut lumen. In some patients acid-fast bacilli are not readily demonstrated, even though caseating granulomata are seen.

7.5.4 DIAGNOSIS

The diagnosis of abdominal tuberculosis may not be suspected clinically, particularly as the presentations of the illness can be so diverse. In two separate series, the diagnosis was not suspected clinically in 64–65% of patients [129,130]. Furthermore, there is a wide differential diagnosis including lymphoma, carcinomatosis, various forms of peritonitis and peritoneal mesothelioma[131].

Routine haematological investigations may reveal non-specific findings such as raised erythrocyte sedimentation rate (ESR) and anaemia. Most patients have a normal white cell count[115]. The tuberculin test is often unhelpful and is commonly falsely negative, particularly in the elderly, those who are undernourished or immunosuppressed, and those with disseminated disease.

Ascitic fluid in tuberculous peritonitis is usually an exudate with a protein content in excess of 3.5 g/dl, most often clear and straw-coloured, and commonly with more than 300 white cells/ml with a lymphocyte predominance. Ziehl-Neelsen staining and culture for *M. tuberculosis* is often negative[132,133]. However *M. tuberculosis* may be seen on smear or can be cultured from a gastric aspirate specimen, often a helpful procedure, especially in children. In those with a pulmonary lesion, smear and culture of sputum can be diagnostic.

Plain abdominal radiographs often demonstrate the presence of ascites or distended small bowel loops, with fluid levels apparent on the erect film. Barium meal examination is rarely helpful, but barium enema examination may reveal features of ileo-caecal involvement, such as those of the ileum passing almost vertically into the colon with the ascending colon appearing to be shortened[107]. Lesions of the colon may be single or multiple and have an annular appearance with shouldering, similar to the features of colonic carcinoma.

Ultrasound and computerized tomographic (CT) scanning have emerged as helpful non-invasive methods of investigation; both methods may show features that are highly suggestive (but not pathognomonic) of tuberculous peritonitis and/or gastro-intestinal involvement. The CT appearances may be those of ascites, usually of high density in the range of 15–30 Houndsfield Units. The thickened mesentery often has a 'stellate' appearance, probably caused by prominent straightened vessels radiating from the base of the mesentery (Fig. 7.6). Bulky mesenteric or retroperitoneal lymph nodes may be seen, which can be mistaken for lymphoma or carcinoma. Tuberculous nodes are more commonly mesenteric or peri-pancreatic, while retroperitoneal nodes are relatively rare. Helpful features include irregular soft-tissue densities in the omentum; central caseation can sometimes be seen in lymph nodes as a well circumscribed central area of low density[134].

In a review of 27 patients with abdominal tuberculosis, 24 patients were detected to have lymphadenopathy on CT scanning. However, eight of these patients also had AIDS and hence may not be representative of all patient groups. In the 24 patients with abdominal tuberculous lymphadenopathy, CT examination showed ten patients with abdominal lymphadenopathy where intra-venous contrast medium had enhanced the inflammatory rim surrounding the caseous centre[101]. This feature is not diagnostic, and is also seen in lymphoma, carcinoma, pyogenic infection and Whipple's disease. In addition to mesenteric adenopathy, CT findings may include thickened bowel wall with nodularity and oedema[101, 126, 131]. Occasionally there may be a disorganized appearance of soft-tissue densities, fluid and bowel loops

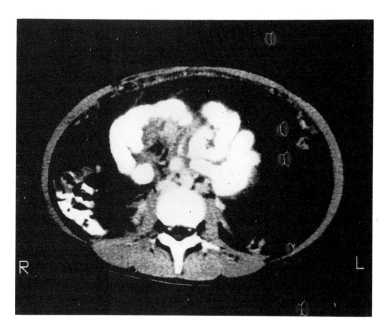

Fig. 7.6 Computerized tomographic (CT) scan in a patient with tuberculous peritonitis with thickened mesentery and marked ascites.

forming a poorly defined mass[131]. Diffuse enlargement or low density masses in the liver and spleen may be visualized, indicative of dissemination. Definitive diagnosis of tuberculous peritonitis requires either culture of the organism or a biopsy specimen of peritoneum, gut or lymph node showing the characteristic histological appearances of caseating granulomata or acid-fast bacilli. Laparotomy will confirm the diagnosis in nearly every patient, but is a major invasive procedure. Blind percutaneous needle biopsy of peritoneum was originally advocated by Levine[135], who achieved a nearly 100% diagnostic yield with minimal complications. Other authors have been unable to match such good results; Singh reported a success rate of 64%[136]. Shukla *et al.*[137] have recommended open peritoneal biopsy as being safer and more reliable, and this avoids the potential risk of perforating bowel during a 'blind' peritoneal biopsy.

However, laparoscopy with target peritoneal biopsy (thus avoiding laparotomy) has been described as effective and safe, and is the current investigation of choice[133,138,139].

In one study, 42 patients with tuberculous peritonitis were diagnosed from 8400 laparoscopies over a 16-year period; 100% were confirmed histologically and there were no complications[138]. The procedure is probably safer if ascites is present, as there is less risk of perforating the bowel. Complications should be minimal if previous ultrasound or CT scanning has been performed to locate the position of the bowel, which occasionally is adherent to the anterior abdominal wall.

The value of colonoscopy to investigate ileo-caecal tuberculosis has also been reported; the collection of adequate specimens for bacteriological and histological examination is emphasized[140], although there are now encouraging reports of colonoscopy and fine-needle aspiration[141].

A number of methods have recently been reported for obtaining rapid diagnosis of abdominal tuberculosis. One method uses an enzyme-linked immunosorbent assay (ELISA) to detect circulating IgG antibodies to *M. tuberculosis*[142]. The method has been shown to be highly sensitive and has a specificity of 85% and 97% respectively in two different patient groups. The method is easy to perform and is undergoing further evaluation (Chapter 17a, p. 368).

The detection of tuberculostearic acid (TBSA) in the cerebrospinal fluid by gas chromatography and mass spectrometry (GCMS) has proven to be a sensitive method of detecting mycobacteria, and has proven to be valuable in the rapid diagnosis of tuberculosis meningitis[81]. The method is currently being evaluated in other manifestations of tuberculosis, including the detection of TBSA in ascites of patients with tuberculous peritonitis. The method has the disadvantage of being expensive and requiring considerable technical expertise. However, studies are in progress to develop a monoclonal antibody to TBSA and to link this to a latex agglutination system. This might provide a rapid and simple test to detect TBSA in serous fluids in the future.

7.5.5 TREATMENT

Before the advent of antituberculosis drugs the mortality of tuberculous peritonitis was reported to be 49% in one series[143]. Since the introduction of effective antituberculosis regimens, survival has been reported to be 100% in one series of 42 patients[139], and one further series reported a mortality of 7% in non-AIDS patients with *M. tuberculosis* infections[144].

Owing to the relative rarity of tuberculous peritonitis, no controlled clinical trials of drug regimens have been conducted and very few studies of long-term follow-up have been reported. With modern treatment the prognosis is generally favourable, provided the patient does not experience potentially lethal complications such as gastrointestinal bleeding, perforation or bowel infarction. Even with these complications, the prognosis is favourable with skilled surgical management. The practice in Hong Kong is to treat patients with four antituberculosis drugs initially for

2 months, namely isoniazid, rifampicin, pyrazinamide and either streptomycin or ethambutol, in dosages that are employed for pulmonary tuberculosis. Isoniazid and rifampicin are given for a total treatment duration of 9 months.

The use of corticosteroid drugs in the treatment of tuberculous peritonitis is controversial. There is the theoretical value of reducing inflammation and fibrosis and promoting prompt resolution of ascitic fluid. However, unlike tuberculous pleural effusion for which corticosteroids have been shown to speed up resolution of serous fluid[145], there are no substantial reports for tuberculous peritonitis. Corticosteroids are therefore not prescribed routinely for patients with tuberculous peritonitis in Hong Kong.

7.6 TUBERCULOSIS OF THE PERICARDIUM

7.6.1 EPIDEMIOLOGY, PATHOGENESIS AND PATHOLOGY

Tuberculous of the pericardium is rare in developed countries. In the USA it occurs in about 1–2% of patients with pulmonary tuberculosis[146], and in England and Wales it accounts for less than 1% of the tuberculosis cases[1]. It is the cause of about 4–7% of all cases of acute pericarditis, cardiac tamponade or chronic constrictive pericarditis in these countries[147,148]. It continues to be important in immunouppressed patients and in some Asian and African populations. For example, in Transkei and the surrounding regions of south-east Africa, it is one of the commonest causes of congestive heart failure[149].

Tuberculous pericarditis is nearly always associated with a focus of tuberculosis elsewhere in the body[150]. The commonest route of infection is from direct extension from adjacent mediastinal lymph nodes, although lympho-haematogenous spread may occur. Acute pericarditis appears to be a primary 'allergic' response to tuberculo-

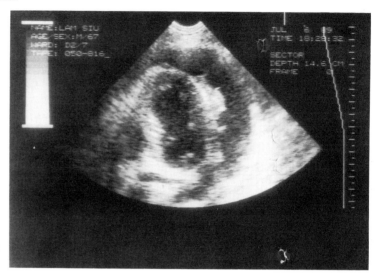

Fig. 7.7 Echocardiogram demonstrating a thickened visceral pericardium and a pericardial effusion in a patient with tuberculous pericarditis.

protein, whereas chronic pericardial effusion and pericardial constriction both reflect granulomatous lesions, often with fibrosis and calcification in the later stage. One autopsy study[151] has shown that in tuberculous pericarditis, all three layers of the heart are in fact involved with varying severity. In the eight heart specimens studied, pericardial thickening and adhesions were present in all cases, and significant endocardial thickening was seen in four, and myonecrosis, lymphohistiocytic cellular infiltration and myofibrosis were observed in seven cases.

7.6.2 CLINICAL FEATURES

Tuberculous pericarditis occurs most commonly in the third to fifth decades of life[152], and usually presents insidiously with fever, night sweats, malaise and weight loss, substernal pain, cough, tachycardia and pericardial friction rub. With pericardial effusion, particularly if tamponade is present, there is dyspnoea, low pulse pressure with pulsus paradoxus, raised jugular venous pressure, hypotension, hepatomegaly and peripheral oedema. Non-specific but widespread T-wave changes and low-voltage QRS complexes are often present on the ECG. The chest radiograph usually shows an enlarged cardiac silhouette (82–98%), with pleural effusions in about 50–70% of the patients [148].

Chronic constrictive pericarditis may occur a few weeks to a few months after the acute stage despite treatment, or may present some years after the pericarditis has healed. In many Asian and African populations, tuberculosis is the leading cause of constrictive pericarditis, accounting for 61% of cases of constrictive pericarditis in one Indian study[153]. It commonly occurs early in the disease, and may be the presenting feature with dyspnoea, weight loss, very high venous pressure, quiet heart sounds, paradoxical pulse, hepatomegaly, ascites and peripheral oedema[149,154]. The cardiac silhouette is often described as normal in size, but in the Indian study[153], it was definitely enlarged in half of the patients.

On echocardiography, pericardial effusion, frank or loculated, or amorphous material may be demonstrated (Fig. 7.7), depending on the predominant lesion. With constrictive pericarditis, pericardial thickening and abnormal septal motion may be detected. The heart is relatively immobile. Haemodynamically, ventricular diastolic filling is impaired. Pericardial effusion and thickening can also be detected by computed tomographic scanning and magnetic resonance imaging[155].

7.6.3 DIAGNOSIS

Tuberculous pericarditis should be suspected in patients with insidious fever and signs of pericardial effusion, particularly those who are susceptible to tuberculosis. Chest radiographs may show active pulmonary tuberculosis in 30% of cases and sputum culture will be positive in 11–30%[156,157]. A positive tuberculin skin test is present in 83–100% of the patients[148]. The characteristics of the pericardial fluid are non-specific, usually showing an exudate with high protein content and increased leucocyte count with lymphocytes and monocytes predominating. Polymorphonuclear leucocytes may predominate in the first 2 weeks. A recent report suggested that assay of adenosine deaminase activity in pericardial fluid could be of value in the early diagnosis of tuberculous pericarditis[158]. The definitive diagnosis of tuberculous pericarditis can be made by pericardial fluid smear or culture, or by pericardial tissue culture or histology. Acid-fast bacilli were found on stained smear of pericardial fluid in 42% of the patients in one study[159]. In the Transkei study, pericardial fluid culture was positive in 59% of cases whereas tuberculous histological lesions were seen in 70% of pericardial biopsy specimens[157]. A new non-surgical technique for multiple pericardial biopsies has recently been described [160]. This technique involves the use of a short catheter introduced under fluoroscopy through the subxiphoid approach, insertion of a bioptome, and outlining of the parietal pericardium by air. The biopsy yielded diagnostic information in nine out of ten patients with a thickened pericardium (six had tuberculosis, three had malignancy), and there were no complications.

7.6.4 TREATMENT

Tuberculous pericarditis was almost invariably fatal before the introduction of antituberculosis chemotherapy. With the advent of effective chemotherapy, mortality from tuberculous pericarditis has fallen to less than 30%. A recent controlled study in Transkei[157,161] has shown that a 6-month regimen consisting of isoniazid plus rifampicin, supplemented by streptomycin and pyrazinamide in the initial 14 weeks, was effective in tuberculous pericarditis. The study has also shed light on the use of prednisolone, which has long been advocated to reduce pericardial inflammation and enhance resorption of pericardial effusion. The controlled study showed that in patients with constriction, prednisolone given in a tapering dose (starting 30–60 mg daily, depending on age) for 11 weeks in addition to antituberculosis chemotherapy increased the speed of improvement, and probably decreased the risk of death (4% versus 11%) and the need for pericardiectomy. In patients with effusion, prednisolone also reduced the risk of death (4% versus 14%) and the need for repeat pericardiocentesis or open surgical drainage. It was therefore recommended that, in the absence of a specific contraindication, prednisolone should be given for an initial period (e.g. 11 weeks) in addition to antituberculosis chemotherapy. Continuing follow-up in the Transkei' study is being assessed to determine whether steroid therapy would reduce late constriction or death in the long term.

Long *et al.*[162] recommended a conservative approach to operative intervention in the treatment of active tuberculous pericarditis, and pericardiectomy was only performed in four of 16 consecutive patients for the relief of cardiac tamponade, all within 2 months of diagnosis. None of the 14 patients who received medical therapy alone was found to have chronic constrictive pericarditis on follow-up. Quale *et al.*[163] recommended placement of a pericardial window for both diagnostic and therapeutic purposes, and if pericardial thickening is present, pericardiectomy is performed. Large recurrent effusions or cardiac compression due to effusive-constrictive disease or constrictive pericarditis are common features presenting early in many Asian and African populations. During this early subacute phase, the response to additional surgical treatment is poor, especially if echocardiography shows fibrocaseous material in the pericardial space[154]. Pericardiectomy would be indicated for life-threatening tamponade in the acute phase, or when deterioration continues at about 6 weeks after starting chemotherapy, that is, when there is persistent elevation of systemic venous pressure unrelieved by pericardiocentesis[146–149, 154]. Overall, it is estimated that about one-third to one-half of patients will eventually require pericardiectomy despite adequate drug therpay.

7.7 GENITOURINARY TUBERCULOSIS

7.7.1 EPIDEMIOLOGY AND PATHOGENESIS

In England and Wales, genitourinary tuberculosis was the third commonest site of extrapulmonary tuberculosis after lymph nodes and orthopaedic tuberculosis respectively in a survey of notifications of tuberculosis in 1983, and the rates were ten times higher in patients of Indian subcontinent (ISC) ethnic origin (4 per 100 000) than White patients (0.4 per 100 000)[1]. In the White patients, tuberculosis of the kidney and urinary tract (54 patients) was reported more frequently than for female genital (20 patients) and male genital (20 patients) tuberculosis, whereas for the ISC patients female genital tuberculosis was relatively more common (Table 7.1).

A more recent survey[2] demonstrated that for White patients, genitourinary tuberculosis was responsible for 28% of all patients with extrapulmonary tuberculosis in that group, whereas for ISC patients with extrapulmonary tuberculosis, only 4% had a genitourinary lesion. The relatively more frequent occurrence of genitourinary tuberculosis in the White patients may reflect the phenomenon of reactivation of a quiescent primary infection contracted in childhood or early adult life.

It is likely that most tuberculous infections of the genitourinary tract are due to secondary blood-borne spread from a primary pulmonary lesion. The majority of foci heal, and are reactivated in later life owing to a change in host defence. This in part explains the phenomenon of *M. bovis* being occasionally isolated from genitourinary lesions[164,165] in addition to the more commonly isolated *M. tuberculosis*.

Reactivation of a renal focus has been reported to occur up to 29 years after the primary infection[164]. Rarely, tuberculosis may be transmitted via a transplanted kidney either by active disease[166] or reactivation of a previous tuberculous infection[167].

Tuberculosis of the urinary tract is often a bilateral disease that commences in the kidneys; the lower portion of the urinary tract is infected by antegrade seeding. Any or a combination of organs can be involved, including male genital organs (testes, epididymis, vas deferens and prostate) and female genital organs (ovaries, vagina and fallopian tubes).

7.7.2 CLINICAL FEATURES

Tuberculosis of the kidney is relatively silent in the initial stages and is occasionally diagnosed as an incidental finding on urine examination. More progressive disease presents with dysuria, haematuria, loin pain, nocturia or abdominal pain. Abdominal (17%) or loin pain (24%) has been reported as a more common presenting symptom in younger patients under the age of 25 years[168].

Constitutional symptoms such as fever, weight loss and night sweats are relatively unusual. Occasionally the diagnosis is revealed during routine investigations for hypertension[168,169].

Tuberculosis may also destroy sufficient renal parenchyma or cause sufficient obstruction through fibrosis to present with renal failure. However, renal failure as a presentation of renal tuberculosis is rare[170,171], and accounts for approximately 1% of patients in Europe who require renal replacement[172]. Diffuse interstitial nephritis has also been documented as an important clinical feature of renal tuberculosis[173], which is probably underdiagnosed, particularly in patients with a relatively high risk of developing tuberculosis. This is an important diagnosis to consider as treatment with corticosteroids in addition to antituberculosis chemotherapy can result in a significant improvement in renal function, thereby avoiding dialysis[174]. Furthermore, tuberculous interstitial nephritis has been reported following kidney transplantation[175].

Bladder involvement can present with cystitis, nocturia and dysuria[176]. Pyuria and haematuria are also presenting features, which is either obvious to the naked eye or is detected on routine urinalysis, particularly if abundant white cells are detected on microscopy and the culture for common urinary pathogens is negative.

The most common genital sites of tuberculous infection are the epididymis and prostate; the testicle is infected less frequently[177]. The usual modes of infection are by antegrade infection from the kidneys, or direct extension from neighbouring foci in the genital tract, and hematogenous seeding. Local symptoms are usually insidious and progressive, and can be confused with other bacterial infections, fungal disease, tumours and cysts as well as with a number of less common illnesses.

Tuberculosis of the female genital tract most commonly presented with infertility (44%) pelvic pain (25%), excessive menstrual loss (18%), amenorrhoea (5%), vaginal discharge (4%) and postmenopausal bleeding (2%) and others (2%), in 710 patients with gynaecological tuberculosis. In most patients there is a focus of tuberculosis elsewhere, dissemination may occur via the blood stream or from tuberculous peritonitis. Primary tuberculosis of the female genital tract is rare. The fallopian tubes are affected in nearly all patients, endometrium in 90%, ovaries in 20% and the cervix in 1%. There is practically no involvement in the vulva or vagina[178].

7.7.3 DIAGNOSIS

For radiological diagnosis the intravenous urogram (IVU) has been the investigation of choice for many years; it is abnormal in 90% of patients with renal tuberculosis. Early in renal tuberculosis, calyceal irregularities may be demonstrated due to oedema and contrast medium extending into the parenchyma of the medulla. The pelviureteric junction may be narrowed and the pelvis dilated. Clearly, to exclude obstruction is critical as prompt treatment may reverse uraemia and prevent further deterioration in renal function[179]. With progression, the pelvis size is reduced and may be obliterated. The presence of small or non-functioning kidneys can also be readily demonstrated. Up to 24% of patients with tuberculous kidneys may be associated with renal calcification[180], hence this feature is an important diagnostic indicator. More recently the contribution of the computerized tomographic (CT) scan has been assessed. In one report of 20 patients with renal tuberculosis, the main CT findings were calyectasis, low parenchymal density, parenchymal retraction and calcification. Three of these abnormal findings were present in two-thirds of the series[181]. Interestingly, total renal volume was normal in 10 of 24 affected kidneys and decreased in only seven. Pelvic dilatation secondary to ureteropelvic junction fibrosis and obstruction, and pelvic contraction, can also be demonstrated, which are important for planning further management[182]. Calcification both within the renal parenchyma and at extra-renal sites may be visualized and intra-renal abscesses are readily demonstrated. Perinephric tuberculous

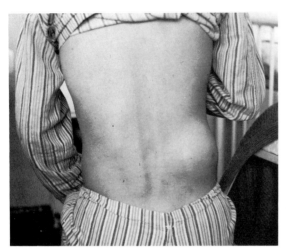

Fig. 7.8   A patient with tuberculosis of the spine and kidney with a large loin abscess.

abscess formation is very rare (Fig. 7.8). CT may also visualize genital tuberculous lesions[183]. An unusual pattern of nephrocalcinosis involving the renal cortex and medulla associated with *M. avium-intracellulare* infection in a patient with AIDS has been reported[184].

Culture of urine for *M. tuberculosis* is a key investigation for any patient suspected to have genitourinary tuberculosis. Early morning urine specimens are preferable, on at least three separate days. The urine can be spun and examined by Ziehl–Neelsen stain, however the yield is low when compared with positive cultures, and *M. smegmatis*, which is morphologically identical to *M. tuberculosis*, can be a source of confusion.

Diagnosis of genitourinary tract tuberculosis is often confirmed on histology from appropriate surgical specimens, and should be pursued by bacteriological culture of tissue.

An abnormal chest radiograph will be present in less than one-half of the patients, but where appropriate sputum samples should be collected for Ziehl–Neelsen staining and also culture for *M. tuberculosis*.

7.7.4 SURGICAL MANAGEMENT

Surgery plays an important role in the management of genitourinary tuberculosis. Essentially surgery can be classified into two types of procedure, namely excision or reconstructive. Unless there is an emergency, surgery is usually delayed until 4–6 weeks after the commencement of appropriate anti-tuberculosis chemotherapy. Irreversibly damaged and non-functioning organs are removed, particularly a damaged kidney as recurrent sepsis and hypertension may result if the kidney is left *in situ*. Partial nephrectomy may be indicated for a tuberculous lesion in one pole that is giving rise to symptoms, for example recurrent bacterial infection. In one series of 1117 patients with genitourinary tuberculosis, 334 (30%) underwent nephrectomy, 80 (7%) partial nephrectomy, 188 (17%) epididymectomy, 42 (4%) orchidectomy[185].

In another series of 631 patients over a 20-year period with urogenital tuberculosis, nephrectomy was performed in 137 (22%) of patients, the most common indication being a destroyed or functionless kidney in 85 (62%) or persistent cystitis in 18 (13%). Non-specific urinary infections were a reason for 16 (12%) of the nephrectomies and pain in 16 (12%) patients. Of the 137 patients, only 3 (2%) had a nephrectomy because of hypertension[186].

Reconstructive procedures include the management of pelviureteric obstruction, bladder reconstruction and ureteric strictures. Of 1117 patients, 65 (6%) underwent reimplantation of the ureter into the bladder, 57 (5%) reconstructive bladder surgery and 24 (2%) ureterocolonic transplantation[185].

Progressive destruction of tissues and fibrosis can occur rapidly, even after the commencement of antituberculosis therapy, and hence the possibility of surgery should be borne in mind[187].

Pelviureteric strictures with obstruction may need urgent treatment to prevent irreversible renal damage. Corticosteroids have been advocated to prevent fibrosis or strictures at the ureterovesical junction, however no controlled studies have ever been performed.

Strictures of the lower ureter may be dilated endoscopically. If this is unsuccessful then ureteric reimplantation may be necessary. Upper ureteric strictures may be treated by ureterotomy at the stricture site, leaving an indwelling ureteric splint[188]. The advantage of a Silastic splint tube is that a nephrostomy is avoided and allows normal voiding of urine.

Bladder augmentation may be required for a small contracted bladder for a patient with intolerable frequency, however augmentation procedures are rarely necessary as such extensive bladder tuberculosis is currently very rare.

7.7.5 MEDICAL TREATMENT

Since the introduction of short course regimens for the treatment of pulmonary tuberculosis there has also been a trend to treat genitourinary tuberculosis for shorter durations. In the UK, the Joint Tuberculosis Committee of the British Thoracic Society recommends a 6-month regimen of 2 months' isoniazid, rifampicin, pyrazinamide and ethambutol followed by 4 months of isoniazid and rifampicin[34]. If pyrazinamide is omitted or cannot be tolerated, treatment should be extended to a total of 9 months. Other authors have advocated longer durations of chemotherapy for patients who have undergone reconstructive surgery[189]. Corticosteroids have been advocated by one author to prevent strictures (which may be due to oedema) developing into ureteric fibrosis[185]. In patients with tuberculous interstitial nephritis the use of corticosteroids has resulted in significantly improved renal function[175].

7.8 TUBERCULOSIS OF THE SKIN

There are a number of forms of cutaneous tuberculosis, all of them are rare[190]. A primary tuberculous skin infection (or primary cutaneous complex) may occur in children and young adults who are inoculated through skin trauma. A nodule develops, which becomes ulcerated and is usually found on the limbs. Lymphangitis and further nodules associated with the lymphatic chain can occur, with regional lymphadenopathy. The lymph nodes may suppurate.

There is also a variety of other forms of inoculation tuberculosis, for example the chronic warty *verrucosa cutis* and the more painful acute *verruca necrogenica*. Those at risk include health care personnel, particularly those involved with post-mortem examinations, and veterinary surgeons, butchers and abattoir workers.

However, the best known form of cutaneous tuberculosis is probably lupus vulgaris, where dull reddish lesions appear on the head, face and extremities. It is generally seen in older patients and is slowly progressive with a presenting history of several years, even decades, before diagnosis (Plate 7). The lesions may be psoriaform in nature with a plaque-like configuration, which disappear after treatment. There is also the mutilans form with progressive destruction of skin, and cartilage of ears and nose with significant deformity. The mouth may be distorted by atrophic or sclerotic scars, and squamous carcinoma of the skin is a recognized complication of chronic lupus vulgaris.

A miliary form of cutaneous tuberculosis has also been recognized, generally in babies, young children or immunosuppressed patients with miliary tuberculosis, and has been described in patients with AIDS, due to both *M. tuberculosis* and *M. avium-intracellulare* [191,192] (see Chapter 13). The lesions are small purplish papules, which are profuse and disseminated over the skin surface.

Tuberculides are a complex subject, about which opinions vary. They are generally considered to be cutaneous manifestations of an immune reaction to tuberculosis elsewhere in the body, usually the lungs. The lesions do not yield *M. tuberculosis* on culture and comprise a variety of forms, including the well-recognized erythema nodosum and Bazin's erythema induratum, to the lesser known papular and papulonecrotic tuberculides. The tuberculid lesions tend to resolve after appropriate antituberculosis chemotherapy.

7.9 ADRENAL TUBERCULOSIS

Tuberculosis is a very rare cause of Addison's disease, however the outcome can be rapidly fatal if undiagnosed[193]. For hypoadrenalism to occur, probably greater than 80% of the adrenal cortices need to be destroyed. Isolated infection of the adrenals is extremely rare, and adrenal involvement will probably be a manifestation of disseminated disease [194]. In one case, large hypodense adrenals were visualized on CT scan[195]. A well-documented phenomenon is when Addisonian crises develop 2–4 weeks after the commencement of antituberculosis chemotherapy[196]. Rifampicin induces hepatic microsomal enzymes resulting in increased elimination of corticosteroids. Rifampicin has been shown to increase the plasma clearance of prednisolone by up to 50%, significantly reducing the amount of drug available to the tissues[197]. Hence, patients with borderline adrenal function can be precipitated into crisis by the commencement of antituberculosis chemotherapy. This is an important finding, and may explain the phenomenon of unexplained sudden death in tuberculosis patients soon after the commencement of antituberculosis chemotherapy[198].

REFERENCES

1. Medical Research Council (1987) National Survey of Tuberculosis Notifications in England and Wales in 1983: characteristics of disease. *Tubercle*, **68**, 19–32.
2. Medical Research Council Cardiothoracic Epidemiology Group (1992) National survey of notifications of tuberculosis in England and Wales in 1988. *Thorax*, **47**, 770–5.
3. Weir, M.R. and Thornton, G.F. (1985) Extrapulmonary tuberculosis. *Am. J. Med.*, **79**, 467–78.
4. Pitchenik, A.E., Fertel, D. and Bloch, A.B. (1988) Pulmonary effects of AIDS: Mycobacterial disease – epidemiology, diagnosis, treatment, and prevention. *Clin. Chest Med.*, **9**, 425–41.
5. Chest Service, Medical and Health Department (1990) *Annual Report*. Hong Kong Government, Hong Kong.
6. Pitchenik, A.E., Cole, C., Russell, B.W. *et al.* (1984) Tuberculosis, atypical mycobacteriosis and the acquired immunodeficiency syndrome among Haitian and non-Haitian patients in South Florida. *Ann. Intern. Med.*, **101**, 641–5.
7. Snider, D.E. and Roper, W.L. (1992) The new tuberculosis (Editorial). *N. Engl. J. Med.*, **326**, 703–5.
8. Berenguer, J., Santiago, M., Laguna, F. *et al.* (1992) Tuberculous meningitis in patients infected with the human immunodeficiency virus. *N. Engl. J. Med.*, **326**, 668–72.
9. Mehta, J.B., Dutt, A., Harvill, L. and Mathews, K.M. (1991) Epidemiology of extrapulmonary tuberculosis. *Chest*, **99**, 1134–8.
10. Citron, K.M. and Girling, D.J. (1987) Tuberculosis. In: *Oxford Textbook of Medicine*, 2nd edn, vol. 1. (eds D.J. Weatherall, J.G.G. Ledingham and D.A. Warrell), Oxford University Press, Oxford, 5.278–5.298.
11. Wolinsky, E. (1988) Tuberculosis. In: *Cecil Textbook of Medicine*, 18th edn, vol. 2., (eds J.B. Wyngaarden, L.H. Smith), W.B. Saunders, Philadelphia 1682–92.
12. Alvarez, S. and McCabe, W.R. (1984) Extrapulmonary tuberculosis revisited: a review of experience at Boston City and other hospitals. *Medicine*, **63**, 25–53.
13. Lau, S.K., Kwan, S., Lee, J. and Wei, W.I. (1991) Source of tubercle bacilli in cervical lymph nodes: a prospective study. *J. Laryngol. Otol.*, **105**, 558–61.
14. Monie, R.D.H., Hunter, A.M., Rocchiccioli, K.M.S. *et al.* (1982) Management of extrapulmonary tuberculosis (excluding miliary and meningeal) in south and west Wales (1976–8). *Br. Med. J.*, **285**, 415–18.
15. British Thoracic Society Research Committee (1985) Short – course chemotherapy for tuberculosis of lymph nodes: a controlled trial. *Br. Med. J.*, **290**, 1106–8.

16. Dandapat, M.C., Mishra, B.M., Dash, S.P. and Kar, P.K. (1990) Peripheral lymph node tuberculosis: a review of 80 cases. *Br. J. Surg.*, **771**, 911–12.

17. Winter, J.H. and Legge, J.S. (1983) Acute tuberculous lymphadenopathy in an immunosuppressed patient. *Br. Med. J.*, **286**, 36–7.

18. Ghimire, M.P. and Walker, R.J. (1985) Painful dysphagia in a case of mediastinal tuberculous lymphadenopathy. *Postgrad. Med. J.*, **61**, 427–8.

19. McNamara, M., Williams, C.E., Brown, T.S. and Gopichandran, T.D. (1987) Tuberculosis affecting the oesophagus. *Clin. Radiol.*, **38**, 419–22.

20. Askari, A., Kyi, T., Patel, J.M. and Chopra, M.P. (1992) Acute arthropathy in mediastinal tuberculosis. *Respir. Med.*, **86**, 57–9.

21. Huhti, E., Brander, E., Ploheimo, S. *et al.* (1975) Tuberculosis of the cervical lymph nodes: a clinical, pathological and bacteriological study. *Tubercle*, **56**, 27–36.

22. Lau, S.K., Wei, W.I., Hsu, C. and Engzell, U.C. (1988) Fine needle aspiration biopsy of tuberculous cervical lymphadenopathy. *Aust. NZ J. Surg.*, **58**, 947–50.

23. Lau, S.K., Wei, W.I., Kwan, S. and Yew, W.W. (1991) Combined use of fine-needle aspiration cytologic examination and tuberculin skin test in the diagnosis of cervical tuberculous lymphadenitis: a prospective study. *Arch. Otolaryngol. Head Neck Surg.*, **117**, 87–90.

24. Lau, S.K., Wei, W.I., Hsu, C. and Engzell, U.C. (1990) Efficacy of fine needle aspiration cytology in the diagnosis of tuberculosis cervical lymphadenopathy. *J. Laryngol-Otol.*, **104**, 24–7.

25. Shaha, A, Webber, C. and Marti, J. (1986) Fine-needle aspiration in the diagnosis of cervical lymphadenopathy. *Am. J. Surg.*, **152**, 420–3.

26. Im, J.G., Song, K.S., Kang, H.S. *et al.* (1987) Mediastinal tuberculous lymphadenitis: CT manifestations. *Radiology*, **164**, 115–19.

27. Farrow, P.R., Jones, D.A., Stanley, P.J. *et al.* (1985) Thoracic lymphadenopathy in Asians resident in the United Kingdom: role of mediastinoscopy in initial diagnosis. *Thorax*, **40**, 121–4.

28. Baron, K.M. and Aranda, C.P. (1991) Diagnosis of mediastinal mycobacterial lymphadenopathy by transbronchial needle aspiration. *Chest*, **100**, 1723–4.

29. Campbell, I.A. and Dyson, A.J. (1979) Lymph node tuberculosis: a comparison of treatments 18 months after completion of chemotherapy. *Tubercle*, **60**, 95–8.

30. British Thoracic Society Research Committee (1988) Short course chemotherapy for lymph node tuberculosis: final report at 5 years. *Br. J. Dis. Chest*, **82**, 282–4.

31. Ormerod, L.P. (1988) A retrospective comparison of two drug regimens RHE2/RH10 and RHZ2/RH10 in the treatment of tuberculous mediastinal lymphadenopathy. *Br. J. Dis. Chest*, **82**, 274–81.

32. McCarthy, O.R. and Rudd, R.M. (1989) Six months' chemotherapy for lymph node tuberculosis. *Respir. Med.*, **83**, 425–7.

33. Jawahar, M.S., Sivasubramanian, S., Vijayan, V.K. *et al.* (1990) Short course chemotherapy for tuberculous lymphadenitis in children. *Br. Med. J.*, **301**, 359–62.

34. Ormerod, L.P. (1990) Chemotherapy and management of tuberculosis in the United Kingdom: recommendations of the Joint Tuberculosis Committee of the British Thoracic Society. *Thorax*, **45**, 403–8.

35. British Thoracic Society Research Committee (1992). Six-months' versus nine-months' chemotherapy for tuberculosis of lymph nodes: preliminary results. *Respir. Med.*, **86**, 15–19.

36. Cheung, W.L., Siu, K.F. and Ng, A. (1988) Tuberculous cervical abscess: comparing the results of total excision against simple incision and drainage. *Br. J. Surg.*, **75**, 563–4.

37. Davies, P.D.O., Humphries, M.J., Byfield, S.P. *et al.* (1984) Bone and joint tuberculosis in a national survey of notifications in England and Wales in 1978/9. *J. Bone Joint Surg.*, **66**B, 326–30.

38. Mann, J.S., and Cole, R.B. (1987) Tuberculous spondylitis in the elderly: a potential diagnostic pitfall. *Br. Med. J.*, **294**, 1149–150.

39. Walker, G.F. (1968) Failure of early recognition of skeletal tuberculosis. *Br. Med. J.*, **1**, 682.

40. Humphries, M.J., Sister Gabriel, M. and Lee, Y.K. (1986) Spinal tuberculosis presenting with abdominal symptoms – a report of two cases. *Tubercle*, **67**, 303–7.

41. Ip, M., Chen, N.K, So, S.Y. *et al.* (1989)

Unusual rib destruction in pleuropulmonary tuberculosis. *Chest*, **95**, 242–4.

42. Gorse, G.J, Pais, J.M, Kurske, J.A and Cesario, T.C. (1983) Tuberculous spondylitis: a report of six cases and a review of the literature. *Medicine (Baltimore)*, **62**, 178–93.

43. Lin-Greenberg, A. and Cholankeril, J. (1990) Vertebral arch destruction in tuberculosis: CT features. *J Comput. Assist. Tomogr.*, **14**(2), 300–2.

44. Bell, G.R, Stearns, K.L, Bonutti, P.M and Boumphrey, F.R. (1990) MRI diagnosis of tuberculous vertebral osteomyelitis. *Spine*, **15**(6), 462–5.

45. Smith, D.F, Smith, F.W and Douglas, J.G. (1989) Tuberculous radiculopathy: the value of magnetic resonance imaging of the neck. *Tubercle*, **70**, 213–16.

46. Angtuaco, E.G.C, McConnell, J.R, Chaddock, W.M and Flannigan, S. (1987) Magnetic resonance imaging of spinal epidural sepsis. *Am. J. Roentgen*, **42**, 1249–53.

47. Allen, B.W, Mitchison, D.A, Darbyshire, J.H *et al*. (1983). Examination of operation specimens from patients with spinal tuberculosis for tubercle bacilli. *J. Clin. Pathol*, **36**, 662–6.

48. Medical Research Council Working Party on Tuberculosis of the Spine (1974) A controlled trial of anterior spinal fusion and debridement in the surgical management of tuberculosis of the spine in patients on standard chemotherapy: a study in Hong Kong. *Br. J. Surg.*, **61**, 853–66.

49. Medical Research Council Working Party on Tuberculosis of the Spine (1973) A controlled trial of ambulant outpatient treatment and inpatient rest in bed in the management of tuberculosis of the spine in young Korean patients on standard chemotherapy. A study in Masan, Korea. *J. Bone Joint Surg.*, **55B**, 678–97.

50. Medical Research Council Working Party on Tuberculosis of the Spine (1973) A controlled trial of plaster-of-Paris jackets in the management of ambulant outpatient treatment of tuberculosis of the spine in children on standard chemotherapy: a study in Pusan, Korea. *Tubercle*, **54**, 261–82.

51. Medical Research Council Working Party on Tuberculosis of the Spine (1974). A controlled trial of debridement and ambulatory treatment in the management of tuberculosis of the spine in patients on standard chemother-

apy. A study in Bulawayo, Rhodesia. *J. Trop. Med. Hyg.*, **77**, 72–92.

52. Medical Research Council Working Party on Tuberculosis of the Spine (1982) A 10-year assessment of a controlled trial comparing debridement and anterior spinal fusion in the management of tuberculosis of the spine in patients on standard chemotherapy in Hong Kong. *J. Bone Joint Surg.*, **64B**, 393–98.

53. Medical Research Council Working Party on Tuberculosis of the Spine (1985) A ten-year assessment of controlled trials of inpatient and outpatient treatment and of plaster-of-Paris jackets for tuberculosis of the spine in children on standard chemotherapy: studies in Masan and Pusan, Korea. *J. Bone Joint Surg.*, **67B**, 103–10.

54. Medical Research Council Working Party on Tuberculosis of the Spine (1986) A controlled trial of six-month and nine-month regimens of chemotherapy in patients undergoing radical surgery for tuberculosis of the spine in Hong Kong. *Tubercle*, **67**, 243–59.

55. Girling, D.J., Darbyshire, J.H., Humphries, M.J. and Sister Gabriel, M. (1988) Extrapulmonary tuberculosis. *Br. Med. Bull.*, **44**, 738–56.

56. Parkinson, R.W., Hodgson, S.P, Noble, J. (1990) Tuberculosis of the elbow: a report of five cases. *J. Bone Joint Surg.*, **72B**(3), 523–4.

57. Valdazo, J.P., Perez-Ruiz, F., Albarracin, A. *et al*. (1990) Tuberculous arthritis. Report of a case with multiple joint involvement and periarticular tuberculous abscesses. *J. Rheumatol.*, **17**(3), 399–401.

58. Ormerod, L.P., Grundy, M. and Rahman, M.A. (1989) Multiple tuberculous bone lesions simulating metastatic disease. *Tubercle*, **70**(4), 305–7.

59. Shannon, F.B., Moore M., Houkom, J.A. and Waeker, N.J. Jr (1990) Multifocal cystic tuberculosis of bone. Report of a case. *J. Bone Joint Surg.* **72**A (7), 1089–92.

60. Kelly, P., Manning, P., Corcoran, P. and Clancy, L. (1991) Hypertrophic pulmonary osteoarthropathy with pulmonary tuberculosis. *Chest*, **99** (3), 769–70.

61. Southwood, T.R., Hancock, E.J., Petty, R.E. *et al*. (1988) Tuberculous rheumatism (Poncet's Disease) in a child. *Arth. Rheum.*, **31** (10), 1311–13.

62. Harries, A.D. (1990) Tuberculosis and human

immunodeficiency virus infection in developing countries. *Lancet*, **i**, 387–90.

63. Watson, J.M. and Gill, O.N. (1990) HIV infection and tuberculosis. *Br. Med. J.*, **300**, 63–5.

64. Bishburg, E., Sunderam, G., Reichman, L.B. and Kapila R. (1986) Central nervous system tuberculosis with the acquired immunodeficiency syndrome and its related complex. *Ann. Intern. Med.*, **105**, 201–13.

65. Fox, W. (1971) The scope of the controlled clinical trial, illustrated by studies in pulmonary tuberculosis. *Bull. WHO*, **45**, 559–72.

66. Rich, A.R. and McCordock, H.A. (1933) The pathogenesis of tuberculous meningitis. *Bull. Johns Hopkins Hosp.*, **52**, 5–37.

67. Medical Research Council Streptomycin in Tuberculosis Trials Committee (1948) Streptomycin treatment of tuberculous meningitis. *Lancet*, **i**, 582–97.

68. Teoh, R., Humphries, M.J. and Chan, J.C.N. *et al.* (1989) Internuclear ophthalmoplegia in tuberculous meningitis. *Tubercle*, **70**, 61–4.

69. Udani, P.M., Parekh, U.C. and Dastur, D.K. (1971) Neurological and related syndromes in CNS tuberculosis. Clinical features and pathogenesis. *J. Neurol. Sci.*, **14**, 317–57.

70. Udani, P.M. and Dastur, P.K. (1970) Tuberculous encephalopathy with and without meningitis: clinical features and pathological correlations. *J. Neurol. Sci.*, **10**, 541–61.

71. Wadia, N.H. and Dastur, D.K. (1969) Spinal meningitis with radiculomyelopathy. Part 1: Clinical and radiological features. *J. Neurol. Sci.*, **8**, 239–60.

72. Teoh, R., Humphries, M.J. and O'Mahoney, G. (1987) Symptomatic intracranial tuberculoma developing during treatment of tuberculosis: a report of 10 cases and review of the literature. *Quart. J. Med.*, **241**, 449–60.

73. Lees, A.J., Macleod, A.F. and Marshall, J. (1980) Cerebral tuberculomas developing during treatment of tuberculous meningitis. *Lancet*, **i**, 1208–11.

74. Ogawa, S.K., Smith, M.A., Brennessel, D.J. and Lowy, F.D. (1987) Tuberculous meningitis in an urban medical centre. *Medicine*, **66**, 317–26.

75. Humphries, M.J., Teoh, R., Lau, J. and Gabriel, M. (1990) Factors of prognostic significance in Chinese children with tuberculous meningitis. *Tubercle*, **71**, 161–8.

76. Snider D.E., Layde P.M., Johnson M.W. and Lyle M.A. (1980) Treatment of tuberculosis during pregnancy. *Am. Rev. Respir. Dis.*, **122**, 65–79.

77. Jeren, T. and Beus, I. (1982) Characteristics of cerebrospinal fluid in tuberculous meningitis. *Acta Cytol.*, **26**, 678–80.

78. Teoh, R., O'Mahoney, G. and Yeung, V.T.F. (1986) Polymorphonuclear pleocytosis in the cerebrospinal fluid during chemotherapy for tuberculous meningitis. *J. Neurol.*, **233**, 237–41.

79. Kennedy, D.H. and Fallon, R.J. (1979) Tuberculous meningitis. *J. Am. Med. Assoc.*, **241**, 264–8.

80. Yu, Y.L., Chow, W.H., Humphries, M.J. *et al.* (1986) Cryptic miliary tuberculosis. *Quart. J. Med.*, **58**, 421–8.

81. French, G.L., Teoh, R., Chan, C.T. *et al.* (1987) Diagnosis of tuberculous meningitis by detection of tuberculostearic acid in cerebrospinal fluid. *Lancet*, **ii**, 117–19.

82. Krambovitis, E., McIllMurray, M.B., Lock, P.E. *et al.* (1984) Rapid diagnosis of tuberculous meningitis by latex particle agglutination. *Lancet*, **ii**, 1229–31.

83. Coovadia, Y.M., Dawood, A., Ellis, M.E. *et al.* (1986) Evaluation of adenosine deaminase activity and antibody to *Mycobacterium tuberculosis* antigen 5 in cerebrospinal fluid and the radioactive bromide partition test for the early diagnosis of tuberculous meningitis. *Arch. Dis. Childh.*, **61**, 428–35.

84. Shankar, P., Manjunath, N., Mohan, K.K. *et al.* (1991) Rapid diagnosis of tuberculous meningitis by polymerase chain reaction. *Lancet*, **2**, 5–7.

85. Editorial (1976) Treatment of tuberculous meningitis. *Lancet*, **i**, 787–788.

86. Ellard, P.T. and Gammon, P.T. (1976) Pharmacokinetics of isoniazid metabolism in man. *J. Pharmacokinet. Biopharm.*, **4**, 83–113.

87. Weber, W.W. and Hein, D.W. (1979) Clinical pharmacokinetics of isoniazid. *Clin. Pharmacokinet.*, **4**, 401–22.

88. Woo, J., Humphries, M.J., Chan, K. *et al.* (1987) Cerebrospinal fluid and serum levels of pyrazinamide and rifampicin in patients with tuberculous meningitis. *Curr. Ther. Res.*, **42**, 235–42.

89. Ellard, G.A., Humphries, M.J. and Allen, B.W. (1993) Penetration of isoniazid, rifampicin and streptomycin into the cerebrospinal

fluid and the treatment of tuberculous meningitis. (In press – *Am. Rev. Respir. Dis*, 1993.)

90. Phuapradit, P. and Vejjajiva, A. (1987) Treatment of tuberculous meningitis: role of short-course chemotherapy. *Quart. J. Med.* **239**, 249–58.

91. Jacobs, R.F., Sunakorn, P., Chotpitayasunonah, T. *et al.* (1992). Intensive short course chemotherapy for tuberculous meningitis. *Pediatr. Infect. Dis. J.*, **11**, 194–98.

92. Horne, N.W. (1966) A critical evaluation of corticosteroids in tuberculosis. *Adv. Tuberc. Res.*, **15**, 1–54.

93. Shaw, P.P., Wang, S.M., Tung, S.G. *et al.* (1984) Clinical analysis of 445 adult cases of tuberculous meningitis. *Chin. J. Tuberc. Respir. Dis.*, **3**(3), 131–2.

94. Teoh, R., Poon, W., Humphries, M.J. and O'Mahoney, G. (1988) Suprasellar tuberculoma developing during treatment of tuberculous meningitis requiring urgent surgical decompression. *J. Neurol.*, **235**, 321–2.

95. Tang, E.S.C., Chau, A., Fong, D. and Humphries, M.J. (1991) The treatment of multiple intracranial tuberculous abscesses: a case report. *J. Neurol.*, **238**, 183–5.

96. Cook, G.C. (1985) Tuberculosis – certainly not a disease of the past! *Quart. J. Med.*, **56**, 519–21.

97. Palmer, K.R., Patil, D.H., Basran, G.S. *et al.* (1985) Abdominal tuberculosis in urban Britain – a common disease. *Gut*, **26**, 1296–305.

98. Schofield, P.F. (1985) Abdominal tuberculosis. *Gut*, **26**, 1275–8

99. Nwokolo, C. (1961) Ascites in Africa. *Br. Med. J.*, **1**, 33.

100. Menzies, R.I., Alsen, H, Fitzgerald, J.M. and Mohapeloa, R.G. (1986) Tuberculous peritonitis in Lesotho. *Tubercle*, **67**, 47–54.

101. Hulnick, D.H., Megibow, A.J., Naidich, D.P. *et al.* (1985) Abdominal tuberculosis – a CT evaluation. *Radiology*, **157**(1), 199–204.

102. Mukerjee, P. and Singal, A.K. (1979) Intestinal tuberculosis: 500 operated cases. *Proc. Asso. Surg. East Afr.*, **2**, 70–5.

103. deMas. R., Lombeck, G. and Rieman, J.F. (1986) Tuberculosis of the oesophagus masquerading as an ulcerated tumour. *Endoscopy*, **18**(4), 153–5.

104. Gupta, S.P., Arora, A. and Bhargava, D.K. (1992) An unusual presentation of oesophageal tuberculosis. *Tuberc. Lung Dis.*, **73**, 174–6.

105. Klimach O E and Ormerod L P. (1985) Gastrointestinal tuberculosis: A retrospective review of 109 cases in a district general hospital. *Quart. J. Med.*, **56**(221), 569–78.

106. Gilinsky, N.H., Marks, I.N., Kottler, R.E. (1983) Abdominal tuberculosis. A 10-year review. *S. Afr. Med. J.*, **64**(22), 849–57.

107. Addison, N.V. (1983) Abdominal tuberculosis – a disease revived. *Ann. R. Coll. Surg. Eng.*, **65**, 105–11.

108. Bastani, B., Shariatzadeh, M.R. and Dehdashti, F. (1985) Tuberculous peritonitis – report of 30 cases and review of the literature. *Quart. J. Med.*, **56**(221), 549–57.

109. Pozniak, A.L. and Dalton-Clarke, H.J. (1985) Colonic tuberculosis presenting with massive rectal bleeding. *Tubercle*, **66**, 295–9.

110. Sherman, S., Rohwedder, J.J., Ravikrishnan, K.P. and Weg, J. G. (1980) Tuberculous enteritis and peritonitis – report of 36 general hospital cases. *Arch. Intern. Med.*, **140**, 506–8.

111. Shukla, H.S. and Hughes, L.E. (1978) Abdominal tuberculosis in the 1970s: a continuing problem. *Br. J. Surg.*, **65**, 403–5.

112. Wolfe, J.H.N., Behn, A.R. and Jackson, B.T. (1979) Tuberculous peritonitis and the role of diagnostic laparoscopy. *Lancet*, **i**, 852–3.

113. Vyravanathan, S. and Jeyarajah, R. (1980) Tuberculous peritonitis: a review of thirty-five cases. *Postgrad. Med. J.*, **56**, 649–51.

114. Coode, P.E., Hossain, J. and Ibrahim, M.B. (1991) Two cases of intestinal obstruction caused by tuberculosis – the role of frozen section diagnosis. *Tubercle*, **72**, 152–4.

115. Das Pritam and Shukla, H.S. (1976) Clinical diagnosis of abdominal tuberculosis. *Br. J. Surg.*, **63**, 941–6.

116. Bhansali, S.K. (1977) Abdominal tuberculosis. Experiences with 300 cases. *Am. J. Gastr.*, **67**, 324–37.

117. Theoni, R.F. and Margulis, A.R. (1979) Gastrointestinal tuberculosis. *Semin. Roentgenol.*, **14**, 283–94.

118. Essop, A.R, Posen, J.A, Hodkinson, J.H. and Segal, I. (1984) Tuberculous hepatitis: a clinical review of 96 cases. *Quart. J. Med.*, **212**, 465–77.

119. Andrew, W.K., Thomas, R.G. and Gollach, B.L. (1982) Miliary tuberculosis the liver – another cause of 'bright liver' on ultrasound examination. *S. Afr. Med. J.*, **62**(22), 808–9.

120. Nagai, H., Shimizu, S., Kawamoto, H. *et al.* (1989) A case of solitary tuberculosis of the liver. *Jpn J. Med.*, **28**(2), 251–5.

121. Gibson, J.A. (1973) Granulomatous liver dis-

ease and portal hypertension. *Proc. R. Soc. Med.*, **66**, 502–3.

122. Sheen-Chen, S.M., Chou, F.F., Tai, D.I. and Eng, H.L. (1990) Hepatic tuberculosis; a rare case of bleeding gastric varices. *Tubercle*, **71**, 225–7.

123. Spiegel, C.T. and Tuazon, C.U. (1984) Tuberculous liver abscess. *Tubercle*, **65**, 127–31.

124. Epstein, B.M. and Leibowitz, C.B. (1987) Ultrasonograpic and computed tomographic appearance of focal tuberculosis of the liver. A case report. *S. Afr. Med. J.*, **71**(7), 461–2.

125. John, E.G., Chan, L., Jonasson, O. *et al.* (1985) Tuberculosis of the liver in end stage renal disease under treatment with haemodialysis. *Int. J. Pediatr. Nephrol.*, **6**(3), 225–6.

126. Denath, F.M. (1990) Abdominal tuberculosis in children: CT findings. *Gastrointest. Radiol.*, **15**(4), 303–6.

127. Crook, L.D. and Johnson, F.P. Jr (1988) Tuberculosis of the pancreas: a case report. *Tubercle*, **69**(2), 148–51.

128. Knowles, K.F., Saltman, D., Robson, H.G. and Lalonde, R. (1990) Tuberculous peritonitis. *Tubercle*, **71**, 65–8.

129. Lambrianides, A.L., Ackroyd, N. and Shorey, B. (1980) Abdominal tuberculosis. *Br. J. Surg.*, **67**, 887–9.

130. al-Hadeedi, S., Walia, H.S. and al-Sayer, H.M. (1990) Abdominal tuberculosis. *Can. J. Surg.*, **33**(3), 233–7.

131. Epstein, B.M. and Mann, J.H. (1982) CT of abdominal tuberculosis. *Am. J. Radiol.*, **139**, 861–6.

132. Rodriguez de Lope, C., San Miguel Joglar, G. and Pons Romero, F. (1982) Laparoscopic diagnosis of tuberculous ascites. *Endoscopy* **14**, 178–9.

133. Sochocky, S. (1967) Tuberculous peritonitis. A review of 100 cases. *Am. Rev. Resp. Dis.*, **95**, 398–401.

134. Hanson, R.D. and Hunter, T.B. (1985) Tuberculous peritonitis: CT appearance. *Am. J. Radiol.*, **144**, 931–2.

135. Levine, H. (1967) Needle biopsy of peritoneum for exudative ascites. *Arch. Intern. Med.*, **120**, 542–5.

136. Singh, M.M., Bhargava, A.N. and Jain, K.P. (1969) Tuberculous peritonitis: an evaluation of pathogenic mechanisms, diagnostic procedures and therapeutic measures. *N. Engl. J. Med.*, **281**, 1091–6.

137. Shukla, H.S., Naitrani, Y.P., Bhatia, S. *et al.*

(1982) Peritoneal biopsy for diagnosis of abdominal tuberculosis. *Postgrad. Med. J.*, **58**, 226–8.

138. Jorge, A.D. (1984) Peritoneal tuberculosis. *Endoscopy*, **16**, 10–12.

139. Manohar, A., Simjee, A.E., Haffejee, A.A., (1990) Symptoms and investigative findings in 145 patients with tuberculous peritonitis diagnosed by peritoneoscopy and biopsy over a five year period. *Gut*, **31**, 1130–2.

140. Kalvaria, I., Kottler, R.E., and Marks, I.N. (1988) The role of colonoscopy in the diagnosis of tuberculosis. *J. Clin. Gastroenterol.*, **10** (5), 516–23.

141. Kochhar, R., Rajwanshi, A., Goenka, M.K. *et al.* (1991). Colonoscopic fine needle aspiration cytology in the diagnosis of ileocaecal tuberculosis. *Am. J. Gastroenterol*, **86** (1), 102–4.

142. Ghandi, B.M., Bhargava, D.K., Irshad, M. (1986). Enzyme linked protein-A. An ELISA for detection of IgG antibodies against *Mycobacterium tuberculosis* in intestinal tuberculosis. *Tubercle* **67**, 219–24.

143. Dineen, P., Homan, W.P., Grafe, W.R. (1976) Tuberculous peritonitis: 43 years experience in diagnosis and treatment. *Ann. Surg.*, **184**, 717–22.

144. Mcmillen, M.A. and Arnold, S.D. (1979) Tuberculous peritonitis associated with alcoholic liver disease. *N Y State J. Med.*, **79**, 922–44.

145. Lee, C.H., Wang, W.J., Lan, R.S. *et al.* (1988). Corticosteroids in the treatment of tuberculous pleurisy. *Chest*, **94**(6), 1256–9.

146. Larrieu, A.J., Tyers, G.F., Williams, E.H., and Derrick, J.R. (1980) Recent experience with tuberculous pericarditis. *Ann. Thorac. Surg.*, **29**, 464–8.

147. Lorell, B.H., and Braunwald, E., (1988) Pericardial disease: tuberculous pericarditis. In: *Heart Disease* – a *Textbook of Cardiovascular Medicine*, 3rd edn (ed. E. Braunwald), W.B. Saunders, Philadelphia, pp. 1509–11.

148. Fowler, N.O. (1991) Tuberculous pericarditis. *J. Am. Med. Assoc.*, **266**, 99–103.

149. Strang, J.I.G. (1984) Tuberculous pericarditis in Transkei. *Clin. Cardiol.*, **7**, 667–70.

150. Silver, M.D. (ed.) (1983) *Cardiovascular Pathology*, Churchill Livingstone, New York, pp. 139–40.

151. Dave, T., Narula, J.P. and Chopra, P. (1990) Myocardial and endocardial involvement in

tuberculous constrictive pericarditis. *Int. J. Cardiol.*, **28**, 245–51.

152. Rooney, J.J., Crocco, J.A. and Lyons, H.A. (1970) Tuberculous pericarditis. *Ann. Intern. Med.*, **72**, 73–8.

153. Bashi, V.V., John, S., Ravikumar, E. *et al.* (1988) Early and late results of pericardiectomy in 118 cases of constrictive pericarditis. *Thorax*, **43**, 637–41.

154. Gibson, D.G. (1987) Pericardial disease. In *Oxford Textbook of Medicine*, 2nd edn, vol. 2, (eds D.J. Weatherall, J.G.G. Ledingham and D.A. Warrell), Oxford University Press, Oxford, pp. 13.304–13.312.

155. Pohost, G.M. and O'Rourke. R.A. (eds) (1991) *Principles and Practice of Cardiovascular Imaging*, Little Brown, Boston, Mass., p. 457.

156. Sagrosta-Sauleda, J., Permanyer-Miralda, G. and Soler-Soler, J. (1988) Tuberculous pericarditis: ten year experience with a prospective protocol for diagnosis and treatment. *J. Am. Coll. Cardiol.*, **11**, 724–8.

157. Strang, J.I.G., Kakaza, H.H.S., Gibson, D.G. *et al.* (1988) Controlled clinical trial of complete open surgical drainage and of prednisolone in the treatment of tuberculous pericardial effusion in Transkei. *Lancet*, **ii**, 759–63.

158. Martinez-Vazquez, J.M., Ribera, E., Ocana, I. *et al.* (1986) Adenosine deaminase activity in tuberculous pericarditis. *Thorax*, **41**, 888–9.

159. Fowler, N.O. and Manitsas, G.T. (1973) Infectious pericarditis. *Prog. Cardiovasc. Dis.*, **16**, 323–36.

160. Endrys, J., Simo, M., Shafie, M.Z. *et al.* (1988) New nonsurgical technique for multiple pericardial biopsies. *Cathet. Cardiovasc. Diagn.*, **15**, 92–4.

161. Strang, J.I.G., Kakaza, H.H.S., Gibson, D.G. *et al.* (1987) Controlled trial of prednisolone as adjuvant in treatment of tuberculous constrictive pericarditis in Transkei. *Lancet*, **ii**, 1418–22.

162. Long, R., Younes, M., Patton, N., Hershfield, E. (1989) Tuberculous pericarditis: Long-term outcome in patients who received medical therapy alone. *Am. Heart J.*, **117**, 1133–9.

163. Quale, J.M., Lipschik, G.Y. and Heurich, A.E. (1987) Management of tuberculous pericarditis. *Ann Thorac. Surg.*, **43**, 653–5.

164. Stoller, J.K. (1985) Late recurrence of *Mycobacterium bovis* genitourinary tuberculosis: case report and review of the literature. *J. Urol.*, **134**(3), 565–6.

165. Yaqoob, M., Goldsmith, H.J. and Ahmad, R. (1990) Bovine genitourinary tuberculosis revisited. *Quart. J. Med.*, **74** (273), 105–9.

166. Peters, T.G., Reiter, C.G. and Boswell, R.L. (1984) Transmission of tuberculosis by kidney transplantation. *Transplantation*, **38**(5), 514–6.

167. Lichtenstein, I.H. and MacGregor, R.R. (1983) Mycobacterial infections in renal transplant recipients: report of five cases and review of the literature. *Rev. Infect. Dis.*, **5**(2), 216–26.

168. Ferrie, B.G. and Rundle, J.S.H. (1985) Genitourinary tuberculosis in patients under twenty five years of age. *Urology*, **XXV**(6), 576–8.

169. Datta, S.K. (1987) Renal tuberculosis presenting as hypertension. *J. Assoc. Physicians India*, **35**(11), 798–9.

170. Tosev, N. and Tabakov, J. (1972) Renal tuberculosis as a reason for chronic renal failure. *Khirurgiya (Sofiya)*, **25**, 370.

171. Benn, J.J., Scoble, J.E., Thomas, A.C. *et al.* (1988) Cryptogenic tuberculosis as a preventable cause of end-stage renal failure. *Am. J. Nephrol.*, **8**(4), 306–8.

172. Broyer, M., Brunner, F.P., Brynger, H. *et al.* (1986) Demography of dialysis and transplantation in Europe 1984. *Nephrol. Dial. Transplant*, **1**, 1–8.

173. Mallinson, W.J.W., Fuller, R.W, Levison, D.A. *et al.* (1981). Diffuse interstitial renal tuberculosis: an unusual cause of renal failure. *Quart. J. Med.*, **50**, 137–48.

174. Morgan, S.H., Eastwood, J.B., Baker, L.R.I. (1990) Tuberculous interstitial nephritis – the tip of an iceberg? *Tubercle*, **71**, 5–6.

175. al-Sulaiman, M.H., Dhar, J.M., al-Hasani, M.K. *et al.* (1990) Tuberculous interstitial nephritis after kidney transplantation. *Transplantation*, **50**(1), 162–4.

176. Weinberg, A.C. and Boyd, S.D. (1988) Short course chemotherapy and role of surgery in adult and pediatric genitourinary tuberculosis. *Urology*, **XXXI**(2), 95–102.

177. Gorse, G.J. and Belshe, R.B. (1985) Male genital tuberculosis: a review of the literature with instructive case reports. *Rev. Infec. Dis.*, **7**(4), 511–24.

178. Sutherland, A.M. (1985) Gynaecological tuberculosis: analysis of a personal series of 710 cases. *Aust. NZ J. Obstet. Gynaecol.*, **25**, 203–7.

179. Lazarus, L. and Peraino, R.A. (1984) Reversible uraemia due to bilateral ureteral obstruction from tuberculosis. *Am. J. Nephrol.*, **4**(5), 322–7.

180. Dolev, E., Bass A. and Nossinowitz, N. (1985) Frequent occurrence of renal calculi in tuberculous kidneys in Israel. *Urology*, **26**(6), 544–5.

181. Okazawa, N., Sekiya T. and Tada, S. (1985) Computed tomographic features of renal tuberculosis. *Radiat. Med.*, **3**(4), 209–13.

182. Goldman, S.M., Fishman, E.K., Hartman, D.S., (1985) Computed tomography of renal tuberculosis and its pathological correlates. *J. Comput. Assist. Tomogr.*, **9**(4), 771–6.

183. Birnbaum, B.A., Friedman, J.P., Lubat E, *et al.* (1990) Extrarenal genitourinary tuberculosis: CT appearance of calcified pipe-stem ureter and seminal vesicle abscess. *J. Comput. Assist. Tomogr.*, **14**(4), 653–5.

184. Falkoff, G.E., Rigsby, C.M. and Rosenfield, A.T. (1987) Partial combined cortical and medullary nephrocalcinosis: US and CT patterns in AIDS-associated MAI infection. *Radiology*, **162**(2), 343–4.

185. Gow, J.G. and Barbosa, S. (1984) Genito urinary tuberculosis. A study of 1117 cases over a period of 34 years. *Br. J. Urol.*, **56**, 449–55.

186. Skutil, V. and Obsitnik, M. (1987) Persistent tuberculous cystitis: the most common indication for nephrectomy in the management of urogenital tuberculosis. *Eur. Urol.*, **13**(1–2), 57–61.

187. Psihramis, K.E. and Donahoe, P.K. (1986) Primary genitourinary tuberculosis: rapid progression and tissue destruction during treatment. *J. Urol.* **135**(5), 1033–6.

188. Osborn, D.E., Rao, N.J. and Blacklock, N.J. (1986) Tuberculous stricture of ureter. A new method of intubated ureterotomy. *Br. J. Urol.*, **58**, 103–4.

189. Wong, S.H., Lau, W.Y., Ho, K.K. *et al.* (1984) The management of urinary tuberculosis – a logical approach. *Br. J. Urol.*, **56**, 349–53.

190. Adriaans, B., Soto, L.D., Canizares, O. *et al.* (1992) Tuberculosis of the skin, in *Clinical Tropical Dermatology*, 2nd edn (eds R. Harman and O. Canizares), Blackwell, Boston, pp. 201–22.

191. Stack, R.J., Bickley, L.K. and Coppel, I.G. (1990) Miliary tuberculosis presenting as skin lesions in a patient with acquired immunodeficiency syndrome. *J. Am. Acad. Dermatol.*, **23**(5, pt 2), 1031–5.

192. Lombardo, P.C. and Weitzman, I. (1990) Isolation of *Mycobacterium tuberculosis* and *M. avium* complex from the same skin lesions in AIDS. *N. Engl. J. Med.*, **323**(13), 916–17.

193. Ward, S. and Evans, C.C. (1985) Sudden death due to isolated adrenal tuberculosis. *Postgrad. Med. J.*, **61**(717), 635–36.

194. Van Kralingen, K.W. and Slee, P.H. (1987) A patient with miliary tuberculosis and acute adrenal failure. *Neth. J. Med.*, **30**(5–6), 235–41.

195. Jagannath, A., Brill, P.W. and Winchester, P. (1986) Addison's disease due to tuberculosis in a 13 year old girl. *Pediatr. Radiol.*, **16**(16), 522–24.

196. Wilkins, E.G.L., Hnizdo, E. and Cope, A. (1989) Addisonian crisis induced by treatment with rifampicin. *Tubercle*, **70**, 69–73.

197. McAllister, W.A.C., Thompson, P.J., Al-Habet, S. *et al.*, (1982) Adverse effects of rifampicin on prednisolone disposition. *Thorax*, **37**, 792.

198. Ellis, M.E. and Webb, A.K. (1983) Cause of death in patients admitted to hospital for pulmonary tuberculosis. *Lancet*, **i**, 665–7.

TREATMENT 8

THE CLINICAL PHARMACOLOGY OF ANTITUBERCULOSIS DRUGS

P.A. Winstanley

8a.1 ISONIAZID

8a.1.1 MODE OF ACTION

Isoniazid (H) inhibits most tubercle bacilli at concentrations above 0.01 mg/l[1], is bactericidal against most rapidly growing tubercle bacilli, but less active against non-dividing organisms. It appears to work by inhibiting the synthesis of mycolic acid constituents of the cell wall. Mutants resistant to H occur in about 1 in 10^7 organisms, probably because of reduced uptake of the drug[2].

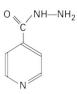

Isoniazid (H)

8a.1.2 PHARMACOKINETICS

(a) Absorption and bioavailability

H may be given orally or intramuscularly (i.m.). Oral H is absorbed completely in the fasted state, even after gastric, duodenal or jejunal surgery[1], but is absorbed less well after food[3] or antacid[4]. When fasted, the time taken to reach maximum plasma concentration (t_{max}) is 1–2 hours[5], but is longer after food. Although oral H is well absorbed its bioavailability (F) is not complete because of extensive first-pass metabolism in gut wall and liver, which is more pronounced in rapid acetylators. After intramuscular administration such first-pass metabolism is not seen.

(b) Distribution

H is distributed to all tissues and reaches similar concentrations both outside and within cells. The drug readily crosses the blood–brain barrier and this is unaffected by concomitant steroids[6]. The apparent volume of distribution (VD) is about 0.6 1/kg (this does not seem to be influenced by acetylator status), and the degree of plasma protein binding is thought to be negligible.

(c) Metabolism and excretion

H is extensively metabolized to a variety of therapeutically inactive metabolites, mainly in the liver and small intestine, predominantly by cytosolic N-acetyl transferase[7,8]. Unchanged drug and metabolites are excreted mainly in the urine. Since metabolism is the principal determinant of H elimination, and since acetylator status is subject to a genetic polymorphism[9], elimination half-life ($t_{1/2}$) can vary from 0.75 to 5 h. Of the various metabolites of H, monoacetyl-

Clinical Tuberculosis. Edited by P.D.O. Davies. Published in 1994 by Chapman & Hall, London. ISBN 0 412 48630 X

hydrazine, though without antitubercular effects, can undergo N-hydroxylation, which generates a reactive and hepatotoxic species, possibly acetyl free radicals[10]. Although fast acetylators produce more monoacetyl-hydrazine than slow acetylators (leading to the suggestion that fast acetylators might be at increased risk of hepatotoxicity), they are also capable of its further acetylation to the non-toxic derivative diacetylhydrazine. It therefore seems that rapid and slow acetyl-ators generate similar amounts of mono-acetylhydrazine, and may have identical risk of liver damage (though this is conten-tious[11]). Up to 2.3% of the daily dose of H may be excreted in breast milk[12].

(d) Influence of age and disease on drug disposition

H $t_{1/2}$ is probably prolonged in neonates[13] because of immaturity of N-acetyltransferase, and dose intervals may need to be length-ened. In both acute and chronic liver disease $t_{1/2}$ and steady-state plasma levels of H may be increased, but renal failure seems to have little effect and the drug may be given in full dosage.

8a.1.3 ADVERSE EFFECTS

(a) Nervous system

Mixed sensory and motor neuropathy is now unusual in the developed world. The risk is higher in slow acetylators[14] and malnour-ished patients[15], is thought to result from perturbation of vitamin B6 metabolism and is prevented by dietary supplementation. Encephalopathy and resultant seizures are very uncommon in the developed world.

(b) Liver

The risk of liver damage, ranging from asymptomatic elevation of transaminases to severe hepatitis, increases with age, and is highest in elderly patients who are slow acetylators[16].

(c) Systemic lupus erythematosus

H induces positive antinuclear antibodies in about 20% of patients during long-term use[17], but only a small fraction of patients develop clinically serious disease. Risk of SLE seems unassociated with age or acetylator status.

(d) Blood

H can cause haemolysis in patients with G6PD-deficiency, and sideroblastic anaemia has been reported. H is considered unsafe in patients with acute porphyria[18].

(e) Drug interactions

See Table 8a.1 for a summary of drug interactions.

8a.2 RIFAMPICIN AND RIFABUTIN

8a.2.1 MODE OF ACTION

Rifampicin (R) and rifabutin (RB) act by interference with DNA transcription through inhibition of RNA-polymerase[19]. Both are bactericidal against most tubercle bacilli at concentrations above 1 mg/l. In most infec-tions, highly resistant mutants occur with a frequency of between 1: 10^7–10^5 organisms. The mechanism of resistance is incompletely understood, but may be due to a combination of reduced permeability of organisms to the drug, and mutation of DNA-dependent RNA-polymerase.

8a.2.2 PHARMACOKINETICS

(a) Absorption and bioavailability

Oral formulations of both R and RB are available, but only R has an intravenous (i.v.) formulation. Both drugs are usually well

Table 8a.1 Important pharmacokinetic drug interactions

Drug X	Drug Y			
	Y increases level of X	Y decreases level of X	X increases level of Y	X decreases level of Y
Isoniazid	Prednisolone Ethionamide	—	Phenytoin Carbamazepine Warfarin Diazepam	Enflurane
Rifampicin	—	PAS	—	Warfarin Sulphonylureas Oral contraceptives Glucocorticoids Phenytoin Diazepam Theophyllines Vitamin D Digitoxin
Ethambutol	—	Al OH	—	—
PAS	—	—	—	Rifampicin
Pyrazinamide	—	—	Probenecid	—
Ethionamide	—	—	Isoniazid	—
Ofloxacin	—	Antacids	—	—
Ciprofloxacin	—	Antacids	Theophyllines Warfarin	—
Norfloxacin	—	Antacids	Theophyllines Warfarin	—

Rifampicin (R)

absorbed when taken orally, even after partial gastrectomy. However, t_{max} of R is delayed by 1–2 h, and maximum plasma concentration (C_{max}) and F are reduced by concomitant food[20]. Oral administration of R with para-amino benzoic acid (PAS) delays the t_{max} of R by 2–4 h, and reduces C_{max} and F by about 50%[21]; reports that R absorption is perturbed by H are contentious. Apart from interactions with other drugs and food, R bioavailability is very dependent on its formulation[22].

(b) Distribution

Both drugs are widely distributed in tissues, and achieve similar intracellular and extracellular concentrations in most sites[23–25]. CSF concentrations of R are usually between 10 and 40% of the plasma value. R has a VD of about 1 l/kg, and is about 80% bound to plasma proteins (both albumin and gamma globulins[26]). RB's VD is larger (8–9 l/kg [25]), and RB is about 70% bound to plasma proteins.

(c) Metabolism and excretion

R and RB are cleared mainly by hepatic metabolism to pharmacologically active, but more water-soluble, desacetylated derivatives [26,27]. Desacetyl-R is principally excreted in bile (where it accounts for about 80% of the microbiological activity), though it is also excreted in urine to a lesser extent. About 20% of desacetyl-R undergoes conjugation with glucuronic acid[28]. In addition, R is hydrolysed to formyl-R, which is mainly excreted in the urine. A minority of the dose is excreted unchanged in the bile and may undergo enterohepatic circulation. Since R metabolism can be saturated at higher doses, the $t_{1/2}$ varies from 2.5 to 5 h[29]. Both R and RB can induce their own metabolism with repeated doses[30,31].

(d) Influence of age and disease on drug disposition

R levels are lower in young children than in adults. R doses need not be altered in renal failure and the drug is dialysable. However, in patients with cirrhosis or hepatitis, R levels may be higher and elimination slower[29].

8a.2.3 ADVERSE EFFECTS

(a) 'Sensitization' during intermittent treatment

When given at weekly intervals or intermittent courses, R can cause haemolytic anaemia, shock and acute renal failure, though these are uncommon.

(b) 'Flu syndrome'

Fever, chills, headache and thrombocytopenic purpura can all occur, more commonly during intermittent therapy.

(c) Liver

Patients with pre-existing liver disease may develop further liver impairment.

(d) Coloration of urine

Since R and RB are strongly coloured, urine, tears and sweat predictably become red or orange during treatment.

(e) Gastrointestinal tract

Some patients develop nausea and abdominal discomfort, which can usually be helped by taking the drugs with meals.

(f) Joints

At high doses, in patients with AIDS-related complex, RB causes arthritis or arthralgia[32].

8a.3 PYRAZINAMIDE

8a.3.1 MODE OF ACTION

Pyrazinamide (Z) is metabolized, by bacterial pyrazinamidase, to pyrazinoic acid, which is the principal bacteriocidal species. Z probably has greater activity against intracellular than extracellular bacilli. Resistance develops rapidly if Z is used as the sole antituberculosis agent.

Pyrazinamide (Z)

8a.3.2 PHARMACOKINETICS

(a) Absorption and bioavailability

Z is available only as an oral formulation. It is completely absorbed[33] and t_{max} is about 1–2 h.

(b) Distribution

The drug is about 50% bound to plasma protein, and is extensively distributed to tissues[34]. CSF concentrations are similar to those in plasma and are unaffected by concomitant steroids[6].

(c) Metabolism and excretion

Z is mainly metabolized to pyrazinoic acid by hepatic microsomal deaminidase, followed by further oxidation of the metabolite, by xanthine oxidase, to pharmacologically inactive derivatives. Metabolites and unchanged drug (which probably accounts for as little as 1% of a dose) are mainly excreted in the urine. Traces of Z are excreted in breast milk. The $t_{1/2}$ of Z is about 9 h in health [35].

(d) Influence of age and disease on disposition

The effect of renal failure on Z kinetics has not been studied, but dose reduction is usually advocated; Z is contraindicated in patients with pre-existing liver disease. The disposition of Z at extremes of age has not been reported.

8a.3.3 ADVERSE EFFECTS

(a) Liver

Z hepatotoxicity is commonest in patients with pre-exisiting liver disease, and risk rises with dose and length of exposure. Liver function should be watched and Z withdrawn if abnormalities develop. Hepatic impairment usually resolves after withdrawal of the drug.

(b) Joints

Z can cause hyperuricaemia and gout, presumably by inhibition of urate secretion[36], and may also cause an arthralgia, of unknown cause. The latter does not require drug withdrawal.

8a.4 ETHAMBUTOL

8a.4.1 MODE OF ACTION

Ethambutol (E) seems to inhibit synthesis of mycobacterial cell walls but the exact mechanism is unknown. The drug is essentially bacteriostatic. E has activity against most strains of *M. tuberculosis*, but if given as monotherapy for tuberculosis, resistance

develops in about 50% of patients within 6 months[37].

$$CH_3\!-\!CH_2\!-\!CH\!-\!CH_2OH$$
$$|$$
$$NH$$
$$|$$
$$(CH_2)_2 \quad \bullet\, 2HCl$$
$$|$$
$$NH$$
$$|$$
$$CH_3\!-\!CH_2\!-\!CH\!-\!CH_2OH$$

Ethambutol (E)

8a.4.2 PHARMACOKINETICS

(a) Absorption and bioavailability

E is well absorbed after oral administration, with t_{max} of about 2 h and *F* of approximately 0.8[38]. Absorption is delayed by aluminium hydroxide and ethanol, but is unaffected by food[39].

(b) Distribution

E is distributed to most body fluids and is about 40% bound to plasma proteins[40]. E does not readily cross the blood–brain barrier and in patients with tuberculous meningitis the CSF:plasma concentration ratio shows great inter-individual variation[41]. However, E does accumulate in lung tissue[42].

(c) Metabolism and excretion

The majority of a dose of E is excreted unchanged in the urine, with pharmacologically inactive metabolites accounting for less than 20% of the dose. The $t_{1/2}$ of E is 10–15 h in patients with normal renal function.

(d) Influence of age and disease on drug disposition

Age has little impact on the pharmacokinetics of E. In patients with renal disease, E levels

Streptomycin (S)

should be estimated regularly since $t_{1/2}$ is likely to be prolonged and there is a risk of drug accumulation[43]. Liver disease does not alter E disposition to a clinically important degree.

8a.4.3 ADVERSE EFFECTS

(a) Eye

Central or peripheral retrobulbar neuritis are related to the dose of E and its duration, may be unilateral or bilateral, but usually resolve when the drug is stopped.

(b) Joints

E may cause hyperuricaemia and gout[36].

(c) Idiopathic reactions

Rashes, thrombocytopenia and jaundice have been reported[11].

8a.5 STREPTOMYCIN AND OTHER AMINOGLYCOSIDES

8a.5.1 MODE OF ACTION

The aminoglycosides are actively transported across bacterial cell membranes, bind to protein constituents of the 30S subunit of ribosomes and interfere with protein synthesis. Of the drugs in this class used for tuberculosis (including kanamycin (Ka) and amikacin (Am)), streptomycin (S) is used

most commonly, particularly in developing countries. There is cross-resistance between each example. S is active against *M. tuberculosis* at concentrations around 10 mg/l *in vivo*.

Kanamycin (Ka)

Amikacin (Am)

8a.5.2 PHARMACOKINETICS

S is given parenterally (usually i.m.) since its oral absorption (like that of all aminoglycosides) is negligible. The drug is about 50% bound to plasma proteins in health (less so in kwashiorkor) and is distributed to most tissues, but crosses the blood–brain barrier poorly. Over 90% is excreted unchanged, mainly in the urine. In health $t_{1/2}$ is about 3 h, but this can reach 100 h in renal failure. S is partly excreted in breast milk[12].

Ka is minimally bound to plasma proteins and excreted unchanged. In patients with normal renal function, $t_{1/2}$ is about 2 h Am, a semisynthetic derivative of Ka, has very similar kinetic properties.

8a.5.3 ADVERSE EFFECTS

(a) VIIIth nerve

Aminoglycosides accumulate in the inner ear and produce concentration-dependent damage; S mainly causes vestibular problems, while kanamycin mainly causes auditory damage. These effects can occur in the fetus during maternal treatment.

(b) Kidney

Concentration-dependent renal impairment can occur, but is unusual with standard doses in patients with normal renal function.

(c) Allergy

Hypersensitivity is common, usually produces mild problems (such as fever and skin rashes), but can be life-threatening. Anaphylaxis and exfoliative dermatitis have been reported.

8a.6 CAPREOMYCIN AND VIOMYCIN

Capreomycin (Cm) and viomycin (Vi) are antibiotics with many similarities to the aminoglycosides, though chemically distinct. Both bind to the 30S and 50S ribosomal subunits and interfere with protein synthesis. Cm and Vi must be given parenterally, and neither penetrates the blood–brain barrier well; it is likely that both are excreted unchanged in the urine. Both are nephrotoxic and ototoxic, and can cause hypersensitivity.

8a.7 CLOFAZIMINE

Clofazimine (Cl) probably works by binding to guanine residues on mycobacterial DNA and interferes with transcription. Absorption of the drug from the gut is highly dependent on formulation. Cl is widely distributed and, because it is highly lipophilic, it penetrates peripheral nerves; data on its concentration within the brain are not available. About 50% of a dose can be recovered from the faeces, but this may represent unabsorbed Cl; coloured metabolites are excreted in the urine. Cl crosses the placenta and is excreted in milk. The elimination half-life is about 10 days. Cl may cause malabsorption, severe gastrointestinal upset, exacerbation of peptic ulcer, and discoloration (red) of the skin, hair, urine and faeces.

8a.8 PARA-AMINOSALICYLIC ACID (PAS)

8a.8.1 MODE OF ACTION

It is likely that PAS competes with para-amino benzoic acid for mycobacterial dihydropteroate synthetase. PAS has little activity against other bacteria, but tubercle bacilli are usually inhibited by concentrations of 1–5 mg/l.

8a.8.2 PHARMACOKINETICS

PAS is readily absorbed after oral dosing, and is often given with food since it may cause gastric irritation; this does not alter drug absorption. PAS is largely unbound in the plasma, and reaches high concentrations in pleural fluid and caseous tissue. Levels in the CSF are lower than in plasma. PAS is mainly cleared by acetylation, and the (pharmacologically inactive) metabolites are mainly excreted in the urine. The $t_{1/2}$ of PAS is about 1 h. Dose alteration is not needed in patients with renal or hepatic disease.

8a.8.3 ADVERSE EFFECTS

(a) Gastrointestinal tract

Nausea, abdominal pain and diarrhoea are common.

Capreomycin

Viomycin (Vi)

(b) Kidney

Very high concentrations of PAS and metabolites occur in the urine, and crystalluria may occur, especially at low pH.

(c) Thyroid

PAS inhibits incorporation of iodine into thyroid hormone. Goitre, with or without hypothyroidism, can occur.

Clofazimine (Cl)

Para aminosalicylic acid (PAS)

(d) Allergy

Drug fever, skin rashes and blood dyscrasias were reported when PAS was in frequent use; all may be due to hypersensitivity.

8a.9 ETHIONAMIDE

8a.9.1 MODE OF ACTION

Ethionamide (Eth) is structurally similar to H and works in the same way.

Ethionamide (Eth)

8a.9.2 PHARMACOKINETICS

Eth is well absorbed after oral administration, its t_{max} being 1–2 h. The drug is widely distributed, 70% unbound in the serum and achieves CSF concentrations similar to the free serum levels. Eth is mainly cleared by hepatic metabolism; ethionamide sulphoxide, the principal metabolite, is equipotent with the parent drug, and is itself metabolized back to the parent drug. The metabolites are mainly excreted in the urine[44]. Eth has $t_{1/2}$ of about 2 h in health. The effects of hepatic or renal disease on Eth disposition are unknown.

8a.9.3 ADVERSE EFFECTS

(a) Allergy

Eth can cause severe allergic cutaneous reactions and drug fever.

(b) Liver

The mechanism of Eth hepatotoxicity is unknown. The drug is contraindicated in patients with pre-existing liver disease.

(c) Gastrointestinal tract

Nausea, diarrhoea and abdominal pain can be severe enough to warrant the drug's withdrawal.

8a.10 FLUORINATED QUINOLONES

8a.10.1 MODE OF ACTION

This group of drugs is thought to act principally by inhibition of topoisomerase II [DNA-gyrase], which mediates the formation of supercoils of DNA[45]. Ciprofloxacin, norfloxacin, perfloxacin and sparfloxacin have all been used for tuberculosis, but most experience has been gained with ofloxacin (Ofx), which is used mainly where the organism is resistant to one or more first-line drugs[46].

Ofloxacin (Ofx)

8a.10.2 PHARMACOKINETICS

Ofx is available in oral and intravenous formulations but, since it is rapidly and completely absorbed after oral administration, parenteral dosing is rarely necessary. The drug is little bound to plasma proteins, and penetrates well into sputum, pleural fluid and many tissues. Ofx is mainly excreted unchanged in the urine with a $t_{1/2}$ of about 5–7 h in patients with normal renal function[47]. Dose regimens of Ofx should be amended in renal failure[48], but hepatic impairment does not alter the drug's kinetics. Unlike ciprofloxacin Ofx is not prone to drug interactions through inhibition of hepatic oxidation.

8a.10.3 ADVERSE EFFECTS

(a) Nervous system

Headache, dizziness, insomnia, tremor, restlessness, confusion and seizures are all reported. The mechanism behind these reactions is unclear, but the drug should be used with caution in epileptic patients.

(b) Gastrointestinal tract

Nausea, vomiting and abdominal pain are reasonably common, but not usually serious.

8a.11 THIACETAZONE.

Thiacetazone (Th) is a cheap bacteriostatic drug used extensively in developing coun-

tries, usually in combination with H and S. Its pharmacokinetics have been reviewed elsewhere[49]. When given to patients with HIV disease, Th causes frequent cutaneous adverse reactions[50].

Thiacetazone (Th)

8a.12 CYCLOSERINE

Cycloserine is an analogue of D-alanine, which works by competing with the amino acid for incorporation into peptidoglycan constituents of the cell wall. It is rarely used because of poor efficacy and frequent adverse effects, which include vertigo, headache, psychosis and convulsions[51].

Cycloserine (Cs)

REFERENCES

1. Robson, J.M. and Sullivan, F.M. (1963) Antituberculosis drugs. *Pharmacol. Rev.*, **15**, 169–223.
2. Youatt, J. (1969) A review of the action of isoniazid. *Am. Rev. Respir. Dis.*, **99**, 729–49.
3. Melander, A., Danielsen, K. and Hanson, A. (1976) Reduction of isoniazid bioavailability in normal men by concomitant intake of food. *Acta Med. Scand.*, **200**, 93–7.
4. Otton, H., Pempel, M. and Siegenthaler, W. (1975) Reaction of isoniazid with antacids and food. In *Antibiotika Fiebel*, George Thieme, Stuttgart.
5. Weber, W.W. and Hein, D.W. (1979) Clinical

pharmacokinetics of isoniazid. *Clin. Pharmacokin.*, **41**, 401–22.

6. Kaojarern, S., Supmonchai K., Phuapradit, P. *et al.* (1991). The effect of steroids on cerebrospinal fluid penetration of antituberculous drugs in tuberculous meningitis. *Clin. Pharmacol. Ther*, **49**, 6–12.

7. Ellard, G.A. and Gammon, P.T. (1976) Pharmacokinetics of isoniazid metabolism in man. *J. Pharmacokinet. Biopharm.*, **4**, 83–113.

8. Price-Evans, D.A. (1992) N-acetyl transferase, in *Pharmacogenetics of Drug Metabolism* (ed. W. Kalow), Pergamon Press, New York and Oxford.

9. Evans, D.A.P, Manley, K.A and McKusik, V.A (1969) Genetic control of isoniazid metabolism in man. *Br. Med. J.*, **2**, 485–91.

10. Timbrell, J.A., Mitchell, J.R., Snodgrass, W.R. and Nelson, S.D. (1980). Isoniazid hepatotoxicity: the relationship between covalent binding and metabolism *in vivo. J. Pharmacol. Exp. Ther.*, **213**, 364–9.

11. Dollery, C. (1991) *Therapeutic Drugs.*, Churchill Livingstone, Edinburgh.

12. Holdiness, M.R. (1984) Breast feeding and antituberculous drugs. *Arch. Intern. Med.*, **144**, 1888.

13. Miceli, J.N., Olson, W.A. and Cohen, S.N. (1981) Elimination kinetics of isoniazid in the newborn infant. *Dev. Pharmacol. Ther.*, **21**, 235–9.

14. Hughes H.B, Biehl J.P, Jones A.P. and Schmidt L.H. (1954) Metabolism of isoniazid in man as related to the occurrence of peripheral neuritis. *Am. Rev. Tuberc.* **70**, 266–73.

15. Krishnamurthy, D.V., Selkon, J.B. and Ramachandran, K. (1967) Effect of pyridoxine on vitamin B6 concentrations and glutamic-oxaloacetate transaminase activity in whole blood of tuberculosis patients receiving high dose isoniazid. *Bull. WHO*, **36**, 853–70.

16. Dickinson, D.S., Bailey, W.C., Hirschowitz, B.I., *et al.* (1981) Risk factors for isoniazid (INH)-induced liver dysfunction. *J. Clin. Gastroenterol.*, **3**, 271–9.

17. Rothfield, N.F., Biere, W.F., and Garfield, J.W. (1978) Isoniazid induction of antinuclear antibodies. *Ann. Intern. Med.*, **88**, 650–2.

18. Goldberg, A., Moore, M.R., McColl, K.E.L. and Brodie, M.J. (1987) Porphyrin metabolism and the porphyrias, in *Oxford Textbook of Medicine* (eds D.J. Weatherall, J.G.G. Ledingham and D.A. Warrell, Oxford Medical Publications, Oxford.

19. Wehrli, W. (1983) Rifampicin: mechanisms of action and resistance. *Rev. Inf. Dis.*, **5** (Suppl. 3), S407–S411.

20. Polasa, K. and Krishnaswamy, K. (1983) Effect of food on bioavailability of rifampicin. *J. Clin. Pharmacol.*, **23**, 433–7.

21. Boman, G. (1974) Serum concentrations and half-life of rifampicin after simultaneous oral administration of aminosalicylic acid or isoniazid. *Eur. J. Clin. Pharmacol.*, **7**, 217–25.

22. Buniva, G., Pagani, V. and Crozzi, A. (1983) Bioavailability of rifampicin capsules. *Int. J. Clin. Pharmacol Ther. Tox.*, **21**; 404–9.

23. Kiss, I.J., Farago E., Juhazs Bacsa, S. and Fabian, E. (1976) Investigation of the serum and lung tissue level of rifampicin in man. *J. Clin. Pharmacol.*, **13**, 42–7.

24. Kiss, I.J., Farago, E., Kiss, B. and Varhelyi, L. (1978) Pharmacokinetic study of rifampicin in biliary surgery. *Int. J. Clin. Pharmacol.*, **16**, 105–9.

25. Skinner, M.H., Hsieh, M., Torseth, J. *et al.* (1989) Pharmacokinetics of rifabutin. *Antimicrob. Agents Chemother.*, **33**, 1237–41.

26. Acocella, G. (1978) Clinical pharmacokinetics of rifampicin. *Clin. Pharmacokin.*, **31**, 108–27.

27. Cocchiara, G., Strolin-Benedetti, M., Vicario, G.P. *et al.* (1989) Urinary metabolism of rifabutin, a new antimycobacterial agent, in human volunteers. *Xenobiotica*, **19**, 769–80.

28. Acocella, G. and Conti, R. (1980) Interaction of rifampicin with other drugs. *Tubercle*, **61**, 171–7.

29. Kenny, M.T. and Strates, B. (1981) Metabolism and pharmacokinetics of the antibiotic rifampicin. *Drug Met. Rev.*, **12**, 159–218.

30. Acocella, G. Pagani, V., Marchetti, M. *et al.* (1971). Kinetic studies on rifampicin. *Chemotherapy*, **161**, 356–70.

31. Strolin-Benedetti, M., Efthymiopoulos, C., Sassella, D. *et al.* (1990) Autoinduction of rifabutin metabolism in man. *Xenobiotica*, **201**, 1113–19.

32. Siegal, F.P., Eilbott, D., Burger, H. *et al.* (1990) Dose-limiting toxicity of rifabutin in AIDS-related complex: a syndrome of arthralgia/arthritis. *AIDS*, **41**, 433–41.

33. Ellard, G.A., Ellard, D.R. and Allen, B.W. (1986) The bioavailability of isoniazid, rifampicin and pyrazinamide in two commercially

available combined formulations designed for use in the short-course treatment of tuberculosis. *Am. Rev. Respir. Dis.*, **133**, 1076–80.

34. Lacroix, C., Phan Hoang, T., Nouveau *et al.* (1989) Pharmacokinetics of pyrazinamide and its metabolites in healthy subjects. *Eur. J. Clin. Pharmacol*, **361**, 395–400.

35. Ellard, G.A. (1969) Absorption, metabolism and excretion of pyrazinamide in man. *Tubercle*, **501**, 144–58.

36. Scott, J.T. (1991) Drug-induced gout. *Ballieres Clin. Rheumatol.*, **5**, 39–60.

37. Donomae, I. and Yamamoto, K. (1966) Clinical evaluation of ethambutol in pulmonary tuberculosis. *Ann. N Y Acad. Sci.*, **135**, 849–81.

38. Place, V.A., Peets, E.A., Buyske, D.A. and Little, R.R. (1966) Metabolic and special studies of ethambutol in normal volunteers and tuberculosis patients. *Ann. N Y Acad. Sci.*, **135**, 775–81.

39. Mattilla, M.J., Lnnoila, M., Seppal, T. and Kroskinen, R. (1978) Effects of aluminium hydroxide and glycopyrronium on the absorption of ethambutol and alcohol in man. *Br. J. Clin. Pharmacol.*, **51**, 161–6.

40. Lee, C.S., Gambertoglio, J.G., Barter, D.C. and Benet, L.Z. (1978) Kinetics of oral ethambutol in the normal subject. *Clin. Pharmacol. Ther.*, **22**, 615–21.

41. Pilheu, J.A., Maglio, F., Cetrangolo, R. and Pleus, A.D. (1971) Concentrations of ethambutol in the cerebrospinal fluid after oral administration. *Tubercle*, **52**, 117–22.

42. Birnberger, A. and Stelter, W.J. (1981) Ethambutol concentrations in lung tissue and serum. *Praxis Pneumologie*, **35**, 1054–5.

43. Strauss, I. and Ehrhardt, F. (1970) Ethambutol absorption, excretion and dosage in patients with renal tuberculosis. *Chemotherapy*, **15**, 148–57.

44. Jenner, P.J., Ellard, G.A., Gruer, P.K., and Aber, V.R. (1984) A comparison of the blood levels and urinary excretion of ethionamide and prothionamide in man. *J. Antimicrob. Chemother.*, **13**, 267–77.

45. Cozzarelli, N.R. (1980) DNA-gyrase and the supercoiling of DNA. *Science*, **207**, 161–3.

46. Yew, W.W., Kwan, S.Y., Ma, W.K. *et al.* (1990). In-vitro activity of ofloxacin against *Mycobacterium tuberculosis* and its clinical efficacy in multiply resistant pulmonary tuberculosis. *J. Antimicrob. Chemother.*, **26**, 227–36.

47. Flor, S. (1989) Pharmacokinetics of ofloxacin. *Am. J. Med.*, **87** (Suppl.6C), 24S–30S.

48. Fillastre, J.P. (1988) Quinolones and renal failure. *Quinolones Bull.*, **41**, 1–8.

49. Holdiness, M.R. (1982) Clinical pharmacokinetics of antituberculous drugs. *Clin. Pharmacokin.*, **91**, 511–44.

50. Nunn, P., Kibuga, D., Gathua, S. *et al.* (1991) Cutaneous hypersensitivity reactions to thiacetazone in HIV-1 seropositive patients treated for tuberculosis. *Lancet*, **337**, 627–30.

51. Dollery C. (1992) Cycloserine, in *Therapeutic Drugs*, Suppl. 1, Churchill Livingstone, Edinburgh, pp. 74–7.

CHEMOTHERAPY OF TUBERCULOSIS 8b

S.L. Chan

8b.1 INTRODUCTION

Bed rest, plenty of food, fresh air and sunshine in sanatoria built on hillsides used to be the only ways to treat tuberculosis. Collapse therapy, including crush of the phrenic nerve, artificial pneumothorax and artificial pneumoperitoneum and then thoracoplasty and lung resection, were practised for some time. Chemotherapy for tuberculosis started after streptomycin (S) was discovered in the 1940s. Sputum conversion, clinical and radiological improvement occurred after 2–3 months of streptomycin treatment of pulmonary tuberculosis. These good responses, however, did not last long, and the disease soon deteriorated as resistance to streptomycin quickly developed[1]. Then it was found that combined chemotherapy with streptomycin plus para-aminosalicylic acid (PAS) prevented the emergence of strains resistant to either of the two drugs and the response to streptomycin plus PAS treatment was better than to single drug treatment[2]. The introduction of isoniazid (H) and its use by itself[3] or in combination with streptomycin or PAS in the treatment of pulmonary tuberculosis[4] further confirmed the inadequacy of monotherapy due to the onset of drug resistance, and led to the development of uniformly successful primary chemotherapy from the 1950s[5–6]. The 'standard' regimen of chemotherapy contained streptomycin plus isoniazid plus PAS and had to be given for a minimum of 18 months to 2 years. PAS could be substituted by ethambutol (E) or thiacetazone (Th) according to their acceptability and availability. Adverse reactions were common, and patients tended to stop treatment prematurely, particularly when they became symptom-free, or to take the treatment irregularly. Therefore failure of chemotherapy and multiple drug resistance occurred. In the early 1960s the Tuberculosis Research Centre, Madras, demonstrated that ambulatory domiciliary treatment was highly effective and did not expose close family contact to additional risk of infection[7]. Sanatorium treatment became less important. Then fully supervised intermittent chemotherapy to ensure drug ingestion was introduced. Streptomycin and isoniazid were given twice a week in the continuation phase of treatment after the triple drug therapy had been given for 3–6 months. For patients who failed the 'standard' regimen, pyrazinamide (Z), ethionamide (Eth) and cycloserine (Cs) given for 6 months followed by pyrazinamide and ethionamide for another 12–18 months were found to be effective. Since the introduction of rifampicin in the 1970s and the re-utilization of pyrazinamide after more experimental studies in animals, short-course chemotherapy[8,9] became the centre of interest in the treatment of tuberculosis.

8b.2 AIMS OF CHEMOTHERAPY

The aims of chemotherapy are:

1. To cure patients with minimum interference with their living in a short period of

Clinical Tuberculosis. Edited by P.D.O. Davies. Published in 1994 by Chapman & Hall, London. ISBN 0 412 48630 X

time, whether the pretreatment organisms are susceptible or resistant to the drugs.
2. To prevent death from active disease or its late effect.
3. To avoid relapse.
4. To prevent emergence of acquired drug resistance.
5. To protect the community from infection.

8b.3 MECHANISM OF DRUG TREATMENT

Antituberculosis drugs vary in their bactericidal action, sterilizing action and their ability to prevent emergence of drug resistance [8–10].

Isoniazid is a very potent bactericidal drug and can kill some 90% of the bacillary population in a patient's lesion during the first few days of chemotherapy. Its action is not influenced by change of pH but takes place after the organisms have been exposed to the drug for 24 h. It also is very effective in preventing the emergence of drug resistance.

Rifampicin is another potent bactericidal drug, which has strong sterilizing activity and can kill the intermittently metabolizing bacilli after a short exposure to the drug. It is very effective in preventing emergence of drug resistance.

Pyrazinamide is a very important sterilizing drug, and can kill the bacilli that are well protected in an acid medium inside the macrophages.

Streptomycin and ethambutol are less potently bactericidal drugs and with slightly less ability to prevent emergence of drug resistance to isoniazid and rifampicin, so their use in short-course chemotherapy is doubtful. They may have some role to play in treating patients with pre-treatment resistant organisms.

PAS and thiacetazone are less potent in bactericidal ability and less effective in preventing emergence of drug resistance, so thiacetazone can be used in the continuation treatment after an initial intensive phase when available resources do not allow the use of rifampicin for the whole course of treatment.

The sterilizing potency and efficacy of regimens containing isoniazid, rifampicin and pyrazinamide are measured by the sputum conversion rate at the end of the second month after starting treatment and the relapse rates after stopping treatment. Short-course regimens containing these drugs can achieve over 90% sputum conversion in 2 months of treatment, and a more than 90% cure rate with a relapse rate less than 5%. A further advantage of regimens containing these drugs is that patients experience fewer adverse reactions to drugs and comply with their treatment more closely. If patients default after having received 3–4 months of treatment with SHRZ, they have up to an 80% chance of cure. Even when relapses occur, the disease is still caused by susceptible organisms and can be re-treated successfully.

8b.4 SMEAR-POSITIVE PULMONARY TUBERCULOSIS

In the past 20–30 years a large number of highly effective regimens with different drug combinations for treating smear-positive pulmonary tuberculosis have been found in clinical controlled trials in both developed and developing countries (Table 8b.1). In some countries the regimens are also found to be highly effective in programme conditions. The relapse rates during 6–30 months follow-up after stopping treatment were low, below 5%. Most regimens are given for 6 months, this being the shortest duration of treatment required. Regimens that do not contain pyrazinamide in the intensive initial phase or rifampicin in the continuation phase have to be given for longer than 6 months[11–19]. Some regimens are entirely oral, given on a daily basis and self-administered. Some regimens are partially intermittent, starting with an initial daily phase followed by two

Table 8b.1   Highly effective short-course regimens

Study	Regimens[a]	Duration (mths)	Patients assessed	Bacteriological relapse (No.)	(%)	No. of doses	Ref.
2BTA 2 French	2 SHR/HR or 3 EHR/HR	9	298	3	1	266	[11,12]
US Trial 21	HR	9	204	6	3	252	[13]
East Africa	2SHRZ/ThH	8	81	0	0	238	[14,15]
	1SHRZ/SHZ$_2$	8	123	4	3	88	
	2SHRZ/H	8	88	2	2	238	[16,17]
Hong Kong	2SHRZ/SHZ$_2$	8	87	3	3	108	[18,19]
	4SHRZ$_3$/SHZ$_2$	8	83	1	1	92	
Singapore	2SHRZ/HRZ	6	78	1	1	182	[20,21]
	2SHRZ/HR	6	80	2	2	182	
	2SHRZ/HR$_3$	6	97	1	1	114	[22,23]
	1SHRZ/HR$_3$	6	94	1	1	96	
	2HRZ/HR$_3$	6	109	1	1	114	
BTA	2SHRZ/HR	6	125	1	1	182	[24]
	2EHRZ/HR	6	132	3	2	182	
Hong Kong	SHRZE$_3$	6	152	1	1	78	[25–27]
	SHRZ$_3$	6	151	2	1	78	
	HRZE$_3$	6	160	4	2	78	
	HRZE	6	163	2	1	182	
	2SHRZ$_3$/ 2SHR$_3$/HR$_3$	6	149	4	3	78	[28]
	4SHRZ$_3$/HR$_3$	6	133	8	6	78	
	4SHRZ$_3$/HRZ$_3$	6	142	2	1	78	
	HRZ$_3$	6	135	6	4	78	
Polish	2HRZ/HR$_2$	6	116	4	4	96	[29]
	2SHRZ/HR$_2$	6	56	1	2	96	
Denver	½SHRZ/ 1½SHRZ$_2$/HR$_2$	6	125	2	2	62	[30]
US Trial 21	2HRZ/HR	6	273	10	4	168	[13]

H, isoniazid; R, rifampicin; Z, pyrazinamide; S, streptomycin; E, ethambutol; Th, thiacetazone.
[a] Number before a group of letters represents number of months in the initial phase of that group of drugs. Number after a group of letters represents number of doses of the drugs per week. A group of letters followed by no number means the group of drugs is given daily.

times or three times weekly in the continuation phase. Some regimens are fully intermittent, given three times a week throughout.

Intermittent treatment with streptomycin, PAS and isoniazid had been studied before the introduction of short-course chemotherapy. Streptomycin and isoniazid twice a week had been used in the continuation phase of the 'standard' treatment[31]. Rifampicin given once a week in high dosage caused various and severe adverse reactions[32], therefore it is recommended that it be used twice or three times a week in a usual dosage of 600 mg and not in any dosage more than 900 mg. Rifampicin, in combination with isoniazid plus or minus other drugs, given in a dosage of 600 mg once a week, was found acceptable and effective in Singapore and Hong Kong[33,34].

The advantages of intermittent short-course regimens are: (i) they are equally or more effective than the daily short-course regimens; (ii) they cause less drug toxicity; (iii) they contain fewer doses of medications than the daily regimens; and (iv) they can be given under full supervision or direct observation. However, there are difficulties in organizing intermittent chemotherapy under direct observation, particularly in large countries, and the large bulk of medicine to be taken in one single dose may not be tolerated by some patients.

The daily 9-month regimen consists of 266 doses, the daily 6-month regimen consists of 182 doses. On the other hand the fully intermittent 6-month regimen consists of 78 doses. The Denver group in the USA[30] also found a 6-month regimen consisting of 62 doses was very effective in treating patients with pulmonary tuberculosis caused by susceptible organisms in places where the level of initial drug resistance is low. Fewer doses of medication are better accepted or preferred by the patients and probably reduce the drug cost of treatment regimens. However, every dose of medication is very important for the efficacy of the treatment regimen and ideally not a single dose should be missed.

The Singapore Study[20–21] comparing 2SHRZ/4HRZ with 2SHRZ/4HR and the Hong Kong Studies[28] on 6-month regimens containing 2 months, 4 months or 6 months of pyrazinamide confirmed that pyrazinamide need only be given for the first 2 months in 6-month regimens with isoniazid and rifampicin used throughout. The Polish Study[29] and the Singapore Study[22–23] showed that streptomycin need not be added to the initial phase of this 6-month regimen of HRZ/HR, and this is confirmed by the Hong

Kong Study[28]. However, Hong Kong still uses streptomycin as the fourth drug in the programme regimen to prevent a small number of chemotherapy failures. The same Hong Kong Study[28] that compared different durations of pyrazinamide, the Singapore Study[35] that compared 1 month and 2 months of SHRZ in the initial phase of treatment followed by HR3 in the continuation phase, and the US Trial 21[36], all compared the efficacy of a fixed-dose combination, Rifater, which contained isoniazid, rifampicin and pyrazinamide in a single preparation, with that of the same three drugs given in separate formulations. The results differed in these studies. The Hong Kong Study[28] showed that the fixed-dose combination for intermittent use was as effective as when the drugs were given in separate formulations but no difference in drug toxicity and patient compliance was found. The Singapore Study[35] showed that the daily preparation of Rifater was not so effective as when the drugs were given in separate formulations, as the relapse rate in patients taking Rifater was slightly higher. The US Trial 21[36] found that the daily preparation of Rifater was as effective as the drugs in their separate formulations. There was no difference in the relapse rate among the two groups, but patients taking Rifater had a quicker conversion of sputum and a higher incidence of drug toxicity. Despite the different findings from different studies in different places, Rifater has its advantages because, by using it, monotherapy with consequent emergence of resistant bacteria can be prevented, adjustment of dosage of drug with body weight is easier, and the bulk of medicine is reduced. However, only the fixed-dose combination whose bioavailability has been tested and assured should be used. It has been found that some preparations are of poor quality[37], and the rifampicin content of the preparations is actually not biologically available.

The 8-month regimen 2SHRZ/6ThH com-

Table 8b.2 Results of treatment in 41,720 new smear-positive patients enrolled on short-course chemotherapy (2SHRZ/6HTh) in IUATLD-assisted National Tuberculosis Programmes in Tanzania, Malawi, Mozambique and Nicaragua, 1983–88

Country	*Percentage of patients*				
	Cured	*Positive*	*Died*	*Absconded*	*Transferred out*
Tanzania	77	2	7	10	4
Malawi	87	1	7	2	2
Mozambique	78	1	2	11	8
Nicaragua	78	2	3	13	5
Total	79	2	6	9	4

bined with hospitalization for the first 2 months has been found to be very effective, not only in clinical controlled trials in East Africa[14,15] but also in programme conditions, as shown in Table 8b.2, by the high cure rate of 80–85% in the International Union Against Tuberculosis and Lung Disease (IUATLD) assisted national tuberculosis control programme[38]. This regimen is therefore recommended to be used in developing countries when resources are not adequate for using rifampicin for 6 months, where thiacetazone is well tolerated and where the level of resistance to isoniazid is low[39].

The British Thoracic Association now recommends, 2HRE/7HR, 2SHRZ/4HR or 2HRZ/4HR to be used in the UK. The former two regimens have been well studied in the country[40–42].

The American Thoracic Society recommends 9HR, or 2HRZ/4HR to be used in the USA, provided that no problem of drug resistance is to be encountered[43].

The IUATLD[39] and the World Health Organization (WHO)[44] recommend 2HRZ/4HR or 2HRZ/4HR$_3$ or 2HRZ/4HR$_2$ for treating smear-positive pulmonary tuberculosis in affluent countries. Streptomycin or ethambutol is used as a fourth drug when there is a high suspicion of initial drug resistance to isoniazid or isoniazid and streptomycin. In less affluent countries 2SHRZ/6ThH or 2SHRZ/6EH is recommended. Whenever

possible, treatment should be given under direct observation. Hospitalization *per se* has no advantage in the treatment of tuberculosis and increases the cost. However, in the IUATLD-assisted programme, hospitalization for the first 2 months can ensure that patients take the drugs and can educate the patients to take the drugs continuously after discharge, when the drugs are self-administered.

8b.5 DISEASE CAUSED BY ORGANISMS INITIALLY RESISTANT TO DRUGS

Initial drug resistance has, for a long time, been recognized as an important factor causing failure in chemotherapy, and in order to prevent further emergence of drug resistance during treatment of tuberculosis, multiple drugs are used[1–4]. Whenever the organisms are found by laboratory sensitivity tests to be resistant to certain drugs, there is a tendency to change the treatment accordingly with no regard to whether the disease is responding to the treatment or to whether the laboratory results are accurate and reliable. A study in Hong Kong[45], a place where initial resistance to one or more of the drugs, isoniazid, streptomycin and PAS, was high at time of study, compared three policies of treatment.

Policy A: Standard chemotherapy with daily streptomycin, isoniazid and PAS was given either for 3 or 6 months at random followed by isoniazid plus PAS, without reference to the results of the pretreatment standard susceptibility tests.

Policy B: Standard chemotherapy with daily streptomycin, isoniazid and PAS was given until the results of the pretreatment standard indirect susceptibility tests were available. Ethionamide was substituted for the period of the triple chemotherapy if pretreatment resistance to any one of the standard drugs was found, and three reserve drugs followed by two reserve drugs were given for resistance to two or all three standard drugs.

Policy C: Before the start of treatment, a slide culture susceptibility test was performed. Treatment was then initiated either with standard chemotherapy with daily streptomycin, isoniazid and PAS if the patient had a fully susceptible strain, or if the patient was found to have a strain resistant to one or more of the standard drugs, with the appropriate combination of standard drug to which the organisms were sensitive plus one or more reserve drugs.

Results of the study showed that for all patients, 89% of Policy A, 92% of Policy B and 94% of Policy C achieved a favourable response. There was no difference in response to the three policies for patients with susceptible strains. For patients with resistant strains, patients in Policy A did less well than in Policy B and C, however the difference was not very great. Despite the fact that 30% of patients in the study had drug resistance to one or more of the three standard drugs – 18% to one drug, 6% to two drugs and 6% to all three drugs – the benefits from acting on the results of accurate indirect susceptibility tests or the direct slide culture susceptibility tests were small, and indeed no greater than that which would have been obtained if the failure of standard chemotherapy, resulting from irregularity in self-administration of oral chemotherapy in patients with fully susceptible organisms, could be avoided. The relative merits of

ignoring the pretreatment susceptibility tests or acting on them must take into consideration the incidence of drug toxicity, the cost of treatment and the reliability of susceptibility test services.

The influence of initial drug resistance on the response to short-course chemotherapy of pulmonary tuberculosis has been fully assessed by Mitchison and Nunn[46] in patients who were admitted into 12 controlled trials carried out in Africa, Hong Kong and Singapore in collaboration with the British Medical Research Council. Among those patients who had pulmonary tuberculosis caused by *Mycobacterium tuberculosis* resistant to isoniazid and/or streptomycin, 17% of patients given a 6-month regimen of isoniazid and rifampicin and 12% of patients given rifampicin in the initial 2-month intensive phase of their regimen failed during chemotherapy. The proportion of failures fell as the number of drugs in the regimen and the duration of treatment with rifampicin were increased, to only 2% of patients who received four or five drugs including rifampicin throughout in 6-month regimens. The sterilizing activity of the regimens, whether these included rifampicin or pyrazinamide, was little influenced by initial resistance, because the sputum conversion rate at 2 months was similar to that in patients with initially sensitive bacilli, and the relapse rates after chemotherapy were only a little higher. However, among the small number of patients with initial rifampicin resistance the response was much less good.

The Hong Kong Studies[25–27] comparing 6-month regimens containing isoniazid, rifampicin, pyrazinamide plus streptomycin or ethambutol or plus streptomycin and ethambutol, and the Hong Kong Study[28] comparing 6-month regimens with isoniazid and rifampicin throughout and pyrazinamide for either 2, 4 or 6 months, showed that all regimens are equally effective in treating patients with pulmonary tuberculosis caused by organisms resistant to isoniazid and/or streptomycin. There were a small number of failures and a low relapse rate. These regimens were less effective in treating patients with rifampicin resistance. When rifampicin or pyrazinamide were not given in the continuation phase of such regimens as 2SHRZ/ThH the relapse rate in patients with initial isoniazid resistance were four to five times higher than in those with initially sensitive bacilli.

It can be assumed that 6-month regimens containing isoniazid, rifampicin and pyrazinamide with or without a fourth and fifth drug such as streptomycin and ethambutol in the initial phase and isoniazid and rifampicin in the continuation phase of treatment are highly effective in treating smear-positive pulmonary tuberculosis whether the disease is caused by organisms fully sensitive to all drugs or resistant to isoniazid and/or streptomycin. Sensitivity tests may not be required before treatment for new patients when resources are limited and need only be done when treatment fails to provide some guidelines for choice of drugs in further treatment. As regimens with four or five drugs are not effective when there is rifampicin resistance, the development of rifampicin resistance has to be avoided by all means in designing treatment regimens and their administration. Treatment of multiple drug-resistant disease is very difficult and costly, with a low success rate. At least three drugs to which the organisms are still susceptible have to be used. The more drugs are available the better the chance of cure. Treatment of such groups of patients should not be given priority in countries with limited resources[44].

8b.6 SMEAR-NEGATIVE PULMONARY TUBERCULOSIS

In many developed and developing countries nearly half of the patients are diagnosed to have active tuberculosis on clinical and radiographic grounds without immediate bacteriological confirmation and are put on treatment. There has always been the question to treat or not to treat this group of patients[47]. It is necessary to determine what proportion of patients with smear-negative disease in different populations do indeed have active tuberculosis requiring treatment, what regimen is effective and what duration of treatment is sufficient. The first Hong Kong Study[48] of 1019 patients with smear-negative, radiographically active pulmonary tuberculosis showed that 36% of patients had one or more initial sputum cultures positive for M. *tuberculosis* and chemotherapy with isoniazid, rifampicin, pyrazinamide and streptomycin given daily for 2 or 3 months was not adequate. Relapse rates of 32% and 13% respectively occurred during 60 months of follow-up in patients with one or more initial cultures positive, even when the organisms were fully sensitive to the four drugs. Relapse rates were 11% and 7% respectively in patients with all their initial cultures negative. In the group of patients who were allocated to the selective chemotherapy series, anti-tuberculosis chemotherapy being witheld until active disease had been confirmed either bacteriologically or radiographically, 57% of the patients were started on treatment within 60 months. The second Hong Kong Study[49] of 1710 patients, again with smear-negative, radiographically active pulmonary tuberculosis but without using the selective chemotherapy series as a control group, showed that 35% of patients had one or more initial sputum cultures positive for *M. tuberculosis*. Over 5 years, the combined relapse rate was 7% for regimens with isoniazid, rifampicin, pyrazinamide and streptomycin given daily or three times a week for 3 months and 4% for the same four-drug regimen given daily or three times weekly for 4-month in patients who were all culture-negative initially. The relapse rate for the 4 month regimen was 2% in patients with drug-susceptible cultures initially and 8% in patients with culture resistant to isoniazid, streptomycin or both drugs but susceptible to rifampicin initially. There was no significant difference between the relapse rates among patients allocated for the 4-month or 6-month regimens of the same four drugs. The Arkansas group in the USA[50] treated a group of patients with positive tuberculin reaction, abnormal chest radiographs and negative bacteriology with isoniazid and rifampicin daily for 1 month, followed by isoniazid and rifampicin twice a week for 3 months (a 4-month regimen), and found that 30% of patients showed radiographic and/or clinical response, suggesting active disease. No resistant organisms were encountered.

Clinical tuberculosis, even in the absence of positive smear and culture, based on the results of the studies mentioned, should be treated whenever available resources allow. Four-month regimens of daily HRZ or HRZ$_3$ for 2 months followed by HR or HR$_3$ for another 2 months are recommended by the World Health Organization for treating such groups of patients[44]. In countries with an expected high level of drug resistance to isoniazid, streptomycin or ethambutol may be added to the initial 2 months, and for developing countries where resources are under constraint, the continuation treatment may be replaced by 6 months of HE or HTh.

8b.7 USE OF OFLOXACIN IN THE TREATMENT OF TUBERCULOSIS

Ofloxacin, an oxazine derivative, has been demonstrated to have antituberculosis activity in laboratories[51,52]. Its therapeutic effect in the treatment of patients with newly diagnosed pulmonary tuberculosis[53] and patients with chronic cavitatory pulmonary tuberculosis[54] were also reported. In a study in Hong Kong on treatment of patients with pulmonary tuberculosis resistant to streptomycin, isoniazid and rifampicin, 17 patients were treated with ofloxacin alone or with companion antituberculosis drugs to which the organisms were still sensitive.

Among 14 patients with strains susceptible to ofloxacin or in whom susceptibility test results were not available, ten showed a response, one to ofloxacin alone; in seven of the ten this was temporary but in the remaining three treated with ofloxacin for 12, 18 and 18 months respectively, the disease was rendered quiescent[55].

The role of ofloxacin in the treatment of new patients requires evaluation. A starting dose of 800 mg followed by 600 mg of ofloxacin was well tolerated with no severe adverse reaction. Ofloxacin can be used for patients with impaired liver function when other hepatotoxic drugs are not allowed.

8b.8 DRUG DOSAGE

For simplicity the dosages of drugs that are commonly used in short-course chemotherapy, either daily or intermittently, are shown in Table 8b.3. It is now agreed that isoniazid 5 mg/kg body weight is adequate for both adults and children, and higher dosages of this drug for children or for tuberculous meningits and miliary tuberculosis is not required but may lead to a more adverse reaction, such as hepatitis.

8b.9 ADVERSE REACTIONS TO DRUGS

The important reactions to the main antituberculosis drugs are listed in Table 8b.4.

In the three Hong Kong clinical studies to evaluate regimens containing isoniazid, rifampicin, pyrazinamide and streptomycin in the treatment of smear-positive or smear-negative pulmonary tuberculosis[25,28,49], 25–60% of a large number of patients reported they had experienced at least one type of adverse reaction. However, most of the reactions were mild and trivial and required no modification of treatment. The most common adverse reactions were gastrointestinal, in the form of nausea and vomiting, and cutaneous; less common were vestibular effects and hepatitis. Adverse re-

Table 8b.3 Dosages of the main antituberculosis drugs

Drug	Daily dosage			Intermittent dosage		
	Adults and children (mg/kg)	Adults		Adults and children (mg/kg)	Adults	
		Weight	Dose		Weight	Dose
Isoniazid	5	—	300 mg	15	—	—
Rifampicin	10	<50 kg	450 mg	15	—	600–900 mg
		≥50 kg	600 mg			
Streptomycin	15–20	<50 kg	750 mg	15–20	<50 kg	750 mg
		≥50 kg	1 g		≥50 kg	1 g
Pyrazinamide	25–35	<50 kg	1.5 g	50	<50 kg	2.0 g
		≥50 kg	2.0 g	3 times/week	≥50 kg	2.5 g
				75	<50 kg	3.0 g
				twice/week	≥50 kg	3.5 g
Ethambutol	25 for 2 months, then 15	—		30 3 times/week	—	—
				45 twice/week		
Thiacetazone	4 (for children)	—	150 mg	—	—	—
Rifater		per 10 kg	1 tablet			
		>60 kg	6 tablets			
Ethionamide	15–20	<50 kg	750 mg			
Prothionamide	(adults)	≥50 kg	1 g			
Cycloserine	15	<50 kg	750 mg			
	(adults)	≥50 kg	1 g			

actions tended to occur in the first 3 months of treatment. Only about 10% or less of patients had treatment interrupted for 7 days or longer and about 8% of patients or less had one or more drugs, more frequently streptomycin and pyrazinamide, terminated. Hepatitis was defined as raised serum alanine aminotransferase with or without jaundice. An overall 2% of patients were reported to have hepatitis and very few patients had jaundice. It is often possible to resume chemotherapy after the liver function has reverted to normal without recurrence of hepatitis.

Peripheral neuropathy caused by isoniazid is usually preventable by an adequate intake of pyridosine (vitamin B6). It is usual practice in some countries to prescribe pyridosine 10 mg/day when isoniazid is given to patients on a poor diet.

Arthralgia can occur during pyrazinamide administration. It is less likely to occur during intermittent than during daily administration and is usually mild and self-limited and responds well to symptomatic treatment.

If a serious reaction to rifampicin occurs, such as thrombocytopenic purpura, shock, haemolytic anaemia or acute renal failure, the drugs should be withdrawn immediately and never given again.

Rifampicin is a powerful enzyme inducer and may therefore cause reduction in serum concentrations of other drugs the patient may be taking. This is of particular importance for

Table 8b.4   Adverse reactions to the main antituberculosis drugs

| Drug | Reactions | | |
	Common	Uncommon	Rare
Isoniazid		Hepatitis Cutaneous hypersensitivity Peripheral neuropathy	Giddiness Convulsion Optic neuritis Mental symptoms Haemolytic anaemia Aplastic anaemia Agranulocytosis Lupoid reactions Arthralgia Gynaecomastia
Rifampicin		Hepatitis Cutaneous reactions Gastrointestinal reactions Thrombocytopenic purpura Febrile reactions 'Flu syndrome'	Shortness of breath Shock Haemolytic anaemia Acute renal failure
Pyrazinamide	Anorexia Nausea Flushing	Hepatitis Vomiting Arthralgia Cutaneous hypersensitivity	Sideroblastic anaemia Photosensitization
Ethambutol		Retrobulbar neuritis Arthralgia	Hepatitis Cutaneous hypersensitivity Peripheral neuropathy
Streptomycin	Cutaneous hypersensitivity Giddiness Numbness Tinnitus	Vertigo Ataxia Deafness	Renal damage Aplastic anaemia Agranulocytosis

Thiacetazone	Gastrointestinal
	  reactions
	Cutaneous
	  hypersensitivity
	Vertigo
	Conjunctivitis
		Hepatitis
		Erythema multiforme
		Exfoliative dermatitis
		Haemolytic anaemia
			Agranulocytosis

women using a contraceptive pill. They should be warned that rifampicin may reduce the efficiency of the pill so that alternative contraception should be used. Rifampicin also reduces serum concentrations of corticosteroids so that the dose should be doubled during rifampicin administration. A full list of drugs that are affected by rifampicin administration is given in Table 8a.1. Patients should be warned that their urine and other body fluids may be turned red.

When a hypersensitivity (allergic) reaction

Table 8b.5 Challenge doses for detecting cutaneous or generalized hypersensitivity to antituberculosis drugs

| Drug | Challenge doses | |
	Day 1	Day 2
Isoniazid	50 mg	300 mg
Rifampicin	75 mg	300 mg
Pyrazinamide	250 mg	1.0 g
Ethambutol	100 mg	500 mg
Thiacetazone	25 mg	50 mg
Streptomycin or other aminoglycosides	125 mg	500 mg

Reproduced with permission from D.J. Girling (1987) *Oxford Textbook of Medicine*, 2nd edn (eds D.J. Weatherall, J.C.G. Ledingham and D.A. Warnell), Oxford University Press, Oxford, p. 5.295.

occurs, all chemotherapy has to be stopped until the reaction has subsided. Once the reaction has subsided the drug or drugs responsible for the reaction have to be identified. The daily challenge doses to the drugs that are least likely to have caused the reaction should be started so that administration of these can be resumed with the minimum delay while (if necessary) challenge doses and desensitizing doses of other drugs are administered. A challenge dose of each drug of the regimen should be given in the sequence in which they are shown in Table 8b.5 until a reaction occurs. If no reaction occurs to either of the challenge doses shown in Table 8b.5, administration of that drug should be continued in full dosage. If the reaction was a particularly severe one, smaller initial challenge doses should be used. These may be approximately one-tenth of the doses shown under day 1.

If a reaction occurs with the first challenge dose, as shown in Table 8b.5, it is known that the patient is hypersensitive to that drug. When starting to desensitize it is usually safe to begin with a tenth of the normal dose. Then the dose is increased by a tenth each day. If the patient has a mild reaction to a dose, the same dose (instead of a higher dose) is given next day. If there is no

reaction, the dose is to be increased again by a tenth each day. If the reaction is severe (which is unusual), a lower dose is used and then increased more gradually.

If a reaction occurs with the second challenge dose as shown in Table 8b.5, desensitization can be started with the first challenge dose and then the dose is increased by the amount equal to the first challenge dose each day.

Some patients may need antihistamine or steroid to control the severe reaction. If steroid is required, prednisolone 15 mg three times a day can be used and then the dose reduced gradually. For very severe drug reactions, hydrocortisone 200 mg or dexamethasone 4 mg i.v. or i.m. have to be given immediately and then substituted by oral steroid. In these cases desensitization should not be attempted.

If other effective drugs are available it is easier to substitute another drug for the one that has caused the reaction.

8b.10 CHEMOTHERAPY IN SPECIAL SITUATIONS

There are special problems that occur from time to time and which may require modification of treatment regimens and the dosage of drugs.

8b.10.1 RENAL IMPAIRMENT AND RENAL FAILURE

Antituberculosis drugs such as isoniazid, rifampicin, pyrazinamide, ethionamide and prothionamide are eliminated almost entirely by other than renal routes, namely by metabolism or by biliary excretion. They can be given in normal dosage to patients in renal failure. Fortunately, the safest antituberculosis drugs for patients with impaired renal function are also the most potent: isoniazid and rifampicin. In severe renal failure, it is recommended that 200 mg isoniazid be given daily with pyridoxine supplement to avoid peripheral neuropathy.

Streptomycin and other aminoglycosides are excreted exclusively and ethambutol predominantly by the kidney. If they are to be given to patients with impaired renal function their dosages must be adjusted according to the degree of impairment. Serum concentration of streptomycin should be monitored and not allowed to exceed 5 μg/ml, and the drug given 8 h before dialysis in severe renal failure. Ethambutol, if necessary, should be given in a dosage of 25 mg/kg three times a week to patients with a creatinine clearance of between 50 and 100 ml/min and twice a week to patients with a creatinine clearance of between 30 and 50 ml/min. In severe renal failure, ethambutol should be given 8 h before dialysis. Whenever possible, serum concentration of ethambutol should be monitored but unfortunately there is no simple way to do it.

Thiacetazone and PAS are partly excreted unchanged in the urine and partly metabolized and both are weak antituberculosis drugs. Moreover, the difference between a toxic and a therapeutically adequate dose of thiacetazone is small, and the gastrointestinal effects of PAS can potentiate or exacerbate acidosis in patients with impaired renal function. Both drugs should be avoided.

8b.10.2 LIVER IMPAIRMENT AND LIVER FAILURE

Isoniazid, rifampicin, pyrazinamide and ethionamide are recognized to be hepatotoxic but there is very little data or evidence to support an increased risk of precipitating or exacerbating acute hepatitis by antituberculosis drugs, particularly in the alcoholic or in persons who are hepatitis B antigen carriers, or who have had hepatitis of some kind in the past. Whenever possible, isoniazid and rifampicin together with one or two other non-hepatotoxic drugs should be used, so that the duration of treatment will not be too long. Streptomycin plus isoniazid plus ethambutol followed by isoniazid plus eth-

ambutol daily or streptomycin and isoniazid twice a week may be the alternate regimen of choice, provided no bleeding tendency is evident.

8b.10.3 PREGNANCY

There is no evidence that isoniazid, rifampicin, pyrazinamide and ethambutol are teratogenic and cause congenital malformations in humans, and these drugs are safe to be used in treating patients who are pregnant. Streptomycin is potently ototoxic and may cause deafness in the babies and therefore should not be given. Ethionamide and prothionamide have been shown to be teratogenic to an important degree and should be avoided in pregnancy. Active tuberculosis in pregnancy needs to be treated because the disease may do more harm than the drugs.

8b.10.4 HIV INFECTION[56–58]

The 6-month regimen of 2HRZ/4HR is quite safe for treating tuberculosis among HIV-infected individuals and the response is expected to be as good as in the non-HIV-infected. However there is some evidence that drug reactions occur more commonly during treatment, particularly to thiacetazone. Higher relapse rates are found among those with HIV infection so that more prolonged treatment may be required. More research in this field needs to be done.

8b.10.5 SILICOSIS

It is recognized that silicotic patients are very prone to develop active pulmonary tuberculosis and are more difficult to treat because in such patients the function of the alveolar macrophages is impaired, and penetration of drugs to the diseased sites may be impaired by the presence of massive fibrosis. In Hong Kong, a rocky island of granite and a place where the building industry prospers, silicosis is a common disease and at one time 40% of the silicotic patients were found to suffer from active pulmonary tuberculosis. A study[59] on such patients showed that with a regimen of HRZS$_3$, ethambutol being added in the first 3 months if there was a history of previous chemotherapy, 6 months' treatment is not adequate. A relapse rate of 22% during 3 years and 33% during 5 years occurred, compared with only 7% during 3 years in patients treated for 8 months. The study also showed slower conversion of sputum in the silicotic patients than in the non-silicotic ones even when the same four- or five-drug regimens were given. Only 80% of the studied group had negative-sputum culture at 2 months after treatment.

8b.11 COMPLIANCE

The most important factor influencing the response to chemotherapy with effective regimens is compliance[60–62]. Whereas bed rest, diet, sanatorium accommodation and nursing are not important, the extent of radiographic disease and initial drug resistance are relatively important[63]. Compliance not only concerns the patients' adherence to treatment but involves all stages from the manufacture to the ingestion of drugs. It has been well recognized that the 'standard' chemotherapy of long duration frequently failed because patients tended to stop treatment prematurely, particularly when they became symptom-free, or took treatment irregularly. This often resulted not only in chemotherapy failure but also in the development of multiple drug-resistant disease, which could be transmitted. Constant and consistent drug supply and appropriate prescription by the practising physicians are as important as the patients' adherence to treatment. Failure is frequently caused by interruption of drug supply. It has also been recognized from different surveys[41] that, despite ample evidence supporting the effectiveness of short-course regimens, a considerable proportion of practising physicians

do not follow the recommendations made by different authorities on drug combination, drug dosage, rhythm of administration and duration of treatment. Not infrequently, drugs are given in divided doses rather than in a single (daily) dose although drugs given in a single dose are found to be more effective in killing the organisms. Wallace Fox concluded in his article on compliance of patients and physicians[64,65], that, 'as with patients' compliance, it is by pooling experience from different disciplines and by combining experimental and observational approaches, that we can best learn how to change the practices of clinicians rather than just informing the medical profession of recent development and current thinking'.

The factors that determine non-compliance of patients are complex and involve poorly understood human behaviours, features of the clinic setting, the type and duration of therapy, adverse effects and costs[60,61]. Directly observed therapy is the only system that assures compliance. The Centers for Disease Control, the American Thoracic Society and the American College of Chest Physicians, WHO and IUATLD strongly recommended directly observed therapy for patients whenever necessary[30,43,66], particularly when using intermittent regimens consisting of fewer doses of medication.

REFERENCES

1. Medical Research Council (1948) A Medical Research Council Investigation. Streptomycin treatment of pulmonary tuberculosis. *Br. Med. J.*, **ii**, 769–82.
2. Medical Research Council (1950) A Medical Research Council Investigation. Treatment of pulmonary tuberculosis with streptomycin and para-aminosalicylic acid. *Br. Med. J.*, **ii**, 1073–85.
3. Medical Research Council (1952) The treatment of pulmonary tuberculosis with isoniazid, an interim report to the Medical Research Council by their Tuberculosis Chemotherapy Trials Committee. *Br. Med. J.*, **ii**, 735–46.
4. Medical Research Council (1955) Various com-

binations of isoniazid with streptomycin or with PAS in the treatment of pulmonary tuberculosis. Seventh report to the Medical Research Council by their Tuberculosis Chemotherapy Trials Committee. *Br. Med. J.,* i, 434–45.

5. Crofton, J. (1960) Drug treatment of tuberculosis. Standard chemotherapy, *Br. Med. J.,* ii, 370–3.

6. British Medical Research Council Co-operative Study (1973) Co-operative controlled trial of a standard regimen of streptomycin, PAS and isoniazid and three alternative regimens of chemotherapy in Britain. *Tubercle,* **54,** 99.

7. Tuberculosis Chemotherapy Centre, Madras (1959) A concurrent comparison of home and sanatorium treatment of pulmonary tuberculosis in South India. *Bull. WHO,* **21,** 51.

8. Fox, W. and Mitchison, D.A. (1975) Short course chemotherapy for pulmonary tuberculosis. *Am. Rev. Respir. Dis.,* **111,** 325–53.

9. Fox, W. (1981) Whither short course chemotherapy? *Bull. Int. Union Tuberc.* **56**(3–4), 135–55.

10. Mitchison, D.A. (1981) Basis of chemotherapy, in *Respiratory Medicine* (eds T.G. Scadding, Gordon Cumming and W.M. Thurbeck, Scientific Foundation, London, pp. 377–9.

11. British Thoracic and Tuberculosis Association (1976) Short course chemotherapy in pulmonary tuberculosis. *Lancet,* ii, 1102–4.

12. British Thoracic Association (1980) Short course chemotherapy in pulmonary tuberculosis. *Lancet,* i, 1182–3.

13. Combs, D.L., O'Brien, R. and Geiter, L. (1990) USPHS tuberculosis short course chemotherapy trial 21. Effectiveness, toxicity and acceptability. The report of final results. *Ann. Intern. Med.,* **112,** 397–406.

14. Third East African/British Medical Research Council Study (1978) First report: Controlled clinical trial of four short course regimens of chemotherapy for two durations in the treatment of pulmonary tuberculosis. *Am. Rev. Respir. Dis.,* **118,** 39.

15. Third East African/British Medical Research Council Study (1980) Second report: Controlled clinical trial of four short course regimens of chemotherapy for two durations in the treatment of pulmonary tuberculosis. *Tubercle,* **61,** 59–69.

16. Fifth East African/British Medical Research Council Study (1983) First report: Controlled clinical trial of four short course regimens

of chemotherapy (three 6-month and one 8-month) for pulmonary tuberculosis. **64,** 153–66.

17. Fifth East African/British Medical Research Council Study (1986) Final report: Controlled clinical trial of four short course regimens of chemotherapy (three 6-month and one 8-month) for pulmonary tuberculosis. *Tubercle,* **67,** 5–15.

18. Hong Kong Chest Service/British Medical Research Council Study (1978) First report: Controlled trial of 6-month and 8-month regimens in the treatment of pulmonary tuberculosis. *Am. Rev. Respir. Dis.* **118** 219–27.

19. Hong Kong Chest Service/British Medical Research Council Study (1979) Controlled trial of 6-month and 8-month regimens in the treatment of pulmonary tuberculosis. The results up to 24 months. *Tubercle,* **60,** 201–10.

20. Singapore Tuberculosis Service/British Medical Research Council (1979) Clinical trial of 6-month and 4-month regimens of chemotherapy in the treatment of pulmonary tuberculosis. *Am. Rev. Respir. Dis.,* **119,** 579–85.

21. Singapore Tuberculosis Service/British Medical Research Council (1981) Clinical trial of 6-month and 4-month regimens of chemotherapy in the treatment of pulmonary tuberculosis. The results up to 30 months. *Tubercle,* **61,** 95–102.

22. Singapore Tuberculosis Service/British Medical Research Council (1985) Clinical trial of three 6-month regimens of chemotherapy given intermittently in the continuation phase in the treatment of pulmonary tuberculosis. *Am. Rev. Respir. Dis.,* **132,** 374–8.

23. Singapore Tuberculosis Service/British Medical Research Council (1988) Five year follow-up of a clinical trial of three 6-month regimens of chemotherapy given intermittently in the continuation phase in the treatment of pulmonary tuberculosis. *Am. Rev. Respir. Dis.,* **137,** 1147–150.

24. British Thoracic Society (1984) A controlled trial of 6-month chemotherapy in pulmonary tuberculosis. Final report: Results during 36 months after the end of chemotherapy and beyond. *Br. J. Dis. Chest,* **78,** 330–6.

25. Hong Kong Chest Service/British Medical Research Council (1981) First report: Controlled trial of four thrice-weekly regimens and a daily regimen all given for 6 months for pulmonary tuberculosis. *Lancet,* i, 171–4.

26. Hong Kong Chest Service/British Medical Research Council (1982) Second report: Controlled trial of four thrice-weekly regimens and a daily regimen all given for 6 months for pulmonary tuberculosis. The results up to 24 months. *Tubercle*, **63** 89–98.

27. Hong Kong Chest Service/British Medical Research Council (1987) Five-year follow up of a controlled trial of five 6-month regimens of chemotherapy for pulmonary tuberculosis. *Am. Rev. Respir. Dis.*, **136**, 1339–42.

28. Hong Kong Chest Service/British Medical Research Council (1991) Controlled trial of 2, 4 and 6 months of pyrazinamide in 6-month, three-times-weekly regimens for smear-positive pulmonary tuberculosis, including an assessment of a combined preparation of isoniazid, rifampicin and pyrazinamide. Results at 30 months. *Am. Rev. Respir. Dis.*, **143**, 700–6.

29. Snider, D.E., Graczyk, J., Bek, E. and Rogowski, J. (1984) Supervised six-months' treatment of newly diagnosed pulmonary tuberculosis using isoniazid, rifampin and pyrazinamide with and without streptomycin. *Am. Rev. Respir. Dis.*, **130**, 1091–4.

30. Cohn, D.L., Catlin, B.J., Peterson, K.L. *et al.* (1990) A 62-dose, 6-month therapy for pulmonary and extrapulmonary tuberculosis. A twice-weekly, directly observed, and cost-effective regimen. *Ann. Intern. Med.* **112**, 407–15.

31. Fox, W. (1971) General considerations in intermittent drug therapy of pulmonary tuberculosis. *Post*grad. *Med. J.*, **47**, 729–36.

32. Aquinas, M., Allan, W.G.L. and Horsfall, P.A.L. (1972) Adverse reactions to daily and intermittent rifampicin regimens for pulmonary tuberculosis in Hong Kong. *Br. Med. J.*, **i**, 765–71.

33. Singapore Tuberculosis Service/British Medical Research Council (1975) Controlled trial of intermittent regimen of rifampicin plus isoniazid for pulmonary tuberculosis in Singapore. *Lancet*, **ii**, 1105–9.

34. Hong Kong Chest Service/British Medical Research Council (1984) Study of a fully supervised programme of chemotherapy for pulmonary tuberculosis given once weekly in the continuation phase in the rural areas of Hong Kong. *Tubercle*, **65**, 5–15.

35. Singapore Tuberculosis Service/British Medical Research Council (1991) Assessment of a daily combined preparation of isoniazid, rifampicin and pyrazinamide in a controlled trial of three 6-month regimens for smear-positive pulmonary tuberculosis. *Am. Rev. Respir. Dis.*, **143**, 707–12.

36. United States Public Health Service Tuberculosis Therapy Trial 21 (1987) Preliminary results of an evaluation of a combination tablet of isoniazid, rifampicin and pyrazinamide. *Tubercle*, **68** (Suppl.), 41–6.

37. Cavenghi, R., Aspesi, F., Acocella, G. *et al.* (1989) Quality control of antituberculosis drugs. Symposium held in Dubrovnik, 6 October 1988. *Bull. Int. Union Tuberc. Lung Dis.*, **64**, 36–42.

38. World Health Organization Tuberculosis Unit, Division of Communicable Disease (1992) Tuberculosis control and research strategies for the 1990s. *Bull. WHO*, **70**(1), 17–21.

39. IUATLD (1988) Antituberculosis regimens of chemotherapy. Recommendation from the committee on treatment of IUATLD. *Bull. Int. Union Tuberc. Lung Dis.*, **63**(2), 60–4.

40. Joint Tuberculosis Committee of the British Thoracic Society (1990) Chemotherapy and management of tuberculosis in the United Kingdom: recommendations. *Thorax*, **45**(5), 403–8.

41. British Thoracic Society Research Committee and the Medical Research Council, Cardiothoracic Epidemiology Group (1991) The management of pulmonary tuberculosis in adults notified in England and Wales in 1988. *Respir. Med.*, **85**, 319–23.

42. Subcommittee of the Joint Tuberculosis Committee of the British Thoracic Society (1992) Guidelines on the management of tuberculosis and HIV infection in the United Kingdom. *Br. Med. J.*, **304**, 1231–3.

43. American Thoracic Society (1986) Treatment of tuberculosis and tuberculosis infection in adults and children. *Am. Rev. Respis. Dis.*, **134**, 355–63.

44. World Health Organization Tuberculosis Unit, Division of Communicable Disease (1991) Guidelines for tuberculosis treatment in adults and children in National Tuberculosis Programmes. WHO/TB/91, 161.

45. Hong Kong Tuberculosis Treatment Service/ British Medical Research Council Investigation (1972) A study in Hong Kong to evaluate the role of pretreatment susceptibility tests in the selection of regimens of chemotherapy for

pulmonary tuberculosis. *Am. Rev. Respir. Dis.*, **106**, 1–22.

46. Mitchison, D.A. and Nunn, A.J. (1986) Influence of initial drug resistance on the response to short-course chemotherapy of pulmonary tuberculosis. *Am. Rev. Respir. Dis.*, **133**, 423–30.

47. Sbarbaro, J.A. (1989) Editorial: To treat or not to treat, that was the question. *Am. Rev. Respir. Dis.*, **139**, 865–6.

48. Hong Kong Chest Service/Tuberculosis Research Centre Madras/British Medical Research Council (1984) A controlled trial of 2-month, 3-month and 12-month regimens of chemotherapy for sputum smear-negative pulmonary tuberculosis. The results at 60 months. *Am. Rev. Respir. Dis.*, **130**, 23–8.

49. Hong Kong Chest Service/Tuberculosis Research Centre Madras/British Medical Research Council (1989) A controlled trial of 3-month, 4-month and 6-month regimens of chemotherapy for sputum smear-negative pulmonary tuberculosis. Results at 5 years. *Am. Rev. Respir. Dis.*, **139**, 871–6.

50. Dutt, A.K., Dory Moers, D. and Stead, W.W. (1989) Smear and culture negative pulmonary tuberculosis, 4-month short-course chemotherapy. *Am. Rev. Respir. Dis.*, **139**, 867–70.

51. Tsukamura, M. (1985) *In vitro* antituberculosis activity of a new antibacterial substance ofloxacin (DL 8280). *Am. Rev. Respir. Dis.*, **131**, 348–51.

52. Tsukamura, M. (1985) Antituberculosis activity of ofloxacin (DL 8280) on experimental tuberculosis in mice. *Am. Rev. Respir. Dis.*, **132**, 915.

53. Tsukamura, M., Yoshii, S., Yasuda, Y. and Saito, H. (1986) Antituberculosis chemotherapy including ofloxacin in patients with pulmonary tuberculosis not treated previously. *Kekkaku*, **61**(1), 15–17.

54. Tsukamura, M., Nakamura, E., Yoshii, S. and Amano, H. (1985) Therapeutic effect of a new antibacterial substance ofloxacin (DL 8280) on pulmonary tuberculosis. *Am. Rev. Respir. Dis.*, **131**, 352–6.

55. Hong Kong Chest Service/British Medical Research Council (1992) A controlled study of rifabutin and an uncontrolled study of ofloxacin in the retreatment of patients with pulmonary tuberculosis resistant to isoniazid, streptomycin and rifampicin. *Tuberc. Lung Dis.*, **73**, 59–67.

56. Nunn, P., Kibuya, D. and Gathua, S. (1991) Cutaneous hypersensitivity reaction due to thiacetazone in HIV seropositive patients treated for tuberculosis. *Lancet*, **337**, 627–30.

57. Perrieus, J.H., Colebunders, R.L. and Karahunga, C. (1991) Increased mortality and tuberculosis treatment failure rate among human immunodeficiency virus (HIV) seropositive compared with HIV seronegative patients with pulmonary tuberculosis treated with 'standard' chemotherapy in Kinshasa, Zaire. *Am. Rev. Respir. Dis.*, **144**, 750–5.

58. Small, M., Schecter, G.F. and Goodman, P.C. (1991) Treatment of tuberculosis in patients with advanced human immunodeficiency virus infection. *N. Engl. J. Med.*, **324**(5), 289–94.

59. Hong Kong Chest Service/Tuberculosis Research Centre Madras/British Medical Research Council (1991) A controlled clinical comparison of 6 and 8 months of antituberculosis chemotherapy in the treatment of patients with silicotuberculosis in Hong Kong. *Am. Rev. Respir. Dis.*, **143**, 262–7.

60. Addington, W.W. (1979) Patient compliance: the most serious remaining problem in the control of tuberculosis in the United States. *Chest*, **76**, 750–6.

61. Snider, D.E. Jr (1985) Improving patient compliance in tuberculosis treatment programme. US Department of Health and Human Services, Atlanta, Ga, pp. 1–18.

62. Sbarbaro, J.A. (1980) Public health aspects of tuberculosis in supervision of therapy. *Clin. Chest Med.*, **1**, 253–63.

63. Fox, W. (1968) Changing concepts in the chemotherapy of pulmonary tuberculosis. The John Barnwell Lecture. *Am. Rev. Respir. Dis.*, **97**, 767–90.

64. Fox, W. (1983) Compliance of patients and physicians: experience and lessons from tuberculosis I. *Br. Med. J.*, **287**, 33–6.

65. Fox, W. (1983) Compliance of patients and physicians: experience and lessons from tuberculosis II. *Br. Med. J.*, **287**, 101–5.

66. Snider, D.E. Jr, Cohn, D.L. and Davidson, P.T. (1985) Standard therapy for tuberculosis 1985. *Chest*, **87** (Suppl.), 117–24.

SURGICAL MANAGEMENT OF PULMONARY TUBERCULOSIS

R.J. Donnelly and P.D.O. Davies

The first successful resection for pulmonary tuberculosis was performed by Tuffler in 1891 and the first successful lobectomy by Friedlorder in 1934.

The early development of thoracic surgery may be attributable to the extensive surgery for the treatment of tuberculosis, which came into use during the 1920s and 1930s[1] (Chapter 1, p. 12). Surgical management of progressive disease provided the only hope of cure or of slowing its process until chemotherapy was developed in the late 1940s. Even during the 1950s and 1960s surgery was often used as adjunct to chemotherapy. Only with the advent of the highly efficient 6- or 9-month short-course chemotherapy regimens did surgery virtually vanish as part of the management of active tuberculosis. However, the emergence of multiple-drug resistant (MDR) organisms together with the increase in tuberculosis world wide and the apparently increasing incidence of infections with drug-resistant environmental mycobacteria, has resulted in an increase in failure of medical treatment alone. The surgical management of active tuberculosis is once again necessary in some cases.

Surgery in tuberculosis may be divided into diagnostic and therapeutic categories.

8c.1 SURGERY IN THE DIAGNOSIS OF TUBERCULOSIS

In the event of doubt in the diagnosis of a pulmonary abnormality, a tissue biopsy obtainable by surgery is often indicated. In the developed world, the usual differential diagnosis of a pulmonary abnormality where there is a possibility of tuberculosis, is a carcinoma. Where doubt remains, even at the time of operation, a lung resection to remove the entire lesion and surrounds may be justifiable.

Tuberculosis, representing single or multiple nodules, which may be well circumscribed, can usually be removed with a wedge excision or segmentectomy. In a recent study from Japan, of 36 patients presenting with a solitary pulmonary nodule on chest radiograph all of whom had a pulmonary tuberculoma on histological diagnosis, 21 (58%) were suspected of having lung cancer. Radiography of these 21 patients showed an ill-defined margin, pleural indentation and radial spiculation[2].

In a 10-year retrospective survey of 31 patients undergoing thoracotomy with pulmonary tuberculosis in England[3], 77% of the operations were performed for a suspected neoplasm. Although preoperative identification of patients with pulmonary tuberculosis may be improved with the introduction of modern diagnostic methods (Chapter 17), it is likely that thoracotomy will remain necessary to obtain a satisfactory diagnosis in a minority of patients.

Recent developments in thoracoscopy have allowed biopsies to be obtained with considerably less trauma to the patient, permitting

Clinical Tuberculosis. Edited by P.D.O. Davies. Published in 1994 by Chapman & Hall, London. ISBN 0 412 48630 X

patients who may be older or more frail or more to undergo a diagnostic procedure than was previously possible[4].

Though CT scanning may provide some help with diagnosis, it cannot provide a tissue diagnosis[5]. A negative transbronchial lung biopsy or percutaneous needle biopsy does not necessarily exclude pathology.

8c.2 THERAPEUTIC SURGERY

Therapeutic surgery of tuberculosis may be divided into surgery for the management of complications of disease and surgery for, or as part of, the treatment of active disease. Both may, however, entail similar procedures.

8c.2.1 SURGERY FOR THE COMPLICATIONS OF RESPIRATORY TUBERCULOSIS

Complications from tuberculosis may arise at any stage during the active phase of disease or after the disease becomes inactive, following treatment. The most common complications are haemoptysis and bronchiectasis. Others include stenosis of the bronchial tree, empyema, formation of a mycetoma in an old cavity, extensive fibrosis with distortion of the bronchial tree or simply loss of lung volume.

(a) Haemoptysis

Haemoptysis during or after active disease is often profuse and may be life-threatening. Common bleeding sites include areas of fibrotic scarring, cavitation with or without mycetoma formation and bronchiectasis. The site of origin of bleeding may be determined by bronchoscopy, in conjunction with the chest radiograph and CT scan if available. Selective pulmonary or bronchial arteriography may also be of value. While an aggressive surgical approach to haemoptysis has been advocated[6], management by selective bronchial artery embolization may

be successful[7,8]. When a patient is fit enough to undergo surgery, lobectomy to remove the source of bleeding is the most effective means of control. If a mycetoma is the cause of bleeding, anti-fungal agents may be tried either intermittently or long term. Recolonization is likely to occur once treatment is stopped. Surgery for removal of a mycetoma is often difficult and associated with much blood loss, but is sometimes indicated for persistent bleeding.

(b) Bronchiectasis

Bronchiectasis can arise in tuberculosis as a result of widespread destruction of the bronchi in one or more lobes of the lung. This may lead to persistent infection with non-mycobacterial organisms resulting in a chronic suppurating lung. If conservative measures such as drainage or prophylactic and therapeutic antibiotics are unsuccessful in controlling the patient's symptoms, segmentectomy or lobectomy may be considered.

(c) Bronchial stenosis

Stenosis of a main or lobar bronchus may occur as a result of surrounding lymph node enlargement, or from distortion during a fibrotic process. If severe, this may be treated by resection, though stenting or endobronchial dilatation using a balloon method may be successful[9,10].

(d) Empyema

The management of empyema, whether caused by tuberculosis infection or by some other organism has been open to some debate. The basic principles of antibiotic therapy and drainage apply, though there is dispute as to when drainage, perhaps by rib resection, should be undertaken in the course of disease. Some surgeons prefer to wait until a full course of antituberculosis chemotherapy has been given, provided adequate drainage can be obtained with intercostal drains in the mean time. Following tuberculosis, empyema causes the lung to shrink, and decortication to enable the lung to reflate and adhere to the inside of the chest wall may be required.

8c.2.2 EXPERIENCE IN SURGERY FOR THE COMPLICATIONS OF TUBERCULOSIS

In a recent retrospective 10-year survey of patients requiring surgery for complications of tuberculosis in the USA, there were 36 complications in 24 patients: in eight because of drug resistance (see later), haemoptysis in 16 patients and bronchiectasis in 12. Bronchiectasis was thought to be a contributing factor in seven of the patients with haemoptysis. Chest cavitation was present in 11, eight also having mycetoma[11]. Surgical resection consisted of lobectomy in 17 patients, bilobectomy in two, pneumonectomy in three and resection of less than a lobe in two.

Postoperative complications occurred in 45% of patients and were bronchopleural fistula (1), empyema (2), pneumonia (1), pleural effusion (1), wound infection (2), atelectasis (3) and mental confusion (1).

In a study of 121 patients with tuberculosis in the University of Washington, ten patients required thoracotomy for complications of tuberculosis[12]. These included resection of parenchymal cavitations unresponsive to medical therapy, closure of bronchopleural fistula and decortication for empyema.

In the recent survey carried out in England[3] of 30 patients with pulmonary tuberculosis who underwent surgery, whether for diagnosis or treatment in a 10-year period, five were operated on for complications of disease: non-functional lung with symptomatic bronchiectasis (1), haemoptysis (1), persistent intrapulmonary cavity (2), and spontaneous bronchopleural fistula and empyema (1). Two patients had a pneumonectomy, one

a lobectomy, one a decortication with lobectomy and one a thoracoplasty. (The remaining patients were diagnosed as a result of surgery.)

8c.2.3 SURGERY IN THE THERAPY OF ACTIVE TUBERCULOSIS

The advent of MDR tuberculosis, and the increasing infection of environmental, or 'atypical' mycobacteria in AIDS, has resulted in an increasing incidence of failure of medical treatment using both first- and second-line drugs[13,14] (Chapter 9). The National Jewish Centre for Immunology and Respiratory Medicine in Denver, Colorado has a large experience of surgical management of drug-unresponsive disease. Between 1983 and 1990, 42 patients with drug-resistant *M. tuberculosis* and 38 patients with environmental mycobacterial infection underwent a total of 85 pulmonary resections[15]. All were either poor candidates for medical therapy alone, or had existing complications. A total of 40 patients underwent pneumonectomies and 45 had lobectomies (left pneumonectomy was more common in multi-drug-resistant *M. tuberculosis*). One operative and six late deaths occurred. Post-operative complications were bronchopleural fistula in 8 patients prolonged air leak or air space in 4, respiratory failure in 2 and recurrent nerve palsy (1), wound breakdown (1), pericardial effusion (1), Horner's syndrome (1) and psychiatric complications (1). The authors recommend that if localized disease is present and prognosis is poor, pulmonary resection should be performed for resistant *M. tuberculosis* infection after at least 3 months of specific drug therapy. Earlier resection should be undertaken in patients with environmental mycobacterial infections before extensive polymicrobial contamination of the lung occurs. Factors influencing morbidity and mortality include sputum smear-positivity, previous chest irradiation, prior pulmonary

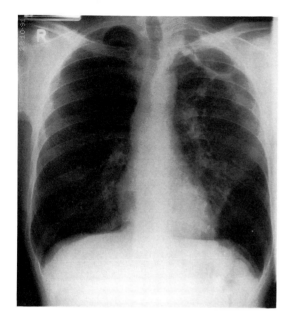

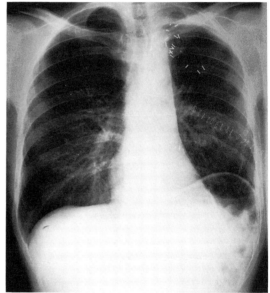

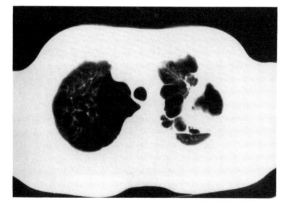

Fig. 8c.1   (a) Chest radiograph of a patient with destruction and cavitation of the left upper lobe infected with *Mycobacterium avium-intracellulare*. (b) CT scan section. (c) Chest radiograph after left upper lobectomy.

resection and polymicrobial contamination of the lung tissue. The overall death rate was 14.2% compared with 22% in a similar group treated medically before the series[16].

Mortality and morbidity from the English series was 0 and 15% respectively[3]. However, when only those patients undergoing thoracotomy for complications of tuber-culosis are considered the morbidity was 2/5 (40%).

8c.3 CONCLUSION

Surgery in the management of tuberculosis, whether for complications or for active disease unresponsive to chemotherapy, must be considered a last resort. Postoperative complications in various series occur in 40–50% of patients. However, it should be seen as having a place for the patient where life-threatening disease or complications are present. Surgery may be indicated at an earlier stage for MDR disease or infection with an environmental organism (Fig. 8c.1).

REFERENCES

1. Naef, A.P., (1991) Tuberculosis – the starting point of thoracic surgery. *Gesnerus*, **49**, pt 3–4, 477–84.
2. Ishida, T., Yokoyama, H., Kaneko, S. *et al.* (1992) Pulmonary tuberculoma and indications for surgery: radiographic and clinico-pathological analysis. *Resp. Med.*, **86**, 431–6.
3. Whyte, R.I., Deegan, S.P., Kaplan, D.K. *et al.* (1989) Recent surgical experience for pulmonary tuberculosis. *Resp. Med.*, **83**, 357–62.
4. Donnelly, R.J., Page, R.D. and Cowen, M.E. (1992) Endoscopy assisted microthoracotomy: intitial experience. *Thorax*, **47**, 490–3.
5. Siegelman, S.S., Zerhouni, E.A., Leo, F.P. *et al.* (1980) CT of the solitary pulmonary nodule. *Am. J. Radiol.*, **135**, 1–13.
6. McLaughlin, J.S., and Hawkins, J.R. (1974) Current aspects of surgery for pulmonary tuberculosis. *Ann. Thorac. Surg.*, **17**, 513–25.
7. Whaley, M.H., Chamorrow, H.A., Rao, G. *et al.* (1976) Bronchial artery embolization for massive haemoptysis. *J. Am. Med. Assoc.*, **236**, 2501–4.
8. Bookstein J.J., Moser K.M., Kalafer M.E. *et al.* (1977), The role of bronchial arteriography and therapeutic embolization in haemoptysis. *Chest*, **72**, 658–61.
9. Simonds, A.K. Irving, J.D., Clarke, S.W. and Dick, R. (1989) Use of expandable metal stents in the treatment of bronchial obstruction. *Thorax*, **44**, 680–1.
10. Bell, J.B., Delaney, J.C., Evans, C.C. *et al.* (1991). Endoscopic bougie and balloon dilatation of multiple bronchial stenosis: 10-year follow up. *Thorax*, **46**, 933–5.
11. Reed, C.E., Parker, E.F., and Crawford, F.A. (1989) Surgical resection for complications of pulmonary tuberculosis. *Ann. Thorac. Surg.*, **48**, 165–7.
12. Langdale, L.A., Meissner, M., Nolan C. and Ashbaugh, D.G. (1992) Tuberculosis and the surgeon. *Am. J. Surg.*, **163**, 505–9.
13. Glassroth, J. (1992) Tuberculosis in the United States. Looking for a silver lining among the clouds. *Am. Rev Respir. Dis.* **146**, 278–9.
14. Chawla, P.K., Klapper, P.J., Kamholy, S.L. *et al.* (1992) Drug resistant tuberculosis in an urban population including patients at risk for human immunodeficiency virus infection. *Am. Rev. Respir. Dis.*, **146**, 280–4.
15. Pomerantz, M., Madsen, L. *et al.* (1991) Surgical management of resistant mycobacterial tuberculosis and other mycobacterial pulmonary infections. *Ann. Thorac. Surg.*, **52**, 1108–12.
16. Globe, M., Hersbury, C.R., Waite, D. *et al.* (1988) Treatment of isoniazid and rifampicin-resistant tuberculosis. *Am. Rev. Respir. Dis.*, **137**, 24.

PROBLEMS IN THE MANAGEMENT OF TUBERCULOSIS 8d

P.D.O. Davies

8d.1 RESPIRATORY DISEASE

8d.1.1 PRESENTATIONS

Most patients presenting with tuberculosis, whether the disease is pulmonary or extra-pulmonary, are well enough to be managed in the outpatient clinic. If the patient is being seen as a contact of a case of smear-positive pulmonary tuberculosis, it is likely that he or she will be completely asymptomatic. The presenting feature will be a shadow on the chest radiograph. In the case of children this may occur anywhere in the lung, but in adults, who are more likely to present with post-primary disease, this is most likely to be in the apices or in the posterior segment of the upper lobes.

A diagnosis of tuberculosis should be considered in any patient presenting with symptoms that include weight loss, malaise, chronic cough, with or without haemoptysis, and the presence of fever, particularly if the patient is elderly or from an ethnic minority group. In the developing world, tuberculosis is the most likely cause of such symptoms.

Physical examination of the patient with pulmonary tuberculosis will often reveal very little in the way of abnormal findings. In severe cases the patient may appear to have lost weight, and may even be cachectic. There may be a continuous irritating cough productive of phlegm. The eyes may appear sunken, but are often unusually bright. Pyrexia may be present but is unlikely to exceed 40°C on any occasion. Characteristically pyrexia is chronic and low-grade.

Examination of the chest may reveal no abnormality or evidence of pneumonia, such as bronchial breathing or diminished breath sounds. In advanced disease, with cavitation, coarse crackles and even amphoteric breathing may be present. Tuberculosis may also cause pleural effusion. Examination of the cardiovascular system, abdomen and central nervous system is unlikely to reveal further abnormalities. In children the presence of erythema nodosum or phlictenular conjunctivitis may occur, though the latter is rare in the developed world. Chest radiography often presents with typical features of disease (Chapter 6, p. 78) – characteristically soft floccular shadowing in the upper lobes with or without cavitation. However, tuberculosis may present with virtually any radiographic abnormality.

8d.1.2 OBTAINING SPECIMENS

Once the diagnosis is suspected every effort should be made to obtain specimens for microbiological analysis by direct smear and culture. Sputum can usually be obtained from the adult patient with post-primary, cavitating disease as he or she can expector-

Clinical Tuberculosis. Edited by P.D.O. Davies. Published in 1994 by Chapman & Hall, London. ISBN 0 412 48630 X

ate into a sputum pot, which can then be sent to the laboratory. At least three specimens should be obtained. If sputum cannot be obtained, further efforts should be made to obtain a specimen. Facilities in developed countries usually enable hospital admission to do this. In the case of infants and small children this may include obtaining gastric washings or specimens by laryngeal swabs. In adults, bronchoscopy for bronchial lavage is the most convenient method to obtain specimens. Bronchoscopy is also of value is helping to exclude other diagnoses, such as bronchogenic carcinoma. Where bronchoscopy is not available, induced sputum may be obtained by getting the patient to inhale twice normal nebulized saline over a period of 5–15 mins. This may often cause distress to the patient through coughing and should preferably be carried out under medical supervision. It is often possible to obtain a sputum specimen by giving a 5 ml injection of normal saline through the trachea, in the midline, mid-way between the larynx and suprasternal notch. This is a technique used for injecting local anaesthesia at bronchoscopy, and may be a convenient way to obtain specimens in the elderly patient who is unable to provide sputum by any other means. Alternatively a fine cannula can be passed through the trachea at this point and aspiration undertaken using saline lavage.

In cases where initial specimens do not provide confirmation of the diagnosis or where doubt remains, further specimens for microbiology may be obtained from early morning urine samples, from bone marrow trephine, or from blood cultures, though the latter are unlikely to be positive except in HIV-positive individuals. Further confirmation may be sought by obtaining biopsy of an abnormal pulmonary lesion either by transbronchial biopsy through a bronchoscope, or by percutaneous needle biopsy, or by thoracoscopic biopsy or by open lung biopsy (Chapter 8c, p. 157). Biopsies should be placed in saline for dispatch to Microbiology for culture testing, as well as sent in formalin to Histopathology for histological diagnosis. The laboratory should be informed if tuberculosis is suspected so that staining can be carried out for acid-fast bacilli.

In the developed world the most likely differential diagnosis in an adult with an abnormal chest radiograph is a lung carcinoma, and if the diagnosis of tuberculosis is in doubt, it is important to obtain a tissue specimen from the abnormality.

The presence of a strongly positive tuberculin test may provide additional evidence for the presence of tuberculosis and is a particularly valuable test in children (Chapter 15d, p. 345). In the HIV-positive individual opportunist infections such as *Pneumocystis carinii* should be excluded. Once specimens have been obtained and if the diagnosis of tuberculosis is suspected, chemotherapy may be started. HIV testing is now advisable for patients aged 15–64, and for others with possible risk factors, provided suitable counselling is undertaken.

8d.1.3 CHEMOTHERAPY

Ideally chemotherapy should comprise isoniazid (H), rifampicin (R) and pyrazinamide (Z) for the first 2 months. If drug resistance is suspected, a fourth drug such as ethambutol (E) or streptomycin (S) should be added. Triple therapy is most conveniently given in the form of the tablet Rifater, which combines HRZ in a single tablet thus precluding self-administered monotherapy with the danger of drug resistance emerging. After 2 months, treatment can be reduced to HR, provided the bacilli are not resistant to either of these drugs. These can also be prescribed conveniently in the combination Rifinah or Rimactazid. (For dosages refer to Chapter 8b, p. 149). Medications should be taken once a day on an empty stomach, preferably half an hour before the first meal of the day. The patient should be warned of possible adverse effects (Chapter 8b, p. 150), of which nausea is the most common. This may be transitory and present little problem to the patient. Occasionally it is severe enough to warrant reassessment of therapy. Nausea may be overcome by giving medication three times a day, or on a full stomach. In either case, this renders the medication less effective and treatment may need to be prolonged. An anti-emetic may be of benefit. Alternatively medication may be stopped and desensitization undertaken (Chapter 8b, p. 150).

It may be necessary to give alternative medication. Again this requires therapy to be prolonged beyond 6 months.

8d.1.4 NURSING MANAGEMENT

For the particularly ill patient or the elderly, admission to hospital for observation during the first days of treatment may be advisable as adverse reactions are common and may occasionally be life-threatening. For reasons not fully understood, mortality tends to be highest in the first few weeks after treatment has started. A smear-positive patient is rendered non-infectious within days of the start of treatment so that isolation is not necessary beyond 2 weeks of treatment. Until this time, such patients should be nursed in a separate cubicle with their own toilet and washing facilities. Barrier nursing is not required and no special precautions need be taken with crockery or personal effects other than usual hygiene. Alternatively, provided the patient agrees to remain at home within this time interval, and avoid meeting new contacts, it is possible for such a patient to be managed on an outpatient basis. Once a smear-positive patient has been undergoing treatment for 2 weeks, segregation on the ward may only be necessary where HIV-positive patients are being nursed.

Though some workers prefer to wear masks when nursing smear-positive patients, there is no evidence that they provide additional protection. No special precautions are required for infection control in the case of patients with sputum smear-negative or extrapulmonary disease, except where they may be in contact with immunocompromised patients.

Often sputum may not convert to smear-negativity for some months after treatment has begun as dead bacilli may continue to be expectorated. Cultures after 2–3 months are almost always negative. However, a full course of treatment is required to prevent relapse (Chapter 8b, p. 143).

8d.1.5 THE SICK PATIENT

Some patients with extensive disease may present with anaemia, hypoxaemia, hyponatraemia or hypoalbuminaemia and require necessary supportive measures. Severe anaemia may be corrected by transfusion but this is not normally necessary. (The absolute level for haemoglobin (Hb) at which transfusion should be given varies with expected normal values. In most developed countries transfusion should be considered for levels of Hb less than 8 g/dl.) If blood gases can be obtained these will provide a guide as to whether oxygen supplementation is required (O_2 less than 60 mmHg). This can be given by using continuous oxygen by face mask or cannulae and the inspired percentage of oxygen may be titrated against blood gas results. Specific measures to correct hyponatraemia are not normally required. Hypoalbuminaemia as a result of prolonged illness is not uncommon, even in the developed world. Providing the patient is able to take an adequate diet this will be corrected during treatment. If the patient is too ill to take food, nasogastric or parenteral feeding should be considered. Addison's disease due to involvement of the adrenal glands is now uncommon in the developed world, but should be considered in the ill, prostrate or comatose patient, and be tested for by hormone assay.

If Addison's disease is suspected, mineralocorticoid and corticosteroid supplements will be required. Hypercalcaemia may occur but is rare. Specific measures to correct this are not usually required.

In the severely ill patient it may be necessary to administer medication parenterally. Parenteral preparations of streptomycin, isoniazid, rifampicin, ethambutol and capreomycin should be available in most countries of the developed world.

Many experienced physicians believe that the addition of corticosteroids to the regimen in the treatment of the severely ill patient is life-saving. Though there is good anecdotal evidence for this, evidence from any controlled trial is lacking. It is postulated that by metabolizing endogenously produced steroids, rifampicin may cause an iatrogenic Addisonian crisis. This may explain the high death rate that has been observed soon after treatment has started. A possible way to avoid this may be to give high-dose mineralo- and corticosteroids to the severely ill patient as the rifampicin-containing antituberculosis regimen is started.

8d.1.6 FEVER

Once antituberculosis treatment is commenced, any fever usually falls to normal in 3–14 days. For disease in which the hypersensitivity response may be high, such as tuberculous pleuritis or meningitis, the course of the fever may be prolonged beyond 2 weeks. In such cases the fever usually responds rapidly to steroids in high doses. Prednisolone in a dose of 0.5mg/kg per day is required for non-rifampicin-containing regimens and twice this dose if a rifampicin-containing regimen is being given. Steroids may be required for 2–4 months of treatment before being reduced gradually.

Alternatively prolonged fever on treatment may be due to a hypersensitivity reaction to one or more of the drugs being given. Other evidence for an adverse reaction should then be looked for, such as a skin rash, abnormal liver function or frank jaundice. If drug hypersensitivity is suspected, medication should be stopped and desensitization should be carried out as detailed in Chapter 8b, (p. 150). Routine liver function testing, once treatment has commenced, is not necessary unless there are other clinical indications to do so.

8d.1.7 INPATIENT CARE

Long-term inpatient care, once the mainstay of antituberculosis therapy, is now no longer necessary except for some non-compliant patients such as alcoholics or those with mental disorders. Recent experience in New York suggests that non-compliance is an increasing problem as many patients default on outpatient regimens. Some health authorities have opened up 'half-way houses', to provide those who would otherwise be discharged into the community with little prospect of returning for outpatient care with directly observed supervised chemotherapy while resident in a home or hostel. An intermittent supervised form of chemotherapy in which the patient attends an outpatient clinic two or three times a week and is observed taking medication is used in a number of countries (Chapter 8b, p. 153). It is suitable for some urbanized communities, such as Hong Kong. If necessary, therapy may be directly administered by district nurses or specialized tuberculosis nurses in the home of patients unable to take medicine on their own, thereby relieving hospital beds.

8d.1.8 FOLLOW-UP

After treatment has started, initial follow-up should be monthly for at least two visits. Sputum may be obtained for culture to ensure conversion is occurring, and is a useful test of patient compliance. Regular weight checks at follow-up are probably the best tests of satisfactory progress. Follow-up chest radiographs are usually unnecessary but can provide a further means of assessing compliance and are often reassuring for the patient. Jaundice, sickness and cutaneous adverse effects, if they occur, usually do so in the first month, forcing the patient to stop therapy, which is why an early appointment is essential. In the event of serious adverse effects the patient should be admitted to a hospital bed, and an alternative regimen given or desensitization to the current regimen carried out (Chapter 8b, p. 150). With good compliance relapse is rare, so that once a course of treatment is completed routine follow-up is not usually necessary. A chest radiograph at completion of treatment is probably of value for comparison in the unlikely event of relapse. Smokers should be given every encouragement to quit the habit.

8d.1.9 FAILURE OF RESPONSE

If a patient fails to respond to treatment five considerations need to be borne in mind.

- Was the initial diagnosis of tuberculosis correct?
- Is the patient taking his or her medications as instructed?
- Is the patient having an adverse drug reaction?
- Is drug resistance a possibility?
- Is there some new disease that has occurred?

At this stage it may be necessary to admit or re-admit the patient to hospital for further assessment. Specimens for microbiology and histology should be obtained if the diagnosis is in doubt. Any evidence of new disease in terms of symptoms, signs or abnormalities in investigations should be considered. If the diagnosis is not in doubt, the patient has been fully compliant with treatment, adverse reaction to drugs is not likely and no new disease is present, then drug-resistant disease is likely (Chapter 9, p. 171). As drug sensitivities may not yet be available at this stage in treatment, an addition or change to the patient's current regimen should be considered. If it is decided to change the regimen

then at least two and preferably three anti-tuberculosis drugs that the patient has never had before should be given. **A single drug should never be added to an apparently failing regimen**.

In such an event, it is likely that the patient may have to be started on second-line chemotherapy, which is often toxic. A period of inpatient observation when starting such a regimen is advisable.

8d.2 STAFF

It is the policy of most centres treating tuberculosis to ensure that those working with potentially infectious patients have been tuberculin tested, and if negative given BCG (Chapter 12a, p. 227). In centres where BCG is not administered it is normal policy to tuberculin test health workers annually, and if the tuberculin test is found to convert or show increased positivity suggestive of an infection, chemoprophylaxis may be given (Chapter 14a, p. 279). If the health worker is likely to be in contact with patients with multi-drug-resistant organisms, prior testing to ensure tuberculin positivity and if this is negative to give BCG is advisable. Routine chest radiography for workers in contact with infectious cases of tuberculosis is not necessary. An early chest radiograph is advised should symptoms suggest disease.

8d.3 THE HIV-POSITIVE PATIENT

The management of the HIV-positive tuberculosis patient is not substantially different from the HIV-negative patient. Positive smear specimens may be more difficult to obtain so that the need for bronchoscopy may be more likely. Appropriate precautions by the bronchoscopist, such as masking and goggles, will be required. The 6-month regimen comprising 2HRZ/4HR usually provides effective cure though some workers recommend continuing isoniazid to provide prophylaxis against subsequent infection.

Follow-up of HIV-positive patients should be life-long.

8d.4 MANAGEMENT OF NON-RESPIRATORY DISEASE

In developed countries non-respiratory disease is likely to be seen relatively infrequently. Joint management of patients between the chest physician, experienced in prescribing antituberculosis drugs, and the appropriate medical or surgical specialist is therefore advisable.

8d.4.1 LYMPH NODE DISEASE
(Chapter 7, p. 94)

In areas where tuberculosis lymphadenitis is very common, many workers commence antituberculosis chemotherapy without microbiological or histological confirmation of disease, on the basis of enlarged lymph nodes alone. Where there is any doubt a biopsy should be taken to provide specimens for culture and histology.

Therapy comprising 2HRZ/4HR is normally sufficient. Lymph nodes may enlarge or discharge during or after therapy. This is normally transient. Where enlarged lymph nodes persist and the diagnosis of tuberculosis is not in doubt, steroids may be of benefit. Rarely, total excision of all enlarged or suppurating glands may be necessary.

8d.4.2 ORTHOPAEDIC TUBERCULOSIS
(Chapter 7, p. 98)

Provided adequate specimens have been obtained from the affected site, the only absolute indication for further surgery in spinal tuberculosis is the development of spinal cord compression as a complication of spinal disease. For these cases an operation as soon as possible after the onset of symptoms is mandatory to prevent paraplegia. Decompression is best undertaken by a surgeon highly experienced in the technique.

The 6-month regimen comprising 2HRZ/4HR has been shown to be as effective as any in orthopaedic tuberculosis. An abscess in conjunction with bone or joint disease rarely requires surgical intervention. In the event of a joint remaining painful or unstable after a full course of chemotherapy, arthrodesis or joint replacement should be considered.

8d.4.3 TUBERCULOUS MENINGITIS
(Chapter 7, p. 102)

It is not uncommon for deterioration to occur in patients with tuberculous meningitis soon after the start of chemotherapy. This may be due to enlargement of meningeal or cerebral tuberculoma. In such cases there is a temptation to tamper with the regimen in the belief that the patient may be infected by drug-resistant organisms. Such a temptation should be resisted.

Computerized tomographic scans, if available, may help in establishing the presence and change in size of tuberculoma. If the patient deteriorates steroids should be added, if they are not being given already. A diagnosis of Addison's disease or other metabolic causes of possible deterioration should be excluded. If these diagnoses are suspected appropriate corrective therapy will be required. It may be necessary to implement parenteral rather than oral therapy in patients who are comatose or restless. Sedation should be avoided.

8d.4.4 ABDOMINAL DISEASE
(Chapter 7, p. 107)

In the developed world, abdominal tuberculosis is possibly the most frequently missed diagnosis of tuberculosis. Carcinoma or inflammatory bowel disease is usually suspected from the presenting symptoms. Diagnosis requires a high index of suspicion and confirmation is made from specimens obtained on biopsy by laparoscopy or laparotomy. Subacute obstruction may persist for many weeks after chemotherapy has been started. Surgical intervention to relieve obstruction is not normally required. Late complications caused by bowel adhesions may occur and though surgery may relieve these temporarily, new adhesions may form subsequently.

8d.4.5 PERICARDITIS (Chapter 7, p. 111)

Tuberculous pericarditis is now so rare in the developed world that it is frequently overlooked. Viral or bacterial pericarditis, myocardial infarction, effusion and even malignancy are commoner causes.

In the absence of any confirmation of the above diagnoses, and if a strongly positive tuberculin test is present even without bacterial confirmation of tuberculosis, a trial of antituberculosis chemotherapy is probably indicated. This should include steroids in the first 2–4 months to speed the reduction in effusion size. The presence of restrictive pericarditis requires surgical intervention to remove the pericardium.

8d.4.6 GENITOURINARY TUBERCULOSIS (Chapter 7, p. 114)

The diagnosis of genitourinary tuberculosis may be suspected on the basis of symptoms and a sterile pyuria. Direct smear of a urine sample will almost invariably be negative in the presence of genitourinary disease because of the high volume of urine in comparison with the number of organisms present. Findings of an IVU may be nonspecific. Diagnosis cannot therefore be confirmed until culture results are available. A trial of antituberculosis chemotherapy is probably indicated until culture results are available.

Regular review of renal function by blood urea and creatinine testing, and of anatomical structure by IVU or ultrasound is required during treatment. Steroids may reduce the incidence of ureteric stricture.

Rarely surgery may be required for partial or total nephrectomy in the case of a severely calcified kidney. Surgery may also be required for ureteric or bladder reconstruction once chemotherapy is completed. Complete obstruction of the urinary tract will require prompt surgical intervention.

THE EXTENT AND MANAGEMENT OF DRUG-RESISTANT TUBERCULOSIS: THE AMERICAN EXPERIENCE

S.W. Dooley, Jr and Patricia M. Simone

9.1 INTRODUCTION

As recently as 10 years ago, tuberculosis was rapidly disappearing in the USA. The number of tuberculosis cases reported to the Centers for Disease Control and Prevention (CDC) declined by approximately 5.6% annually from more than 84 000 cases in 1953 to 22 255 cases in 1984. However, in 1985 this steady decline ended, and from 1985 to 1991 there was an 18.4% increase in reported cases. This change in tuberculosis morbidity trends has been attributed to a number of factors, including the human immunodeficiency virus (HIV) epidemic, tuberculosis occurring in foreign-born persons from countries with a high prevalence of tuberculosis, transmission of tuberculosis in congregate settings (e.g. health care facilities, correctional facilities, drug-treatment facilities, shelters for the homeless), and a deterioration of the health care infrastructure[1,2].

Coincident with the increase in tuberculosis cases, large outbreaks of multi-drug-resistant tuberculosis have occurred. Resistance to antituberculosis drugs has been noted since the drugs were introduced[3], and outbreaks of drug-resistant tuberculosis have occasionally been reported. However, the size of the recent multi-drug-resistant outbreaks, the rapidity with which they have propagated and their occurrence in institutional settings, are suggestive of a new phenomenon. This chapter reviews available information on drug-resistant tuberculosis in the USA and discusses approaches to its control.

9.2 MECHANISMS AND TYPES OF DRUG RESISTANCE

Drug-resistant *M. tuberculosis* develops from random mutations of the bacterial chromosome, which occur spontaneously in wild-type strains even before contact with an antituberculosis drug. These mutations occur at a low rate, which varies depending on the drug. In a bacterial population that has not been exposed to antituberculosis drugs, the highest proportions of drug-resistant mutants that will occur have been estimated to be 3.5×10^{-6} for isoniazid, 3.8×10^{-6} for streptomycin, 0.5×10^{-4} for ethambutol, and 3.1×10^{-8} for rifampin*[4]. The probability of a randomly occurring mutant being resistant to more than one drug is equal to the probabilities of resistance for each individual drug. Since mutants resistant to a single drug make up only about 1 in 10^{6} bacilli, mutants resistant to two drugs should occur only once in a population of 10^{12} organisms. Most types of pulmonary tuberculosis involve only 10^{2} to

Clinical Tuberculosis. Edited by P.D.O. Davies. Published in 1994 by Chapman & Hall, London. ISBN 0 412 48630 X
* Rifampin is known as rifampicin in most countries outside the USA.

10^4 bacilli, whereas pulmonary cavities contain about 10^7 to 10^9 bacilli[5]. Thus, *cavitatory* lesions are likely to contain a small number of bacilli resistant to any single drug.

Drug resistant tuberculosis occurs when drug-resistant mutants are selected because of inadequate therapy. If a large number of bacilli are present, as in cavitatory disease, treating tuberculosis with only one drug eliminates the organisms susceptible to that drug but selects for organisms resistant to the drug. Eventually the resistant bacilli make up a substantial proportion of the bacterial population, and clinical drug resistance occurs. However, the likelihood that cavitatory lesions contain mutants resistant to more than one drug is extremely low. Therefore, by treating tuberculosis with two or more drugs in combination, mutants resistant to any single drug are killed by one of the other drugs in the regimen, and the selection of drug-resistant organisms can be prevented.

Drug resistance in tuberculosis is usually divided into two types: primary resistance and secondary (acquired) resistance. Primary resistance occurs in persons who are initially infected with drug-resistant organisms because of exposure to a person with drug-resistant tuberculosis. Secondary (acquired) resistance develops when drug-resistant organisms are selected because patients are treated with an inadequate regimen or fail to take a regimen appropriately. Primary and secondary drug resistance can coexist if primary drug resistance is present but not suspected, and an inadequate regimen is prescribed. In this situation, mutants resistant to additional drugs will be selected.

One of the major causes of drug resistance is non-adherence to therapy. Many patients fail to adhere to a prescribed regimen during the treatment of tuberculosis because of the adverse effects associated with antituberculosis drugs and because of the necessarily long duration of therapy. If a patient is prescribed isoniazid and rifampin but does not take the rifampin because of gastrointestinal upset or urine discoloration, isoniazid-resistant mutants may be selected. Inappropriate prescribing practices by clinicians can also lead to the selection of drug-resistant organisms. For example, if resistance to isoniazid is not suspected in a patient with isoniazid-resistant disease, therapy with isoniazid and rifampin is equivalent to therapy with rifampin alone. In this situation, most of the bacilli will be susceptible to rifampin and be killed; however, random mutations in the population of isoniazid-resistant bacilli may eventually result in a few mutants resistant to both isoniazid and rifampin. With continued inadequate treatment, these multi-drug-resistant mutants may eventually make up a large proportion of the bacterial population.

9.3 EPIDEMIOLOGY OF DRUG-RESISTANT TUBERCULOSIS

The national surveillance system for tuberculosis in the USA has not routinely collected information on the drug susceptibility of reported cases. However, information on the epidemiology of drug-resistant tuberculosis in the USA is available from two large national surveys of drug resistance that have been conducted at repeated intervals over the years, and from a number of studies by individual investigators. When interpreting data on drug resistance, it is necessary to recognize two important limitations[6]. First, it may be difficult to distinguish primary from secondary drug resistance because reliable histories of previous treatment are often hard to obtain. The primary drug-resistance rate will be falsely elevated if patients who have received previous therapy and developed secondary resistance are inadvertently misclassified as having primary drug-resistance. Conversely, the primary drug resistance rate will be falsely lowered if patients with primary drug resistance are misclassified as having secondary resistance. Second, technical and methodological differences in performing and interpreting susceptibility tests in different studies may limit the comparability of the data reported by different investigators. However, studies of drug resistance can provide valuable information if interpreted carefully.

9.3.1 NATIONAL TRENDS IN DRUG-RESISTANT TUBERCULOSIS

Hobby and associates conducted a series of surveys of primary drug resistance in tuberculosis patients hospitalized in Veterans Administration hospitals throughout the USA from 1962 to 1973[7–10]. The data from these surveys suggest that in this population, which was limited to adult male veterans, the incidence of primary drug resistance was low and there was no clear trend towards an increase in resistance to any of the drugs tested (Table 9.1). Data from the surveys was not analysed by geographical region or by demographic variables such as age.

The CDC has also conducted a series of surveys of primary drug resistance. The first of the CDC surveys was conducted among patients admitted to 22 participating hospitals in the USA from 1961 to 1968[11,12]. Of 9380 strains tested, 331 (3.5%) were resistant to at least one of the drugs tested – isoniazid, streptomycin, or para-aminosalicylic acid (PAS). No significant increase in the rates of resistance to the three drugs was observed during this period (Table 9.2). Of interest, of 470 persons with drug-resistant organisms who were initially classified as previously untreated, 132 (28%) were later found to have actually received previous chemotherapy. This highlights the difficulty of distinguishing primary and secondary drug resistance in surveys of this kind.

A second CDC survey of primary drug resistance was conducted between 1975 and 1982[13–15]. This survey initially included 16 public health laboratories located throughout the USA, and later incorporated four additional state and city laboratories. *Mycobacterium tuberculosis* organisms resistant to one or more of the ten antituberculosis drugs tested were isolated from 6.9% of the 12 157 cases surveyed. The overall resistance rate in this survey was higher than in the 1961–1968 CDC survey[11,12]; however, significant technical and methodological differences between the surveys make such comparisons difficult. Nevertheless, there was a marked decline in the rate of primary drug resistance during the period of the 1975–1982 survey[15].

A third CDC survey of primary drug resistance was conducted between 1982 and 1986 in co-operation with 31 public health laboratories located throughout the USA[16]. Of 3760 isolates tested, 9.0% were resistant to at least one of the ten drugs tested, and the percentage of primary resistance decreased significantly during the course of the survey. The higher level of primary drug resistance in this survey compared with the previous survey (6.9%) was again attributed to methodological differences.

In summary, the three CDC surveys differed from one another in the absolute percentages of primary drug resistance, apparently because of technical and methodological differences. However, in all three of the surveys there was a relatively low rate of primary drug resistance, and within the period of each survey there was a stable or decreasing trend in the percentage of primary resistance. For this reason, and because of resource constraints and competing priorities, the CDC discontinued surveillance of drug resistance in 1986.

Recently, because of the occurrence of several outbreaks of multi-drug-resistant tuberculosis, the CDC conducted a survey of drug resistance among tuberculosis cases reported from January to March 1991 [CDC, unpublished data]. Provisional analyses have found that, of 4051 culture-positive cases reported during the study period, results of susceptibility testing for at least one drug were available for 3352 (82.7%). The overall rate of resistance to at least one drug

Table 9.1 Primary drug resistance in tuberculosis in a veteran population in the USA

Study year	Total no. strains	% of strains resistant to				
		S	*PAS*	*H*	*R*[a]	*E*[a]
1962–1963	1204	3.1	2.9	3.9		
1963–1964	1400	2.6	8.0	3.3		
1964–1965	1373	2.1	4.9	2.7		
1965–1966	1175	2.5	4.3	2.7		
1966–1967	856	3.2	2.1	1.5		
1967–1968	651	1.5	5.0	2.2		
1968–1969	501	1.6	7.2	4.2	0.4	15.8
1969–1970	405	2.2	1.7	3.5	0.0	1.0
1970–1971	365	4.4	3.6	4.4	1.6	1.6
1971–1972	267	5.6	4.5	4.1	1.9	2.2
1972–1973	248	3.2	4.4	2.8	0.8	9.7
		S alone	*PAS alone*	*H alone*	*R alone*	*E alone*
1962–1963	1204	1.9	2.1	2.4		
1963–1964	1400	1.7	6.5	1.9		
1964–1965	1373	1.0	3.8	1.5		
1965–1966	1175	1.4	2.9	1.4		
1966–1967	856	1.8	1.5	0.7		
1967–1968	651	0.8	3.8	0.9		
1968–1969	501	0.6	5.0	1.8	NS	12.6
1969–1970	405	1.5	1.0	2.5	0.0	0.5
1970–1971	365	1.1	0.8	0.8	0.0	0.0
1971–1972	267	4.1	2.6	2.6	1.5	1.9
1972–1973	248	1.6	2.4	1.2	0.4	8.1
		Streptomycin and		*H and*	*H and*	*H*
		PAS	*H*	*PAS*	*PAS*	*and R*[b]
1962–1963	1204	0.08	0.70	0.40	0.30	
1963–1964	1400	0.43	0.21	0.14	0.93	
1964–1965	1373	0.36	0.22	0.44	0.29	
1965–1966	1175	0.26	0.34	0.60	0.51	
1966–1967	856	0.00	0.70	0.00	0.15	
1967–1968	651	0.30	0.15	0.30	0.75	
1968–1969	501	0.00	0.20	0.80	1.40	NS
1969–1970	405	0.00	0.49	0.00	0.49	0.00
1970–1971	365	0.27	0.82	0.00	0.55	1.64
1971–1972	267	1.12	0.00	0.40	0.37	0.37
1972–1973	248	0.81	0.40	0.00	0.40	0.00

Adapted from G.L. Hobby, P.M. Johnson and V. Boytar-Papirnyik (1970) *Am. Rev. Respir. Dis.*, **102**, 347–55.
S, streptomycin; PAS, para-aminosalicylic acid; H, isoniazid; R, rifampin; E, ethambutol. NS, not specified.
[a] Testing for rifampin and ethambutol was first included in 1968–1969.
[b] May be resistant to additional drugs.

Table 9.2 Rates of drug resistance to isoniazid, streptomycin, and para-aminosalicylic acid among newly diagnosed, untreated tuberculosis cases, 1961–1968

Year	Total strains tested	% of strains resistant to		
		H	S	PAS
1961	767	0.8	2.0	0.8
1962	2940	1.8	3.0	1.0
1963	998	2.1	2.8	0.8
1964	936	1.7	2.6	0.6
1965	988	2.3	1.3	0.7
1966	1065	2.0	2.3	0.8
1967	866	1.4	1.4	0.2
1968	820	1.3	0.9	0.2
Total	9380	1.8	2.3	0.7

Adapted from B. Doster, G.J. Caras and D.E. Snider Jr, (1967) *Am. Rev. Respir. Dis.*, **113**, 419–25.
Abbreviations as Table 9.1.

among these 3352 cases was 13.9%. Of new cases, 13.0% were reported as being resistant to at least one antituberculosis drug, and 3.2% were reported as being resistant to both isoniazid and rifampin. Of recurrent cases, 26.2% were reported as being resistant to at least one drug, and 6.8% were reported as being resistant to both isoniazid and rifampin.

The methodology used in the 1991 survey differed significantly from that of the previous CDC surveys. First, in the previous surveys, isolates were sent to a single laboratory for susceptibility testing, whereas in the 1991 survey susceptibility testing was performed in local laboratories. Second, the previous surveys included isolates from a sample of areas, whereas the 1991 survey attempted to collect results on all cases reported during the study period. Third, in the previous surveys a concerted effort was made to determine which patients had a history of previous chemotherapy and to exclude them from the study. In the 1991 survey, no attempt was made to verify this information; cases reported as 'new' were assumed to have had no previous chemo-

therapy, and cases reported as 'recurrent' were assumed to have received previous chemotherapy. Finally, underreporting of drug susceptibility results in the 1991 survey could have biased some of the findings. In spite of these limitations, this study provides the most current available information on rates of drug resistance in the USA.

Although it is not possible to conclude from these data that there has been a significant change in the rates of drug resistance nationwide, local data from New York City indicates a substantial increase in drug resistance. In a survey of all patients with positive cultures for *M. tuberculosis* in New York City in April 1991, Frieden *et al.* found that, among patients with no history of prior treatment, 23% had organisms resistant to at least one drug and 7.0% had organisms resistant to both isoniazid and rifampin[17]. In contrast, in the 1982–1986 CDC survey, 9.7% of the cases from New York City had organisms resistant to at least one drug, and 3.0% had organisms resistant to both isoniazid and rifampin [CDC, unpublished data]. The possibility that local increases have occurred in other areas cannot be ruled out on the basis of available data.

9.3.2 FACTORS ASSOCIATED WITH DRUG RESISTANCE

During the past three decades, a number of investigations have attempted to determine risk factors for drug-resistant tuberculosis in the USA. Most of these studies have been retrospective; thus, data usually was not collected systematically to evaluate specific risk factors, and the information collected might be incomplete or inaccurate. Also, since most of the studies have been hospital-based, they may not be representative of all tuberculosis cases in the community. Finally, only a few studies differentiate primary and secondary resistance before analysing potential risk factors, which may obscure important associations, and the small number of patients in some studies limits meaningful comparisons of subgroups. Nevertheless, these studies provide some useful information on the relationship between drug resistance and certain epidemiological factors.

Investigators have consistently found a strong association between drug resistance and a history of prior treatment with anti-tuberculosis drugs[16–27]. Furthermore, in a study of drug resistance among previously treated tuberculosis patients, Costello *et al.* found that, while 41% of such patients overall were excreting drug-resistant organisms, resistance rates increased significantly with increasing length of previous therapy[19]. Frieden *et al.* found a similar relationship between drug resistance and duration of previous therapy; drug resistance was present in 7% of patients treated for less than 2 months, in 19% of patients treated for 2–14 months, and in 39% of patients treated for more than 14 months[17].

It is often assumed that drug resistance occurring in persons with a history of prior treatment with antituberculosis drugs is acquired resistance. The relationship between duration of previous therapy and rate of drug resistance supports this assumption. However, Frieden *et al.* found that of 91 previously treated patients who had drug-resistant isolates in April 1991, 55 (60%) had had isolates resistant to at least one drug on their initial susceptibility test, suggesting that these patients had primary, rather than acquired, drug resistance[17]. Furthermore, Nardell *et al.* have demonstrated that persons previously treated for drug susceptible tuberculosis may subsequently be reinfected with drug-resistant strains of *M. tuberculosis* [28,29]. Thus, drug-resistant disease in a person with a history of previous treatment may be caused by acquired resistance, but may also occur because the patient initially had primary drug-resistant disease, or because a patient with previous drug-susceptible disease was reinfected with drug-resistant organisms.

Contact with a person who has infectious, drug-resistant tuberculosis is a major risk factor for the occurrence of primary drug-resistant disease, although a history of the occurrence of such exposure may be difficult to obtain. In a prospective study of primary drug-resistant tuberculosis among children, Steiner *et al.* documented a very close correlation between the drug susceptibility patterns of isolates from children and those from their presumed adult source cases[30]. In several recent nosocomial outbreaks of tuberculosis, the occurrence of multi-drug-resistant tuberculosis has been strongly associated with prior exposure to a patient with infectious, multi-drug-resistant tuberculosis[31–35].

Traditionally, drug resistant tuberculosis was thought to be less infectious than drug-susceptible tuberculosis. Based largely on animal studies[36], this notion was widely accepted, despite reports of apparent transmission of drug resistant tuberculosis. However, a study by Snider *et al.* compared the contacts of previously untreated drug-resistant cases with the contacts of drug-susceptible cases and found that the risk of infection did not differ significantly between the two groups[37]. On the other hand, the risk of infection was higher for contacts exposed to previously treated patients with drug-resistant bacilli, probably because of repeated exposure during recurrent episodes of disease in patients who were non-adherent to therapy and infectious for longer periods of time.

Several investigators have examined the relationship between drug resistance and country of origin. In a prospective study of tuberculosis patients in Los Angeles, California, Barnes found that of previously treated patients, those from Latin America, Asia or Africa were significantly more likely than those from the USA, Canada or Europe to have drug-resistant organisms[25]. Of patients with no history of prior therapy, recent immigrants (10 years or less in the USA) from Latin America, Asia or Africa were significantly more likely to have drug-resistant organisms than those from the USA, Canada or Europe, or than Latin American, Asian or African immigrants who had been in the USA for more than 10 years. In a community-based study of drug-resistant tuberculosis in Santa Clara County, California, Riley *et al.* found that resistance rates varied markedly by country of origin (19% for patients born in the USA, 33% for patients from Vietnam, 35% for patients from the Philippines, 15% for patients from Mexico, 39% for patients from China, 45% for patients from South Korea, 0% for patients from Cambodia, and 23% for patients from other countries)[27].

A CDC report of four independent surveys from Santa Clara County, California (1975–1979), San Francisco, California (1978–1980), Washington State (1980), and the CDC (1980) noted that about 33% (range 23–44%) of all culture-positive Indochinese refugee patients had organisms resistant to at least one drug[38]. However, it was not possible in these surveys to differentiate between primary and acquired drug resistance. In the 1982–1986 CDC survey of primary drug resistance, both primary and acquired drug resistance were about twice as likely in foreign-born patients than in patients born in the USA[16]. Finally, Pitchenik *et al.* found that the rate of primary drug resistance was higher among newly arriving Haitians in Florida (32%) than among Haitians already living in Florida (12%) or among non-Haitian patients (4.5%)[39]. Thus, considerable evidence indicates higher rates of both primary and secondary drug resistance among recent immigrants from areas of the world with a high prevalence of tuberculosis, such as Latin America, South East Asia and China, the Philippines and Haiti. The higher rates of primary resistance in immigrants may result from transmission of drug-resistant organisms in areas of the world where drug resistance is prevalent, or from the misclassification of patients with unrecognized or unacknowledged prior treatment as having primary resistance, or both.

Rates of primary drug resistance have been found to vary markedly among the various geographical areas of the USA[13–16]. These geographical differences have persisted even after adjustment for country of origin, race and ethnicity, and age: adjusted rates ranged from 2.4% in Indiana to 16.4% in New Mexico [CDC, unpublished data]. Specific reasons for this geographical variation are unclear, but the variation suggests that the frequency of transmission of drug-resistant organisms is different from place to place.

Some investigators have reported an association between drug resistance and the age of the patient. In New York City, Steiner *et al.* noted that the rates of primary drug resistance among children were higher than among adults in New York City[40]. The three CDC surveys of primary drug resistance found that younger persons had significantly higher resistance rates than older persons[12–15] [CDC, unpublished data]. In contrast to these studies, other investigators have found no association between drug resistance and patient age[11,21,23–25]. Variation in resistance rates by age may occur because adult cases include many individuals who were infected before the advent of antituberculosis chemotherapy, whereas many children with tuberculosis were infected after the introduction of these drugs. Thus, these childhood cases reflect more accurately the current transmission of drug-resistant organisms[40]. An alternative explanation is that the age distribution of tuberculosis cases in immigrants from Latin American and Asian countries, who have higher rates of drug resistance, differs from that of patients born in the USA, in that the immigrant cases tend to be younger. The higher primary resistance rates in young patients may therefore reflect the disproportionate percentage of foreign-born patients in the younger age groups[25]. Either or both of these explanations may apply in different areas, depending on local circumstances.

Data on the relationship between drug resistance and race or ethnicity are also conflicting. In the 1961 to 1968 CDC survey, no relationship was found between race and the risk of primary drug resistance[11,12]. The 1975–1982 CDC survey found that overall rates for Asian and Hispanic persons were significantly higher than for persons from other racial or ethnic groups [13–15]. However, when the data from each individual geographical area were analysed separately, no significant differences in rates by race or ethnicity were found[13]. Data on country of origin were not available in either of these surveys, which makes interpretation of the rates in Asian and Hispanic persons difficult. The 1982–1986 CDC survey again found variations in primary resistance rates by race and ethnicity; the higher rates found in Hispanic persons were explainable, in part, on the basis of geographical variation and country of origin [CDC, unpublished data]. Several other investigators have found no association between drug resistance rates and race or ethnicity[17,21,24,25]. Thus, the relationship between drug resistance and race or ethnicity remains undefined. No association between drug resistance rates and gender has been observed[11–13,16,17,21] [CDC, unpublished data].

Recent outbreaks of drug-resistant tuberculosis among HIV-infected persons have suggested a possible association between HIV infection and drug resistance. Three investigations of drug resistance conducted at Kings County Hospital Center in New York City failed to show a relationship between HIV infection or HIV risk factors and drug-resistant tuberculosis[20,21,41]. However, Frieden *et al* found that among 227 patients with no history of prior treatment, drug resistance was significantly more common in patients with documented HIV infection or acquired immunodeficiency syndrome (AIDS) than in patients without docu-

mented HIV infection or AIDS[17]. The HIV and AIDS status was not known for many of the patients in this study; thus, the group without documented HIV infection or AIDS could have included patients with these conditions. On the other hand, the study was conducted during a time when outbreaks of multi-drug-resistant tuberculosis were occurring among HIV-infected patients at several New York City hospitals; thus, it may reflect a more recent pattern of transmission of drug-resistant organisms, with rapid progression of new infection to active disease in those contacts who were HIV-infected.

Finally, the social instability associated with substance abuse and homelessness could lead to a higher prevalence of acquired drug resistance in patients with these characteristics. This could, in turn, lead to higher rates of primary drug resistance because of transmission of drug-resistant organisms in shelters for homeless persons and other congregate settings where homeless persons and substance abusers converge. Although some investigators have reported an association between drug resistance and substance abuse[17] or homelessness[42], others have not found such an association[17,21,25,41]. This is remarkable, considering the high rate of non-adherence to therapy that is often observed among homeless persons and substance abusers.

In summary, factors associated with drug-resistant tuberculosis have not been studied systematically and analysed rigorously. However, the available data indicate that history of prior treatment for tuberculosis, country of origin, and known contact with a person who has drug-resistant tuberculosis are consistently associated with an increased risk of drug-resistant disease. Rates of drug resistance vary considerably according to geographical area. Data on other factors, such as age, race or ethnicity, HIV and AIDS, homelessness and substance abuse are variable, and may differ substantially from area to area. These data suggest that the rates of drug resistance observed for the nation as a whole might not be generalizable to specific localities, and illustrate the importance of conducting ongoing local surveillance for drug resistance and associated factors.

9.3.3 OUTBREAKS OF DRUG-RESISTANT TUBERCULOSIS

Reports of drug-resistant tuberculosis outbreaks have been uncommon until recently. An extensive review of community and school-based tuberculosis outbreaks published in 1965 found none in which drug-resistant strains were involved[43]. From 1970 to 1990, two outbreaks of isoniazid-resistant tuberculosis and five outbreaks of multi-drug-resistant disease were reported [28,29,44–49]. These outbreaks generally involved small numbers of cases among family members and close social contacts in households, schools and communities; one involved a shelter for homeless persons. The outbreaks also usually involved prolonged or repeated exposure to the source cases, who often were symptomatic for several months before diagnosis, or who developed acquired drug resistance and remained infectious for long periods of time because of non-adherence to therapy. Finally, these outbreaks propagated relatively slowly, sometimes persisting for several years.

Recently, several large outbreaks of multi-drug-resistant tuberculosis have occurred. These differ from the previously described outbreaks in that they have spread rapidly, have involved larger numbers of patients, and have occurred in institutional settings. From 1990 to August 1992, the CDC, in collaboration with state and local health departments and hospital and prison officials, conducted investigations of outbreaks of multi-drug-resistant tuberculosis in seven hospitals in Florida, New York and New Jersey, and in the New York State correctional system[31–35,50–54] [CDC, unpublished data]. The number of cases in each of the hospital outbreaks ranged from 7 to 70 (Table 9.3). In the correctional system, there

have been approximately 42 cases, although some of these cases were also included in one of the hospital outbreaks in New York City. The total number of cases for all the outbreaks combined is now approximately 253. All of these outbreaks involve transmission of multi-drug-resistant tuberculosis from patient to patient or from patient to health care worker. In each instance, compelling epidemiological evidence of nosocomial transmission has been corroborated by laboratory evidence showing that epidemiologically linked cases had *M. tuberculosis* isolates with identical restriction fragment length polymorphism (RFLP) patterns.

All but six of the patients in these outbreaks had disease caused by organisms resistant to both isoniazid and rifampin. Most patients had isolates that were also resistant to additional drugs; in three hospitals and the correctional system, the outbreak strain was resistant to seven drugs (isoniazid, rifampin, streptomycin, ethambutol, ethionamide, kanamycin and rifabutin). Because many of the patients were severely immuno-suppressed by HIV infection or other causes, and because of the difficulty of rapidly determining an effective treatment regimen, the mortality among patients in these outbreaks has been very high (60–89%), with rapid progression from diagnosis to death (median interval 4–16 weeks).

In all but one of the recent multi-drug-resistant tuberculosis outbreaks, more than 80% of the cases have occurred in persons infected with HIV. This is likely to be a consequence of the outbreaks occurring on hospital units providing care to HIV-infected persons or in other settings with a high prevalence of HIV-infected persons (e.g. outpatient clinics for HIV-infected persons or correctional facilities), where most of those exposed were HIV-infected. In addition, active tuberculosis is highly likely to develop rapidly – within weeks to months from the time of infection – in HIV-infected persons who become newly infected with *M. tubercu-*

Table 9.3   HIV-associated multi-drug-resistant tuberculosis outbreaks January 1990 to August 1992

Facility	Location	Year of investigation	Total cases[a]	Resistance pattern[b]	HIV infection[c] (%)	Mortality[c] (%)	Median interval TB diagnosis to death (wk)[c]
Hospital A	Miami	1990	65	H, R (E, Eth)	93	72	7
Hospital B	New York City	1990	35	H, S (R, E)	100[d]	89	16
Hospital C	New York City	1991–1992	70[f]	H, R, S (E, Eth, Ka, B)	94	82	4
Hospital D	New York City	1991	29	H, R (E, Eth)	91	83	4
Hospital E[e]	New York State	1991	7	H, R, S (E, Eth, Ka, RB)	20	60	4
Hospital F	New York City	1992	16	H, R, S, (E, Eth, Ka, RB)	82	82	4
Hospital G	New Jersey	1992	13	H, R (E)	100	85	4
Prison system	New York State	1991–1992	42[f]	H, R (S, E, Eth, Ka, RB)	91	74	4
Total cases			253[f]				

Adapted from M.E. Villarino, L.J. Geiter and P.M. Simone (1992) *Publ. Hlth. Rep.*, **107**, 616–25.
[a] Includes cases found during initial investigation plus cases found through follow-up surveillance.
[b] Nonparenthetical = all cases resistant to these; parenthetical = many cases also resistant to these. H, isoniazid; R, rifampin; S, streptomycin; E, ethambutol; Eth, ethionamide; Ka, kanamycin; RB, rifabutin.
[c] Denominator includes only cases for which outcome information has been ascertained, as follows: Hospital A, n = 29; Hospital B, n = 18; Hospital C, n = 51; Hospital D, n = 23; Hospital E, n = 5; Hospital F, n = 17; Hospital G, n = 13; Prison system, n = 42.
[d] HIV infection was part of case definition.
[e] Investigated by the New York State Department of Health.
[f] 24 prison cases are also counted with Hospital C.

losis[55,56]. In these outbreaks, active tuberculosis has often developed in patients within a few weeks of their exposure to the disease. These patients have then become sources of transmission themselves, so that multiple generations of transmission occurred within a relatively short period of time. Although persons not infected with HIV might have become infected with *M. tuberculosis* in these outbreaks, active tuberculosis is considerably less likely to develop in them. Also, these persons would have a longer interval between infection and onset of disease. Thus, HIV infection is a factor that has both amplified and accelerated the outbreaks.

Health care workers have also been affected by the recent multi-drug resistant-tuberculosis outbreaks. At two hospitals, 13 (33%) out of 39 and 9 (39%) out of 23 workers had documented tuberculin skin test conversions following exposure to patients with multi-drug resistant tuberculosis. At a third hospital, more than 50 health care workers had skin test conversions following exposure to hospitalized prison inmates with multi-drug-resistant tuberculosis. Active, multi-drug-resistant tuberculosis has developed in at least 16 health care workers and one correctional worker who guarded hospitalized inmates; Seven of the health care workers were known to be HIV-seropositive, and the correctional worker was immunocompromised because of a malignancy. At least six of these workers have died, including five health care workers (four of whom were known to be HIV-seropositive) and the correctional worker.

9.3.4 FACTORS CONTRIBUTING TO MULTI-DRUG-RESISTANT OUTBREAKS

Several conditions have contributed to the outbreaks of drug-resistant tuberculosis in health care facilities and other congregate settings. First, some tuberculosis control programmes have difficulty ensuring adequate management of all patients with tuberculosis. Tuberculosis programme management data collected by the CDC indicate that only about 74–78% of patients nationwide complete a full course of therapy within 12 months. Poor adherence to therapy contributes to the development of drug-resistant disease, which can then be transmitted to other persons. Second, the increasing incidence of tuberculosis in some areas and the high prevalence of HIV infection in some institutional and congregate settings results in a convergence of people with infectious tuberculosis and immunocompromised persons, who are extremely vulnerable to tuberculosis if exposed and infected. Finally, in many institutional settings, infection-control practices and isolation facilities are insufficient for preventing transmission of tuberculosis.

In some of the multi-drug-resistant outbreaks, the diagnosis of tuberculosis in HIV-infected patients was delayed because of a low index of suspicion, unusual clinical and radiographic features, co-infection with other pulmonary pathogens (e.g. *Pneumocystis carinii*) to which their symptoms were ascribed, or delays in completing and reporting results of acid-fast bacillus (AFB) smears and mycobacterial cultures. Recognition of drug resistance was often delayed because of the length of time taken to perform and report results of drug susceptibility tests. Consequently, it was difficult to determine effective therapeutic regimens, and patients sometimes remained infectious for prolonged periods.

Initiation of AFB isolation precautions was also sometimes delayed because of the lags in diagnosis of tuberculosis. Even when tuberculosis was suspected, inadequate isolation facilities and lapses in infection control procedures facilitated transmission. In addition, some facilities discontinued isolation after an arbitrary number of days, without awaiting signs of decreased infectiousness, such as decreasing cough and decreasing numbers of AFB on sputum smears. In one outbreak, transmission in an outpatient clinic was associated with the administration of aerosolized pentamidine to patients who had active tuberculosis. The rooms used for pentamidine administration had positive air pressure relative to the adjacent clinic areas [35,50]. In the correctional system outbreak, the transfer of clinically ill inmates from facility to facility probably contributed to the spread of multi-drug-resistant tuberculosis between correctional facilities and the transmission of multi-drug-resistant tuberculosis within at least one facility. Finally, the lack of consistent follow-up of patients after discharge sometimes resulted in repeated hospital admissions of patients with infectious tuberculosis, as well as the potential transmission of drug-resistant tuberculosis in the community.

In addition to hospitals and correctional facilities, outbreaks of multi-drug-resistant tuberculosis have also occurred in a shelter for homeless persons and a substance-abuse treatment facility[28,29,57]. An outbreak of drug-susceptible tuberculosis has occurred in a congregate living facility for persons with HIV infection[55]. The factors leading to these outbreaks have been similar to those mentioned above.

9.4 APPROACHES TO PREVENTING, MANAGING, AND CONTROLLING DRUG-RESISTANT TUBERCULOSIS

Several areas must be addressed if drug-resistant tuberculosis is to be controlled and outbreaks of drug-resistant tuberculosis are to be prevented. Steps should be taken to ensure that patients with drug-susceptible tuberculosis adhere to the prescribed treatment regimen so that they do not develop drug-resistant disease. Patients with drug-resistant tuberculosis should be appropriately managed so that they have the best chance of cure and are rendered non-infectious. Current CDC guidelines for preventing the transmission of tuberculosis in health care settings should be rapidly implemented. Finally, tuberculosis control programmes should conduct ongoing surveillance to track trends in, and risk factors associated with, drug-resistant tuberculosis.

9.4.1 PATIENT MANAGEMENT

The most effective method of dealing with drug-resistant tuberculosis is to prevent it by ensuring that drug-susceptible tuberculosis is treated appropriately. The Advisory Council for the Elimination of Tuberculosis, a national advisory committee to the United States Secretary of Health and Human Services, has recently developed the following new recommendations for the initial management of patients with tuberculosis in the USA[58]:

1. *In vitro* drug susceptibility testing should be performed on the initial *M. tuberculosis* isolates from all patients with tuberculosis;
2. The initial treatment regimen should generally include four antituberculosis drugs to ensure that patients with unsuspected drug resistance are adequately treated while drug-susceptibility results are pending.
3. Directly observed therapy should be used to ensure that patients adhere to their medication regimen.

Early diagnosis and appropriate treatment of persons with active tuberculosis offer the best chance of cure, reduce the likelihood of drug-resistant disease, and prevent transmission of disease to other susceptible persons. Early diagnosis of active tuberculosis, and of drug resistance, requires a high clinical index of suspicion for tuberculosis and use of the most rapid and sensitive laboratory methods available (e.g. fluorescence microscopy for AFB smears and radiometric methods for culture and drug-susceptibility testing).

Initiating appropriate chemotherapy is the most effective way to decrease the infectiousness of a patient. Drug therapy should be started as soon as tuberculosis is suspected, before laboratory confirmation. In most cases, initial therapy should include four drugs: isoniazid, rifampin, pyrazinamide and either ethambutol or streptomycin. In areas where resistance rates are very low (i.e. less than 4%), a three-drug regimen (isoniazid, rifampin and pyrazinamide) may be adequate, whereas in areas with high rates of drug resistance, more than four drugs may be necessary for initial therapy. When susceptibility results are known, the drug therapy can be adjusted accordingly.

Prescribing appropriate chemotherapy does not ensure that the medications will be ingested by the patient. Tuberculosis clinicians have used various methods, such as pill counting and testing urine for isoniazid metabolites or colour changes caused by rifampin, in an attempt to assess patient adherence. But patients who throw out their pills instead of swallowing them or patients who only take their medications before clinic appointments would not be recognized as non-adherent with these methods. Thus, directly observed therapy is recommended to ensure adherence.

Directly observed therapy should be accomplished by a health care provider or other person who can assist the patient, in a manner that is individualized and based on a thorough assessment of each patient's unique needs, constraints and preferences, while ensuring patient confidentiality. Patients can receive directly observed therapy in the tuberculosis clinic. Adherence to directly observed therapy can be improved by the use of a variety of incentives provided by the clinic, such as providing transportation to the clinic, food, childcare, toiletries or other articles or services that are valuable to patients[59]. Alternatively, directly observed therapy can be provided by a health worker or other person at a patient's residence or place of employment. By using one of several regimens that can be given two or three times weekly, this method is also cost-effective. Other settings, such as methadone clinics and correctional facilities, may lend themselves to the effective use of directly observed therapy. These methods may appear costly, but ensuring completion of therapy is cost-effective in the long run.

Once drug-resistant tuberculosis has developed, it is much more difficult to treat than drug-susceptible tuberculosis. Tuberculosis resistant to both isoniazid and rifampin can be cured in only 45% to 56% of cases[60,61]. Despite the lack of controlled clinical trials of the treatment of multi-drug-resistant tuberculosis, there are several principles of treatment that should be followed[62,63]. First, a drug regimen should be used that includes at least three drugs for which the patient's organisms have proven *in vitro* susceptibility, and preferably that have not been used to treat the patient before. Generally, an injectable medication is included in the regimen. Secondly, a single drug should never be added to a failing regimen, because doing so may select for organisms that are resistant to progressively more drugs. Drugs should be added in combinations of two or three to avoid development of further drug resistance. Finally, the therapy of all patients with multi-drug-resistant tuberculosis should be observed directly.

Because of the high risk of relapse, treatment for multi-drug-resistant tuberculosis is usually continued for 24 months after cultures have converted to negative. Since most patients cannot tolerate therapy with an injectable drug for that length of time, injectable drugs are usually discontinued 4 months after culture conversion. Surgical resection of a major pulmonary focus of tuberculosis may be a useful adjunct to chemotherapy in some cases of drug-resistant disease[64] (Chapter 8c, p. 157).

The medications currently available for the treatment of drug-resistant tuberculosis are less effective, more costly, and associated with greater toxicity than the first-line anti-tuberculosis drugs (Table 9.4)[62,63,65–67].

The dosage of **ethionamide** is 250 mg two to four times a day. Ethionamide often causes adverse gastrointestinal effects, including abdominal pain, nausea and anorexia. Gastrointestinal intolerance may be reduced by starting with a low dose and increasing to a full dose over several days, using anti-emetics and antacids or bedtime dosing. Hypersensitivity reactions and hepatitis may occur. Rarely, endocrine disturbances such as hypothyroidism, menstrual irregularities and impotence have been associated with ethionamide administration.

Cycloserine commonly causes neurological and psychiatric disturbances ranging from minor reactions such as headache, tremor, memory problems and insomnia to more serious reactions such as psychosis or convulsions. The usual dosage is 250–750 mg a day in divided doses. Most reactions are dose-related and disappear when the medication is discontinued. Concomitant use of pyridoxine and monitoring of serum drug levels may help prevent most serious reactions. The dosage of cycloserine must be adjusted for renal impairment.

Capreomycin, kanamycin and **amikacin** must be given parenterally, usually by intramuscular injection. Even at the usual dosage of 15 mg/kg 5 days a week, these medications may cause ototoxicity, such as hearing loss, tinnitus or vestibular disturbances, especially in elderly patients or patients with pre-existing renal disease. Patients should have a baseline audiogram and be monitored with monthly audiograms and for vestibular problems during therapy. Because of potential renal toxicity, blood urea nitrogen (BUN) and

Table 9.4   Second-line antituberculosis drugs

Drug	Daily dose	Adverse effects	Monitoring	Other
Ethionamide	500–1000 mg p.o. (in divided doses if necessary for tolerance)	GI intolerance, hepatitis, endocrine disturbances, hypersensitivity	SGOT	Consider antiemetics or bedtime dosing
Cycloserine	250–750 mg p.o. (in divided doses) (adjust for renal impairment)	Neurological and psychiatric disturbances	Serum levels	Administer pyridoxine (vitamin B6)
Capreomycin Amikacin Kanamycin	15 mg/kg i.m. 5 days a week (adjust for renal impairment	Hearing loss, vestibular damage, renal toxicity, electrolyte disturbances	Audiogram, vestibular exam. BUN and creatinine	
Para-aminosalicylic acid (PAS)	10–20 g p.o. (in divided doses for tolerance)	GI intolerance, hepatitis, hypersensitivity	SGOT	Consider antacids or dosing at mealtime
Ciprofloxacin	500–1000 mg q.d., p.o.	GI intolerance, headache, restlessness, hypersensitivity, drug interactions	Monitor for drug interactions	Avoid antacids, iron, zinc and sucralfate, which decrease absorption
Ofloxacin	400–800 mg q.d., p.o.			
Clofazimine	100–300 mg q.d., p.o.	Abdominal pain skin discoloration (both dose-related) photosensitivity		Consider dosing at mealtime; avoid sunlight; efficacy unproven

creatinine levels should be monitored and if elevated, the dose should be adjusted accordingly.

P-aminosalicylic acid (PAS) frequently causes gastrointestinal complaints. The usual dosage is 12g (or 24 tablets of 500 mg each) a day given in divided doses. Gastrointestinal intolerance can be decreased by beginning with a low dose and gradually increasing to a full dose over 7–10 days, taking the medication on a full stomach or using antacids. Infrequently, PAS may cause hypersensitivity reactions, hypothyroidism or haemolytic anaemia.

Ciprofloxacin and **ofloxacin** appear to have excellent *in vitro* activity against *M. tuberculosis*, however there are no controlled clinical trials of their use for tuberculosis. These medications are generally well tolerated. Significant drug interactions may occur with cimetidine, cyclosporin, non-steroidal anti-inflammatory agents, warfarin, theophylline and even caffeine [68]. The most frequently reported adverse reactions are nausea, diarrhoea, abdominal discomfort, headache, restlessness and rash. Antacids and iron supplements reduce the absorption of these drugs and should be avoided within 2 h of the dose (Chapter 8a, p. 131).

Clofazimine has been used for many years to treat leprosy. The efficacy of this medication for the treatment of tuberculosis is unknown. The drug deposits in various tissues of the body including the skin, producing an orange or brown discoloration. Gastrointestinal complaints are common. Clofazimine has a very long half-life. The usual starting dosage is 200–300 mg a day, decreasing to 100 mg a day once there is evidence of tissue saturation such as skin discoloration.

9.4.2 INFECTION CONTROL FOR HEALTH CARE SETTINGS

To prevent transmission of tuberculosis in health care settings, appropriate infection control procedures must be used[69]. The highest priority is controlling transmission at the source by diagnosing persons with tuberculosis early, beginning appropriate therapy, and initiating isolation. Patients with suspected or confirmed infectious tuberculosis should be placed promptly in tuberculosis (acid-fast bacillus, AFB) isolation in a private room with negative air pressure relative to adjacent areas, with air exhausted directly to the outside of the building, to prevent the spread of infectious droplet nuclei to other areas of the facility. The role of other potential adjunctive measures, such as germicidal ultraviolet irradiation, is not well defined. Isolation precautions should be maintained until the patient improves clinically, until cough has decreased substantially, and until there is a progressive decrease in the number of acid-fast bacilli on sequential sputum smears. When drug-resistant tuberculosis is suspected or confirmed, AFB isolation precautions should be maintained until the sputum smear is negative for acid-fast bacilli. When cough-inducing procedures (e.g. bronchoscopy, sputum induction, administration of aerosol treatments) are done in patients who may have tuberculosis, they should be carried out in rooms or booths with negative air pressure and with air exhausted directly to the outside or through high-efficiency particulate air (HEPA) filters.

Finally, patients and health care workers who are exposed to infectious tuberculosis patients for whom adequate isolation precautions have not been instituted should be identified and evaluated for tuberculosis infection or active disease. Routine, active surveillance should be conducted by health care facilities to identify tuberculin skin test conversions among health care workers. A screening programme should include testing at the time of employment as well as retesting every 6–24 months, depending on the prevalence of tuberculosis in the institution. This type of programme enables infection control personnel to identify workers for whom preventive therapy may be indicated, and to evaluate the effectiveness of current infection control practices by detecting transmission through monitoring skin test conversions.

9.4.3 SURVEILLANCE

Tuberculosis control programmes should conduct surveillance for drug-resistant tuberculosis and associated risk factors for several reasons[6]. Information on the epidemiology of drug-resistant tuberculosis can be used to help determine the appropriate initial therapy regimen for patients in a given area or for individual patients. The current recommendation for the initial therapy of tuberculosis patients in the USA includes isoniazid, rifampin and pyrazinamide, plus either ethambutol or streptomycin. However, in some geographical areas this regimen may be inadequate for a significant proportion of patients, and in other areas an initial regimen with fewer than four drugs may be acceptable. Analysis of epidemiological data can help determine whether modifications in the recommendations for the initial treatment regimen are warranted. In addition, epidemiological data may be useful in determining characteristics of persons at increased risk for drug-resistant tuberculosis so that the initial treatment regimen prescribed for these persons can be modified appropriately. Furthermore, data from ongoing or periodic epidemiological surveys of drug resistance can be used to track trends in the rates of drug resistance and to guide tuberculosis-control activities. The occurrence of primary resistance may reflect ongoing transmission, suggesting a need for improved case-finding and containment. On the other hand, the occurrence of secondary drug resistance may indicate the need to improve the programme's effectiveness in managing cases and ensuring that patients adhere to and complete therapy.

9.5 FUTURE DIRECTIONS

Future efforts to control drug-resistant tuberculosis will need to focus on several areas. Epidemiological studies are needed to better define risk factors for drug-resistant tuberculosis. Improved use of currently available tools for diagnosing, treating and preventing tuberculosis is needed. Additional research is needed to identify more sensitive and rapid diagnostic techniques, new drugs that require a shorter therapeutic course and new preventive measures for tuberculosis. Evaluation of supplemental infection control measures, such as germicidal ultraviolet irradiation, would help clarify the role of these measures in infection control programmes. Finally, coalitions should be developed between health departments and community organizations to address the specific needs of the community, especially those community members at highest risk for tuberculosis. Tuberculosis control efforts will be more successful as tuberculosis education is expanded and community awareness is raised.

REFERENCES

1. Jereb, J.A., Kelly, G.D., Dooley Jr, S.W. *et al.* (1991) Tuberculosis morbidity in the United States: Final Data, 1990. *Morbid. Mortal. Weekly Rep.*, **40** (SS-3), 23–6.
2. Brudney, K. and Dobkin, J. (1991) Resurgent tuberculosis in New York City. Human immunodeficiency virus, homelessness and the decline of tuberculosis control programs. *Am. Rev. Respir. Dis.*, **144**, 745–9.
3. Youmans, G.P., Williston, E.II., Feldman, W.H. *et al.* (1946) Increase in resistance of tubercle bacilli to streptomycin. A preliminary report. *Proc. Mayo Clin.*, **21**, 126–7.
4. David, H.L. (1970) Probability distribution of drug-resistant mutants in unselected populations of *Mycobacterium tuberculosis*. *Appl. Microbiol.*, **20**, 810–14.
5. Canetti, G. (1965) The J. Burns Amberson Lecture. Present aspects of bacterial resistance in tuberculosis. *Am. Rev. Respir. Dis.*, **92**, 687–703.
6. Gangadharam, P.R.J. (1984) *Drug Resistance in Mycobacteria*, CRC Press, London.
7. Hobby, G.L., Johnson, P.M., Lenert, T.F. *et al.* (1964) A continuing study of primary drug resistance in tuberculosis in a veteran population within the United States I. *Am. Rev. Respir. Dis.*, **89**, 337–49.
8. Hobby, G.L., Johnson, P.M. and Boytar-Papirnyik, V. (1970) Primary drug resistance: A continuing study of drug resistance in tuberculosis in a veteran population within the United States VII. September 1965 –

September 1969. *Am. Rev. Respir. Dis.*, **102**, 347–55.

9. Hobby, G.L., Johnson, P.M. and Boytar-Papirnyik, V. (1971) Primary drug resistance: A continuing study of drug resistance in tuberculosis in a veteran population within the United States IX. September 1969 – September 1970. *Am. Rev. Respir. Dis.*, **103**, 842–4.

10. Hobby, G.L., Johnson, P.M. and Boytar-Papirnyik, V. (1974) Primary drug resistance: A continuing study of drug resistance in tuberculosis in a veteran population within the United States X. September 1970–September 1973. *Am. Rev. Respir. Dis.*, **110**, 95–8.

11. US Public Health Service Cooperative Investigation (1964) Prevalence of drug resistance in previously untreated patients. *Am. Rev. Respir. Dis.*, **89**, 327–36.

12. Doster, B., Caras, G.J. and Snider Jr, D.E. (1976) A continuing survey of primary drug resistance in tuberculosis, 1961 to 1968. A US Public Health Service cooperative study. *Am. Rev. Respir. Dis.*, **113**, 419–25.

13. Kopanoff, D.E., Kilburn, J.O., Glassroth, J.L. *et al.* (1978) A continuing survey of tuberculosis primary drug resistance in the United States: March 1975 – November 1977. A United States Public Health Service cooperative study. *Am. Rev. Respir. Dis.*, **118**, 835–42.

14. Centers for Disease Control (1980) Primary resistance to antituberculosis drugs – United States. *Morbid. Mortal. Weekly Rep.*, **29**, 345–6.

15. Centers for Disease Control (1983) Primary resistance to antituberculosis drugs – United States. *Morbid. Mortal. Weekly Rep.*, **32**, 521–3.

16. Snider Jr., D.E., Cauthen, G.M., Farer, L.S. *et al.* (1991) Drug-resistant tuberculosis (letter). *Am. Rev. Respir. Dis.*, **144**, 732.

17. Frieden, T.R., Sterling, T., Pablos-Mendez, A. *et al.* (1993) The emergence of drug-resistant tuberculosis: New York City. *N. Engl. J. Med.*, **328**, 521–6.

18. Aswapokee, P., Aswapokee, N., Neu, C.O. *et al.* (1980) Drug-resistant tuberculosis: serious problem. *NY State J. Med.*, **80**, 1541–5.

19. Costello, H.D., Caras, G.J. and Snider Jr., D.E. (1980) Drug resistance among previously treated tuberculosis patients, a brief report. *Am. Rev. Respir. Dis.*, **121**, 313–16.

20. Shafer, R.W., Kim, D.S., Weiss, J.P. and Quale, J.M. (1991) Extrapulmonary tuberculo-sis in patients with human immunodeficiency virus infection. *Medicine*, **70**, 384–97.

21. Chawla, P.K., Klapper, P.J., Kamholz, S.L. *et al.* (1992) Drug-resistant tuberculosis in an urban population including patients at risk for human immunodeficiency virus infection. *Am. Rev. Respir. Dis.*, **146**, 280–4.

22. Arango, L., Brewin, A.W. and Murray, J.F. (1973) The spectrum of tuberculosis as currently seen in a metropolitan hospital. *Am. Rev. Respir. Dis.*, **108**, 805–12.

23. Schiffman, P.L., Ashkar, B., Bishop, M. *et al.* (1977) Drug resistant tuberculosis in a large southern California hospital. *Am. Rev. Respir. Dis.*, **116**, 821–5.

24. Ben-Dov, I. and Mason, G.R. (1987) Drug-resistant tuberculosis in a southern California hospital: trends from 1969 to 1984. *Am. Rev. Respir. Dis.*, **135**, 1307–10.

25. Barnes, P.F. (1987) The influence of epidemiologic factors on drug resistance rates in tuberculosis. *Am. Rev. Respir. Dis.*, **136**, 325–8.

26. Page, M.I. and Lunn, J.S. (1984) Experience with tuberculosis in a public teaching hospital. *Am. J. Med.*, **77**, 667–70.

27. Riley, L.W., Arathoon, E. and Loverde, V.D. (1989) The epidemiologic patterns of drug resistant *Mycobacterium tuberculosis*: A community-based study. *Am. Rev. Respir. Dis.*, **19**, 1282–5.

28. Centers for Disease Control (1985) Drug resistant tuberculosis among the homeless – Boston. *Morbid. Mortal. Weekly Rep.*, **34**, 429–31.

29. Nardell, E., McInnis, B., Thomas, B. and Weidhaas, S. (1986) Exogenous reinfection with tuberculosis in a shelter for the homeless. *N. Engl. J. Med.*, **315**, 1570–5.

30. Steiner, M., Zimmerman, R., Park, B.H. *et al.* (1968) Primary tuberculosis in children: 2. Correlation of susceptibility patterns of *M. tuberculosis* isolated from children with those isolated from source cases as an index of drug-resistant infection in a community. *Am. Rev. Respir. Dis.*, **98**, 201–9.

31. Centers for Disease Control (1990) Nosocomial transmission of multidrug resistant TB to health-care workers and HIV-infected patients in an urban hospital – Florida. *Morbid. Mortal. Weekly Rep.*, **39**, 718–22.

32. Centers for Disease Control (1991) Nosocomial transmission of multidrug resistant tuberculosis among HIV-infected persons – Florida and

New York, 1988–1991. *Morbid. Mortal. Weekly Rep.*, **40**, 585–91.

33. Edlin, B.R., Tokars, J.I., Grieco, M.H. *et al.* (1992) An outbreak of multidrug resistant tuberculosis among hospitalized patients with the acquired immunodeficiency syndrome. *N. Engl. J. Med.*, **326**, 1514–21.

34. Pearson, M.L., Jereb, J.A., Frieden, T.R. *et al.*, (1992) Nosocomial transmission of multidrug resistant *Mycobacterium tuberculosis*. A risk to patients and health care workers. *Ann. Intern. Med.*, **117**, 191–6.

35. Beck-Sague, C., Dooley, S.W., Hutton, M.D. *et al.* (1992) Outbreak of multidrug resistant *Mycobacterium tuberculosis* infections in a hospital: transmission to patients with HIV infection and staff. *J. of the Am. Med. Assoc.*, **268**, 1280–6.

36. Riley, R.L., Mills, C.C., O'Grady, F. *et al.* (1962) Infectiousness of air from a tuberculosis ward. *Am. Rev. Respir. Dis.*, **85**, 511–25.

37. Snider, D.E., Kelly, G.D., Cauthen, G.M. *et al.* (1985) Infections and disease among contacts of tuberculosis cases with drug resistant and drug susceptible bacilli. *Am. Rev. Respir. Dis.*, **132**, 125–32.

38. Centers for Disease Control (1981) Drug resistance among Indochinese refugees with tuberculosis. *Morbid. Mortal. Weekly Rep.*, **30**, 273–5.

39. Pitchenik, A.E., Russell, B.W., Cleary, T. *et al.* (1982) The prevalence of tuberculosis and drug resistance among Haitians. *N. Engl. J. Med.*, **307**, 162–5.

40. Steiner, M. and Cosio, A. (1966) Primary tuberculosis in children: 1. Incidence of primary drug resistant disease in 332 children observed between the years 1961 and 1964 at the Kings County Medical Center of Brooklyn. *N. Engl. J. Med.*, **274**, 755–9.

41. Shafer, R.W., Chirgwin, K.D., Glatt, A.E., *et al.* (1991) HIV prevalence, immunosuppression and drug resistance in patients with tuberculosis in an area endemic for AIDS. *AIDS*, **5**, 399–405.

42. Pablos-Mendez, A., Raviglione, M.C., Battan, R. and Ramos-Zuniga, R. (1990) Drug resistant tuberculosis among the homeless in New York City. *NY State J. Med.*, **90**, 351–5.

43. Lincoln, E.M. (1965) Epidemics of tuberculosis. *Adv. Tubercs. Res.*, **14**, 157–201.

44. Centers for Disease Control (1980) INH-resistant tuberculosis in an urban high school

– Oregon. *Morbid. Mortal. Weekly Rep.*, **29**, 194–6.

45. Centers for Disease Control (1983) Interstate outbreak of drug resistant tuberculosis involving children – California, Montana, Nevada, Utah. *Morbid. Mortal. Weekly Rep.*, **32**, 516–18.

46. Steiner, M., Chaves, A.D., Lyons, H.A. *et al.* (1970) Primary drug resistant tuberculosis. Report of an outbreak. *N. Engl. J. Med.*, **283**, 1353–8.

47. Reeves, R., Blakey, D., Snider Jr., D.E. and Farer, L.S. (1981) Transmission of multiple drug resistant tuberculosis: Report of a school and community outbreak. *Am. J. Epidemiol.*, **113**, 423–35.

48. Centers for Disease Control (1987) Multi-drug resistant tuberculosis – North Carolina. *Morbid. Mortal. Weekly Rep.*, **35**, 785–7.

49. Centers for Disease Control (1990) Outbreak of multidrug resistant tuberculosis – Texas, California, and Pennsylvania. *Morbid. Mortal. Weekly Rep.*, **39**, 369–72.

50. Fischl, M.A., Uttamchandani, R.B., Daikos, G.L. *et al.* (1992) An outbreak of tuberculosis caused by multiple-drug resistant tubercle bacilli among patients with HIV infection. *Ann. Intern. Med.*, **117**, 177–83.

51. Fischl, M.A., Daikos, G.L., Uttamchandani, R.B. *et al.* (1992) Clinical presentation and outcome of patients with HIV infection and tuberculosis caused by multiple-drug resistant bacilli. *Ann. Intern. Med.*, **117**, 184–90.

52. Centers for Disease Control (1992) Transmission of multidrug resistant tuberculosis among immunocompromised persons in a correctional system – New York, 1991. *Morbid. Mortal. Weekly Rep.*, **41**, 507–9.

53. Dooley, S.W., Jarvis, W.R., Martone, W.J. (1992) Multidrug resistant tuberculosis (Editorial). *Ann. Intern. Med.*, **117**, 257–8.

54. Villarino, M.E., Geiter, L.J. and Simone, P.M. (1992) The multidrug resistant tuberculosis challenge to public health efforts to control tuberculosis. *Publ. Hlth Rep.*, **107**, 616–25.

55. Daley, C.L., Small, P.M., Schecter, G.F. *et al.* (1992) An outbreak of tuberculosis with accelerated progression among persons infected with the human immunodeficiency virus. An analysis using restriction-fragment-length polymorphisms. *N. Engl. J. Med.*, **326**, 231–5.

56. Di Perri, G., Cruciani, M., Danzi, M.C. *et al.*

(1989) Nosocomial epidemic of active tuberculosis among HIV-infected patients. *Lancet*, **2**, 1502–4.

57. Centers for Disease Control (1991) Transmission of multidrug-resistant tuberculosis from an HIV-positive client in a residential substance-abuse treatment facility – Michigan. *Morbid. Mortal. Weekly Rep.*, **40**, 129–31.

58. Centers for Disease Control (1993) Initial therapy for tuberculosis in the era of multidrug resistance: Recommendations of the Advisory Council for the Elimination of Tuberculosis. *Morbid. Mortal. Weekly Rep.*, **42** (RR-7), 1–8.

59. Snider Jr, D.E. and Hutton, M.D. (1989) Improving patient compliance. *Centers for Disease Control*, Atlanta, Ga.

60. Mitchison, D.A. and Nunn, A.J. (1986) Influence of initial drug resistance on the response to short course chemotherapy of pulmonary tuberculosis. *Am. Rev. Respir. Dis.*, **133**, 423–30.

61. Goble, M., Horsburgh Jr, C.R., Waite, D. *et al.* (1988) Treatment of isoniazid and rifampin-resistant tuberculosis. *Amer. Rev. Respir. Dis.*, **137** (Suppl.), 24.

62. Iseman, M.D. and Madsen, L.A. (1989) Drug-resistant tuberculosis. *Clin. Chest Med.*, **10**, 341–53.

63. Goble, M. (1986) Drug resistant tuberculosis. *Semin. Respir. Infect.*, **1**, 220–9.

64. Iseman, M.D., Madsen, L., Goble, M. and Pomerantz, M. (1990) Surgical intervention in the treatment of pulmonary disease caused by drug resistant *Mycobacterium tuberculosis*. *Am. Rev. Respir. Dis.*, **141**, 623–5.

65. Girling, D.J. (1982) Adverse effects of anti-tuberculosis drugs. *Drugs*, **23**, 56–74.

66. Moulding, T. and Davidson, P.T. (1974) Tuberculosis II: Toxicity and intolerance to antituberculosis drugs. *Drug Therapy*, 39–43.

67. Lefkowitz, M.S. (1981) The antimycobacterial drugs. *Semin. Respir. Med.*, **2**, 196–201.

68. Stein, G.E. (1991) Drug interactions with fluoroquinolones. *Am. J. Med.*, **91** (Suppl. 6A) 81S–86S.

69. Centers for Disease Control. (1990) Guidelines for preventing the transmission of tuberculosis in health-care settings, with special focus on HIV-related issues. *Morbid. Mortal. Weekly Rep.*, **39** (RR-17), 1–29.

TUBERCULOSIS IN IMMIGRANTS, ETHNIC MINORITIES AND THE HOMELESS

P.D.O. Davies

10.1 INTRODUCTION

Wherever people have migrated in the world they have carried their diseases with them. Tuberculosis is no exception. Until the middle of this century the trend was for the (present) developed Western world to export tuberculosis to the developing nations. Migrants and convicts sent to Australia took the disease to the native Aborigines[1] and the British were also responsible for infecting the native Maori in New Zealand[2]. Explorers and possibly missionaries and traders carried the organism to Africa[3] during the last century and even earlier to India[4]. As recently as the 1940s and 1950s the White man appears responsible for transmitting the disease to the natives in the relatively isolated areas of Central New Guinea[5] (Chapter 1, p. 6). In exploration of the New World, Europeans have also spread disease to South and Central America, to the native Indians of North America and the Eskimos of Canada[6]. In all cases the initial spread of disease to a previously non-infected and therefore non-immune population resulted in devastating consequences in terms of mortality and morbidity.

Rates of disease in Europe reached a peak in the early half of the nineteenth century when approximately one death in four was caused by tuberculosis. By 1850 this had fallen to 12% of deaths and by the beginning of the twentieth century to 9%.

Accurate estimates of data from the developing world are even now unreliable but, until the 1980s as rates of disease declined in the developed world, rates appeared to remain high or be declining only slowly in the developing world. Movement of individuals or populations from the developing to the developed world inevitably resulted in high rates of disease in the immigrant population from developing countries. The experience of the UK, with immigration mainly from its former colonies since the end of the Second World War, has been particularly closely documented (Fig. 10.1).

10.2 EXPERIENCE OF IMMIGRATION AND TUBERCULOSIS IN THE UK

10.2.1 IMMIGRATION IN THE 1950s

The problem of certain minority ethnic groups who have recently immigrated to the UK and who appear to be more susceptible to tuberculosis, has been well described. Among the first such minorities to come under scrutiny were the Irish[7]. In a study of tuberculosis hospital patients in London, a higher proportion of Irish immigrants were found to be tuberculin-negative than the English. The immigrant Irish had higher rates

Clinical Tuberculosis. Edited by P.D.O. Davies. Published in 1994 by Chapman & Hall, London. ISBN 0 412 48630 X

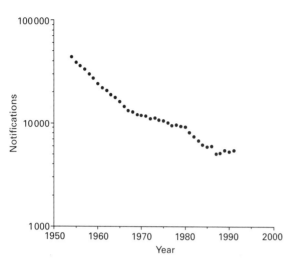

Fig. 10.1 Notifications of tuberculosis (all forms) in England and Wales from 1954 to 1991. The exponential decline slowed from approximately 10% per annum to 3% per annum from 1965 to 1980 as a result of immigration. The reason for the increase since 1987 is not yet clear.

the West Indies. In 1965, in a paper drawing a parallel between the incidence of tuberculosis and sarcoidosis in London, Brett pointed to a decline of rates of disease among the Irish between the years 1958 and 1963, but an increase in rates among West Indian immigrants[10].

10.2.2 TUBERCULOSIS IN IMMIGRANTS FROM THE INDIAN SUBCONTINENT

(a) First reports

The first to draw attention to the increasing incidence of tuberculosis in immigrants born in India or Pakistan was Springett in Birmingham in 1958[11]. In a review of notifications in Birmingham he showed that there had been a steady rise in the proportion of notifications among immigrants from these countries and calculated rates of disease in the group to be four to six times the rates for the White population. He suggested immigrants brought their disease with them and higher rates reflected rates in the countries of origin.

Nicol Roe in Uxbridge in 1959[12] showed a steadily rising incidence of notifications of Indian immigrants since 1954. He found that the majority did not develop disease until a year or more after entry to the UK and a large proportion of contacts were tuberculin-negative. He concluded the disease was acquired mainly in the UK.

Aspin in Wolverhampton[13] and Stevenson in Bradford in 1962 [14] also showed that there were increasing numbers of individuals of Indian and Pakistani ethnic origin developing tuberculosis from 1954 onwards. Rates among Indians in Wolverhampton were four times higher and in Pakistanis in Bradford 30 times higher than in the indigenous White population. Both workers suggested that the majority of patients developed tuberculosis after entry to the UK. Aspin recommended BCG and chest radiograph for all Asian* immigrants on arrival to the UK.

of tuberculosis than those born to Irish parents in the UK. Also, there was a higher incidence of pleural effusion and primary disease in the Irish than in the English patients of similar age. The authors suggest that tuberculosis had passed through the UK in a 'wave-like epidemic' affecting the English population first, and at that time resulted in a more resistant English and a more susceptible Irish population.

In 1961 evidence was published of high rates in immigrant workers in Soho, particularly the Chinese[8]. Rates were found to be twice as high in immigrant workers compared with the indigenous population and more than ten times as high in workers from Hong Kong. Brett, in 1958[9] in a mass miniature radiography (MMR) study, emphasized the high rates in the Irish. He also drew attention to higher rates in immigrants from

* The MRC attempted to introduce the term 'Indian subcontinent ethnic origin' to define the population originating from India, Pakistan and Bangladesh, rather than the less accurate term 'Asian', which would describe those originating in any part of Asia. This has now become important as Chinese and others from South-East Asia are presenting in increasing numbers.

The Tuberculosis Disease Committee of the Chest Group of the British Medical Association[15] came to the same conclusion and pointed out that if rates of immigration from the New Commonwealth continued the numbers of cases of tuberculosis in this group would exceed 1000 per year, a prediction that proved to be a gross under-estimate.

(b) Immigration to Birmingham

Springett, and later Innes, in a number of further publications[16–19], continued to trace the development of tuberculosis in immigrants in Birmingham. By comparing notification numbers around the times of the national censuses in 1961 and 1971[18], Springett was able to make accurate calculations of rates of disease by sex and country of birth. Whereas annual rates for males born in the UK had declined from 0.68 to 0.28 per 1000 per year, and for females from 0.39 to 0.18 in the 10-year period between the censuses, rates among Indian-born males had increased from 4.5 to 5.1, and for Indian-born females from 4.2 to 8.3 per 1000 per year. Rates for Indians were, therefore, seven times those for the White population in 1961 but 20 times in 1971. Rates for Pakistani-born patients, though much higher than rates for Indians in 1961, showed a relative decline to levels similar to the Indian-born patients by 1971.

Rates were highest in the young adult group in which large-scale immigration was taking place. Springett concluded that the increase in the number of notifications of ISC immigrants would cease when the immigration of dependants was completed. He also showed that though non-respiratory tuberculosis accounted for 11% of cases among those born in the UK, it accounted for 40% of those of ISC origin. Rates in the West Indian population were not appreciably different from those born in the UK.

(c) Further local reports

A number of further reports from areas with a large Asian population have been published. Rowland *et al.*[20], in a tuberculin survey of commonwealth immigrant children in Bradford, showed higher tuberculin positivity rates among immigrant children than among those born in the UK. McNicol in Brent in 1971[21] also showed a rising trend in notification rates in the Asian population from 1964 to 1970. However, they also showed that immigrants had less extensive disease than the White population and were more likely to be sputum smear-negative.

A rise in notification rates from 1963 to 1970 among the Asian population was reported from Blackburn in 1972[22] and from East London in 1976[23]. Casemore reported that an increasing proportion of bacteriological confirmation of all forms of tuberculosis was found among Asian patients in South Cleveland in 1968, accounting for 0.7% of cases in 1968 but 8% in 1974[24].

Grenville-Mathers and Clark from North West London in 1979[25] reported seeing large numbers of Asian patients with disease in their Chest Clinic. They suggested that relatively few patients arrive with overt disease. The highest frequency of new cases occurred between 3 months and 1 year after immigration into the country. They concluded that patients arrive with tuberculosis infection but only develop overt disease after entry to the UK. Clarke *et al.* in 1979[26] reported high rates of tuberculosis among the Asian population of Leicester.

10.2.3 TUBERCULOSIS AMONG VAGRANTS

The problem of tuberculosis among vagrants has also been well documented. Scott *et al.* [27] in a prevalence study of those residing in common lodging houses in Edinburgh showed tuberculosis to be present in 10.3% of 310 subjects examined. Caplin, in 1978 [28,29] in East London, showed a very high association between alcoholism and tuberculosis, 42% of 227 admissions to Bethnal Green tuberculosis ward over 3 years being classified as alcoholic and 80% of these were homeless. These people required special facilities for follow-up and were provided with an intermediate house for resettling in the community.

Patel in Glasgow[30] and Shanks in Manchester[31] have also drawn attention to the high prevalence of tuberculosis in, and difficulty of following-up, individuals residing in common lodging houses.

10.2.4 NATIONAL SURVEYS

In 1965 a national survey was undertaken by the British Tuberculosis Association[32]. A total of 285 chest physicians in 488 chest clinics agreed to co-operate. Details requested on patients included place of birth, site of disease and date of first entry to the UK. No attempt was made to ascertain the extent or activity of disease.

During the 3-month period of the survey 3806 notifications were received by the survey co-ordinator, representing 87% of all notifications in England and Wales according to figures published by the Ministry of Health.

Persons born outside the UK provided 16.5% of the notifications, although they formed only 4% of the population in 1965. Notifications for those born in India and Pakistan were 9% of the total, though they comprised only 1% of the population. Compared with those born in the UK, tuberculosis notification rates were 12 times higher among those born in India and 26 times higher among those born in Pakistan.

A second national survey using the same methods as the 1965 survey was undertaken by the British Thoracic and Tuberculosis Association in 1971[33]. In a 4-month period, a total of 3521 notifications were received representing 85% of all notifications during the survey period. In this second survey persons born outside the UK provided 32%

of notifications but comprised only 5% of the population. Notification rates were 27 times for the Indian and 54 times for the Pakistani population over the rate for those born in the UK. Except for genitourinary disease, non-respiratory tuberculosis rates also increased substantially in the ISC-born individuals between the two surveys.

(a) Rates related to length of stay

A finding from the 1971 survey[34] was that notification rates for immigrant groups tended to be highest for recent arrivals, becoming progressively lower for immigrants who had been in the UK for a longer period. The highest rate of 1109 per 100 000 per annum was in the Pakistani/Bangladeshi females, of whom 80% had immigrated within the previous 2 years, whereas the lowest rate was 414/100 000 among Indian males, only 65% of whom had immigrated within 2 years.

(b) Non-respiratory disease

The high rates of extrapulmonary disease in the Asian immigrant group had been noted since 1961 when Silver and Steel[35] pointed to the high incidence of mediastinal gland involvement in Asians. They suggested that this was due to a failure of acquired resistance at the time of primary infection leading to a combined picture of primary and chronic pulmonary disease simultaneously. Corruthers and Lang in 1970[36] from Bradford showed that though Asians provided 61% of pulmonary and 78% of extrapulmonary tuberculosis cases, they only comprised 13% of the genitourinary cases. Andrews and MacMillan in 1975[37] in Smethwick, giving figures for the incidence of intracranial tuberculosis, pointed out that in ten cases over 20 years, the last five had occurred in the most recent 5 years, all in Asian immigrants.

Williams and Hetzel in 1978[38] showed that the recent rise in cases of tuberculous pericarditis in South West London was due to the high numbers of Asians.

Among patients with gastrointestinal disease in Bradford[39] from 1967 to 1977, Findlay *et al.* found 45 of 52 were Asians. They presented with disease between 6 months and 16 years from immigration. The authors suggested that 'stress of immigration may modify the immune status'. Data on superficial lymph node tuberculosis was provided by Summers and McNicol from Brent in 1980[40]. Of 239 cases reported from 1972 to 1976, 79% were in patients of Asian origin, 75% of whom developed disease within 5 years of entry. In 93% of these cases the disease affected the cervical or supraclavicular nodes. A *Lancet* leader[41] in 1983 referred to the continuing problem of scrofula.

Bone and joint disease has received reviews from Bradford[42] (1974), Manchester[43] (1982) and East London[44] (1982). All showed higher rates among the Asian population. They also suggested that the disease may be more acute in Asian patients and have a greater systemic component, though this may be related to the younger average age of Asian patients.

Evidence of tuberculous meningitis[45] in 1983 showed it to be a continuing problem but not greatly affected by the Asian immigrant population. Innes, when reviewing non-respiratory disease[46] in 1981, showed that there had been no decline in non-respiratory disease in the past 16 years, a period when the decline for respiratory disease was continuing at between 5 and 10% per annum.

10.2.5 THE NEED TO DEFINE ETHNIC ORIGIN

During the 1970s it became apparent that national notification surveys, using date of birth to determine the national origin of patients, was insufficient to provide accurate data, as a new generation of children were growing up who had been born in the UK to immigrant parents[32,33]. Further notification surveys would need to include a question on ethnic origin. The first such survey was undertaken by the Medical Research Council Tuberculosis and Chest Diseases Unit, and included all notifications in England and Wales from 1 October 1978 to 31 March 1979[47]. Estimation of rates of disease from this and subsequent surveys was complicated by the fact that, for political reasons, a question on ethnic origin was not included in the National Censuses of 1981. Population estimates by ethnic origin were, however, obtained from a national dwelling and housing survey, for England alone[48].

The main findings from this survey were:

1. Of patients with 'new' disease (patients not previously treated for disease), 57% were White and 35% of ISC ethnic origin, though the latter formed only 2% of the population.
2. Rates of disease were 30 times higher for respiratory disease and 80 times higher for non-respiratory disease among those of ISC ethnic origin than the White population.
3. Rates for respiratory disease were higher in White men than White women, whereas the sex incidence for respiratory disease was equal in the ISC population. Rates for non-respiratory disease were approximately equal between White men and women, but were much higher in ISC females compared with males. Rates increased progressively with age.
4. Non-respiratory disease at any site was much more common in the ISC than the White group, but lymph node disease was by far the most common in the ISC group (56% of those with non-respiratory disease) while GU disease was more common in the White group (30%).
5. Radiographic extent of disease was, on average, less extensive in the ISC group compared with the White group, and cavitation less frequent.

Table 10.1 Annual notification rates for newly notified previously untreated patients per 100 000 population in England and Wales and by ethnic group for England

| Country | Ethnic origin | 1978/9 | | 1983 | | 1988 | |
		Popn. estimate (000)	Rate per 100 000	Popn. estimate (000)	Rate per 100 000	Popn. estimate (000)	Rate per 100 000
England	White	43 320	9.4	42 994	6.9	43 938	4.7
	Indian	525	354.0	773	178.0	800	134.6
	Pakistani/Bangladeshi	248	353.0	422	169.0	541	100.5
	West Indian	514	30.0	494	30.0	464	29.2
	Other	425	97.0	634	47.0	792	25.9
	All	45 779[a]	16.4	46 164[a]	12.2	46 829[a]	8.6
Wales	All	2768	13.5	2778	8.7	2823	5.3
England and Wales	All	48 547	16.3	48 942	12.0	49 652	8.4

[a] Includes 747 000 in 1978/9, 847 000 in 1983 and 296 000 in 1988 whose ethnic origin was unclassified.

6. Patients with pulmonary disease were more likely to be sputum smear- and culture-positive in the White compared with the ISC group.
7. Drug resistance in the White group was 1.6% of isolates, ten to a single drug (7S, 3H) and three to both, compared with 7.5% of strains from the ISC patients, 12 to a single drug (4S, 8H) and three to both.
8. Children born to ISC parents in the UK had rates three times those of White children. ISC children born abroad had rates that were tenfold greater.

Further notification surveys, including a question on ethnic origin, have been carried out for a 6-month period in 1983, and again in 1988[49,50]. This has enabled accurate estimates to be made of the decline in the rate of disease in the different ethnic groups (Table 10.1). Over the 10 years between the first and the third MRC Notification Surveys, rates have declined in all groups, except the West Indian. Rates among the White population have halved, and those among the ISC group decreased threefold, the decline being greater in the Pakistani/Bangladeshi group than the Indian group. However, the overall picture has shown little change; the White popula-

tion now accounts for 53% of notifications, the ISC group 39%, the West Indian group 3% and others 5%. The pattern of non-respiratory disease also remains similar, though more White patients presented with lymph node disease (31% of those with a non-respiratory site in 1978/9, but 37% in 1988).

Drug resistance, which had increased in the ISC group from 7.5% in 1978/9 to 12.8% in 1983, fell to 3% in 1988. Drug resistance in the White population has remained at approximately 1% throughout.

The impact on tuberculosis in England and Wales made by immigration from the Indian subcontinent during the 1960s and 1970s has been substantial (Fig. 10.1). A 9.5% annual decline from 1954 to the mid 1960s suddenly changed to a 3% annual decline. However, for a short period, from 1980, the 9.5% annual decline resumed, as predicted by Springett[18].

10.2.6 FURTHER LOCAL REPORTS

The findings from the three national surveys of tuberculosis undertaken by the Medical Research Council have been substantiated by local reports published over the same time period. Clarke *et al.* reported that the rate of disease in Asians in Leicestershire was 70 times that for the non-Asian population. Rates were much higher for non-respiratory disease among Asian women. Using Hospital Activity Analysis they also found that only 68% of non-Asians, but 92% of Asians were actually being notified[51]. In a retrospective study tracing cases of tuberculosis who entered the country through Heathrow Airport, Khogali found that the majority developed disease after entry[52].

Screening for tuberculosis at ports of entry found 0.96 cases per 1000 in 1970 and 3.85 per 1000 in 1979[53]. Bone and joint disease increased as a result of much higher rates in the increasing ISC population[54,55]. Even so, other workers suggest that screening at entry was ineffective[56].

In a study to determine the effect of visiting their country of origin on disease in Asians, McCarthy found that 20% of his patients developed disease as a result of a visit to Asia. He also showed that the great majority presented with disease soon after arrival, and the great majority within 5 years of their last visit[57] to Asia.

A register of tuberculosis drug resistance from Birmingham showed that immigrants presenting prior to 1970 had an incidence of drug resistance of 7%, but this had since declined to between 1% and 4%[58]. Drug resistance in Blackburn was shown to be higher (11%) in earlier years, but has fallen subsequently[59,60].

Infection in Asian patients can frequently lead to disease if the immune system becomes compromised, as occurs in renal failure[61]. The author of this paper recommended that patients from the Indian subcontinent should receive antituberculosis chemoprophylaxis when starting a dialysis programme.

10.2.7 SOUTH-EAST ASIA

The lease back of Hong Kong to mainland China in 1997 may result in increased immigration from South-East Asia to developed countries such as Australia, Canada and the UK. A small retrospective study of patients of Hong Kong and South-East Asian ethnic origin in Liverpool showed that patients were more likely to present with extrapulmonary disease, when presenting in the UK, than when presenting in Hong Kong[62,63]; a phenomenon similar to that seen in those of ISC ethnic origin presenting to chest services in the UK. The incidence of drug resistance (14%) was similar to that in the country of origin.

10.2.8 SUMMARY OF EXPERIENCE OF ETHNIC MINORITIES IN THE UK

The present UK population includes two relatively large ethnic minority groups, those of West Indian (Caribbean) and Indian subcontinent (South Asian) ethnic origin, which now comprise over 5% of the population. The former have had rates of disease of 30/100 000 per year consistently since accurate data became available, but rates in this group are not falling[50]. There is little evidence that rates of non-respiratory disease are higher in this group. Rates amongst the ISC group are very much higher, at one time being 30 times the White rate for respiratory disease, and 80 times the White rate for non-respiratory disease. Rates in this group have been declining steadily[50]. In the past 5 years tuberculosis notifications in the UK have been increasing[64,65]. This may be partly as a result of immigration from new areas, such as South East Asia, the horn of Africa, Eastern Europe and Western Asia[66].

10.3 EXPERIENCE OF IMMIGRATION IN THE USA

The problem of immigration from high-incidence countries represented by Southern Europe, the West Indies and Asia to the USA, has been known for many years[67–69]. High rates of tuberculosis in those from Haiti,

Central and Southern America, Africa, the Philippines and Indo-China have also been highlighted[70–72]. In particular, high rates of disease and drug resistance have been described in refugees[73,74].

Unusual extrapulmonary presentations have been observed[75]. Powell and others pointed out that 50% of foreign-born persons presented with tuberculosis within 5 years of entering the USA. They refer to the 'stress' of life in a new cultural environment as being a risk factor for tuberculosis in these groups [76].

Passes reported that 80% of immigrants from South-East Asia, including Vietnam, Cambodia and Laos, had a positive tuberculin test. About 50% of those from other countries, such as Iran, Afghanistan, Ethiopia and Central Africa, had a positive test[77].

High rates of disease and drug resistance in Haitian immigrants were reported by Pitchneck and others in 1982[78]. The high incidence of HIV infection in this group of immigrants to the USA has resulted in particularly high rates of disease[79,80]. Extrapulmonary disease was found to be very significantly more common in Haitian patients with AIDS. High rates of disease and tuberculin positivity (53%) have been reported in the foreign-born Latino population of San Francisco (El Salvador, Mexico, Nicaragua, Guatemala) compared with 9% of the USA-born. Conversion rates for the Latinos were 15 to 30 times that of the USA general population[81,82].

A number of recent reports have underlined the problem of tuberculosis in migrant farm workers, a large number of whom are Black, Hispanic or Haitian. Tuberculosis was found in 0.47% of Hispanics and 3.6% of USA-born Blacks. Tuberculin positivity was present in 37% of Hispanics, 62% of USA-born Blacks and 76% of Haitians. A high proportion had been in prison or were from shelters for the homeless[83–87].

In a review of tuberculosis in the USA in

1989, Bloch and others reported that 11 002 of 22 517 (49%) of tuberculosis cases occurred in racial minorities, rising to 64% of cases if Hispanics were included[88]. The largest increase from 1985 to 1987 occurred in Blacks and Hispanics, aged 25–44 years. Although AIDS is likely to be a major contributor, other factors, such as immigration or poverty, may be implicated. Eight countries accounted for 63% of the 5261 foreign-born cases for whom the country of origin was known: Mexico, Cambodia, Laos, Vietnam, the Philippines, Haiti, South Korea and the People's Republic of China. The obverse of these rather worrying statistics is that in the 25 years before publication of this report, the number of USA counties reporting no cases had doubled.

Extrapulmonary tuberculosis continued to occur more frequently in ethnic minorities and the foreign-born, the most common site being lymphatic[89].

In contrast to the UK, where individuals from ethnic minorities originating from the Indian subcontinent and the West Indies account for the great majority of high-risk individuals, in the USA, because of its greater proximity to the impoverished Central American and Caribbean states, ease of immigration from South-East Asia and its own large indigenous Black population, high-risk groups in the USA are more diverse and may be more difficult to identify. Screening of populations for tuberculosis control may therefore be more complex and require, proportionately, more resources.

10.4 EXPERIENCE IN CANADA

The original native population of Canada, comprising Indians and Inuit, were infected by arrivals from Europe in the sixteenth and seventeenth century. The result was decimation of the (then) native population by diseases, including tuberculosis. High rates in the aboriginal people continue[90]. In 1965 restriction on immigration to Canada was eased and a fresh wave of migration began.

High rates of tuberculosis were described in Chinese immigrants. Prevalence of disease was as high as 68 per 1000 in Chinese immigrants from 1964 to 1968[91]. As part of the British Commonwealth, Canada received a number of Ugandan Asians in the early 1970s, among whom tuberculosis prevalence was also high. In 1974 a report from Ontario showed that there was a high risk of succumbing to disease after immigration and an abundance of lymphadenitis in the Asian-born[92]. The prevalence of drug-resistant bacteria appeared to increase as a result of immigration. In 1975 drug resistance among Asians was 11.7% and in Southern Europeans 16.7%[93]. Increased drug resistance and lymphadenitis in the Asian group have been reported elsewhere[94].

The problem of analysing the effect of immigration on rates of tuberculosis in an immigrant population to a developed country is hampered by lack of precise data on rates in the country of origin. In a study examining rates of disease in Finnish immigrants to Canada, Enarson *et al.* were able to compare rates in newly arrived immigrants to rates in the country of origin. They showed that rates of disease in Scandinavian immigrants, even after a long duration of residence in their country of adoption, were very similar to rates in the country of birth. They concluded that the early experience of tuberculosis predetermines future susceptibility throughout the life span of the immigrant group. The question 'where did you live in your childhood?' is the most important[95]. This reflected the likelihood of them becoming infected prior to the age of 20 years[96].

More recent reports show that lymphadenitis and drug resistance continues to be a problem in immigrants from Asia to Canada, particularly from the Philippines[97,98].

As in the USA, Canada has experienced an increase in tuberculosis in the foreign-born since 1975. Disease rates are highest in the years immediately after immigration. Almost 50% of foreign-born cases were from Asia [99].

10.5 EXPERIENCE IN SCANDINAVIAN COUNTRIES

A review of tuberculosis in Scandinavian countries in 1978 showed only very small numbers from minority ethnic groups. However, more recent reports from Denmark show that immigrants mainly from Pakistan, the Philippines and the former Yugoslavia had higher rates of disease than native Danes, particularly extrapulmonary disease, including bone and joint involvement [100,101]. Rates of disease were between 13 and 40 times higher in immigrant than Danish children[102,103].

10.6 OTHER EUROPEAN COUNTRIES

Over the past three decades it is estimated that about 15 million people have migrated to Central and Northern Europe[104]. Virtually every country reports higher rates of disease in immigrant groups, whether in Switzerland, the former Federal Republic of Germany, France or the Netherlands[105]. More recent data from Germany and Switzerland show a much greater incidence of lymphadenitis in immigrants[106,107].

However, there was no evidence that disease was being passed on to the indigenous population. From 1989 to 1990 Switzerland experienced a 15% increase in notifications, half of whom were foreign-born[108].

10.7 EXPERIENCE IN ISRAEL

Israel, with its diversity of ethnic grouping, represents a unique situation. Experience of tuberculosis is broadly similar to patterns seen elsewhere. High rates of disease, particularly extrapulmonary, have been found in immigrants from Ethiopia, who had a prevalence of 19/1000 in 1979[109]. The incidence rate of the population of the host community is very low at 4.5/100 000[110]. Other high-rate groups within the country include the Bedouin[111]. One problem for the tuberculosis services was that groups with the highest rates are least compliant with treatment.

10.8 EXPERIENCE IN AUSTRALIA AND NEW ZEALAND

As in Canada, New Zealand and Australian natives suffered large-scale fatality from tuberculosis when the countries were first colonized by Europeans. Within the past two decades, immigration from the Third World has tended to reverse the otherwise downward trend in the number of cases reported.

Referring to the increased rate of disease in Asians, one report talks of stress being responsible for the progression of infection to disease[112]. A certain degree of xenophobia is communicated in some of the publications relating to tuberculosis in immigrants to these countries[113,114]. About 15% of immigrants are given prophylaxis on arrival [115].

A high incidence of drug resistance in immigrants, particularly from Vietnam and the Philippines, is confirmed[116,117]. Within New Zealand rates for all groups, European, Maouri and Pacific Islanders, appear to have been declining progressively over the past two decades (personal communication, M. Wilsher).

10.9. EXPERIENCE IN HONG KONG

Low prevalence countries with immigration from the Third World are not the only countries to experience a rise in cases as a result of immigration. For a period from the late 1970s the numbers of cases of tuberculosis in Hong Kong increased due to the influx of refugees from Vietnam. In 1980, 712 of 8065 cases in Hong Kong were in Vietnamese people[63].

10.10 TUBERCULOSIS IN THIRD WORLD NATIONS

Accurate data on the incidence of tuberculosis in many Third World countries is difficult to obtain. Latest estimates suggest that the highest incidence is in the African region, with rates of over 250/100 000 per annum [118]. It is probable that rates in most of the Indian subcontinent, South-East Asia and the Pacific exceed 100/100 000. These figures compare with rates between 4 and 10/100 000 in the indigenous population of Western Europe, Canada, the USA, Australia and New Zealand.

Twenty years prior to this, a report on world tuberculosis suggested rates as high as 500/100 000 in Macau and Burma, 350/100 000 in the Philippines, 250/100 000 as the highest in African countries and 200/100 000 in some South American countries. Rates amongst certain age groups may exceed 1000/100 000[119].

10.11 AIDS AND IMMIGRATION

Although AIDS-related tuberculosis may not impact the developed world directly except in certain small-risk groups in the immediate future, as suggested by Styblo[120], its effect on rates in Africa, India and South-East Asia is likely to be appreciable within the next decade (Chapter 12), causing rises in rates of disease in the developing world. With continued immigration this is likely to cause cases in the developed world to increase as well. Indeed this may already be occurring.

Besides the knowledge that rates of disease in immigrant groups and ethnic minorities are invariably higher than in the indigenous population of developed nations, three main conclusions about the experience of immigration and ethnic minorities can be made:

1. Tuberculosis tends to arise in immigrants relatively soon after immigration, usually within the first 5 years.
2. Disease is much more likely to present

with an extrapulmonary site than in the indigenous population.

3. Disease is not passed on to other ethnic groups.

What are the causes of these phenomena?

10.12 TRANSMISSION OF DISEASE

The fact that there seems to be little evidence for transmission between ethnic groups should not be a matter for surprise. The nature of the infectivity of tuberculosis is such that only household contacts or close associates of a sputum smear-positive case are at any appreciable risk of disease.

A study from the UK suggested that the infection rate of Whites by a White index case may be higher than that of Asian contacts from an Asian case[121], perhaps because pulmonary disease in Asians in the UK tends to be less extensive than in Whites and less often smear-positive[47]. It may be that health professionals in the UK recognize symptoms of tuberculosis earlier in the immigrant population than in the White population.

10.13 RATES AND PATTERNS OF DISEASE IN IMMIGRANTS

Theories as to why immigrants and ethnic minorities suffer from high rates and a non-respiratory pattern of disease may be divided broadly into two groups – genetic and environmental.

10.13.1 GENETIC CAUSES

An experimental basis for the evidence for a genetic resistance to tuberculosis is outlined in Chapter 3. In a study of twins with tuberculosis, it has been shown that concordance for tuberculosis was significantly higher among monozygotic than dizygotic twin pairs, indicating that inherited susceptibility is an important risk factor[122]. The strongest case made recently using epidemiological researchers for a genetic cause for the apparent racial differences to susceptibility to tuberculosis has been made by Stead in a study of nursing homes in Arkansas[123]. Using repeat skin testing of 25 398 initially tuberculin-negative nursing home residents, he found that 13.8% of Black residents, but only 7.2% of Whites, had evidence of new infection. However, among those infected there was no racial difference in those later found to have clinical tuberculosis. These findings are consistent with other studies, which show increased tuberculin conversion rates in Blacks compared with Whites, with similar degrees of exposure to an infectious case[124]. Stead believes his data suggest heritable differences between individuals and groups with respect to defence mechanisms, which function before infection develops as distinct from the cell-mediated immunity that develops after initial infection.

A heritable basis for protection against or susceptibility towards tuberculosis has had many advocates. Motulsky, believed that the ability of an organism to phagocytose the tuberculous organism was inherited[125].

A 20-year follow-up of 12 000 tuberculin-positive subjects described by Comstock showed a significant difference between Blacks and Whites in terms of numbers developing disease only in the 20–39-year age groups, largely because of the high rates among Black females[126].

In contrast, among naval recruits infected by the tubercle bacillus, case rates were three times greater among men at least 10% underweight for their height than among those at least 10% overweight. In a separate study, Comstock describes an excess of cases among the very thin. He concluded that, whereas the risk factors of developing disease after infection, such as age, sex, race and body build, are intrinsic or inherited characteristics, risk factors for acquiring infection are all extrinsic.

However, from Stead's work in homes for the elderly showing that though Black residents had a greater chance of initial infection than White residents, they had a similar chance of going on to develop disease, it may be that though inherited characteristics predispose to disease after infection, race may not be one of them.

Though no definitive studies have been carried out, experience from the UK, however, suggests that infected individuals from the Indian subcontinent have a much greater chance of developing disease than White individuals.

10.13.2 A WORLD PANDEMIC

A theory that combines the genetic with the environmental is one that may be loosely termed the pandemic theory of tuberculosis[7,127]. It is postulated that high rates of disease in individuals from the developing world and low rates in the developed world are a consequence of the fact that the epidemic of tuberculosis passed through the mainly White population of Western Europe towards the end of the eighteenth century, peaked towards the beginning of the nineteenth century, when mortality from tuberculosis was 25% of all causes, and has been on the decline since. The population remaining are therefore relatively resistant to the bacillus because of natural selection. The very high rates in Africa, the Indian subcontinent, South-East Asia and Australasia are evidence of the pandemic currently being near or approaching its peak in this section of the globe. High rates in immigrant groups simply reflect the high rates in the countries of origin where tuberculosis is still causing large-scale fatalities among a largely susceptible population. The problem with this theory is that it takes no account of the relative wealth and poverty of the two worlds. Europe in the early nineteenth century, newly industrialized and urbanized, was a ripe breeding ground for the bacillus. Similar situations have now developed in parts of the Third World, where conditions favour the bacillus, but with improved living standards in the West, the disease has declined.

Even in the developed world, tuberculosis remains strongly associated with poverty [128].

10.13.3 ENVIRONMENTAL FACTORS

One phenomenon that does not appear to be explained by the genetic account is the way disease seems to be accelerated by immigration resulting in high rates of non-respiratory disease. The parallel between the way AIDS-related tuberculosis and migration-related tuberculosis present has been pointed out[129].

It is suggested that vitamin D deficiency may play a part in this AIDS-like development of disease in ISC immigrants to the UK, an 'acquired immune deficiency of immigration'[130]. *In vitro* work has shown that vitamin D3 has a role in activating macrophages to destroy mycobacteria[131,132]. It is also well established that ISC immigrants in the UK are severely vitamin D-deficient. ISC subjects acquire infection within their country of origin, but with plentiful sunlight vitamin D remains high and the individual's immune system is able to contain the infection. However, on migration to a temperate climate where sunlight is less frequent, particularly in the winter months, serum vitamin D concentrations fall, the specific cell-mediated immune system is compromised and the previously contained infection flares into overt disease.

This sudden fall in serum vitamin D concentrations on immigration may explain why disease occurs soon, usually within 5 years, after immigration. The relative immune deficiency resulting from macrophage deactivation by vitamin D deprivation may also explain why non-respiratory disease, is more prevalent in the immigrant group. A small number of bacilli may disperse from the lung to distant sites via the blood stream, the blood-borne macrophages being too immunodeficient to engulf or kill the organisms.

An alternative explanation is that immuno-deficiency is actually acquired due to vegetarianism and associated vitamin deficiency [133]. It seems unlikely that the pattern of disease is related to different bacteriological typing[134,135]. Thus the 'stress' of immigration referred to by a number of authors [25,39,76,112] may in fact be due to sunlight or diet-induced vitamin deprivation compromising the immune system.

It should be said that this hypothesis remains untested and therefore unproven.

10.14 TUBERCULOSIS CONTROL IN IMMIGRANTS

It is important to screen immigrants from countries with high rates of tuberculosis for active disease and for infection. In addition to pre-immigration screening undertaken by such countries receiving migrants as South Africa, Canada and Australia, there are, in practice, three points at which this can be carried out.

10.14.1 AT THE PORT OF ENTRY

This may be the least satisfactory site to screen, as large numbers of individuals may suddenly arrive and medical as well as immigrant screening may delay families for hours or even days. Nevertheless, a simple chest radiograph of symptomatic individuals to exclude active disease, likely to be infectious, would seem appropriate.

10.14.2 AS THE IMMIGRANT TAKES UP RESIDENCE

Screening as the immigrant becomes resident depends on close co-operation between authorities at the port of entry and community health care in the local authority of residence. In the UK, the port of arrival (POA) is supposed to inform the local Consultant in Communicable Disease Control (CCDC) of the name and address of the immigrant on arrival in the area for which the CCDC is responsible. The CCDC is then responsible for ensuring that screening is undertaken, usually through a visit to the immigrants' home by a specialist nurse. The immigrant can then by referred to the local chest clinic where screening can take place[136].

Screening should include a chest radiograph of all adults to exclude disease, and a tuberculin test of all children. In the event of a positive test, radiography should be performed. Chemoprophylaxis is indicated in the event of a strongly positive tuberculin test and a normal chest radiograph[137], and BCG in the event of a negative tuberculin test.

A problem frequently arises when the address provided by the POA to the CCDC is only temporary, so that when the health visitor arrives at the given address, the newly arrived immigrants cannot be traced. In practice less than 50% of new immigrants are adequately screened.

This system also requires an adequate supply of health visitors, able to see the immigrants in their homes, appropriate translation facilities and provision of a chest clinic to provide screening facilities. In short, a fully comprehensive public health system at street level is essential.

10.14.3 AS THE IMMIGRANT ENTERS THE COMMUNITY THROUGH SCHOOL, COLLEGE OR EMPLOYMENT

The third point at which immigrants may be screened is on entry to school, college or place of employment. Some authorities in the UK, where a high proportion of immigrants reside, have instituted a certificate, which the immigrant must obtain from a chest clinic to provide proof to the school, college or employers that he or she has been screened for tuberculosis. If the individual does not possess such a certificate, an early referral to the chest clinic is made. As many immigrants remain unemployed for long periods this option may not apply to all.

Even if the immigrant has been adequately screened, health professionals should be aware of the high incidence of tuberculosis developing within 5 years of arrival. Chemoprophylaxis in children with a positive tuberculin test has considerably reduced the incidence of tuberculosis in recent immigrants[137].

10.15 SUMMARY

Immigrants from developing countries to the developed world are at greatly increased risk of tuberculosis. Suitable facilities, both community and hospital-based, need to be targeted to areas where these individuals live. Experience in the UK has shown them to be easily identifiable and generally co-operative to health care workers. Disease is therefore containable. There seems to be no reason why this should not be the case in other developed countries, provided resources are made available.

10.16 THE FUTURE

Until 1985 tuberculosis appeared to be a declining problem in all parts of the globe. With the increase in disease in many countries since then, the picture has radically changed. A number of factors may lead to a further increase in rates of disease as a result of immigration.

First, case rates in many developing countries are increasing dramatically, mainly due to HIV. Secondly, the end of the 'Iron Curtain' division between East and West has resulted in large-scale migration from the poorer Eastern Europe to the West. The numbers of asylum seekers to Western Europe has increased considerably in the past few years[138]. Thirdly, the possible political strains in South-East Asia as a result of Hong Kong reverting to Chinese control in 1997 may increase immigration from that part of the world, across the Pacific Ocean and towards Europe. Countries receiving migrants and refugees should be aware of the potential problem and plan resources accordingly.

REFERENCES

1. O'Brien, E.M. (1950) *The Foundation of Australia*, Angus and Robertson, Sydney.
2. Proust, A.J. (ed.) (1991) *History of Tuberculosis in Australia, New Zealand and Papua New Guinea*, Brolga Press, Canberra.
3. Metcalf, C. (1991) A history of tuberculosis, in: *A Century of Tuberculosis. South African Perspectives*, (eds H.M. Covadia and S.R. Benator), Oxford University Press, Capetown.
4. Cummins, S.L. (1920) Tuberculosis in primitive tribes and its bearing on tuberculosis of the civilized communities. *Int. J. Publ. Health*, **1**, 10–171.
5. Wiggley, S. (1977) The first hundred years of tuberculosis in New Guinea, in *The Melanesia Environment* (ed. J.H. Windslow), ANU Press, Canberra.
6. Grzybowski, S., Styblo, K. and Dorken, E. (1976) Tuberculosis in Eskimos. *Tubercle*, **57** (Suppl. 4).
7. Hess, E.V. and MacDonald, N. (1954) Pulmonary tuberculosis in Irish immigrants in Londoners. Comparison of hospital patients. *Lancet*, **ii**, 132–7.
8. Emerson, P.A., Beath, G., and Tomkins, J.G. (1961) Tuberculosis in Soho. *Br. Med. J.*, **i**, 148–52.
9. Brett, G.Z., (1958) Pulmonary tuberculosis in immigrants: a mass radiography study survey in 1956. *Tubercle*, **39**, 24–8.
10. Brett, G.Z. (1965) Epidemiology trends in tuberculosis and sarcoidosis in a district of London between 1958 and 1963. *Tubercle*, **46**, 412–16.
11. Springett, V.H., Adams, J.C.S., D'Costa, T.B. and Hemming, M. (1958) Tuberculosis in immigrants in Birmingham. *Br. J. Prev. Soc. Med.*, **12**, 135–40.
12. Nicol Roe, J.T. (1959) Tuberculosis in Indian immigrants. *Tubercle*, **40**, 387–8.
13. Aspin, J. (1962) Tuberculosis among Indian immigrants to Midland industrial areas. *Br. Med. J.*, **i**, 1386–8.
14. Stevenson, D.K. (1962) Tuberculosis in Pakistanis in Bradford. *Br. Med. J.*, **i**, 1382–6.
15. Tuberculosis Disease Committee of the Chest Group of the British Medical Association (1961) *Br. Med. J.*, **2** (Suppl. 2), 253–4.

16. Springett, V.H. (1964) Tuberculosis in immigrants. *Lancet*, **i**, 1091–5.

17. Springett, V.H. (1969) The changing pattern of tuberculosis. Notifications in Birmingham. *Tubercle*, **50**, 313–17.

18. Springett, V.H. (1973) Tuberculosis in immigrants in Birmingham 1970–72. *Br. J. Prev. Soc. Med.*, **27**, 242–6.

19. Innes, J.A. (1981) Tuberculosis in Asians. *Postgrad. Med. J.*, **57**, 779–80.

20. Rowland, A.J. and Bell, G.A. (1966) Control of tuberculosis in immigrants: a tuberculin survey of commonwealth immigrant children in Bradford. *Publ. Hlth (Lond.)*, **80**, 179–87.

21. McNicol, M.W., Mikhail, J.R. and Sutherland, I. (1971) Tuberculosis in Brent. *Postgrad. Med. J.*, **47**, 591–3.

22. Gardner, P.A., Moss, P.D. and Stalker, R. (1972) Tuberculosis and the immigrant in Blackburn. *Publ. Hlth (Lond.)*, **86**, 189–96.

23. Fullner, I.W. and Hall, C.J. (1976) Tuberculosis in East London: an analysis of notifications. 1970–74 in the City and East London Area Health Authority (teaching). *Publ. Hlth (Lond.)*, **90**, 157–63.

24. Casemore, D.P. (1978) Tuberculosis in South Cleveland 1968–74. Laboratory based survey. *Publ. Hlth (Lond.)*, **92**, 264–71.

25. Grenville-Mathers, R. and Clark, J.B. (1979) The development of tuberculosis in Afro-Asian immigrants. *Tubercle*, **60**, 25–9.

26. Clarke, M., Somani, N. and Diamond, P. (1979) Tuberculosis morbidity amongst immigrants: notification and hospitalization. *Comm. Med.*, **1**, 23–8.

27. Scott, R., Gaskell, P.G. and Morrell, D.C. (1966) Patients who reside in common lodging houses. *Br. Med. J.*, **ii**, 1561–4.

28. Caplin, M. and Rehahn, M. (1978) Alcoholism and tuberculosis, in *Topics in Therapeutics 4* (ed. D.W. Vare), Royal College of Physicians, London, pp. 136–49.

29. Anonymous (Leader) (1978) Tuberculosis and the alcoholic. *Lancet*, **ii**, 460–1.

30. Patel, K.R. (1984) Pulmonary tuberculosis in residents of lodging houses, night shelters and common hostels in Glasgow: a 5 year prospective survey. *Br. J. Dis. Chest*, **79**, 60–5.

31. Shanks, N.J. and Caswal, K.B. (1984) Persistent tuberculosis disease among inmates of common lodging houses. *J. Epidemiol. Commun. Hlth*, **38**, 66–7.

32. British Tuberculosis Association (1966) Tuberculosis among immigrants to England and Wales: a national survey in 1965. A report from the Research Committee of the British Tuberculosis Association. *Tubercle*, **47**, 145–6.

33. British Thoracic and Tuberculosis Association (1973) A tuberculosis survey in England and Wales 1971; the influence of immigration and county of birth upon notifications. A report from the Research Committee of the British Thoraic and Tuberculosis Association. *Tubercle*, **54**, 249–60.

34. British Thoracic and Tuberculosis Association (1975) Tuberculosis among immigrants related to length of residence in England and Wales. A report from the Research Committee of the British Thoracic and Tuberculosis Association. *Br. Med. J.*, **ii**, 698–9.

35. Silver, C.P. and Steel, S.J. (1961) Mediastinal lymphatic gland tuberculosis in Asian and coloured immigrants. *Lancet*, **i**, 1254–6.

36. Corruthers, R.K. and Lang, S.V. (1970) Genito-urinary tuberculosis in an area with a large Asian immigrant population. *Br. J. Urol.*, **42**, 535–9.

37. Anderson, J.M. and Macmillan, J.J. (1975) Intracranial tuberculoma – an increasing problem in Britain. *J. Neurol. Neurosurg. Psychiat.*, **38**, 194–201.

38. Williams, I.P. and Hetzel, M.R. (1978) Tuberculosis pericarditis in South-West London: an increasing problem. *Thorax*, **33**, 816–17.

39. Findlay, J.M., Stevenson, D.K., Addison, N.V. and Mirza, Z.A. (1979) Tuberculosis of the gastrointestinal tract in Bradford 1967–77. *J. Roy. Soc. Med.*, **72**, 587–91.

40. Summers, G.D. and McNicol, M.W. (1980) Tuberculosis of superficial lymph nodes. *Br. J. Dis. Chest*, **74**, 369–73.

41. Editorial (1983) Scrofula today. *Lancet*, **i**, 335–6.

42. Nicholson, R.A. (1974) Twenty years of bone and joint tuberculosis in Bradford – a comparison of the disease in the indigenous and Asian populations. *J. Bone Joint Surg.*, **56B**, 760–5.

43. Newton, P., Sharp, I. and Barnes, K.L. (1982) Bone and joint tuberculosis in Greater Manchester 1969–79. *Ann. Rheum. Dis.*, **41**, 1–6.

44. Halsy, J.P. Rubach, J.S. and Barnes, C.G. (1982) A decade of skeletal tuberculosis. *Ann. Rheum. Dis.*, **41**, 7–10.

45. Bateman, D.E., Newman, R.K. and Foster,

J.B. (1983) A retrospective survey of proven cases of tuberculosis meningitis in the Northern Region 1970–80. *J.Roy. Coll. Phys. Lond.*, **17**, 106–10.

46. Innes, J.A. (1981) Non-respiratory tuberculosis. *J. Roy. Coll. Phys.*, **15**, 227–31.

47. Medical Research Council Tuberculosis and Chest Diseases Unit (1980) National survey of tuberculosis notifications in England and Wales 1978–9. *Br. Med J.*, **281**, 895–8.

48. Department of the Environment (1979) *National Dwelling and Housing Survey*, HMSO, London.

49. Medical Research Council Tuberculosis and Chest Diseases Unit (1985) National survey of tuberculosis notifications in England and Wales 1983. *Br. Med. J.*, **291**, 658–61.

50. Medical Research Council Cardiothoracic Epidemiological Group (1992) National survey of notifications of tuberculosis in England and Wales 1988. *Thorax*, **47**, 770–5.

51. Clarke, M., Samani, N. and Diamond, P. (1979) Tuberculosis morbidity amongst immigrants: notification and hospitalization. *Comm. Med.*, **1**, 23–8.

52. Khogali, M. (1979) Tuberculosis among immigrants in the United Kingdom: the role of occupational health servies. *J. Epidemiol. Comm. Hlth*, **33**, 134–7.

53. Helliwell, C.J.V. and Turner, A.C. (1980) Imported disease at point of entry. *The Practitioner*, **224**, 793–6.

54. Halsey, P., Reeback, J.S. and Barnes, G.C. (1982) A decade of skeletal tuberculosis. *Ann. Rheum. Dis.*, **41**, 7–10.

55. Davies, P.D.O., Humphries M.J., Byfield, S.P. *et al.* (1984) A survey of notifications in England and Wales. *J. Bone Joint Surg.*, **66B**, 326–30.

56. Markey, A.C., Forster, S.M., Mitchell, R. *et al.* (1986) Suspected cases of pulmonary tuberculosis referred from port of enty into Great Britain 1980–3. *Br. Med. J.*, **292**, 378.

57. McCarthy, O.R. (1984) Asian immigrant tuberculosis – the effect of visiting Asia. *Br. J. Dis.*, **78**, 248–53.

58. Thomas, H.E. and Ayres, J.G. (1986) The Birmingham tuberculosis drug resistance register 1956–1983. *Tubercle*, **67**, 179–88.

59. Ormerod, L.P. Harrison, J.M.L. and Wright, P.A. (1986) Drug resistance in *Mycobacterium tuberculosis*: a survey of 25 years in Blackburn. *Thorax*, **41**, 946–50.

60. Ormerod, L.P., Harrison, J.M.L. and Wright, P.A. (1990) Drug resistance trends in *M. tuberculosis*: Blackburn 1985–1989. *Tubercle*, **71**, 283–5.

61. Kwan, J.T.C., Hart, P.D., Raftery, M.J. *et al.* (1991) Mycobacterial infection is an important infective complication in British Asian dialysis patients. *J. Hosp. Infect.*, **19**, 249–53.

62. Nisar, M., Williams, C.S.D. and Davies, P.D.O. (1991) Experience of tuberculosis in immigrants from South East Asia – implications for the imminent lease back of Hong Kong. *Resp. Med.* **85**; 219–22.

63. Chest Service of the Government Medical and Health Department (Hong Kong) (1990) *Annual Report*, 1988.

64. Office of Population Censuses and Surveys (1992) Communicable Diseases (area) (Series MB2), HMSO, London.

65. Davies, P.D.O. and Williams, C.S.D. Tuberculosis is increasing in England and Wales. *Tuberc. Lung Dis.* (in press).

66. Gilbertson, K., Stork, D., Taw, K. and Morre-Gillon, J. (1991) Use of community organisations to assess immigrant populations at risk of tuberculosis. *Thorax*, **46**, 311P.

67. Massachusetts Department of Public Health (1971) Tuberculosis and the new citizen. *N. Engl. J. Med.*, **285**, 919–20.

68. Massachusetts Department of Public Health (1975) Importing tuberculosis – a paradox. *N. Engl. J. Med.*, **293**, 357.

69. American Thoracic Society (1977) Tuberculosis in the foreign born. *Am. Rev. Respir. Dis.*, **116**, 561–4.

70. Abeles, H. (1978) Tuberculosis in the foreign born (Correspondence). *Am. Rev. Respir. Dis.*, **117**, 185.

71. Breitenbucher, R. (1979) Detection and chemoprophylaxis of tuberculosis in South East Asian immigrants. *Minn. Med.*, **62**, 805–6.

72. Powell, K.E., Brown, E.D. and Farer, L.S. (1983) Tuberculosis among Indo-Chinese refugees in the United States. *J. Am. Med. Assoc.*, **249**, 1455–60.

73. Byrd, R.B., Fisk, D.E., Roethe, R.A. *et al.* (1979) Tuberculosis in oriental immigrants. *Chest*, **72**, 136–9.

74. Snider, D.E. and Farer, L.S. (1980) Tuberculosis in oriental immigrants (Correspondence). *Chest*, **77**, 812.

75. Ellis, J.G. (1979) Extrapulmonary tuberculosis in immigrants. (Editorial). *Lancet*, **i**, 621.

76. Powell, K.E., Meader, M.P. and Farer, L.S. (1981) Foreign-born persons with tuberculosis in the United States. *Am. J. Publ. Hlth*, **71**, 1223–7.

77. Passes, H.I. (1981) Isoniazid prophylaxis in new immigrants. (Editorial). *Ann. Intern. Med.*, **95**, 657.

78. Pitchenick, A.E., Russell, B.W., Cleary, T. *et al.* (1987) The prevalence of tuberculosis and drug resistance among Hiatians. *N. Engl. J. Med.*, **307**, 162–5.

79. Vieira, H., Frank, E., Sira, T.J. and Landesman, S.H. (1983) Opportunistic infections in previously healthy Hiatian immigrants. *N. Engl. J. Med.*, **308**, 125–9.

80. Pitchenick, A.E., Cole, C., Russell, B.W. *et al.* (1984) Tuberculosis, atypical mycobacteriosis, and the acquired immunodeficiency syndrome among Hiatian and non-Hiatian patients in South Florida. *Ann. Intern. Med.*, **101**, 641–5.

81. Perez-Stable, E.J., Levin, R., Pineda, A. and Slutkin, G. (1985) Tuberculin skin test reactivity and conversions in United States – and foreign-born latino children. *Paed. Infect. Dis.*, **4**, 476–9.

82. Perez-Stable, E.J., Slutkin, G., Paz, A. *et al.* (1986) Tuberculin reactivity in United States and foreign-born latinos: results of a community-based screening program. *Am. J. Publ. Hlth*, **76**, 643–5.

83. Leads from the MMWR (1986) Tuberculosis among migrant farm workers – Virginia. *J. Am. Med. Assoc.*, **256**, 977–81.

84. Jacobson, M.L., Mercer, M.A., Miller, L.K. and Simpson, T.W. (1987) Tuberculosis risk among migrant farm workers on the Delmarva Peninsula. *Am. J. Publ. Hlth*, **77**, 29–31.

85. Gross, T.P., Silverman, P.R., Bloch, A.B. *et al.* (1989). An outbreak of tuberculosis in rural Delaware. *Am. J. Epidemiol.*, **129**, 362–71.

86. Ciesielski, S.D., Seed, J.R., Esposito, D.H. and Hunter, N. (1991) The epidemiology of tuberculosis among North Carolina migrant farm workers. *J. Am. Med. Assoc.*, **265**, 1715–19.

87. Snider, D.E. and Hutton M.D. (1991) Tuberculosis and migrant farm workers (Editorial). *J. Am. Med. Assoc.*, **265**, 1732.

88. Bloch, A.B., Rieder, H.L., Kelly, G.D. *et al.* (1989) The epidemiology of tuberculosis in the United States. Implications for diagnosis and treatment. *Clin. Chest Med.*, **10**, 297–313.

89. Rieder, H.L., Snider, D.E. and Cauthen, G.M. (1990) Extrapulmonary tuberculosis in the United States. *Am. Rev. Respir. Dis.*, **141**, 347–51.

90. Enarson, D.A., Wang, J.S. and Grzybowski, S. (1990) Case-finding in the elimination phase of tuberculosis: tuberculosis in displaced people. *IUATLD*, **65**, 71–2.

91. Willis, J.S. and Duncan, R.A. (1972) Medical status of Chinese immigrants 1964–1968. *Can. J. Publ. Hlth*, **63**, 237–47.

92. Barr, J.W.B. (1979) Arrival of Uganda Asians (Editorial). *Can. Med. Assoc. J.*, **107**, 1062.

93. Ashley, M.L., Anderson, T.W. and Le Riche, W.H. (1974) The influence of immigration on tuberculosis in Ontario. *Am. Rev. Respir. Dis.*, **110**, 137–46.

94. Hershfield, E.S., Eidus, L. and Helbecque, D.M. (1979) Canadian survey to determine the rate of drug resistance to isoniazid, PAS, streptomycin in newly detected untreated tuberculosis patients and retreatment cases. *Intern. J. Clin. Pharmacol.*, **17**, 387–93.

95. Enarson, D., Ashley, M.J. and Grzybowski, S. (1979) Tuberculosis in immigrants to Canada. *Am. Rev. Respir. Dis.*, **119**, 11–18.

96. Enarson, D., Sjogren, I. and Grzybowski, S. (1980) Incidence of tuberculosis among Scandinavian immigrants in Canada. *Eur. J. Respir. Dis.*, **61**, 139–42.

97. Wang, J.S., Allen, E.A., Chao, C.W. *et al.* (1989) Tuberculosis in British Columbia among immigrants from five Asian countries 1982–1985. *Tubercle*, **70**, 179–86.

98. Orr, P.H., Manfreda, J. and Hershfield, E.S. (1990) Tuberculosis surveillance in immigrants to Manitoba. *Can. Med. Assoc. J.*, **142**, 453–8.

99. Orr, P.H., Hershfield, E.S. and Manfreda, J. (1992) The epidemiology of tuberculosis in the foreign-born in North America. *Am. Rev. Respir. Dis.*, **145**, A104.

100. Daddi, G. and Riska, N. (1978) Tuberculosis situation in the Scandinavian countries. *Scand. J. Respir. Dis.*, **102**, 19–35.

101. Lange, P., Mortensen, J. and Viskum, K. (1986) Tuberculosis in a developed country. *Acta Med. Scand.*, **219**, 481–7.

102. Autzen, B. and Elberg, J.J. (1988) Bone and joint tuberculosis in Denmark. *Acta Orthop. Scand.*, **59**, 50–2.

103. Mortensen, J., Lange, P., Storm, H.K. and Viskum, K. (1989) Childhood tuberculosis in a developed country. *Eur. Respir. J.*, **2**, 985–7.

104. Tala, E. (1989) Migration, ethnic minorities and tuberculosis (Editorial). *Eur. Respir. J.*, **2**, 492–3.

105. Lundguist, J. (1965) Tuberculosis in immigrants and foreign workers. *Bull. Int. Union Tuberc.*, **36**, 105–41.

106. Ferlinz, R. (1988) Antituberculous measures for displaced persons in the Federal Republic of Germany. *IUATLD*, **63**, 27–28.

107. Rieder, H.L. (1992) Misbehaviour of a dying epidemic: a call for less speculation and better surveillance. *Tubercle Lung Dis.*, **73**, 181–3.

108. Zellweger, J.P., and Vejdovsky, R. (1988) Tuberculosis among refugees: study of a population screening at the tuberculosis clinic in Lausanne (Switzerland) between 1983 and 1988. *IUATLD*, **63**, 29–31.

109. Oren, S., Jamal, J., London, D. and Viskoper, J.R. (1991) Extrapulmonary tuberculosis: five case reports. *Israel J. Med. Sci.*, **27**, 390–3.

110. Wartski, S.A. (1991) Tuberculosis in Ethiopian immigrants. *Israel J. Med. Sci.*, **27**, 288–91.

111. Dolberg, O.T., Alkan, M. and Schlaeffer, F. (1991) Tuberculosis in Israel: A 10 year survey of an immigrant society. *Israel J. Med. Sci.*, **27**, 886–9.

112. Proust, A.J. (1974) The Australian screening programme for tuberculosis in prospective migrants. *Med. J. Aust.*, **2**, 35–7.

113. Australia Communicable Diseases Intelligence (1979) The wog and us. *Med. J. Aust.*, **2**, 234.

114. Sapolu-Fuimaono, I. (1986) The immigration plague (Editorial). *NZ Med. J.*, **99**, 959.

115. Streeton, J.A. (1987) Paradise lost? *Med. J. Aust.*, **146**, 1–3.

116. Plant, A.J., Rushworth, R.L., Wan, Q. and Thomas, M. (1991) Tuberculosis in New South Wales. *Med. J. Aust.*, **154**, 86–9.

117. Chest Service of the Government Medical and Health Department (Australia) (1988) *Annual Report*, 1987.

118. Kochi, A. (1991) The global tuberculosis situation and the new control strategy of the World Health Organization. *Tubercle*, **72**, 1–6.

119. Hershfield, E.S. (1979) Tuberculosis in the world. *Chest*, **76**, 805–11.

120. Styblo, K. Overview and epidemiologic assessment of the current global tuberculosis situation with an emphasis on control in developing countries. *Rev. Infect. Dis.*, **11**, S339–S346.

121. BTS Research Committee (1978) A study of standardised contact procedure in tuberculosis. *Tubercle*, **59**, 245–59.

122. Comstock, G.W. (1978) Tuberculosis in twins: a re-analysis of the Prophit Survey. *Am. Rev. Respir. Dis.*, **117**, 621–4.

123. Stead, W.W., Senner, J.W., Reddick, W.T. and Lofgren, J.P. (1990) Racial differences in susceptibility to infection by *Mycobacterium tuberculosis*. *N. Engl. J. Med.*, **322**, 422–7.

124. Trump, D.H. and Distasio, A.J. (1990) Racial differences in susceptibility to infection by *Mycobacterium tuberculosis*. *N. Engl J. Med.*, **322**, 1671–2.

125. Motulsky, A.G. (1960) Metabolic polymorphisms and the rate of infectious diseases in human evolution. *Hum. Biol.*, **32**, 28–62.

126. Comstock, G.W. (1975) Frost revisited: the modern epidemiology of tuberculosis. *Am. J. Epidemiol.*, **101**, 363–82.

127. Grzybowski, S. and Enarson, D. Tuberculosis, in *Current Pulmonology* (ed. D.H. Simmons) Year Book Medical Publishers, Chicago, pp. 75–96.

128. Spence, D.S., Williams, C.S.D., Hotchkis, J. and Davies, P.D.O. (1993) Tuberculosis and poverty. *Br. Med. J.*, **307**, 759–61.

129. Davies, P.D.O. (1989) The role of vitamin D in tuberculosis. *Am. Rev. Respir. Dis.*, **139**, 1571.

130. Davies, P.D.O. (1985) A possible link between vitamin D deficiency and impaired host defence to *Mycobacterium tuberculosis*. *Tubercle*, **66**, 301–6.

131. Rook, G.A.W., Steele, J., Fraher, L. *et al.* (1986) Vitamin D3, gamma interferon, and control of proliferation of *Mycobacterium tuberculosis* by human monocytes. *Immunology*, **57**, 159.

132. Crowle, A.J., Ross, E.J. and May, M.H. (1987) Inhibition by 1,25(OH)2-vitamin D3 of the virulent tubercle bacilli in cultured human macrophages. *Infect. Immun.*, **55**, 2945–50.

133. Finch, P.J., Millard, F.J.C. and Maxwell, J.D. (1991) Risk of tuberculosis in immigrant Asians: culturally acquired immunodeficiency? *Thorax*, **46**, 1–5.

134. Grange, J.M., Aber, V.R., Allen, B.W. *et al.* Comparison of strains of *Mycobacterium tuberculosis* from British, Ugandan and Asian immigrant patients: A study in bacteriophage typing, susceptibility to hydrogen peroxide and sensitivity to thiophen-2-carbonic acid hydrazide. *Tubercle*, **58**, 207–15.

135. Jones, W.D. and Woodley, C.L. (1983) Phage-type patterns of *Mycobacterium tuberculosis* from South East Asian immigrants. *Am. Rev. Respir. Dis.*, **127**, 348–9.

136. Ormerod, L.P. (1990) Tuberculosis screening and prevention in new immigrants 1983–1988. *Resp. Med.*, **84**, 269–71.

137. Ormerod, L.P. (1987) Reduced incidence of paediatric tuberculosis following prophylactic chemotherapy in strongly tuberculin-positive children. *Arch. Dis. Child.*, **62**, 1005–8.

138. Layton-Henry, Z. (1992) Crowded corner of a troubled world. *The Times* (London), 6 November 1992, p. 19.

G.W.K. Wong and S.J. Oppenheimer

11.1 INTRODUCTION

Although the incidence of tuberculosis has declined dramatically in most developed countries over the past century, tuberculosis remains a disease resulting in significant morbidity and mortality in children of many developing countries[1]. Children are typically infected by prolonged, close contact with an adult who has untreated open pulmonary tuberculosis. Although the incidence of tuberculosis is low in developed countries, migrants from developing countries provide a constant source of new cases of tuberculosis[1]. It is important that infected children are diagnosed and treated, as those with untreated or inadequately treated primary infection may still become 'new' cases of tuberculosis if their disease reactivates during adult life.

The diagnosis of active tuberculosis in adults can usually be confirmed by isolation of the organism from a symptomatic patient. Positive bacterial isolation in children is difficult because the disease is frequently asymptomatic and paucibacillary. The diagnosis of TB in children, therefore, is more dependent on case contact-tracing and supportive tests such as the tuberculin skin test. In several recent studies of childhood tuberculosis, a large percentage of cases were diagnosed simply through case contact-tracing and investigation[2–4]. Accurate diagnosis of tuberculosis in children without positive bacterial isolation is enhanced by the recent development of new diagnostic techniques such as polymerase chain reaction (PCR) and enzyme-linked immunosorbent assay (ELISA) (Chapter 17, p. 382 and p. 368). As childhood tuberculosis becomes less common, it may be easy to miss the diagnosis as the index of suspicion may be low. There are many types of childhood tuberculosis, but the common and important clinical forms are pulmonary tuberculosis, tuberculous meningitis, tuberculous lymphadenitis and miliary tuberculosis.

Chemotherapy is the mainstay of treatment and is very effective so long as compliance can be maintained. Children in general tolerate antituberculosis treatment better than the adults. The duration of treatment has been significantly shortened by the rational use of three- and four-drug regimens in the past two decades. Until recently most recommendations for treatment of childhood tuberculosis have, however, been based on adult experience. In this chapter, the epidemiology, clinical spectrum, diagnosis, treatment and prevention of childhood tuberculosis will be discussed. The differences between adult and childhood tuberculosis will be emphasized.

11.2 THE EPIDEMIOLOGY OF CHILDHOOD TUBERCULOSIS

The incidence of tuberculosis in developed countries has declined steadily over the past 30 years. The current annual case rate in England and the USA is under 10 per 100 000 population[5,6]. The number of cases in

Clinical Tuberculosis. Edited by P.D.O. Davies. Published in 1994 by Chapman & Hall, London. ISBN 0 412 48630 X

children below the age of 15 years is 5–6% of the total number of cases[7,8]. The period between the ages 5 and 14 years has been termed 'the favourable school age period' as children in this age group have a consistently lower active case rate than any other age group of the population. Many factors are responsible for the decline of the incidence of tuberculosis in the developed countries. These factors include improvement of socio-economic conditions, accurate diagnosis, effective treatment of the infected individuals, comprehensive case contact-tracing programmes and possibly the use of BCG vaccination. After three decades of consistently declining incidence, however, a resurgence of tuberculosis is occurring in the USA. Between 1987 and 1990, there has been a 39% increase in reported cases of childhood tuberculosis under 5 years in the USA[5]. Tuberculosis currently remains a major public health problem in Africa, Latin America and Asia, with annual case rates varying from 200 to over 400 per 100 000 population. Of the total number of cases in these developing countries, 15% are children under 15 years [9]. Despite being a highly urbanized and modern city, Hong Kong still has a very high case rate of tuberculosis, at over 100 per 100 000.

Children younger than 4 years of age have a higher risk of mortality and morbidity since tuberculous meningitis and miliary tuberculosis are most common in this age group. Of deaths from tuberculosis in the developed and developing countries, 10–20% are among children under 15 years of age[9]. There are many factors responsible for the differences of morbidity and mortality among different countries and different population groups. Natural resistance to tuberculosis is greater among Whites and Jews than among Africans, Eskimos, American Indians, Polynesians and Melanesians, possibly because generations of exposure to the disease during the eighteenth to twentieth centuries in Whites and Jews have selected in favour of the more resistant individuals (Chapter 10, p. 190).

11.3 THE CLINICAL FORMS OF CHILDHOOD TUBERCULOSIS

Tuberculosis has been classically described in the following forms: primary tuberculosis, progressive primary tuberculosis, post-primary tuberculosis and generalized tuberculosis. However, the distinction between different forms is often blurred. Primary infection occurs when a child is exposed to tubercle bacilli. During the initial infection, bacilli are disseminated to different organs and tissues resulting in different clinical forms of tuberculosis at varying periods after the primary infection. Early massive lympho-haematogenous dissemination of tubercle bacilli can result in miliary tuberculosis and/or tuberculous meningitis. Such early massive dissemination occurs most commonly in children under 4 years of age. The usual primary route of infection of tuberculosis in children is by inhalation of contaminated droplets produced by coughing, sneezing or laughing of untreated adults. Tuberculosis can also be acquired by direct inoculation through the skin, and bovine tuberculosis can be acquired by ingestion of unpasteurized and contaminated milk. Children who are under prolonged exposure to adult household contacts with sputum-positive disease are at the highest risk. The majority of children with primary pulmonary tuberculosis are asymptomatic. Tubercle bacilli are disseminated to other extrapulmonary sites by haematogenous and lymphatic routes. Other than generalized lymphohaematogenous forms of tuberculosis, other important foci of tuberculous infection in children include superficial lymph nodes, bones, joints and the gastrointestinal tract.

11.3.1 PULMONARY TUBERCULOSIS

Primary pulmonary infection in children is frequently asymptomatic. If a child has been exposed to a person who has active tubercu-

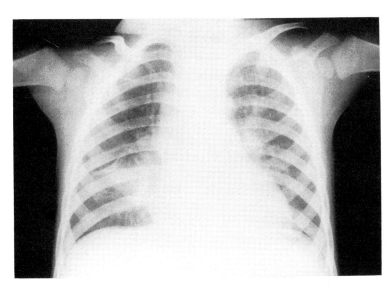

Fig. 11.1 Anteroposterior radiograph of a 2-year-old child with tuberculosis showing enlargement of the right hilar and paratracheal glands and segmental collapse in the mid zone.

losis and the tuberculin skin test is positive, tuberculosis should be suspected and appropriate investigations should be instituted. The infected patient may have occasional cough or low-grade fever. In childhood pulmonary tuberculosis, the radiological hallmark is hilar or paratracheal lymphadenopathy. There may or may not be any parenchymal changes. In a recent review, lymphadenopathy was identified in 92% of the chest radiographs of 191 children under 16 years with primary tuberculosis[10]. All patients under 3 years in this series had lymphadenopathy. In younger children and infants, the hilar lymph nodes can be large enough to cause bronchial obstruction resulting in localized hyperaeration and eventually atelectasis (Fig. 11.1). Such radiographic changes have been termed 'epituberculosis', 'collapse–consolidation' and 'segmental lesions'[11]. Occasionally, hilar lymphadenitis can erode and cause perforation of the bronchus. Subcarinal nodes can be involved and impinge on the oesophagus, causing dysphagia. Perforation of the oesophagus can further result in the formation of a broncho-oesophageal fistula. Pleural effusion is a common finding in children with pulmonary tuberculosis. It is usually serous and localized but bilateral and generalized effusions can occur. Calcification, a result of caseation of the primary complex, usually involves the lymph nodes. Calcification has been seen within 2 months but usually takes 6 or more months to develop[8]. Progressive primary tuberculosis and chronic pulmonary tuberculosis or 'adult-type' tuberculosis are rare in the paediatric population. The yield from sputum cultures or gastric washings in children varies from 15 to 40%[3,4,12]. Aspiration of pleural fluid can be performed with or without ultrasound guidance depending on the location and the size of the effusion. Pleural fluid is usually clear but may be bloodstained; glucose is low and protein is increased. Cell count will tend to show lymphocyte predominance. Culture of pleural fluid is positive in 50% of patients. Pleural punch biopsy is a useful diagnostic procedure as the tissue may show acid-fast bacilli as well as the typical histological features of tuberculosis. Biopsy material should also be sent for mycobacterial culture.

11.3.2 GENERALIZED LYMPHOHAEMATOGENOUS SPREAD

During the initial phase of the infection, tubercle bacilli from the lymphadenitis of the primary complex are disseminated to various organs or tissues in the body. The spread is usually occult and the child remains asymptomatic. Massive lymphohaematogenous spread, however, occurs more frequently in young children and infants, probably due to reduced host resistance in this age group. Miliary tuberculosis usually occurs within the first few months of the initial infection. The presenting signs and symptoms are rather non-specific. Constitutional symptoms such as fever, weight loss and night sweats are common. With more advanced involvement, patients may present with dyspnoea and cyanosis. Meningitis is found in about 20–30% of children with miliary tuberculosis[13]. The tuberculin skin test is frequently negative at presentation but most patients will convert during the illness[14]. A documented history of contact with an adult with tuberculosis aids in the diagnosis. Chest radiography usually shows uniform distribution of tubercles throughout the lungs. Bacteriological confirmation may be obtained by culturing urine, gastric aspirate or bone marrow aspirates. Liver or lymph node biopsy specimens may show typical histological features. Although the response to treatment is slow, most patients recover without any long-term sequelae. In a recent series of 94 cases of miliary tuberculosis reviewed by Hussey and colleagues[13], the only significant predictor of mortality in the group was concurrent tuberculous meningitis. The case fatality rate in this series was 14%.

11.3.3 CENTRAL NERVOUS SYSTEM TUBERCULOSIS

About 5% of children with tuberculosis have central nervous system involvement[15]. Central nervous system tuberculosis occurs as a result of lymphohaematogenous spread of tubercle bacilli during the initial phase of the primary infection. The different forms of CNS tuberculosis include tuberculous meningitis and tuberculoma. The spinal cord can also be infected locally, resulting in spinal tuberculous leptomeningitis. Tuberculous meningitis (TBM) occurs most commonly in young children and frequently accompanies miliary tuberculosis. The majority of patients with TBM are under 4 years of age[16–18]. The onset is insidious and the presenting features are non-specific. The course of meningitis can be divided into three clinical stages[19]. The first stage is characterized by personality changes, anorexia, listlessness as well as fever, although the patient is fully conscious. The first stage usually lasts for 1–2 weeks. Subsequently patients will develop signs and symptoms of increased intracranial pressure, hemiplegia, focal or generalized convulsions, and cranial nerve palsies commonly affecting the IIIrd, VIth and VIIth nerves. These focal or generalized neurological deficits are the hallmark of the second stage. In addition to focal or generalized neurological deficits, the third stage is characterized by coma and irregular respiration and pulse.

The classic CSF findings include an elevated cell count in the range of 100–400 mm^3 with lymphocyte predominance, a low glucose level and a high protein level. Computerized tomographic brain scans will frequently show hydrocephalus, basal enhancement, subdural effusion or tuberculoma[15]. Ziehl–Neelsen staining of the CSF may show tubercle bacilli. A positive CSF culture occurs in about 20–40% of cases[16–18]. Initial Mantoux test may be negative in up to 50% of patients[20]. The two significant prognostic factors in TBM are age and clinical stage. Younger age and more advanced stage predict a poor neurological outcome[18]. Long-term sequelae include recurrent seizures, ophthalmoplegia, hemiplegia, quadraplegia, deafness, intracranial calcification and mental retardation as well as hyperactivity.

Clinical response to therapy is usually quite slow and it takes months for the CSF changes to normalize. The key to successful

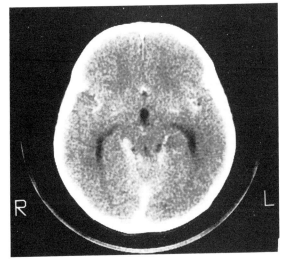

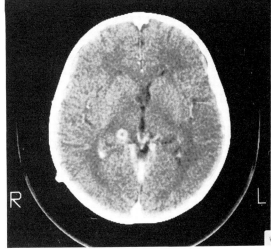

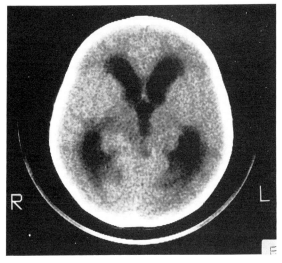

Fig. 11.2 (a) CT scan of a patient with tuberculous meningitis (reported normal). (b) CT scan of the same patient after one month showing extensive ventricular enlargement causing hydocephalus. (c) CT scan of the same patient after shunting operations to correct hydrocephalus showing development of a tuberculoma despite 2 months' therapy.

management of TBM is early diagnosis and institution of appropriate antituberculosis treatment. If there is a clinical suspicion of TBM and the child has been in contact with a case of tuberculosis, antituberculosis treatment should be started while awaiting confirmatory laboratory results.

Tuberculoma is not common in children. As with TBM, younger children are more prone to develop tuberculoma. The presenting features are similar to those of a space-occupying lesion. Headache, vomiting and convulsions are common. The presence of

fever may suggest the diagnosis of brain abscess. **Occasionally, tuberculoma can develop during the course of treatment in patients with tuberculous meningitis** (Fig. 11.2). Tuberculoma without concurrent meningitis, however, has a better prognosis than TBM[21] (Chapter 7, p. 102).

11.3.4 SUPERFICIAL LYMPH NODE TUBERCULOSIS

Tuberculosis of the superficial lymph nodes in children usually occurs in the cervical or supraclavicular region. Other lymph nodes, including the tonsillar, submandibular, preauricular, axillary and inguinal nodes, can also be affected. The typical presentation is a gradual painless enlargement of the lymph nodes. The infected nodes are discrete, rubbery and non-tender. The overlying skin may appear shiny and erythematous. Acute onset with abscess formation resulting in a fluctuant mass may occasionally occur. For any child presenting with cervical or supraclavicular lymphadenopathy, it is advisable to perform a tuberculin skin test as well as a chest radiograph[22]. If aspiration of lymph nodes is performed, specimens should be sent for Ziehl-Neelsen staining and mycobacterial culture. Without proper antituberculosis treatment, needle aspiration or incision and drainage may result in sinus tract formation. Clinical features of atypical mycobacterial lymph node infection are similar. Excisional biopsy and culture of biopsy material are necessary to differentiate tuberculosis from other non-tuberculous mycobacterial infection.

11.3.5 SKELETAL TUBERCULOSIS

Skeletal tuberculosis is an uncommon form of childhood tuberculosis. It occurs in children whose primary tuberculosis is either inadequately treated or untreated. The tubercle bacilli reach the skeletal structures through lymphohaematogenous spread during the primary infection. The most frequently affected bones are the vertebrae, in particular, the thoracic vertebrae. Other classic sites include the hips, knees and the small bones of the hands and feet.

Tuberculous spondylitis usually starts in the metaphyseal portions of the epiphyses due to their rich blood supply. Gradual destruction of bony cortex will result in the formation of a cold abscess. The initial symptoms include 'night cries' and restless sleep due to the pain. Physical examination reveals guarding due to dorsal muscle spasm.

The patient may have an abnormal neck posture or gait. Progressive destruction of the vertebral bodies will result in collapse producing kyphosis, also known as gibbus. If the disease is untreated, paraplegia can arise as a result of spinal cord compression and destruction.

Tuberculous dactylitis is characterized by cystic bony lesions occurring in infants and young children[23]. The basic pathology is endarteritis and the patient usually presents with painless swelling of the small bones. Tuberculous arthritis is uncommon in children and may present as limping or refusal to walk. The definitive diagnosis of skeletal tuberculosis is by bacterial culture and histological examination of specimens obtained by means of aspiration or open biopsy[24].

11.3.6 PERINATAL TUBERCULOSIS

Tuberculosis can be transmitted from the mother to the fetus prenatally or to the newborn postnatally. Congenital tuberculosis is a rare form of childhood tuberculosis. It is thought to be acquired either by haematogenous dissemination transplacentally or by aspiration or swallowing of infected material *in utero*. Newborns with congenital tuberculosis invariably present within the first few weeks of life with non-specific signs and symptoms such as respiratory distress, fever, poor feeding, hepatosplenomegaly, lymphadenopathy and failure to thrive[25,26]. Diagnosis, unfortunately, is frequently made at autopsy. Tuberculin skin testing is rarely positive in the newborn during the early stages of the disease. Early treatment with antituberculosis drugs can be very successful[26]. Prevention of this rare entity requires careful examination of pregnant mothers from high-risk populations. Uninfected infants born to mothers with untreated active disease are at high risk of acquiring infection postnatally[27]. Postnatal infection can be just as devastating as congenital tuberculosis. Sometimes, the distinction between the two entities in an infant is difficult. Appropriate measures should be instituted to treat the mother and the infant to prevent transmission of the disease.

11.3.7 OTHER RARE FORMS OF CHILDHOOD TUBERCULOSIS

Tuberculosis of the urinary tract is rare in the paediatric population. It is a late complication and is hence usually diagnosed during adolescence. Tubercle bacilli are disseminated to the highly vascular renal cortex during lymphohaematogenous spread of the initial infection. In the early course of the illness, renal tuberculosis is asymptomatic but persistent 'sterile' pyuria may suggest the diagnosis[28,29]. Symptoms such as frequency, dysuria and haematuria will develop when the bladder is involved. Diagnosis is confirmed by positive mycobacterial culture of the urine. Chemotherapy is effective but long-term urological follow-up is necessary to monitor the development of complications such as ureteric stricture and hydronephrosis.

Tuberculous infections of the abdominal lymph nodes (Fig. 11.3) and tuberculous peritonitis are occasionally encountered in the paediatric population. Tubercle bacilli can reach the abdominal lymph glands either by

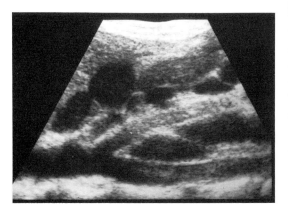

Fig. 11.3 Ultrasound image of the aorta at its bifurcation showing massive periaortic lymph node enlargement due to tuberculosis.

direct penetration of the gastrointestinal wall after being ingested or by lymphohaematogenous dissemination. Symptoms and signs of abdominal tuberculosis are non-specific and include abdominal pain, fever and abdominal distension. Definitive confirmation is by bacteriological and histological examination of specimens from biopsy or paracentesis. There is one report of the successful use of percutaneous abdominal fine-needle biopsy of peritoneal lymph nodes under ultrasound guidance[30].

Cutaneous tuberculosis is caused either by direct inoculation of tubercle bacilli or by haematogenous dissemination. The most prominent clinical feature of cutaneous tuberculosis caused by direct inoculation is the associated regional lymphadenitis. Diagnosis is confirmed by needle aspiration of the affected lymph glands. Erythema nodosum, characterized by painful reddish or violaceous nodules, usually located on the skins, is a common manifestation of hypersensitivity to tuberculin. Erythema nodosum, however, is not specific for tuberculosis, as it can occur in many other types of infection (Plate 8).

Other rare sites of infection include the pericardium, middle ear, mastoids, eye, tonsils, adenoids, buccal mucosa and the genital tract. Involvement of these sites may be caused by direct contact of infected foci or by lymphohaematogenous dissemination of tubercle bacilli. Early diagnosis is difficult as the signs and symptoms are rather non-specific. Confirmation is usually by mycobacterial culture and histological examination of surgical specimens.

11.4 DIAGNOSIS OF TUBERCULOSIS IN CHILDREN

Since tuberculous infection in children is usually paucibacillary and the infection is frequently silent, bacteriological confirmation is difficult to obtain. Up to 50% of children who have been exposed to an adult with open disease may become infected and up to 20% of these children will later develop progressive disease. Detailed examination and investigation of exposed children is thus mandatory. The importance of case contact investigation cannot be overemphasized as up to 50% of children with tuberculosis in developed countries are diagnosed as a result of case contact investigations[2–4]. Supportive investigations for the diagnosis of tuberculosis include the tuberculin skin test and a chest radiograph.

The most widely available tuberculin skin test is the Mantoux test. It involves an intradermal injection of a fixed amount of purified protein derivative. The immunophysiological basis and interpretation of this test are discussed in Chapter 5 (p. 61 and Chapter 15d, p. 345). Similarly to adults, approximately 10% of children with culture-proven tuberculosis do not react initially to the tuberculin skin test[31]. Some patients with tuberculosis may have persistently negative tuberculin reactions[32]. The use of BCG vaccination can result in positive tuberculin skin testing (Chapter 15d, p. 345). Furthermore, mycobacterial cultures are positive in only 15–40% of paediatric patients with a clinical diagnosis of tuberculosis[1]. Given these limitations, other methods are required for the early and accurate diagnosis of childhood tuberculosis.

With the advances in immunochemistry and genetic engineering, new techniques are now available for the rapid and accurate diagnosis of tuberculosis. Enzyme-linked immunosorbent assays (ELISA) utilizing specific mycobacterial antigens can detect antibodies in serum as well as cerebrospinal fluid[33]. Detection of tuberculostearic acid, a structural component of mycobacteria, in sputum, serum and CSF has also been used for diagnosis[34]. This procedure, however, requires complicated laboratory equipment and is not widely available. The use of polymerase chain reaction techniques for the detection of DNA or RNA base sequences

specific for mycobacteria has also been developed for the diagnosis of tuberculous infection[35]. These new diagnostic techniques will be of particular importance for the diagnosis of paediatric tuberculosis (Chapter 17).

11.5 THE CONTROL OF CHILDHOOD TUBERCULOSIS

The prevention, early identification and adequate treatment of individuals with tuberculosis are the cornerstones for the control of childhood tuberculosis. Bacillus Calmette–Guerin (BCG) vaccine is the oldest of the vaccines in routine use today (Chapter 14b, p. 297). The organism was derived by *in vitro* attenuation of an isolate of *M. bovis* at the Pasteur Institute of Lille, France. The currently available BCG vaccines are all derived from the original strain but their antigenicities and efficacies are different. There has been considerable controversy regarding the efficacy of BCG vaccination. The reported efficacy of BCG vaccines in many large well-controlled studies ranges from 0–80%[36]. The proposed reasons for such wide variations include differences in the quality and characteristics of the different BCG vaccines, the interaction of vaccines with different environmental mycobacteria, the regional differences in prevalence of tuberculosis, the nutritional or genetic differences in trial populations, and the methodological differences in the different trials. Despite the controversy, there is evidence that BCG vaccination is effective in the prevention of meningitis and miliary tuberculosis in children[37,38]. To complement these efficacy studies, the experience in Hong Kong has also shown the practical effect of BCG vaccination on infant mortality: with the introduction of BCG vaccination, the infant TB mortality rate in Hong Kong dropped by 90% between 1954 and 1962 while over the same period the overall notification rate only dropped by 40% (Fig. 11.4). Such a reduction

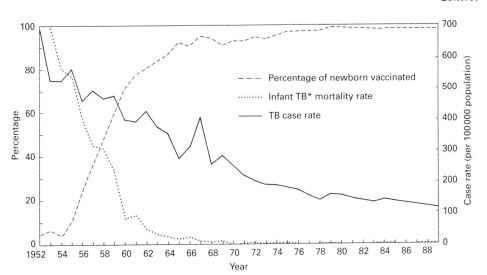

Fig. 11.4 Graph showing infant morbidity and mortality rates to tuberculosis in Hong Kong (1952–1989) together with the percentage of newborns vaccinated. *Expressed as percentage of the corresponding mortality rates in 1952. TB mortality rate in 1952 = 168.07; infant mortality rate in 1952 = 3.50.

of infant mortality is unlikely to be explained by a reduction of transmission of disease from adults to infants and children.

The major disadvantage of BCG vaccination is that it may produce a positive tuberculin skin test in vaccinated individuals. Previous vaccination with BCG, however, usually causes an induration of 10 mm or less. In a recent study of 1945 children in Saudi Arabia who had BCG at birth, only 7.8% were Mantoux-positive with greater than or equal to 10 mm induration at 5 years of age[39]. If there is epidemiological evidence of exposure and clinical suspicion of tuberculosis, it is reasonable to treat children and adolescents with positive tuberculin skin tests regardless of their vaccination status.

Chemotherapy is discussed in detail in Chapter 8, but there are differences in the principles of chemotherapy between adults and children. In general, children tolerate antituberculosis drugs better than adults. Isoniazid (H), rifampicin, streptomycin and pyrazinamide have been widely used in the treatment of childhood tuberculosis. Ethambutol has the unique toxic adverse effect of

retrobulbar neuritis. Periodic monitoring of visual acuity, visual fields and colour vision is required when ethambutol is used. Its use is thus limited since such monitoring is not reliable in young children. Historically most clinical trials of tuberculosis chemotherapy have been carried out in adults. Although most trials of short-course chemotherapy documenting effectiveness have been carried out in adults, the literature on short-course chemotherapy in children is accumulating and it appears that the use of three- to four-drug regimens for 6 months is just as effective as a 9–12 month course in the treatment of pulmonary tuberculosis and tuberculous lymphadenitis[40–44]. The recommended schedules and dosages of tuberculosis chemotherapy in children are listed in Tables 11.1 and 11.2. Twice-weekly regimens can replace daily regimens if direct supervision of drug administration is available.

Newborns are particularly vulnerable to tuberculous infection if the mother has active disease. These infants should be examined carefully for any evidence of congenital tuberculosis and they should be separated

Table 11.1 Recommended treatment regimens for tuberculosis in children[a]

Tuberculous infection	Regimens
TB meningitis/ miliary TB	2 months of H, R, Z and S daily followed by 10 months of H and R daily; steroids for second and third stage TBM
Bone/joint	2 months of H, R, Z and S daily followed by 10 months of H and R daily
Pulmonary and extrapulmonary (other than meningitis, miliary TB, bone/joint)	1. Standard: 6-month regimen 2 months of H, R and Z daily followed by 4 months of H and R daily 2. Alternative: 9-month regimen 9 months of H and R daily

H, isoniazid; R, rifampicin; Z, pyrazinamide; S, streptomycin.
[a] Summarized from several sources, see references [40–44].

from the mother until she is non-infectious. If these infants do not have any evidence of congenital tuberculosis, isoniazid should be started at 5 mg/kg daily. By 2–3 months of age, these infants should be skin-tested and isoniazid can be stopped provided that the infant is tuberculin-negative and the chest radiograph is normal. Isoniazid should be continued for 1 year if the infant is tuberculin-positive[11].

In addition to antituberculosis drugs, corticosteroids have been shown to be useful in clinical situations where suppression of inflammatory reaction is beneficial. There is considerable evidence that corticosteroids are beneficial in patients with second- and third-stage tuberculous meningitis. Corticosteroids not only reduce the severity but also the mortality of patients with TBM[45,46]. Other clinical situations where corticosteroids are beneficial include miliary disease with alveolocapillary block and respiratory dis-

tress due to bronchial obstruction associated with significant hilar lymphadenopathy [47,48]. Prednisone is commonly used at the dose of 1–2 mg/kg per day for 4–6 weeks.

Preventive therapy (a preferred term to chemoprophylaxis) is a well-established form of treatment for adults and children with asymptomatic tuberculous infection. In children, 1 year of isoniazid treatment has been demonstrated to be effective in preventing active disease for at least 30 years[49]. Currently the optimal duration of isoniazid therapy is being re-evaluated. The American Academy of Pediatrics recommends a 9-month period of isoniazid preventive therapy in children, although a high degree of protection may be achieved with a 6-month course[50]. Rifampin should be given if isoniazid-resistant infection is suspected. It cannot be over-emphasized that compliance is extremely important in order to ensure the effectiveness of antituberculosis treatment.

11.6 CONCLUSION

Childhood tuberculosis remains a challenge for clinicians and other health care professionals both in developing and developed countries. As the disease becomes rarer in the developed countries, paediatricians are becoming less familiar with the clinical presentation of the disease and accurate diagnosis and treatment may be delayed. In developing countries, many children are still dying of miliary tuberculosis and tuberculous meningitis although these conditions are readily manageable if resources are available. In contrast to the diagnosis of tuberculosis in adults, the diagnosis of childhood tuberculosis is more frequently made on epidemiological and clinical grounds supported by tuberculin skin test and chest radiograph than by bacteriological methods. Bacteriological isolation is difficult owing to the paucibacillary nature of the disease in children. With the introduction of new diagnostic techniques, an earlier and more accurate

Table 11.2 Drugs used for treatment of childhood tuberculosis

Drugs	Daily dose (mg/kg per day)	Twice weekly dose[a] (mg/kg per dose)	Maximum dose	Adverse reactions
Isoniazid	10–15	20–40	Daily: 300 mg Twice weekly: 900 mg	Hepatitis, hypersensitivity, peripheral neuritis
Rifampicin	10–20	10–20	600 mg	Hepatitis, thrombocytopenia, orange staining of urine
Pyrazinamide	20–40	50–70	2 g	Hepatotoxicity, hyperuricaemia
Streptomycin	20–40	20–40	1 g	Nephrotoxicity, ototoxicity

[a] If direct supervision of drug administration is available, daily regimens can be replaced by twice-weekly regimens.

diagnosis can be made. Although there has been a dramatic reduction of mortality of childhood tuberculosis in endemic countries such as Hong Kong, where BCG vaccination is practised at birth and effective case contact-tracing exists, the overall burden of the disease in children will continue to be dependent on the control of active adult disease.

REFERENCES

1. Fox, E. (1991) Mycobacterial infections, in *Hunter's Tropical Medicine*, 7th edn (ed. G.M. Strickland), W.B. Saunders, Philadelphia, pp. 458–63.
2. Nemir, T.L. and O'Hare, D. (1991) Tuberculosis in children 10 years of age and younger: three decades of experience during the chemotherapeutic era. *Pediatrics*, **88**, 236–41.
3. Starke, J.R. and Taylor-Watts, K.T. (1989) Tuberculosis in the pediatric population of Houston, Texas. *Pediatrics*, **84**, 28–35.
4. Toppet, M., Malfroot, A., Hofman, B. *et al.* (1991) Tuberculosis in children: A 13 year follow-up of 1714 patients in a Belgian home care centre. *Eur. J. Pediatr.*, **150**, 331–5.
5. Starke, J.R., Jacobs, R.F. and Jereb, J. (1992) Resurgence of tuberculosis in children. *J. Pediatr.*, **120**, 839–55.
6. Rieder, H., Cauthen, G., Kelly, G., *et al.* (1989) Tuberculosis in the United States. *J. Am. Med. Assoc.*, **262**, 385–9.
7. US Department of Health and Human Services, Centers for Disease Control (1987) 1985 Tuberculosis Statistics – States and Cities. HHS Publication no. (CDC) 87–8249.
8. Starke, J. (1988) Modern approach to the diagnosis and treatment of tuberculosis in children. *Pediat. Clin. North Am.*, **35**, 441–64.
9. Murray, C., Styblo, K. and Rouillon, A. (1990) Tuberculosis in developing countries: burden, intervention and cost. *Bull. Int. Union Tuberc. Lung Dis.*, **65**, 6–38.
10. Leung, A., Muller, N., Pineda, P. and FitzGerald, J (1992) Primary tuberculosis in childhood: radiographic manifestations. *Radiology*, **182**, 76–91.
11. Smith, M.H.D. and Marquis, J.R. (1987) Tuberculosis and other myobacterial infections, in *Textbook of Pediatric Infectious Disease*, 2nd edn (eds R.D. Feigin and J.D. Cheng), Saunders, Philadelphia, pp. 1342–87.
12. International Union Against Tuberculosis and Lung Disease (1991) Tuberculosis in children: guidelines for diagnosis, prevention and treatment. *Bull. Int. Union Tuberc. Lung Dis.*, **66**, 61–7.
13. Hussey, G., Chisholm T. and Kibel, M. (1991) Miliary tuberculosis in children: a review of 94 cases. *Pediatr. Infect. Dis. J.*, **10**, 832–6.
14. Schuit, K.E. (1979) Miliary tuberculosis in children. *Am. J. Dis. Child.*, **133**, 583–5.
15. Curless, R.G. and Mitchell, C.D. (1991) Central nervous system tuberculosis in children. *Pediatr. Neurol.*, **7**, 270–4.

16. Sumaya, V.C., Simek, M., Smith, M. and Seidemann, M.F. (1975) Tuberculous meningitis in children during the isoniazid era. *J. Pediatr.*, **87**, 43–9.

17. Donald, P.R., Schoeman, J.G., Cotton, M.F. and Vanzyl, L.E. (1991) Cerebrospinal fluid investigations in tuberculous meningitis. *Ann. Trop. Pediatr.*, **11**, 241–6.

18. Humphries, M.J., Teoh, R., Lau, J. and Gabriel, M. (1990) Factors of prognostic significance in Chinese children with tuberculous meningitis. *Tubercle*, **71**, 161–8.

19. Medical Research Council (1948) Streptomycin treatment of tuberculous meningitis. *Lancet*, **i**, 582–96.

20. Steiner, P. and Portugaleza, C. (1973) Tuberculous meningitis in children. *Am. Rev. Respir. Dis.*, **107**, 22–9.

21. Wallace, R.C., Burton, E.M., Banett, F.F. *et al.* (1991) Intracranial tuberculosis in children. *Pediatr. Radiol.*, **21**, 241–6.

22. Barton, L.L. and Feigin, R. (1974) Childhood cervical lymphadenitis: a reappraisal. *J. Pediatr.*, **84**, 846–52.

23. Hardy, J.B. and Hartmann, J.R. (1947) Tuberculous dactylitis in childhood. *J. Pediatr.*, **30**, 146–56.

24. Berney, S., Goldstein, M. and Bishko, F. (1972) Clinical and diagnostic features of tuberculous arthritis. *Am. J. Med.*, **53**, 36–42.

25. Hageman, J. Shulman, S. and Schreiber, M. (1980) Congenital tuberculosis: critical reappraisal of clinical findings and diagnostic procedures. *Pediatrics*, **66**, 980–4.

26. Nemir, R.L. and O'Hara, D. (1985) Congenital tuberculosis – review and diagnostic guidelines. *Am. J. Dis Child*, **139**, 284–7.

27. Light, I.J., Saidleman, M. and Sutherland, J. (1974) Management of newborns after nursery exposure to tuberculosis. *Am. Rev. Respir. Dis.*, **109**, 415–19.

28. Ehrlich, R.M. and Lattimer, J. (1971) Urogenital tuberculosis in children. *J. Urol*, **105**, 461–5.

29. Smith, A.M. and Lattimer, J.K. (1983) Genitourinary tract involvement in children with tuberculosis. *NY State J. Med.*, **73**, 2325–8.

30. Liu, K.W., Chan, Y.L., Tseng, R. and Oppenheimer, S.J. (1992) Abdominal tuberculosis in children. *HK J. Pediatr.*, **1**, 96–9.

31. Hsu, K. (1983) Tuberculin reaction in children treated with isoniazid. *Am. J. Dis. Child*, **137**, 1090–2.

32. Steiner, P., Rao, M. and Victoria, M. (1980) Persistently negative tuberculin reactions. *Am. J. Dis. Child.*, **134**, 747–50.

33. Daniel, T. and Debanne, S. (1987) The serodiagnosis of tuberculosis and other mycobacterial diseases by enzyme-linked immunosorbent assay. *Am. Rev. Respir. Dis.*, **135**, 1137–51.

34. French, G.L., Chan, C.Y., Cheung, S.W. *et al.* (1987) Diagnosis of pulmonary tuberculosis by detection of tuberculostearic acid in sputum by using gas chromatography-mass spectrometry with selected ion monitoring. *J. Infect. Dis.*, **156**, 356–62.

35. Daniel, T. (1989) Rapid diagnosis of tuberculosis: laboratory techniques applicable in developing countries. *Rev. Infect. Dis.*, **11**, S471-S478.

36. Fine, P. (1989) The BCG story: lessons from the past and implication for the future. *Rev. Infect. Dis.*, **11**, S353-S359.

37. Miceli, I., Kantor, I., Colaiacoro, D. *et al.* (1988) Evaluation of effectiveness of BCG vaccination using case-control method in Buenos Aires, Argentina. *Int. J. Epidemiol.*, **17**, 629–34.

38. Sirinavin, S., Chotpitayasunondh, T., Suwanjuthas, *et al.* (1991) Protective efficacy of neonatal Bacillus Calmette–Guerin vaccination against tuberculosis. *Pediatr. Infect. Dis. J.*, **10**, 359–65.

39. Al-Kassimi, F.A., Abdullah, A.K., Al-Orainey, I.O., *et al.* (1991) The significance of positive Mantoux reactions in BCG-vaccinated children. *Tubercle*, **72**, 101–4.

40. Starke, J.R. and Taylor-Watts, K.T. (1989) Six-month chemotherapy of intrathoracic tuberculosis in children. *Am. Rev. Respir. Dis.*, **139**, (Suppl.), A314.

41. Biddulph, J. (1990) Short-course chemotherapy for childhood tuberculosis. *Pediatr. Infect. Dis. J.*, **9**, 794–801.

42. Jawahar, M.S., Sivasubramanian, S., Vijavan, V.K. *et al.* Short course chemotherapy for tuberculous lymphadenitis in children. *Br. Med. J.*, **301**, 359–61.

43. Kumar, L., Dhand, R., Singhi, P.D. *et al.* (1990) A randomized trial of fully intermittent VS daily followed by intermittent short course chemotherapy for childhood tuberculosis. *Pediatr. Infect. Dis. J.*, **9**, 802–6.

44. Stark, J.R. (1990) Multidrug chemotherapy for tuberculosis in children. *Pediatr. Infect. Dis. J.*, **9**, 785–93.

45. Escobar, J.A., Belsey, M.A., Ovenas, A. *et al.* (1975) Mortality from tuberculous meningitis reduced by steroid therapy. *Pediatrics*, **56**, 1050–5.

46. Girgis, N.I., Farid, Z., Kilpatrick, M.E. *et al.* (1991) Dexamethasone as an adjunct to treatment of tuberculous meningitis. *Pediatr. Infect. Dis. J.*, **10**, 179–83.

47. Nemir, R.L., Cardona, J., Vaziri, F. *et al.* (1967) Prednisone as an adjunct in the chemotherapy of lymph node-bronchial tuberculosis in childhood: a double-blind study. *Am. Rev. Respir. Dis.*, **95**, 402–10.

48. Smith, M.H.D. and Matsaniotis, N. (1958) Treatment of tuberculosis pleural effusions with particular reference to adrenal corticosteroids. *Pediatrics*, **22**, 1074–87.

49. Hsu, K.H.K. (1984) Thirty years after isoniazid: its impact on tuberculosis in children and adolescents. *J. Am. Med. Assoc.*, **251**, 1283–5.

50. American Academy of Pediatrics (1992) Chemotherapy for tuberculosis in infants and children. *Pediatrics*, **89**, 161–5.

HIV-RELATED TUBERCULOSIS 12

TUBERCULOSIS AND HUMAN IMMUNODEFICIENCY VIRUS INFECTION IN INDUSTRIALIZED COUNTRIES

H.L. Rieder

12a.1 INTRODUCTION

At the first international conference on the acquired immunodeficiency syndrome (AIDS) in 1985, epidemiologists from New York City reported on the geographical association of the increasing incidence of tuberculosis in the city with AIDS[1]. Six months later, the Centers for Disease Control (Atlanta, USA) reported that ongoing surveillance suggested that tuberculosis cases during the first 39 weeks of 1985 had failed to decline as was expected from previous years[2]. Subsequently, the Centers for Disease Control in collaboration with state and local health authorities initiated several studies, including in Florida[3,4] and in New York City[5], to determine better the relationship between AIDS and tuberculosis and to gain better knowledge of the demographic and clinical characteristics of tuberculosis patients with and without AIDS. These descriptive, retrospective studies confirmed what had earlier been suggested in smaller studies[6,7], that

1. Tuberculosis was common among patients with AIDS from populations with a recognized high prevalence of infection with tubercle bacilli.

2. Tuberculosis often preceded conditions constituting the then valid surveillance definition of AIDS[8].
3. In patients with AIDS, clinical forms of tuberculosis often deviated from the accustomed manifestations of the disease in non-compromised hosts.

Among all the factors that have been identified as allowing the progression from subclinical infection with *Mycobacterium tuberculosis*, infection with the human immunodeficiency virus (HIV) has now emerged to be by far the most potent[9–11] (Chapter 14a, Table 3, p. 290). The Centers for Disease Control has accordingly long changed its case definition for AIDS and now includes in the currently applicable definition pulmonary tuberculosis in the presence of infection with HIV as an AIDS-defining condition[12].

The purpose of this chapter is to highlight salient features of the epidemiology of HIV-associated tuberculosis in industrialized countries, its impact on tuberculosis control and the role of various intervention strategies to stem adverse effects of the HIV epidemic on the course of the tuberculosis epidemic in these countries.

Clinical Tuberculosis. Edited by P.D.O. Davies. Published in 1994 by Chapman & Hall, London. ISBN 0 412 48630 X

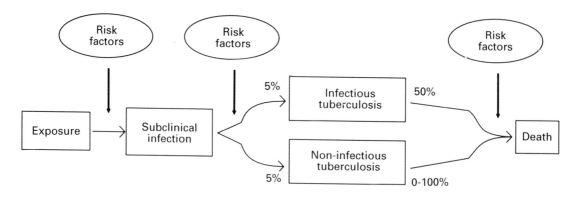

Fig. 12a.1 Diagrammmatic presentation of the pathogenesis of tuberculosis. Reprinted from *Tuberculosis – A comprehensive international approach,* p. 168, edited by L.B. Reichman and E.S. Hershfield, by courtesy of Marcel Dekker, Inc., NY, 1993.

Table 12a.1 Tuberculosis among AIDS patients in Florida by ethnic group

Ethnicity group	Total AIDS patients (n)	AIDS patients with tuberculosis (n)	(%)
White	881	16	(1.8)
Hispanic	242	14	(5.8)
Black, American	446	52	(11.7)
Haitian	282	77	(27.3)

Adapted from Rieder *et al., Arch. Intern. Med.,* 1989, **149**, 1268–73.

12a.1.1 EPIDEMIOLOGY OF HIV-ASSOCIATED TUBERCULOSIS

As trivial it may appear, it needs to be re-emphasized that the most important risk factor for tuberculosis is infection with *M. tuberculosis* (Fig. 12a.1). Only persons infected with tubercle bacilli can develop tuberculosis. In the retrospective study in Florida[4], the frequency of tuberculosis among AIDS patients ranged considerably in different race/ethnicity groups (Table 12a.1). While only about 2% of White American AIDS patients had tuberculosis, almost 30% of Haitian AIDS patients were known to have had tuberculosis in Florida. Taking into account that even among Haitians not all young adults are infected with tubercle bacilli[13], it is likely that dually infected persons have a risk of at least 30% of developing tuberculosis during the course of HIV infection.

The occurrence of HIV-associated tuberculosis is thus critically dependent on three factors:

1. The prevalence of infection with *M. tuberculosis*.
2. The prevalence of infection with HIV.
3. The extent to which these two segments of the population overlap.

In most industrialized countries the risk of becoming infected with tubercle bacilli during the course of 1 year (annual risk of infection) has decreased very rapidly since 1945[11,14–17] (Fig. 12a.2). As a result, the prevalence of infection in the general indigenous population has become very small among those under 50 years of age, but is still very high in the oldest segments of the population, as can be shown for Western Europe[18] (Fig. 12a.3). However, the population segments within different industrialized countries are often non-homogeneous in respect to infection with tubercle bacilli. This has been mirrored in different levels of tuberculosis incidence in different population segments before the advent of the HIV

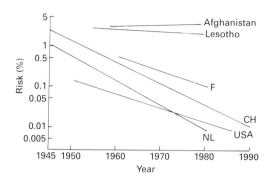

Fig. 12a.2 Secular trend in the annual risk of infection with tubercle bacilli in selected countries (CH, Switzerland; NL, the Netherlands; F, France; USA, United States). (Data drawn from several sources: see references 11, 14–17.)

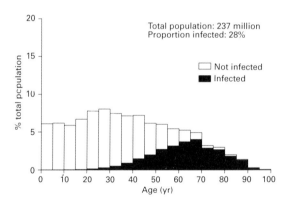

Fig. 12a.3 Prevalence of infection with *M. tuberculosis* in Western Europe. (Data from Sudre *et al.* (1991), World Health Organization.)

epidemic. In the USA, racial/ethnic minorities are well recognized to have a much higher incidence of tuberculosis than non-Hispanic Whites[19–23]. Intravenous drug users were also known to have had a higher tuberculosis incidence than would be expected from the general population[24]. An increasingly important segment of the population in industrialized countries is comprised of immigrants, refugees and asylum seekers from resource-poor countries with a high incidence of tuberculosis[25–27]. HIV infection is also apparently unequally distributed within different population segments[28,29]. It is thus not surprising that HIV-associated tuberculosis has emerged early in USA prison populations where both ethnic/racial minorities and disenfranchised groups such as injection drug users – both with excess tuberculous and HIV infection prevalence in comparison to the general population – are over-represented[30–32].

In several metropolitan areas in the USA, but also in Europe, tuberculosis has recently increased. Particularly notable is the case of New York City, where tuberculosis has increased almost steadily since 1979[33]. In 1978, cases in the city comprised 4.6% of the national morbidity, while by 1991 this proportion had increased to 14.0%[26,34]. This increase has been attributed to a deterioration in public services and increased poverty, all complicated by the HIV epidemic[33]. In Europe, increases have also been noted in several countries[27]. In many of the European countries, however, it is not association with HIV but rather increased immigration of people from high incidence countries that is causally related to the observed levelling of tuberculosis notifications[27].

12a.1.2 IMPACT OF HIV-ASSOCIATED TUBERCULOSIS

HIV may alter the epidemiology of tuberculosis in three ways[35]:

- Endogenous reactivation of pre-existing infection with *M. tuberculosis* in persons who become infected with HIV.
- Progression from infection with *M. tuberculosis* to tuberculosis in persons with pre-existing HIV infection.
- Transmission of tubercle bacilli to the general population from tuberculosis patients who developed tuberculosis because of HIV infection.

The retrospective study in Florida[4] indirectly and the prospective study in New York City[9] directly demonstrated that the proportion of tuberculosis cases that developed by endogenous reactivation was of over-riding importance. That primary progression to tuberculosis and transmission of tubercle bacilli to susceptible individuals can become of major importance has been particularly well documented in numerous investigations of outbreaks of tuberculosis in health care facilities[36–48]. From a public health perspective, it is of particular concern if increased transmission occurs, because this will almost certainly lead to an increase in the pool of infected persons from which future cases will arise. It has been estimated that in recent years the risk of infection in the USA has increased by more than 10% per year, if the increase of tuberculosis in US-born children under 5 years of age is taken as indicative of recent transmission[49]. The increase in infection risk in the general population is likely to be less, because children from ethnic/racial minorities are disproportionately frequently affected by tuberculosis in the USA[50]. Nevertheless, since tuberculosis in children is a sensitive sentinel for the tuberculosis epidemiology[51], the USA surveillance data suggest that excess transmission of tubercle bacilli might be occurring at a considerable scale in that country.

Available data suggest that HIV has a much less spectacular impact on tuberculosis morbidity in Europe[27]. However, certain areas can be identified where HIV does impact on tuberculosis morbidity. This is the case in certain areas where a large proportion of AIDS patients are found among injection drug users, such as in certain areas in Spain and Italy[27,52,53]. That the overall impact is relatively small is not particularly surprising, because prevalence of infection with *M. tuberculosis* is low in the more homogenous autochthonous population in those countries of Western Europe from which such data are available[15,16,54] and it is likely that other countries with similar morbidity patterns have a similar underlying prevalence of infection.

12a.2 INTERVENTIONS

In line with the pathogenesis of tuberculosis, three major points of intervention are possible (Fig. 12a.4). **Vaccination** with BCG, if given before infection, can prevent progression from infection with *M. tuberculosis* to tuberculosis to various degrees under different circumstances[55,56]. **Preventive therapy** can prevent progression from infection to disease in a considerable proportion of asymptomatically infected people[57]. **Chemotherapy** of tuberculosis can prevent death and interrupt transmission. Additionally, although less investigated, prophylactic therapy is often recommended for strongly exposed, still tuberculin-negative contacts, particularly small children[58].

12a.2.1 PREVENTION OF DISEASE BY VACCINATION IN HIV-INFECTED PERSONS

The issue of efficacy of BCG vaccination remains clouded. Nevertheless, there is general agreement that BCG protects against severe haematogenous complications of tuberculosis in children in a large proportion of cases[59]. Little is known of the extent to which BCG vaccination may protect (HIV-uninfected) adults who were vaccinated at birth. Nothing is known about the protective efficacy of BCG in persons infected with HIV. It is unlikely that BCG will be capable of conferring considerable protection against tuberculosis in HIV-infected persons should they become infected with *M. tuberculosis*, because HIV destroys those very cells that are in the chain of cellular protection and immunity.

A few case reports about complications from BCG vaccination have been published. A boy born to an HIV-seropositive mother developed mycobacterial meningitis due to

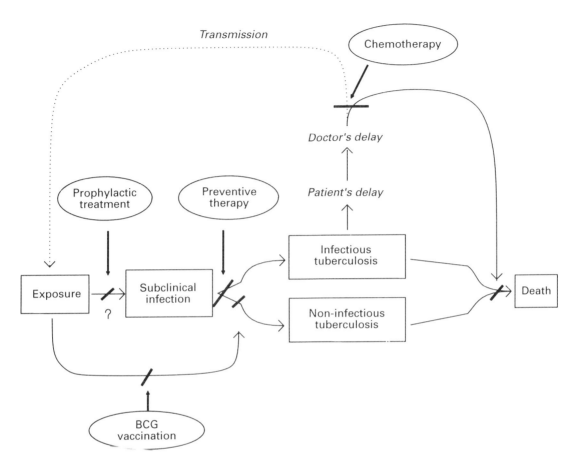

Fig. 12a.4 Diagrammatic presentation of the pathogenesis of tuberculosis and points of intervention.

BCG at the age of 4 months after receiving BCG at birth[60]. Bilateral cervical axillary adenopathy due to BCG was reported in an AIDS patient 30 years after vaccination[61] and disseminated BCG disease developed in another, also 30 years after vaccination[62]. Other isolated reports of adverse reactions in HIV-infected children who were BCG-vaccinated have been reported[63,64]. In larger investigations, such as the study in Rwanda, no difference in the frequency of complications was seen between BCG-vaccinated children with and without HIV infection[65]. Intuitively one might expect to observe complications more frequently with

BCG vaccination in HIV-infected children. It has not been satisfactorily resolved why this is not the case. Among various possible explanations, the most disturbing possibility is that complications, particularly disseminated BCG disease, may be too difficult to diagnose in those countries where both HIV infection is common and BCG vaccination is widely used[66].

The World Health Organization's finding in 1987 that the evidence for an increased frequency of adverse reactions after BCG immunization of asymptomatic HIV-infected individuals remains inconclusive[67] is still valid. For countries with a high risk of tuberculosis, BCG is recommended at birth or as soon as possible, unless the children are symptomatically infected with HIV. In areas where BCG is still recommended but the risk of tuberculosis is low (e.g. several European countries), BCG may be withheld from individuals known or suspected to be infected with HIV[67]. It has become accepted policy in the USA and Europe to withhold BCG from known HIV-infected individuals, even if they do not have symptoms[68–71].

12a.2.2 PREVENTIVE THERAPY FOR HIV-INFECTED INDIVIDUALS CO-INFECTED WITH *M. TUBERCULOSIS*

Preventive therapy with isoniazid given for 12 months for infection with *M. tuberculosis* can substantially reduce the risk of progression to tuberculosis[57]. The efficacy depends critically on adherence of patients to the prescribed regimen[72]. Preventive therapy of infection can rationally be prescribed only if infection with tubercle bacilli can be identified. There is a direct correlation between the CD4/CD8 ratio and delayed-type hypersensitivity reactions[73]. In patients with HIV and tuberculous infection, the tuberculin skin test becomes falsely negative with increasing frequency as immunosuppression progresses[4] and identification of infection with *M. tuberculosis* thus may become very difficult[74–79]. This is particularly worrisome because anergic patients who are infected with tubercle bacilli have a particularly high risk of developing tuberculosis[79].

There is general agreement that patients with dual infection should be given preventive therapy[68–70]. Difficulties arise in determining what diameter of the tuberculin skin test reaction size should be taken as indicative for infection. In the USA, where BCG has not been used, the cut-off for HIV-infected individuals is set at 5 mm induration using 5 TU PPD (equivalent to 2 TU PPD RT23 in Europe)[70,80]. In Europe, where the majority of the young adult population is still

vaccinated with BCG, recommendations are more difficult to make. The British Thoracic Society has developed such recommendations[69], which are useful in countries with a large coverage of BCG and might be adapted until more knowledge accumulates (Fig. 12a.5). Both the Centers for Disease Control [80] and the British Thoracic Society[69] recommend that HIV-infected individuals with small tuberculin reactions who are not BCG-vaccinated should be tested with at least two other recall antigens (such as *Candida*, mumps, or tetanus toxoid) to aid in the interpretation of tuberculin skin test results in HIV-infected persons.

A multitude of trials is in progress to assess the efficacy of preventive therapy among HIV-infected individuals co-infected with tubercle bacilli[81,82], but little has been published. One of these studies, already generating tangible results, is being conducted in Lusaka, Zambia[83]. HIV-infected individuals are randomly assigned without prior tuberculin skin testing to either 30 months of vitamin B complex or 6 months of treatment with isoniazid followed by 24 months of vitamin B complex. The preliminary data suggest an almost 90% lower incidence of tuberculosis during follow-up among the preventive therapy group than in the placebo group. Although anecdotes of preventive therapy failure have been reported[84], the ongoing trial in Zambia suggests that preventive therapy is in general also highly effective in HIV-infected individuals. There is a clear need for more data on feasibility and efficacy studies of preventive therapy[85].

12a.2.3 CHEMOTHERAPY OF TUBERCULOSIS

Several factors have emerged that impede curative treatment of tuberculosis among HIV-infected patients. These include difficulties in establishing the diagnosis, poor tolerance of antituberculosis drugs, resistance to antituberculosis drugs and failure of patients to adhere to prescribed regimens.

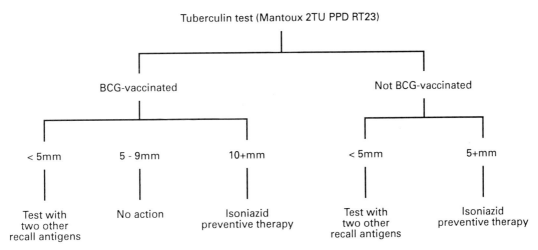

Fig. 12a.5 Recommendations for tuberculin skin test interpretation and preventive therapy in HIV-infected individuals. (Adapted from British Thoracic Society guidelines on the management of tuberculosis, see reference 69.)

The clinical manifestation of tuberculosis often differs in HIV-infected patients from that commonly observed in patients without HIV infection[86]. A multitude of specimens thus may need to be taken to establish the diagnosis of tuberculosis[70]. It appears, however, that one of the most common pitfalls lies in the failure to consider the possibility of the disease[87–89].

Tuberculosis patients with AIDS do also appear to tolerate antituberculosis drugs less well than non-compromised patients[90]. Adverse reactions manifesting as rashes appear to be particularly common and may be attributable to any of the drugs used. At least one case of Lyell's syndrome attributable to rifampicin in an HIV-seropositive patient has been reported[91]. Rashes, hepatitis and gastrointestinal distress appear to be the most common adverse reactions that may be seen in HIV-infected tuberculosis patients, and rifampicin appears to be most commonly the culprit, requiring discontinuation in perhaps some 10% or more of patients[92].

Generally, the treatment regimen recommended for non-compromised hosts also appears to be effective in achieving sputum conversion in HIV-infected tuberculosis patients[92]. Nevertheless, cases of failure have been reported in a patient with a susceptible strain[93], and less surprisingly, in a patient with a drug-resistant strain[94]. The Centers for Disease Control recommends that patients with HIV infection should be treated with isoniazid, rifampicin and pyrazinamide during the first 2 months. Ethambutol should be added if drug resistance is suspected[70]. The continuation phase with rifampicin and isoniazid should be continued for a minimum of 9 months and for at least 6 months beyond documented culture conversion as evidenced by three negative cultures. Given the emergence of drug resistance, it might be wise to begin treatment generally with four drugs (isoniazid, rifampicin, pyrazinamide, ethambutol), irrespective of prior probability of drug susceptibility patterns or immunodeficiency.

Drug resistance, particularly multiple-drug resistance including resistance to rifampicin and isoniazid, has become a major problem in the USA[40–42, 44–47, 95–101] and is thus threatening the efficacy of antituberculosis treatment. It is not HIV infection *per se* that is at the root of the problem of emergence of drug resistant tubercle bacilli. Clearly, patients treated insufficiently in the past have a higher probability of harbouring drug-resistant bacilli if they have recurrent disease than patients previously never treated for tuberculosis. A recent report from Central Harlem, New York City, sheds some light on possible reasons for the epidemic of drug resistance[33]. In that area, the majority of newly diagnosed tuberculosis patients were lost alreay during hospitalization or within the first 3 months after the initiation of treatment. After recurrence of symptoms, many of the defaulters were re-admitted only to be lost again. Insufficient and inadequate treatment is not only conducive to drug resistance, but is also likely to keep patients discharging and transmitting tubercle bacilli beyond the natural course of untreated disease[102]. The deterioration of public health services in New York City and spreading poverty, all complicated and accelerated by HIV infection, have allowed tuberculosis to get out of control in that City. There is apparently a high price to pay for the damage caused by inaction[49]. In other areas of the USA, the problem has been less spectacular. Nevertheless, the impact of HIV on tuberculosis is becoming a major problem, almost throughout the country, but to a different extent in different geographic locations[103]. In Seattle–King County, for example, a quarter of all tuberculosis cases are estimated to be attributable to HIV infection[104].

To address the newly emerging problems in tuberculosis control, the USA federal government has formed a Tuberculosis Task Force, which aims to co-ordinate control efforts and research[105].

12a.3 CONCLUSIONS

The impact the HIV epidemic exerts on the tuberculosis situation depends on the prevalence of infection with *M. tuberculosis* in the respective segments of the population most susceptible to HIV infection. In the USA the impact of HIV infection on tuberculosis morbidity has been painfully registered in the large proportion of the large segments of the population of African Americans and Hispanics who are infected with both microorganisms with a disproportionately high frequency. In Europe, the indigenous population is relatively more homogenous in respect to infection with tubercle bacilli and the prevalence of infection with *M. tuberculosis* in the population under the age of 50 years has become very low. Notable exceptions include injection drug users. Although tuberculosis may emerge, or has already done so in some areas, as a significant problem in this segment of the indigenous population, the overall impact of HIV infection on the epidemiology of tuberculosis is likely to remain limited. Of utmost importance is what happens to children today, because the prevalence of tuberculous infection among them will determine the future size of the tuberculosis problem. As the generation of parents in Europe, and parents among the White population in the USA have, in general increasingly less tuberculosis, the chain of transmission to the next generation becomes severed. Injection drug users may increasingly transmit tubercle bacilli among themselves, but their relative isolation from the greater community will generally prohibit significant transmission to the general population and to school-age children in particular.

Among the available interventions, timely diagnosis of infectious (and other) cases of tuberculosis followed by adequate chemotherapy until the patient is cured remain the most efficient. The danger of missing the diagnosis increases as the frequency of tuberculosis decreases, and atypical manifestations of tuberculosis among HIV-afflicted patients may delay the diagnosis. This puts not only the patient's life at risk, it also provides ample opportunity for tubercle bacilli to be transmitted unchecked.

Drug resistance, in particular resistance to isoniazid and rifampicin, threatens tuberculosis control. The emergence of drug resistance points to serious deficiencies in the health care system. It has long been recognized that compliance with long-term medication poses serious problems of adherence among patients with a prescribed regimen. There is no excuse for neglecting the issue. The International Union Against Tuberculosis and Lung Disease has developed principles on how to combat tuberculosis in high-incidence, resource-poor countries[106]. These principles have aided the achievement of a cure ratio in excess of 75%[49]. Because compliance is a major issue and because irregular drug intake may lead to acquisition of drug resistance, measures that may be costly per patient treated, such as directly observed treatment, must be taken. If such basic principles are being neglected, tuberculosis will continue to take its toll, and in some areas ever increasingly so. Above all, disregard for the need to cure a patient who is diagnosed can indeed be very costly[49].

Vaccination with BCG is unlikely to stem HIV-associated tuberculosis because its main effect is on non-transmissible forms of the disease in children. Preventive therapy of dually infected persons might have considerable impact on unnecessary individual suffering and may be able to prevent transmission. Problems arise in identifying dually infected persons. It should nevertheless become adopted policy that individuals known to be infected with HIV should be offered tuberculin skin testing as early as possible, and if found to have dual infection be given preventive therapy against tuberculosis.

Tuberculosis can be controlled and plans for its elimination[68,107] can be implemented if complacency about the bottom line in tuberculosis control can be overcome. A patient diagnosed as having tuberculosis must be cured from his or her disease with one single course of effective chemotherapy and close contacts must be promptly identified and be offered preventive therapy if found to be infected with tubercle bacilli.

REFERENCES

1. Stoneburner, R.L. and Kristal, A. (1985) Increasing tuberculosis incidence and its relationship to acquired immunodeficiency syndrome in New York City. International Conference on Acquired Immunodeficiency Syndrome (AIDS), Atlanta, Georgia, 14–17 April.
2. Centers for Disease Control (1985) Tuberculosis – United States, first 39 weeks, 1985. *Morbid. Mortal. Weekly Rep.*, **34**, 625–7.
3. Centers for Disease Control (1986) Tuberculosis and acquired immunodeficiency syndrome – Florida. *Morbid. Mortal. Weekly Rep.*, **35**, 587–90.
4. Rieder, H.L., Cauthen, G.M., Bloch, A.B. *et al.* (1989) Tuberculosis and acquired immunodeficiency syndrome – Florida. *Arch. Intern. Med.*, **149**, 1268–73.
5. Centers for Disease Control (1987) Tuberculosis and acquired immunodeficiency syndrome – New York City. *Morbid. Mortal. Weekly Rep.*, **36**, 785–95.
6. Pape, J.W., Liautaud, B., Thomas, F. *et al.* (1983) Characteristics of the acquired immunodeficiency syndrome (AIDS) in Haiti. *N. Engl. J. Med.*, **309**, 945–50.
7. Pitchenik, A.E., Cole, C., Russell, B.W. *et al.* (1984) Tuberculosis, atypical mycobacteriosis, and the acquired immunodeficiency syndrome among Haitian and non-Haitian patients in south Florida. *Ann. Intern. Med.*, **101**, 641–5.
8. Centers for Disease Control (1985) Revision of the case definition of acquired immunodeficiency syndrome for national reporting – United States. *Morbid. Mortal. Weekly Rep.*, **34**, 373–5.
9. Selwyn, P.A., Hartel, D., Lewis, V.A. *et al.* (1989). A prospective study of the risk of tuberculosis among intravenous drug users with human immunodeficiency virus infection. *N. Engl. J. Med.*, **320**, 45–50.
10. Braun, M.M., Badi, N., Ryder, R.W. *et al.* (1991) A retrospective cohort study of the risk of tuberculosis among women in childbearing age with HIV infection in Zaire. *Am. Rev. Respir. Dis.*, **143**, 501–4.
11. Rieder, H.L., Cauthen, G.M., Comstock,

G.W. *et al.* (1989) Epidemiology of tuberculosis in the United States. *Epidemiol. Rev.*, **11**, 79–98.

12. Centers for Disease Control (1993) 1993 revised classification system for HIV infection and expanded surveillance case definition for AIDS among adolescents and adults. *Morbid. Mortal. Weekly Rep.*, **41** (No. RR–17), 1–19.

13. Pitchenik, A.E., Russell, B.W., Cleary, T. *et al.* (1982) The prevalence of tuberculosis and drug resistance among Haitians. *N. Engl. J. Med.*, **307**, 162–5.

14. Cauthen, G.W., ten Dam, H.G. and Pio, A. (1988) Annual risk of tuberculosis infection. WHO/TB/88.154. World Health Organization, Geneva.

15. Rieder, H.L., Zimmermann, H., Zwahlen, M. and Billo, N.E. (1990) Epidemiologie der Tuberkulose in der Schweiz (English abstract). *Schweiz. Rundschau. Med. (Praxis)*, **79**, 675–9.

16. Lotte, A. and Uzan, J. (1973) Evolution of the rates of tuberculous infection in France and calculation of the annual risk by means of a mathematical model. *Intern. J. Epidemiol.*, **2**, 265–82.

17. Styblo, K. and Enarson, D.A. (1991) The impact of infection with human immunodeficiency virus on tuberculosis in *Recent Advances in Respiratory Medicine*, No. 5 (ed. D.M. Mitchell), Churchill Livingstone, Edinburgh, pp.147–62.

18. Sudre, P., ten Dam, G., Chan, C. and Kochi, A. (1991) Tuberculosis in the present time: a global overview of the tuberculosis situation. WHO/TUB/91.158. World Health Organization, Geneva.

19. Centers for Disease Control (1987) Tuberculosis in minorities – United States. *Morbid. Mortal. Weekly Rep.*, **36**, 77–80.

20. Centers for Disease Control (1987) Tuberculosis in blacks – United States. *Morbid. Mortal. Weekly Rep.*, **36**, 212–20.

21. Centers for Disease Control (1987) Tuberculosis among Asians/Pacific Islanders – United States, 1985. *Morbid. Mortal. Weekly Rep.*, **36**, 331–4.

22. Centers for Disease Control (1987) Tuberculosis among American Indians and Alaskan Natives – United States, 1985. *Morbid. Mortal. Weekly Rep.*, **36**, 493–5.

23. Centers for Disease Control (1987) Tuberculosis among Hispanics – United States, 1985. *Morbid. Mortal. Weekly Rep.*, **36**, 568–9.

24. Reichman, L.B., Felton, C.P. and Edsall, J.R. (1979) Drug dependence, a possible new risk factor for tuberculosis disease. *Arch. Intern. Med.*, **139**, 337–9.

25. Office fédéral de la santé publique (1991) Tuberculose, Suisse 1990. *Bulletin de l'Office fédéral de la santé publique*, No. 35, 546–51.

26. Rieder, H.L. (1992) Misbehaviour of a dying epidemic: a call for less speculation and better surveillance (Editorial). *Tuberc. Lung Dis.*, **73**, 181–3.

27. Raviglione, M., Sudre, P., Rieder, H.L. *et al.* (1992) Secular trends of tuberculosis in Western Europe. *Tuberculosis Surveillance Research Unit Progress Report 1992*, vol. 2, KNCV, The Hague, pp.1–33.

28. Wiley, J.A. and Samuel, M.C.(1989) Prevalence of HIV infection in the USA. *AIDS*, **3** (Suppl.) S71–S78.

29. European Centre for the epidemiological monitoring of AIDS (1992) AIDS surveillance in Europe. *Quarterly Report*, No. 33, 31 March.

30. Braun, M.M., Truman, B.I., Maguire, B. *et al.* (1989) Increasing incidence of tuberculosis in a prison inmate population. *J. Am. Med. Assoc.*, **261**, 393–7.

31. Salive, M.E., Vlahov, D. and Brewer, T.F. (1990) Coinfection with tuberculosis and HIV-1 in male prison inmates. *Publ. Hlth Rep.*, **105**, 307–10.

32. Darbyshire, J.H. (1989) Tuberculosis in prisons. Possible links with HIV infection (Editorial). *Br Med J.*, **299**, 874.

33. Brudney, K. and Dobkin, J. (1991) Resurgent tuberculosis in New York City. Human immunodeficiency virus, homelessness and the decline of tuberculosis control programs. *Am. Rev. Respir. Dis.* **144**; 745–9.

34. Centers for Disease Control. (1991) *1991 Final Tuberculosis Data*. Public document, Division of Tuberculosis Elimination, Centers for Disease Control, Atlanta, Ga.

35. Sutherland, I. (1990) The epidemiology of tuberculosis and AIDS. *Communicable Disease Report* [UK], 90/10, 9 March.

36. Di Perri, G., Cruciani, M., Danzi, M.C. *et al.* (1989) Nosocomial epidemic of active tuberculosis among HIV-infected patients. *Lancet*, **2**, 1502–4.

37. Centers for Disease Control (1991) Tuberculosis outbreak among persons in a residential

facility for HIV-infected persons – San Francisco. *Morbid. Mortal. Weekly Rep.*, **40**, 649–52.

38. Centers for Disease Control (1989) *Mycobacterium tuberculosis* transmission in a health clinic – Florida, 1988. *Morbid, Mortal. Weekly Rep.*, **38**, 256–64.

39. Dooley, S.W., Villarino, M.E., Lawrence, M. *et al.* (1992) Nosocomial transmission of tuberculosis in a hospital unit for HIV-infected patients. *J. Am. Med. Assoc.*, **267**, 2632–5.

40. Centers for Disease Control (1991) Transmission of multidrug resistant tuberculosis from an HIV-positive client in a residential substance-abuse treatment facility – Michigan. *Morbid. Mortal, Weekly Rep.*, **40**, 129–31.

41. Centers for Disease Control. (1992) Transmission of multidrug resistant tuberculosis among immunocompromised persons, correctional system – New York, 1991. *Morbid. Mortal. Weekly Rep.*, **41**, 507–9.

42. Centers for Disease Control (1991) Nosocomial transmission of multidrug resistant tuberculosis among HIV-infected persons – Florida and New York, 1988–1991. *Morbid. Mortal. Weekly Rep.*, **40**, 585–91.

43. Daley, C.L., Small, P.M. and Schecter, G.F. (1992) An outbreak of tuberculosis with accelerated progression among persons with the human immunodeficiency virus. An analysis using restriction-fragment-length polymorphisms. *N. Engl. J. Med.*, **326**, 231–5.

44. Edlin, B.R., Tokars, J.I., Grieco, M.H. *et al.* (1992) An outbreak of multidrug resistant tuberculosis among hospitalized patients with the acquired immunodeficiency syndrome. *N. Engl. J. Med.*, **326**, 1514–21.

45. Fischl, M.A., Uttamchandani, R.B. and Daikos, G.L. (1992) An outbreak of tuberculosis caused by multiple-drug resistant tubercle bacilli among patients with HIV infection. *Ann. Intern. Med.*, **117**, 177–83.

46. Pearson, M.L., Jereb, J.A., Frieden, T.R. *et al.* (1992) Nosocomial transmission of multidrug-resistant *Mycobacterium tuberculosis*. A risk to patients and health care workers. *Ann. Intern. Med.*, **117**, 191–6.

47. Beck-Sagué, C., Dooley, S.W., Hutton, M.D. *et al.* (1992) Hospital outbreak of multidrug-resistant *Mycobacterium tuberculosis* infections. Factors in transmission to staff and HIV-infected patients. *J. Am. Med. Assoc.*, **268**, 1280–6.

48. Iseman, M.D. (1992) A leap of faith. What can we do to curtail intrainstitutional transmission of tuberculosis? *Ann. Intern. Med.*, **117**, 251–3.

49. Bloom, B.R. and Murray, C.J.L. (1992) Tuberculosis: commentary on a re-emergent killer. *Science*, **257**, 1055–64.

50. Snider, D.E. Jr, Rieder, H.L., Combs, D. *et al.* (1988) Tuberculosis in children. *Pediatr. Infect. Dis. J.*, **7**, 271–8.

51. Bloch, A.B. and Snider, D.E. Jr (1986) How much tuberculosis in children must we accept? (Editorial). *Am. J. Public Hlth*, **76**, 14–15.

52. Laguna, F., Adrados, M., Diaz, F. *et al.* (1991) AIDS and tuberculosis in Spain. A report of 140 cases. *J. Infect.*, **23**, 139–44.

53. Antonucci, G., Armignacco, O., Giardi, E. *et al.* (1991) Tuberculosis and human immunodeficiency virus infection in Italy. Preliminary results from a multicenter study (Correspondence). *Chest*, **100**, 586.

54. Styblo, K. (1990) The global aspects of tuberculosis and HIV infection. *Bull. Int. Union Tuberc. Lung Dis.*, **65**, 28–31.

55. ten Dam, H.G. (1984) Research on BCG vaccination. *Adv. Tuberc. Res.*, **21**, 79–106.

56. Rodrigues, L.C. and Smith, P.G. (1990) Tuberculosis in developing countries and methods for its control. *Trans. Roy. Soc. Trop. Med. Hyg.* **84**, 739–44.

57. Ferebee, S.H. (1969) Controlled chemoprophylaxis trials in tuberculosis. A general review. *Adv. Tuberc. Res.*, **17**, 28–106.

58. American Thoracic Society / Centers for Disease Control (1986) Treatment of tuberculosis and tuberculosis infection in adults and children. *Am. Rev. Respir. Dis.*, **133**, 431–6

59. ten Dam, H.G. and Hitze, K.L. (1980) Does BCG protect the newborn and young infants? *Bull. WHO*, **58**, 37–41.

60. Ninane, J., Grymonprez, A., Burtonboy, G. *et al.* (1988) Disseminated BCG in HIV infection. *Arch. Dis. Child.*, **63**, 1268–9.

61. Reynes, J., Perez, C., Lamaury, I. *et al.* (1989). Bacille Calmette–Guérin adenitis 30 years after immunization in a patient with AIDS (Correspondence). *J. Infect. Dis.*, **160**, 727.

62. Armbruster, C., Junker, W., Vetter, N. and Jaksch, G. (1990) Disseminated Bacille Calmette–Guérin infection in an AIDS

patient 30 years after BCG vaccination (Correspondence). *J. Infect. Dis.*, **162**, 1216.

63. Boudes, P., Sobel, A., Deforges, L. and Leblic, E. (1989) Disseminated *Mycobacterium bovis* infection from BCG vaccination and HIV infection (Correspondence). *J. Am. Med. Assoc.*, **262**, 2386.

64. Lallement-Le Coeur, S., Lallement, M., Cheynier, D. *et al.* (1991) Bacille Calmette-Guérin immunization in infants born to HIV-1-seropositive mothers. *AIDS*, **5**, 195–9.

65. Centers for Disease Control (1991) BCG vaccination and pediatric HIV infection – Rwanda, 1988–1990. *Morbid. Mortal. Weekly Rep.*, **40**, 833–6.

66. Reichman, L.B. (1989) Why hasn't BCG proved dangerous in HIV-infected patients? (Correspondence). *J. Am. Med. Assoc.*, **261**, 3246.

67. World Health Organization (1987) Special Programme on AIDS and Expanded Programme on Immunization Joint Statement. Consultation on human immunodeficiency virus (HIV) and routine childhood immunization. *Weekly Epidem. Rec.*, **62**, 297–304.

68. Clancy, L., Rieder, H.L., Enarson, D.A. and Spinaci, S. (1991) Tuberculosis elimination in the countries of Europe and other industrialized countries. Based on a workshop held at Wolfheze, Netherlands, 4–9 March 1990, under the joint auspices of the IUATLD (Europe region) and WHO. *Eur. Respir. J.*, **4**, 1288–95.

69. Subcommittee of the Joint Tuberculosis Committee of the British Thoracic Society (1992) Guidelines on the management of tuberculosis and HIV infection in the United Kingdom. *Br. Med. J.*, **304**, 1231–3.

70. Centers for Disease Control (1989) Tuberculosis and human immunodeficiency virus infection: recommendations of the Advisory Committee for the Elimination of Tuberculosis (ACET). *Morbid. Mortal. Weekly Rep.*, **38**, 236–50.

71. Quinn, T.C. (1989) Interactions of the human immunodeficiency virus and tuberculosis and the implications for BCG vaccination. *Rev. Infect. Dis.*, **11** (Suppl. 2), S379–S384.

72. International Union Against Tuberculosis Committee on Prophylaxis (1982) Efficacy of various durations of isoniazid preventive therapy for tuberculosis: 5 years of follow-up. *Bull. WHO*, **60**, 555–64.

73. Borleffs, J.C.C., Vrehen, H.M., Bosboom-Kalsbeek, K.C. *et al.* (1991). Delayed-type hypersensitivity skin testing in patients with HIV infection (Correspondence). *AIDS*, **5**, 110–12.

74. Robert, C.F., Hirschel, B., Rochat, T. and Deglon, J.J. (1989) Tuberculin skin reactivity in HIV-seropositive intravenous drug addicts (Correspondence). *N. Engl. J. Med.*, **321**, 1268.

75. Canessa, P.A., Fasano, L., Lavecchia, M.A. *et al.* (1989) Tuberculin skin test in asymptomatic HIV seropositive carriers (Correspondence). *Chest*, **96**, 1215–16.

76. Johnson, M.P., Coberly, J.S., Clermont, H.C. *et al.* (1992) Tuberculin skin test reactivity among adults infected with human immunodeficiency virus infection. *J. Infect. Dis.*, **166**, 194–8.

77. Graham, N.M.H., Nelson, K.E., Solomon, L. *et al.* (1992) Prevalence of tuberculin positivity and skin test anergy in HIV-1-seropositive and -seronegative intravenous drug users. *J. Am. Med. Assoc.*, **267**, 369–73.

78. Huebner, R.E., Villarino, M.E. and Snider, D.E. Jr (1992) Tuberculin skin testing and the HIV epidemic (Editorial). *J. Am. Med. Assoc.*, **267**, 409–10.

79. Selwyn, P.A., Sckell, B.M., Alcabes, P. *et al.* (1992). High risk of active tuberculosis in HIV-infected drug users with cutaneous anergy. *J. Am. Med. Assoc.*, **268**, 504–9.

80. Centers for Disease Control (1991) Purified protein derivative (PPD)-tuberculin anergy and HIV infection: guidelines for anergy testing and management of anergic persons at risk of tuberculosis. *Morbid. Mortal. Weekly Rep.*, **40**, (Suppl. RR-5), 27–33.

81. World Health Organization Tuberculosis Programme and Global Programme on AIDS (1990) Preventive tuberculosis chemotherapy among persons infected with human immunodeficiency virus. Report of the informal consultation, Geneva, 6–8 February 1990. WHO/TUB/AIDS/90.1. World Health Organization, Geneva.

82. World Health Organization Tuberculosis Programme and Global Programme on AIDS (1992). Tuberculosis/HIV research. Report of a WHO review and planning meeting, Geneva, 24–26 February 1992. WHO/TB/92.167. World Health Organization, Geneva.

83. Wadhawan, D., Hira, S., Mwansa, N. *et al.*

(1991) Preventive tuberculosis chemotherapy with isoniazid among persons infected with human immunodeficiency virus. VII International Conference on AIDS, Florence 16–21 June 1991, Abstract W.B. 2261.

84. Johnson, S.C., Stamm, C.P. and Hicks, C.B. (1990) Tuberculous psoas muscle abscess following chemoprophylaxis with isoniazid in a patient with human immunodeficiency virus infection. *Rev. Infect. Dis.*, **12**, 754–6.

85. Narain, J.P., Slutkin, G., ten Dam, H.G. and Kochi, A. (1992) Preventive tuberculosis chemotherapy in HIV infection: a priority for study (Correspondence). *AIDS*, **6**, 744–6.

86. Barnes, A.B., Bloch, A.B., Davidson, P.T. and Snider, D.E. Jr (1991) Tuberculosis in patients with human immunodeficiency virus infection. *N. Engl. J. Med.*, **324**, 1644–50.

87. Flora, G.S., Modilevsky, T., Antoniskis, D. and Barnes, P.F. (1990) Undiagnosed tuberculosis in patients with human immunodeficiency virus infection. *Chest*, **98**, 1056–9.

88. Kramer, F., Modilevsky, T., Waliany, A.R. *et al.* (1990) Delayed diagnosis of tuberculosis in patients with human immunodeficiency virus infection. *Am. J. Med.*, **89**, 451–6.

89. Hill, A.R., Kramer, F. and Barnes, P.F. (1991) Delayed diagnosis of HIV-related tuberculosis (Correspondence). *Am. J. Med.*, **91**, 319–20.

90. Chaisson, R.E., Schecter, G.F., Theuer, C.P. *et al.* (1987), Tuberculosis in patients with the acquired immunodeficiency syndrome. Clinical features, response to therapy, and survival. *Am. Rev, Respir. Dis.*, **136**, 570–4.

91. Prazuck, T., Fisch, A., Simonnet, F. and Noat, G. (1990) Lyell's syndrome associated with rifampicin therapy of tuberculosis in an AIDS patient (Correspondence). *Scand. J. Infect. Dis.*, **22**, 629.

92. Small, P.M., Schecter, G.F., Goodman, P.C. *et al.* (1991). Treatment of tuberculosis in patients with advanced human immunodeficiency virus infection. *N. Engl. J. Med.*, **324**, 289–4.

93. Sunderam, G. Mangura, B.T., Lombardo, J.M. and Reichman, L.B. (1987) Failure of 'optimal' four-drug short-course tuberculosis chemotherapy in a compliant patient with human immunodeficiency virus. *Am. Rev. Respir. Dis.*, **136**, 1475–8.

94. Dylewski, J. and Thibert, L. (1990) Failure of tuberculosis chemotherapy in a human immunodeficiency virus-infected patient (Correspondence). *J. Infect. Dis.*, **162**, 778–9.

95. Centers for Disease Control. (1992) Preliminary results of first quarter 1991 susceptibility survey. Memorandum to State and Territorial TB Control Officers and New York City and Washington DC TB Control Officers, Atlanta, 1 June 1992.

96. Pitchenik, A.E., Burr, J., Laufer, M. *et al.* (1990) Outbreaks of drug-resistant tuberculosis at AIDS Centre (Correspondence). *Lancet*, **336**, 440–1.

97. Shafer, R.W., Chirgwin, K.D., Glatt, A.E. *et al.* (1991) HIV prevalence, immunosuppression, and drug resistance in patients with tuberculosis in an area endemic for AIDS. *AIDS*, **5**, 399–405.

98. Monno, L., Angarano, G., Carbonara, S. *et al.* (1991) Emergence of drug-resistant *Mycobacterium tuberculosis* in HIV-infected patients (Correspondence). *Lancet*, **337**, 852.

99. Dooley, S.W., Jarvis, W.R., Martone, W.J. and Snider, D.E. Jr (1992) Multidrug-resistant tuberculosis (Editorial). *Ann. Intern. Med.*, **117**, 117–18.

100. Chawla, P.K., Klapper, P.J., Kamholz, S.L. *et al.* (1992) Drug-resistant tuberculosis in an urban population including patients at risk for human immunodeficiency virus infection. *Am. Rev. Respir. Dis.*, **146**, 280–4.

101. Fischl, M.A., Daikos, G.L., Uttamchandani R.B. *et al.* (1992) Clinical presentation and outcome of patients with HIV infection and tuberculosis caused by multiple drug-resistant bacilli. *Ann. Intern. Med.*, **117**, 184–90.

102. Grzybowski, S. and Enarson, D.A. (1978) The fate of cases of pulmonary tuberculosis under various treatment programmes. *Bull. Int. Union Tuberc.*, **53**, 70–5.

103. Onorato, I.M., McCray, E. and the Field Services Branch (1992) Prevalence of human immunodeficiency virus infection among patients attending tuberculosis clinics in the United States. *J. Infect. Dis.*, **165**, 87–92.

104. Heckbert, S.R., Elarth, A. and Nolan, C.M. (1992) The impact of human immunodeficiency virus infection on tuberculosis in young men in Seattle–King County, Washington. *Chest*, **102**, 433–7.

105. Snider, D.E. Jr and Roper, W.L. (1992) The new tuberculosis (Editorial). *N. Engl. J. Med.*, **326**, 703–5.

106. International Union Against Tuberculosis and Lung Disease (1991) *Tuberculosis Guide for High Prevalence Countries*. Misereor/ International Union Against Tuberculosis and Lung Disease, Aachen/Paris.

107. Advisory Committee for the Elimination of Tuberculosis (1989) A strategic plan for the elimination of tuberculosis in the United States. *Morbid. Mortal. Weekly Rep.*, **38** (Suppl.3), 1–25.

THE ASSOCIATION BETWEEN HIV AND TUBERCULOSIS IN THE DEVELOPING WORLD

A.D. Harries

12b.1 INTRODUCTION

Tuberculosis has for a long time caused considerable morbidity and mortality in tropical countries of the world. The human immunodeficiency virus (HIV) arrived in the 1970s, and the first cases of AIDS were reported in 1981. The subsequent devastating spread of the virus, particularly in Africa, during the past decade is having a profound effect on the epidemiology, clinical features and management of tuberculosis. This chapter attempts to address the important issues that arise from this interaction in the developing world.

12b.2 THE HUMAN IMMUNODEFICIENCY VIRUS (HIV) AND THE AIDS PANDEMIC

The World Health Organization estimates that at least 10 million people are infected with the human immunodeficiency virus world wide. By 1 April 1992, 484 148 AIDS cases had been reported to the WHO by 164 countries in the world[1]. The cumulative number of AIDS cases reported from tropical countries is shown in Table 12b.1. Owing to underdiagnosis, under-reporting and delays in notification, the figures reported in Table 12b.1 are a gross underestimate of the true picture. WHO predicts that by the year 2000, there will be an accumulated total number of

Table 12b.1 Cumulative number of AIDS cases reported in the tropics (World Health Organization, 1 April 1992)

	No. of cases	Countries
Africa	144 863	52
Latin America	45 766	21
Caribbean	3499	21
Asia	1442	28
Oceania (not Aus/NZ)	102	9
Total	195 672	131

10 million AIDS cases, with 90% of them in developing countries[2]. The greatest impact of HIV infection and AIDS has been in sub-Saharan Africa. HIV seroincidence and seroprevalence studies[3] indicate the magnitude of the problem in some African countries: in Uganda, for example, urban HIV seropositivity rates are 8–30% and rural rates are 7–12%[4]. AIDS is responsible for an increasing proportion of medical admissions to hospital, particularly in persons aged 20–40 years. In some African cities, such as Abidjan, Ivory Coast, AIDS is now recognized as the leading cause of adult death[5]. Although small numbers of AIDS patients have been reported from Asia, the explosive epidemic of HIV infection in intravenous drug users and

Clinical Tuberculosis. Edited by P.D.O. Davies. Published in 1994 by Chapman & Hall, London. ISBN 0 412 48630 X

prostitutes in Thailand and the increasing HIV infection rates in prostitutes in India[6] are the harbinger of a rapidly worsening AIDS epidemic. HIV-1 accounts for the majority of global HIV infection. HIV-2 occurs in epidemic form only in Africa, principally West Africa.

Some useful reviews on the global epidemiology of AIDS have been published, with special reference to developing countries[6–8]. In sub-Saharan Africa and Haiti, virus transmission is principally by heterosexual intercourse with equal numbers of males and females affected; specific risk factors include frequent sexual contact with prostitutes, lack of circumcision and the presence of genital ulcer disease. Perinatal transmission and transmission by blood transfusion is relatively common, and the use of unsterilized syringes/ needles and other skin-piercing methods outside health services represent potential risks. In most of Latin America and parts of the Caribbean, virus transmission is more akin to that observed in Europe and the USA (i.e. through homosexuality, bisexuality and intravenous drug use).

12b.3 TUBERCULOSIS IN THE TROPICS

The World Health Organization (WHO) Tuberculosis Unit estimated that, in 1990, there were 8 million new cases of tuberculosis (TB) in the world: 7.6 million (95%) in developing countries and 400 000 (5%) in industrialized countries[9]. The largest numbers were in the WHO's Western Pacific Region (2.6 million), the South-East Asian Region (2.5 million) and the African Region (1.4 million). The estimated incidence of tuberculosis (all forms and smear-positive) in developing countries in 1990 is shown in Table 12b.2; the highest incidence of the disease is in sub-Saharan Africa[10]. It was further estimated that tuberculosis caused 2.9 million deaths in 1990, making this disease the largest cause of death from a single

Table 12b.2 Estimated incidence of tuberculosis in developing countries, 1990

	Incidence rates per 100 000	
	All forms TB	Smear-positive TB
Sub-Saharan Africa	229	103
Asia	174	79
North Africa	120	54
Western Asia	120	54
South America	120	54
Central America	120	54
Caribbean	120	54
Total	171	77

Adapted from C.J.L. Murray, K. Styblo and A. Rouillon, *Bull. Int. Union Tuberc. Lung Dis.*, 1990, **65**, 2–20.

Table 12b.3 Estimated deaths from all forms of tuberculosis in developing countries, 1990

	Deaths per 100 000 (per annum)
Sub-Saharan Africa	104
Asia	58
Central America	57
Caribbean	57
South America	42
Western Asia	37
North Africa	37
Total	61

Adapted from C.J.L. Murray, K. Styblo and A. Rouillon, *Bull. Int. Union Tuberc. Lung Dis.*, 1990, **65**, 2–20.

pathogen in the world. Table 12b.3 shows the estimated deaths from tuberculosis in 1990 in the developing world; the highest incidence again is in sub-Saharan Africa. While 1.3 million cases and 450 000 deaths from tuberculosis in developing countries occur in children under the age of 15 years[11], the greatest incidence and mortality is concentrated in the economically most productive age group of the population, those aged 15–

50 years. Over 75% of the tuberculosis toll in developing countries falls in this age group, and 26% of avoidable adult deaths are calculated to be a result of tuberculosis[10].

Since the 1950s, tuberculin skin test surveys in developing countries have given epidemiologists an approximate picture of the annual risk of infection in different regions of the world. A review of survey data in 1988[12] shows that risk of infection is highest in sub-Saharan Africa (1.5–2.5%), followed closely by South and East Asia (1.0–2.0%). Thus, in some countries over half of the adult population aged 15–50 years have been infected with *Mycobacterium tuberculosis*, which may reactivate and cause disease if cell-mediated immune defences decline. Recent estimates of tuberculous infection in the age group 15–50 years are 54% for Africa and 52% for South-East Asia[13].

Up until the mid-1980s there had been a dramatic decrease in the incidence of tuberculosis in most industrialized countries. However, over the same time internal in many low-income developing countries in sub-Saharan Africa and the Indian subcontinent there has been no observable decline and the absolute number of cases has probably been increasing because of population growth. This has occurred despite tuberculosis control programmes whose principal technical activities include BCG vaccination of children, active case finding and chemotherapy of those known to be infected. The failure of many such programmes is multifactorial. Firstly, the epidemiological impact of BCG vaccination has been overestimated. Although BCG greatly reduces childhood tuberculosis, it does not prevent transmission of the infection and its effects on the infectious types of adult tuberculosis have been limited[9]. Secondly, most case detection in developing countries relies on a passive strategy of sputum smear examination to detect smear-positive cases (i.e. those who transmit the disease). In theory it should be successful because 90% of smear-positive

Table 12b.4 Examples of 'short-course' and 'standard' tuberculosis treatment regimens in Africa

	Course (mth)	Regimen[a]
Short course		
Sputum-positive		
PTB	8	2SRHZ/6ThH(ThE)
Standard		
Sputum-negative		
PTB; EPTB	12	1SThH/11ThH(ThE)

S, streptomycin; H, isoniazid; Th, thiacetazone; R, rifampicin; Z, pyrazinamide; E, ethambutol.
PTB, pulmonary tuberculosis; EPTB, extrapulmonary tuberculosis.
[a] Regimens are an initial intensive phase (usually in hospital) and a maintenance phase (usually at home). The number before the first letter of the initial and maintenance phase of the regimen is the duration in months of that phase.

pulmonary tuberculosis patients develop a productive cough soon after the onset of disease, and this persuades patients to seek medical advice. However, it is estimated that over half of the existing tuberculosis patients in developing countries are not covered by TB services; between 1988 and 1989, in Africa tuberculosis service coverage was estimated at 24%, and in South-East Asia at 44%[9]. Furthermore, at the peripheral level health workers often do not consider the diagnosis of tuberculosis in patients with a chronic cough, and patients may attend health units several times before a diagnosis is made [14,15]. Only a third to a half of smear-positive cases therefore are routinely diagnosed. Thirdly, under routine conditions the success rate of 'standard anti-tuberculosis chemotherapy regimens' (Table 12b.4) is often below 50%[16]. The reasons for this include:

1. Non-adherence to treatment, particularly when the supervised daily injections have been completed and the patient feels better.
2. High rates of treatment failure in the

presence of primary isoniazid resistance, which is a major problem in many developing countries[17].

3. Hypersensitivity reactions to the drugs, which leads to interrupted courses of treatment.
4. Overall failure of health workers to manage the disease properly[18].

Although 'short-course chemotherapy' (Table 12b.4) costs US$30–40 per patient compared with 'standard chemotherapy' costing US$15, operations research in three African countries with good monitoring systems (Malawi, Mozambique and Tanzania) has shown that short-course treatment is more cost-effective in terms of deaths averted and years of life saved[19]. This is because short-course treatment secures patient compliance with high cure rates, is associated with lower relapse rates and therefore less need for expensive retreatment, and prevents the emergence of drug-resistant bacilli. Improved case detection and the introduction of short-course chemotherapy have been proposed as the key to improved tuberculosis control in developing countries.

12b.4 ASSOCIATION OF TUBERCULOSIS AND HIV INFECTION

The impact of HIV on tuberculosis depends on the degree of overlap between the two infections. This varies considerably in different parts of the world and even between different population groups within the same country. Tuberculosis was not mentioned as a manifestation of AIDS in early descriptions of the disease from the USA and Europe. First reports of tuberculosis were in Haitian patients with AIDS in Florida[20] and in Haiti[21], and also in intravenous drug abusers[22]. The association between the two infections soon became recognized, and in 1990 it was estimated that more than 3 million persons globally were dually infected[13]. Given the high prevalence of *M. tuberculosis* and HIV infection in adults from sub-Saharan

Africa, it is not surprising to find that in 1990 the vast majority (78%) of those with dual infection lived in this part of the world[13].

12b.4.1 THE ASSOCIATION IN AFRICA

Initial reports of HIV-associated tuberculosis in Africa were in immigrants receiving treatment overseas. For example, HIV infection was reported in 17% of African immigrants with tuberculosis who were being treated in Brussels[23]. In Zaire, and later in many other African countries, the strong association between the two infections became recognized and reported. In Ethiopia[24], Zimbabwe[25], Malawi[26] and Zambia[27], tuberculosis was found at presentation in approximately one-third of patients infected with HIV. A more recent study from Kenya [28] found that of 500 consecutive admissions to a Nairobi hospital, tuberculosis was diagnosed in 18% of HIV-seropositive patients compared with 6% of HIV-seronegative patients. These results in HIV-seronegative patients are similar to previous studies carried out before the AIDS epidemic: 8% of acute general medical admissions in Nairobi[29] and 6% in Mombasa[30] had tuberculosis. HIV infection has also been found to be highly prevalent in tuberculosis patients[31–53] (Table 12b.5). From countries in East and Central Africa, HIV-seropositivity refers to infection with HIV-1, but in some West African countries HIV-seropositivity indicates infection with HIV-1, HIV-2 or both. In Abidjan, Ivory Coast, 4.7% of adult tuberculosis was associated specifically with HIV-2[50]; similar associations between tuberculosis and HIV-2 have been found in Guinea–Bissau[54]. The studies summarized in Table 12b.5 are heterogeneous, and include populations with different ages and therefore different degrees of risk for HIV infection; with bacteriologically proven disease or with suspected disease; with newly diagnosed disease (Table 12b.6) or who have been inpatients receiving treatment in tuber-

Table 12b.5 HIV-seroprevalence rates in tuberculosis patients in Africa

Year	Country	No. TB patients	%HIV +ve	Ref.
1985	Zaire	159	33	[31]
1985–1986	Burundi	328	55	[32]
1985–1987	Zaire	231	40	[33]
1985–1987	Uganda	150	45	[34]
1985–1987	Uganda	31	30	[34]
1986	Malawi	125	26	[35]
1986–1987	CAR	72	54	[36]
1987	Zambia	131	58	[37]
1987	Zaire	509	17	[38]
1987	Zaire	287	36	[39]
1987	Zambia	54	50	[40]
1987	CAR	55	55	[41]
1987	CAR	220	28	[42]
1987	Ivory Coast	193	51	[43]
1987–1988	Ivory Coast	259	24	[44]
1988–1989	Kenya	196	25	[45]
1988–1989	Kenya	195	18	[45]
1988–1990	Burkina-Faso	310	12	[46]
1988–1989	Malawi	152	52	[47]
1988–1989	Zambia	346	60	[48]
1989	Rwanda	61	31	[49]
1989–1990	Ivory Coast	2043	40	[50]
1990	Zimbabwe	591	41	[51]
1990	Zaire	1011	20	[52]
1990	Uganda	59	66	[53]
Total		7768	35	

Year, Year in which the study was carried out.
CAR, Central African Republic.

Table 12b.6 HIV-seroprevalence in new tuberculosis patients in Africa

Year	Country	No. TB patients	%HIV +ve	Ref.
1987	Zambia	131	58	[37]
1987	Zaire	509	17	[38]
1987	Zambia	54	50	[40]
1987	CAR	220	28	[42]
1988–1989	Kenya	168	26	[45]
1988–1989	Malawi	152	52	[47]

culosis sanatoria; and from urban and rural areas. This heterogeneity may explain partly some of the variations in HIV-seropositivity rates. Many of the studies in Table 12b.5 were carried out in urban areas where HIV-seroprevalence rates among the general population can vary from 5 to 20%[3,8]. In rural areas HIV infection rates tend to be lower than in the towns and cities[4,55], and rural patients with tuberculosis have lower HIV infection rates than their urban counterparts[40]. However, when tuberculosis patients are compared and matched with healthy persons according to area of residence, HIV-seroprevalence is significantly higher in those with tuberculosis. It is also clear from these studies that there are countries such as Burundi, Malawi, Uganda and Zambia where HIV seroprevalence in tuberculosis patients is 50% or higher, whereas there are other countries such as Burkina–Faso, Kenya and Zaire where the rates are generally lower at 15–25%.

12b.4.2 RISK OF TUBERCULOSIS IN HIV-INFECTED PERSONS

In most people exposed to *M. tuberculosis*, infection is contained and tuberculosis does not develop, although small numbers of dormant acid-fast bacilli may remain in the body. Clinically apparent tuberculosis develops in approximately 10% of infected subjects, either soon after primary infection (3–5%) or years later (3–5%) as a result of reactivation[56]. In HIV infection, the progressive depletion and dysfunction of CD4 T lymphocytes, coupled with defective macrophages and monocytes, places the patient at high risk for primary and reactivation tuberculosis. It is generally believed that reactivation of dormant tuberculous infection is the principal pathogenetic mechanism. A prospective study[57] among intravenous drug users with HIV infection in New York found that the risk of developing active tuberculosis was 7.9% per year in those with a prior positive Mantoux test compared with only 0.3% per year in those with a negative skin reaction. Of the eight patients who developed active tuberculosis in this study,

six had pulmonary disease (three were sputum smear-positive, all were sputum culture-positive) and two had extrapulmonary disease. Two other studies have demonstrated that HIV-seropositive patients who are exposed to *M. tuberculosis* may not be able to contain the new infection, and may rapidly develop clinical features of primary tuberculosis. In Italy, 38% of 18 HIV-infected inpatients developed active tuberculosis within 60 days of exposure to the index case[58]. In San Francisco, 37% of 30 HIV-infected persons in a residential facility developed active tuberculosis within 106 days of exposure to the index case[59]; restriction fragment length polymorphisms (RFLP) of cultured organisms were similar to those of the index case, demonstrating that the same strain was causative of disease in the group.

In Africa there have been three studies investigating the incidence of tuberculosis in HIV-infected individuals. In Zambia, the incidence of active tuberculosis in placebo-treated HIV-seropositive subjects enrolled in an isoniazid chemoprophylaxis trial was 4.4% per year[60]. In Rwanda, the incidence of tuberculosis was 4.2% in HIV-seropositive subjects compared with 0.1% in HIV-seronegative subjects followed for 2 years[61]. In Zaire, a retrospective study of women of childbearing age showed that the incidence of tuberculosis was 3.1% per year in HIV-seropositive compared with 0.12% per year in HIV-seronegative women; the incidence of smear-positive PTB was 1.2% per year in HIV-seropositive women compared with 0.12% per year in HIV-seronegative women[62]. These studies almost certainly underestimate the true incidence of tuberculosis because of default from follow-up, unexplained deaths (which may be due to tuberculosis), and because diagnosis of tuberculosis in Africa relies on sputum smear microscopy without the additional back-up of culture facilities. These studies also do not address the question as to whether active tuberculous disease is a result of primary, reactivated or secondary exogenous infection. This question could be determined by surveilling household contacts of index cases and 'fingerprinting' cultured organisms using RFLP to see if the strains are similar or different (Chapter 17c).

Tuberculosis usually occurs in HIV-infected patients without pre-existing AIDS, presumably because *M. tuberculosis* is more virulent than other HIV-associated pathogens, such as *Pneumocystis carinii* or *M. avium* complex. Studies in developed countries show that, in general, infections such as tuberculosis and oral candidiasis supervene at CD4 lymphocyte counts of between 250 and 500/mm^3, while infections such as *P. carinii*, *M. avium* complex, or cryptococcosis occur at CD4 counts of 50–125/mm^3[63]. In San Francisco, tuberculosis was the first clinical manifestation of immunosuppression in 88% of HIV-seropositive subjects, occurring at a median CD4 cell count of 326/mm^3[64]. In a French study, which included 50% of patients from developing countries, tuberculosis was the first symptomatic disease in 66% of patients, occurring at a median CD4 count of 281/mm^3, which contrasted with median CD4 counts of 129/mm^3 in those with an AIDS-defining illness[65]. There is only limited data at present on CD4 counts in patients with tuberculosis in sub-Saharan Africa. In Zaire, 70% of HIV-positive pulmonary TB patients had CD4 counts < 200/mm^3[66]. More information from Africa is required, comparing CD4 counts in tuberculosis patients and healthy controls, and relating CD4 counts to clinical features of tuberculous disease (pulmonary, extrapulmonary and disseminated disease).

12b.4.3 INCREASE IN TUBERCULOSIS IN AFRICA

An unfortunate consequence of the strong association between tuberculosis and HIV in Africa is an upsurge of tuberculosis: several African countries (e.g. Tanzania, Malawi,

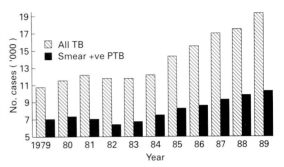

Fig. 12b.1 Tuberculosis cases in Tanzania, 1979–1989. (Source: International Union against Tuberculosis and Lung Disease, Dr K. Styblo [67,68].)

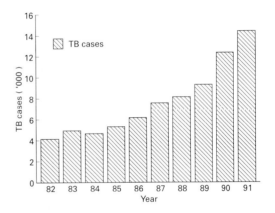

Fig. 12b.2 Tuberculosis (all forms) in Malawi, 1982–1991. (Source: Malawi National Tuberculosis Programme.)

Burundi, Uganda and Zaire) have reported increases in tuberculosis incidence in the past 5–10 years. IUATLD-assisted National Tuberculosis Programmes in Tanzania and Malawi have allowed accurate surveillance of the situation. Fig. 12b.1 shows the increase in all forms of tuberculosis and new smear-positive cases in Tanzania between 1979 and 1989[67,68], and Fig. 12b.2 shows similar increases in Malawi from 1982 to 1991. Although HIV infection undoubtedly contributes significantly to the increase in tuberculosis, other factors play a part. For example, in Tanzania the reporting system for tuberculosis became national in 1979 and complete by 1982; short-course chemotherapy was introduced in 1983, and the favourable influence of good results of such treatment resulted in increased attendance and increased self-referrals. A similar pattern was seen in Malawi when short-course chemotherapy was introduced in 1984, and this was compounded by the influx of refugees from Mozambique from 1986 onwards. In Uganda, the annual number of confirmed tuberculosis cases doubled from 1984 to 1987[4], and the numbers continue to rise dramatically. Mathematical models have been used to predict the estimated incidence rates of tuberculosis in sub-Saharan African countries by the year 2000[69]. In a sexually active population aged 15–49 years, assuming a 2% annual risk of tuberculous infection, 60% prevalence for tuberculous infection and 20% HIV-seroprevalence rate, tuberculosis incidence rates would increase to 4218 per 100 000. Extrapolating this scenario to the whole population would give a tuberculosis incidence rate of 1875 per 100 000 – nearly 2% of the population developing tuberculosis every year.

12b.4.4 TUBERCULOSIS AND HIV INFECTION IN OTHER DEVELOPING COUNTRIES

In Latin America a high proportion (up to 60%) of Haitian AIDS patients present with tuberculosis[70]. In Haiti itself, high HIV-seroprevalence rates are found in patients with tuberculosis[71,72] – similar findings to those in sub-Saharan Africa. There are also urban/rural differences of HIV infection in the general population (9% versus 3%); this is reflected in patients with tuberculosis, in whom urban patients have HIV-sero-prevalence rates of 45%, compared with rates of 15% in patients from rural areas. In Mexico city, tuberculosis is found in 14% of AIDS patients[73]. In Brazil between 20 and

25% of patients with AIDS have tuberculosis[74]. However, in Brazil, lower HIV-seropositivity rates are found in tuberculosis patients in comparison to Africa; 3.1% in patients with pulmonary tuberculosis and 2.3% in those with extrapulmonary disease[75,76].

In Asia, the HIV epidemic has been relatively limited, apart from the dramatic increase seen in intravenous drug users and prostitutes in Thailand in the past 4 years[8]. However, given the huge reservoir of tuberculous infection in this region, extensive spread of HIV in the general population would almost certainly lead to a large upsurge of tuberculosis, similar to the situation being seen in Africa. A decrease in the risk of tuberculous infection in Asian countries needs urgent attention in order to combat the effects of future HIV infection.

12b.5 CLINICAL FEATURES

12b.5.1 AFRICAN TUBERCULOSIS BEFORE AIDS

Large surveys carried out in Kenya and Tanzania between 1964 and 1984 by the British Medical Research Council (MRC) and East African Research Centres[77–80] provide excellent data on the pattern of African tuberculosis prior to the AIDS epidemic. Altogether 8741 TB patients were studied; the pattern of disease and main types of extrapulmonary disease are shown in Table 12b.7. Almost 90% of all patients had pulmonary disease. Of those with extrapulmonary tuberculosis lymphadenopathy (mainly cervical in distribution), bone/joint disease and pleural effusion were responsible for 85% of the total (Plates 9 and 10). In Kenya, pericardial/peritoneal disease was seen in 5% of patients with extrapulmonary tuberculosis. Among adults and children older than 15 years with pulmonary tuberculosis, 78% had positive sputum smears for acid-fast bacilli on Ziehl-Neelsen stain and 66% had cavitation on

Table 12b.7 Tuberculosis in East Africa before AIDS

	Year	No.	Pattern of disease (%)		
			PTB	PTB + EPTB	EPTB
Kenya	1964	1164	89.8	2.5	7.7
	1974	1490	88.5	3.0	8.5
	1984	1961	85.4	2.5	12.1
Tanzania	1970	1884	87.4	2.5	10.1
	1980	2242	91.5	0.6	7.9
Total		8741	88.5	2.1	9.4

	Year	No.	Extrapulmonary disease (%)		
			Lymphadenopathy	Bone/joint	Pleura
Kenya	1964	132	48	21	15
	1974	172	51	25	9
	1984	286	52	22	8
Tanzania	1970	237	54	28	7
	1980	191	40	26	19
Total		1018	49.5	24.5	10.9

Data from East African/MRC Co-operative Studies [77–80].
PTB, pulmonary tuberculosis; EPTB, extrapulmonary tuberculosis.

chest radiography (Fig. 12b.3). There were highly significant associations in the different surveys between extent of cavitation and sputum smear-positivity; these findings are in accord with the observation that in cavitatory tuberculosis 98% of patients have positive sputum smears for acid-fast bacilli[81]. Extensive disease involving more than three radiographic zones was found in 30% of patients. Miliary disease was uncommon, and in Kenyan adults it was present in only 1.7% of 1722 TB patients.

12b.5.2 AFRICAN TUBERCULOSIS IN ASSOCIATION WITH HIV INFECTION

With the advent of HIV infection in Africa, experienced clinicians began to notice a change in the pattern of tuberculosis. More patients presented who either produced no sputum, or who had negative sputum smears on microscopy; on chest radiography had pulmonary infiltrates without cavitation (Fig. 12b.4); had extrapulmonary disease, especially in forms previously uncommon, such as pericarditis, peritonitis (Plate 11) or miliary in distribution. Clinical studies on the interaction between TB and HIV infection have confirmed these initial impressions.

(a) General features

Formal studies[39,45,48,53] have shown that certain social variables and clinical features are significantly more common in HIV-positive TB patients compared with HIV-negative TB patients. HIV infection is associated with good full-time education, good housing, a divorced or widowed marital state, history of herpes zoster and a history of previous treatment for sexually transmitted diseases. Symptoms and signs strongly associated with HIV infection include: diarrhoea for longer than 1 month, dysphagia (related to oesophageal candidiasis), oral candidiasis, generalized papular itchy rash and lymphadenopathy in more than one extrainguinal site.

Many patients with tuberculosis have

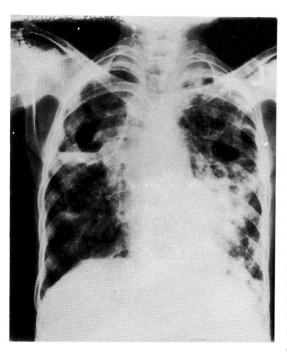

Fig. 12b.3 Typical chest radiograph of pulmonary tuberculosis in Africa. HIV-negative, sputum smear-positive patient.

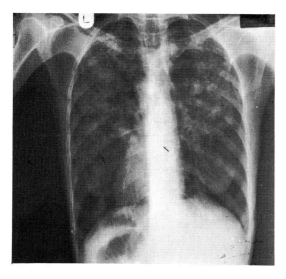

Fig. 12b.4 Chest radiograph of HIV-positive patient with pulmonary tuberculosis.

weight loss, irrespective of HIV state[45,48]. Significant malnutrition as judged by anthropometry is also a common observation[82] (Plate 12). This is one of the factors that has rendered the WHO case definition for AIDS in Africa unreliable and of low specificity in TB patients. However, protein-calorie malnutrition is worse in TB patients co-infected with HIV[83], and severe weight loss – >20% or more than 10 kg – seems to predict HIV-seropositivity in TB patients[39,53]. These observations have led to suggestions that HIV-seropositive TB patients in Africa may only be reported as cases of AIDS if tuberculosis is accompanied by features of the wasting syndrome, i.e. pronounced weight loss or cachexia[84]. In the Ivory Coast, of 82 patients diagnosed with AIDS because of the HIV wasting syndrome, 44% had disseminated tuberculosis at autopsy, which suggests that in a substantial proportion of cases, 'slim disease' may actually be caused by tuberculosis (K. De Cock, personal communication).

(b) Pattern of tuberculous disease

There have been several recent studies in different African countries examining the pattern of tuberculosis in relation to HIV status in consecutive patients attending hospital (Table 12b.8). The findings show that extrapulmonary disease is more common in HIV-seropositive patients. The proportion of HIV-seronegative patients with pulmonary/extrapulmonary disease is in general similar to that observed in the MRC studies carried out in East Africa in the pre-AIDS era. Prevalences of pulmonary and extrapulmonary TB in HIV-seropositive Africans are similar to those observed in the USA[64,85].

(c) Pulmonary disease

Initial impressions were that HIV infection in Africa was associated with a large increase in smear-negative pulmonary tuberculosis[86].

Table 12b.8 Pattern of tuberculosis in association with HIV infection

Country	No. HIV+ve	PTB (%)		EPTB (%)		Ref.
Zambia	239	116	(49)	123	(51)	[27]
Zaire	176	154	(87)	22	(13)	[39]
Kenya	70	50	(71)	20	(29)	[45]
Malawi	80	34	(42)	46	(58)	[47]
Zambia	229	133	(58)	96	(42)	[48]
Ivory Coast	821	662	(81)	159	(19)	[50]
Total	1615	1149	(71)	466	(29)	

PTB, pulmonary tuberculosis; EPTB, extrapulmonary tuberculosis.

Table 12b.9 Confirmed and suspected pulmonary tuberculosis in relation to HIV status

Country	No.	HIV-positive			Ref.
		Confirmed PTB (%)		Suspected PTB (%)	
Zaire	154	94	(61)	60	(39)	[39]
Zambia	35	8	(23)	27	(77)	[40]
Kenya	64	46	(72)	18	(28)	[45]
Zambia	133	73	(55)	60	(45)	[48]
Ivory Coast	662	609	(92)	53	(8)	[50]
Total	1048	830	(79)	218	(21)	

Country	No.	HIV-negative			Ref.
		Confirmed PTB (%)		Suspected PTB (%)	
Zaire	265	193	(73)	72	(27)	[39]
Zambia	37	10	(27)	27	(73)	[40]
Kenya	287	237	(83)	50	(17)	[45]
Zambia	117	76	(65)	41	(35)	[48]
Ivory Coast	1068	1001	(94)	67	(6)	[50]
Total	1774	1517	(86)	257	(14)	

However, it is apparent from systematic studies that the majority of HIV-positive PTB is sputum smear-positive, although the proportion of patients with smear-negative, suspected PTB is greater in those with HIV infection compared with those who are HIV-negative (Table 12b.9). For patients with a positive smear, there is a tendency for HIV-seropositive patients to have a lower count of acid-fast bacilli[48]. Sputum culture in HIV-positive patients improves the diagnostic rate[45,48], although this facility is not available in most African hospitals.

Typical radiographic features of reactivation tuberculosis in immunocompetent adults include cavitation and upper lobe infiltrates. Two studies from East Africa[53,87] found radiographs to be atypical in 49% and 41% of HIV-seropositive compared with 26% and 14% of HIV-seronegative patients. The proportion of those with cavitation and upper lobe infiltrates in relation to HIV status is

Table 12b.10 Radiographic changes of pulmonary tuberculosis in relation to HIV status

Country	No.	Cavitation (%)		Upper zones involved (%)		Ref.
HIV-positive						
Zambia	67	32	(48)	46	(69)	[48]
Zaire	85	29	(34)	55	(59)	[39]
Kenya	48	27	(56)	—		[45]
Total	200	88	(44)	101/152	(66)	
HIV-negative						
Zambia	72	49	(68)	66	(92)	[48]
Zaire	149	66	(44)	107	(72)	[39]
Kenya	241	166	(69)	—		[45]
Total	462	281	(61)	173/221	(78)	

shown in Table 12b.10. Mediastinal and hilar lymphadenopathy is also more common in HIV-infected patients[39,42,87]. Some HIV-positive patients may have normal findings on chest radiography[37].

Among HIV-infected patients with relatively preserved immune function, radiographic findings and sputum smear microscopy are very similar to those found in immunocompetent individuals; as immune function deteriorates so the features become less typical and resemble more those seen in primary tuberculosis. Many African hospitals do not have facilities to culture mycobacteria and rely on sputum smears and plain chest radiography for diagnosis. Patients with chronic cough, fever and weight loss who are sputum-negative but have pulmonary infiltrates on chest radiography are often diagnosed as having pulmonary tuberculosis and are given antituberculosis chemotherapy. However, there are many other diseases associated with HIV (particularly as immune function deteriorates) that affect the lower respiratory tract and give rise to radiographic pulmonary infiltrates[88,89]. In a study in Rwanda on 92 patients with chronic respiratory symptoms and radiographic pulmonary infiltrates, tuberculosis was confirmed in only 20% using fibre-optic bronchoscopy combined with bronchoalveolar lavage and transbronchial biopsy[90].

These data suggest that pulmonary tuberculosis may be overdiagnosed in HIV-positive patients in Africa. There are a number of possible solutions to this problem. Firstly, it may be reasonable to insist on a more stringent case definition for presumed pulmonary tuberculosis: e.g. a patient with repeatedly negative sputum smears for acid-fast bacilli **plus** fever, weight loss and cough for at least 1 month **plus** pulmonary infiltrates on chest radiograph, not resolving with antibiotics, but improving within 8 weeks of treatment for tuberculosis. Secondly, it may be possible to utilize better simple techniques for improving diagnosis, such as the induction of sputum with hypertonic nebulized saline[91]. Of 82 Malawian adults with clinically suspected tuberculosis, but either unable to produce sputum or sputum smear-negative, induced sputum smears showed positive acid-fast bacilli in 22% (C. Parry *et al.*, unpublished obser-

Table 12b.11 Pattern of extrapulmonary disease in HIV-positive tuberculosis patients

| | Number of patients in study | | | | | | | |
	Zambia 1989 [27]	Zambia 1990 [48]	Malawi 1989 [26]	Malawi 1990 [47]	Kenya 1992 [45]	Kenya 1991 [28]	Total (%)	
Pleural	61	67	44	34	11	—	217	(60)
Lnode	21	7	13	3	6	3	52	(14)
Pcard	10	16	8	5	1	—	40	(11)
Miliary	25	—	7	—	2	3	37	(10)
Other	6	—	1	4	—	2	13	
							359	(100)

Lnode, lymphadenopathy; Pcard., pericardial.

vations). Thirdly, the efficacy of serology in this group of patients needs to be explored. New, competitive monoclonal antibody ELISA tests have shown high sensitivity and specificity in Western countries[92], but how well these will perform in Africa where there is such a high background of tuberculous exposure needs evaluation. Other diagnostic techniques can be mentioned, if only to be discarded as unsuitable for use in Africa. The use of high technology such as fibre-optic bronchoscopy or polymerase chain reaction on sputum is outside the reach of most hospitals in Africa. The response to purified protein derivative PPD is unreliable in HIV-positive tuberculosis patients, and it contributes nothing to diagnosis in the adult patient. For example, in Zaire[31] and the Central African Republic[42], between 29 and 57% of HIV-positive tuberculosis patients had cutaneous anergy to 5 tuberculin units compared with 19–22% of HIV-negative tuberculosis patients.

(d) Extrapulmonary tuberculosis

The commonest forms of extrapulmonary disease in HIV-positive patients are pleural, pericardial, lymph node enlargement and miliary/disseminated tuberculosis (Table 12b.11). Pleural and pericardial tuberculosis are diagnosed mostly by radiography, without microbiological or histological evidence, and confirmation of the diagnosis is based on response to treatment (Fig. 12b.5). In Tanzania, a large increase in the number of pericardial effusions was documented at one medical centre between 1987 and 1989; in over 90% a tuberculous aetiology was suspected and antituberculosis treatment commenced, and over 70% of the patients were HIV-seropositive[93].

Tuberculous lymphadenopathy is relatively easy to diagnose by lymph node biopsy. In Uganda, tuberculous lymphadenopathy used to be uncommon; in 1983, only six of 120 new patients with tuberculosis seen at Mulago hospital, Kampala, over 6 months, had lymphadenopathy, whereas in 1986, 16 patients with tuberculous lymphadenopathy were diagnosed over 6 weeks – all of whom were HIV-seropositive[94]. Symmetrical generalized lymphadenopathy is common in HIV infected patients usually due to follicular hyperplasia. In such patients, lymph node biopsy is generally not indicated; one study from Zimbabwe in 100 such patients found follicular hyperplasia in 97 and *M. tuberculosis* in three[95]. Where tuberculous lymphadenitis is suspected on clinical grounds (because of asymmetrical or rapid lymph node enlargement, marked systemic disturbance or hilar lymph node enlargement), lymph node biopsy shows tuberculosis in 85%[96]. It has been shown that lymph node aspiration smears, smears from the cut surface of a

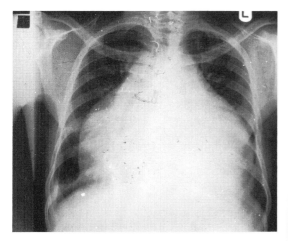

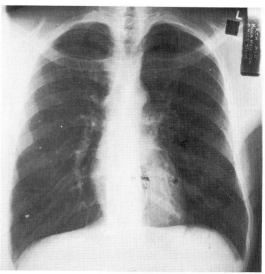

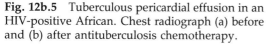

Fig. 12b.5 Tuberculous pericardial effusion in an HIV-positive African. Chest radiograph (a) before and (b) after antituberculosis chemotherapy.

biopsied lymph node and examination of the lymph node for macroscopic caseation give a diagnostic yield of 15%, 15% and 68% respectively[96]. The combination of macroscopical examination of a lymph node in combination with a direct smear from the cut surface gives a diagnostic yield of 79%, and this approach may be very useful in areas where histopathological facilities are lacking. In AIDS patients, *Nocardia* spp. have been found in lymph node biopsies associated with *M. tuberculosis*[97]; this dual infection needs to be remembered especially as *Nocardia* can cause pulmonary cavitation, pericarditis etc., and responds to sulphonamides or co-trimoxazole.

Although disseminated disease and *M. tuberculosis* bacteraemia is not uncommon in AIDS patients investigated in Western institutions[98], the diagnosis in Africa is uncommonly made ante mortem. However, a study in Abidjan, Ivory Coast, found that 40% of 203 consecutive autopsied AIDS patients had disseminated tuberculosis (K. De Cock, personal communication), which suggests considerable underdiagnosis of this condition during life. Other types of extrapulmonary

tuberculosis in HIV infection, such as peritoneal TB, renal TB or cerebral tuberculomas, are difficult to diagnose reliably, and this may be one of the reasons for low reporting of these forms in Africa. Although the diagnosis of extrapulmonary tuberculosis is not important for African TB control programmes, the difficulties in accurate diagnosis in many HIV-positive patients probably result in significant untreated morbidity and mortality. In this regard, supplementary investigations for use in Africa, such as serology, adenosine deaminase or DNA amplification of serous fluid, and mycobacterium blood cultures, need to be explored.

12b.5.3 TUBERCULOSIS AND HIV INFECTION IN OTHER DEVELOPING COUNTRIES

Haitians show similar disease patterns to those found in Africans. Haitians with pulmonary disease are more likely to have a chest radiograph consistent with primary disease, and intrathoracic adenopathy is common[99]. Extrapulmonary disease is more common in HIV-positive patients, and the pattern differs in relation to HIV status: in

HIV-negative patients, pleural effusion, lymphadenopathy and bone/joint disease are most common (84% of the total); in those with AIDS, lymphadenopathy and miliary TB are most common, and pericardial, peritoneal and meningeal disease account for the remainder[70]. Similar HIV-related disease patterns are found in Brazil[100].

12b.6 MANAGEMENT OF TUBERCULOSIS, WITH SPECIAL REFERENCE TO AFRICA

In developed countries the evidence is that HIV-positive tuberculosis responds well to chemotherapy[101]. In Haiti[70] and Brazil[102] the response of tuberculosis to treatment is good. Reports from Africa also show that tuberculosis in HIV-positive patients responds almost as well to chemotherapy as tuberculosis in HIV-negative patients [36,39,47,53,103]. The time to clearance of AAFB in sputum and improvement of radiographic abnormalities is similar in both groups. However, in Africa a number of problems occur in the management of HIV-positive tuberculosis patients that are generally not seen in HIV-negative patients.

(a) The use of intramuscular streptomycin

Several African countries, especially those supported by IUATLD, use 'short-course chemotherapy' for smear-positive pulmonary tuberculosis and reserve 'standard treatment' for smear-negative and extrapulmonary tuberculosis (Table 12b.4). These regimens all include daily intramuscular injections of streptomycin for the initial 1–2 months. Epidemiological evidence from central Africa has implicated use of injections with increased transmission of HIV infection[104]. Although as yet there is no evidence to incriminate i.m. streptomycin in increasing HIV-seroprevalence in hospitalized patients [45], nevertheless the use of daily injections in patients with a high prevalence of HIV infection is a cause for concern, and it is vital

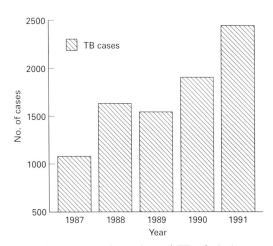

Fig. 12b.6   Annual number of TB admissions to the tuberculosis ward, Queen Elizabeth Central Hospital, Malawi, 1987–1991. (Source: District TB Officer, Queen Elizabeth Central Hospital, Blantyre, Malawi.)

to ensure adequate supplies/sterilization of syringes and needles for tuberculosis wards and clinics.

(b) In-hospital stay with tuberculosis treatment regimens

The initial intensive phase of short-course and standard treatment often involves the patient staying in hospital for 1–2 months; this improves compliance and allows health education of the patient and time to screen household contacts, especially young children. However, the upsurge in tuberculosis (resulting in many more admissions) has lead to overcrowding and congestion on TB wards (Fig. 12b.6). This has necessitated a review of existing treatment policies, and a consideration of new regimens that involve less time spent in hospital for smear-positive tuberculosis, and full ambulatory treatment for smear-negative and extrapulmonary tuberculosis[105]. Research studies in a few designated centres to assess compliance, cure rates and risk of relapse will be needed before these new regimens can be recommended for routine use.

(c) Associated complications and mortality

The weight gain that usually accompanies effective chemotherapy in tuberculosis patients may be less apparent if there is HIV infection[39]. HIV-positive patients more often run a stormy course on treatment with recurrent fevers, intermittent diarrhoea, chest infections and mucosal candidiasis. Bacteraemia, particularly due to *Salmonella typhimurium*, is common in African patients with HIV infection[106] and it is important not to simply ascribe fever in a tuberculosis patient to a complication of antituberculosis chemotherapy. Undiagnosed and untreated bacteraemia may in part be responsible for the excess mortality seen in HIV-positive tuberculosis patients during and after chemotherapy.

Nunn and colleagues (personal communication) in Nairobi followed 107 HIV-positive and 174 HIV-negative patients for 12 months after the start of treatment. Thirty-five (33%) HIV-positive patients died: ten from tuberculosis, six from bacteraemia and the remainder from other causes. Thirteen (7%) HIV-negative patients died: six from tuberculosis, none from bacteraemia and six from other causes. Among HIV-positive patients, there were significantly fewer deaths during the first 6 months of treatment in those on regimens containing rifampicin, probably because rifampicin protects against bacterial infections. These results are similar to those obtained in other countries. In Zambia, 27% of HIV-positive tuberculosis patients died during a 2-year follow-up[27]. In Zaire, in patients given 'standard chemotherapy' for 1 year, 31% of HIV-positive and 4% of HIV-negative patients had died 1 year after diagnosis, and during the subsequent year the mortality rate was 26% in HIV-positive patients compared with 2% in HIV-negative patients[107]. There is also evidence to sug-

gest that HIV-positive patients with tuberculosis fare worse than HIV-positive patients without tuberculosis; in Zairian women, 26% with HIV-positive tuberculosis died during a 2-year follow-up compared with 11% with HIV infection and no diagnosed tuberculosis[62].

(d) Reactions to chemotherapy

HIV-positive patients experience a high incidence of cutaneous adverse effects associated with therapy. In the pre-AIDS era, cutaneous hypersensitivity reactions to standard chemotherapy regimens (streptomycin, isoniazid and thiacetazone) were reported with low frequency (2–4%) from several African countries[108,109] and from Papua New Guinea in Melanesians[110]. Thiacetazone was the drug most often implicated. The incidence of severe reactions such as exfoliative dermatitis and Stevens–Johnson syndrome was very low (0–0.5%). With the advent of HIV in Africa, there has been a big increase in the incidence of cutaneous reactions, particularly in patients receiving 'standard chemotherapy' (Table 12b.12). These reactions generally occur during the first 2 months of treatment (Plate 13). Most studies have found these reactions to be rare in regimens using streptomycin, isoniazid, rifampicin and pyrazinamide for the initial 2 months[53,111], but reactions may occur in 22% of those starting the continuation phase with isoniazid and thiacetazone[111]; this suggests that thiacetazone is to blame. Indeed, in patients in Nairobi who had cutaneous reactions[111], none of the patients rechallenged with streptomycin or isoniazid reacted, while six of seven challenged with thiacetazone had a reaction. Similarly, in Zambia[27] 21 out of 30 reactions in HIV-positive patients were attributed to thiacetazone. These reactions may be life-threatening[112], and in one series the mortality rate for cutaneous reactions due to thiacetazone in HIV-positive tuberculosis patients was 3%[111]. These findings have

Table 12b.12 Cutaneous reactions in tuberculosis patients receiving 'standard treatment': relation to HIV status

Country	No.	HIV-positive Reaction		Severe		No.	HIV-negative Reaction		Severe		Ref
Kenya	52	10	(19)	7	(13)	144	16	(11)	4	(3)	[45]
Zaire	50	10	(20)	2	(4)	95	7	(7)	—		[39]
Uganda	25	8	(32)	3	(12)	15	—		—		[53]
Zaire	66	18	(27)	—		281	34	(12)	—		[107]
Kenya	93	18	(19)	5	(5)	134	1	(1)	—		[111]
Zambia	239	30	(13)	13	(5)	—	—		—		[27]
Zambia	206	15	(7)	8	(4)	140	5	(4)	—		[48]
Total	731	109	(15)	38	(5)	809	63	(8)	4	(0.5)	

Numbers in parenthesis are percentages.
Severe reaction = Stevens–Johnson syndrome or exfoliative dermatitis.

some major implications for National Tuberculosis Control Programmes that utilize thiacetazone. One option is to substitute ethambutol for thiacetazone in the treatment regimens, but this will increase the cost of chemotherapy. The second option is to screen all tuberculosis patients for HIV infection, and to give thiacetazone only to those who are HIV-negative and ethambutol to those who are HIV-positive. The third option is to continue to use thiacetazone, but to educate health workers and patients to stop treatment immediately a skin reaction occurs.

Although skin reactions are uncommon in Africa with short-course chemotherapy regimens, in one study such reactions were found ten times more commonly in HIV-positive compared with HIV-negative patients during the first 2 months of treatment[66]. Incidence of other reactions, such as hepatitis, appears to be low[66].

(e) Relapse rates

The relapse rate of TB after completing chemotherapy is not well documented in Africa. In Zaire, 18% of HIV-positive patients relapsed with positive sputum smears 12 months after completing standard chemotherapy compared with 6% of HIV-negative patients[107]. In Kenya [113, and Nunn, personal communication] relapse rates of tuberculosis based on sputum cultures, after an average of 6 months post-treatment follow-up, were nine times higher in HIV-positive patients; this appeared to be related to a break of therapy and change to ethambutol from thiacetazone in those experiencing cutaneous reactions. Other possible reasons for increased relapse rates are poor compliance, insufficient length of treatment or the development of drug resistance in those taking standard treatment. It is also not clear whether such relapse is due to relapse of the original infection or a second infection. Many African countries cannot afford short-course chemotherapy for smear-positive disease. However, given that short-course chemotherapy in Africa has much better effective cure rates than standard treatment and that for each year of life saved it is in fact cheaper[19], it may be better to consider more widespread use of short-course chemotherapy. Alternatively, following standard treatment patients could be given secondary prophylaxis with isoniazid. These options require evaluation in carefully controlled studies.

(f) Prevention

Despite the limitations of BCG in reducing transmission of infection, it is effective in preventing the lethal forms of childhood tuberculosis, such as TB meningitis and miliary disease. In many African countries, BCG is administered to infants as early in life as possible. In theory, the administration of a live, albeit attenuated, vaccine to immunodeficient subjects would seem hazardous, and there have been isolated reports of disseminated *M. bovis* in HIV-infected infants following BCG vaccination, including one from Zaire[114]. However, the evidence is that in general BCG is safe. In Zaire none of 19 children with BCG abscesses was HIV-seropositive[115]. A large prospective study in the Congo[116] on 64 babies at risk of perinatal HIV infection found no chronic or deep ulcerations at the site of injection, no disseminated forms of BCG infection and no increased frequency of BCG-related lymphadenopathy (24%) compared with a group of uninfected children (19%). This confirms previous reports from Zaire[117]. These studies support the WHO guidelines that BCG vaccination be given to HIV-seropositive infants (unless they have symptoms of HIV infection) (see also Chapter 14b).

Preliminary evidence suggests that primary chemoprophylaxis with isoniazid prevents the onset of active tuberculosis in HIV-positive patients with *M. tuberculosis* infection[57,118]. In Zambia, no cases of active tuberculosis developed in 190 HIV-positive patients who received 300 mg isoniazid per day for 6 months and who were then followed for an average of 6 months; in contrast, among 220 HIV-positive patients who received placebo, active tuberculosis developed in 4.4%[60]. However, in this study there were a number of unexplained deaths in each group, and confirmatory studies in Africa need to be done. Primary chemoprophylaxis, if effective, has some obvious benefits: it prevents tuberculous reactivation in the individual; it can limit the spread of tuberculosis from index cases to the community; and it can slow the progression of HIV infection to AIDS – *M. tuberculosis* can activate T helper lymphocytes[119], which, if infected with HIV, may lead to viral multiplication. However, primary chemoprophylaxis for widespread use in Africa is fraught with difficulties and problems, such as the potential for increasing drug resistance and the considerable logistic and financial difficulties that will arise if such policy is implemented (see also Chapter 14a, p.286)

12b.7 TB AND HIV: IMPLICATIONS FOR TUBERCULOSIS CONTROL

The efficacy of a tuberculosis control programme depends on the case detection rate (particularly of smear-positive cases), the proportion of detected cases who start and complete treatment, and the proportion of those completing treatment who are cured. As previously discussed, in many African countries, even before the advent of AIDS, the success rate of case detection and effective treatment was poor. Increased case detection is the least amenable of the factors to improvement, and the relative increase in smear-negative and extrapulmonary tuberculosis with HIV infection threaten to make it worse. However, improved chemotherapy (through the introduction of short-course chemotherapy for smear-positive disease) is undoubtedly one of the most important successes of the IUATLD-assisted National Tuberculosis Programmes[68], and it is believed that this will be cost-effective even in HIV-seropositive patients[19]. The achievement of the global target of tuberculosis control – 70% detection of all new cases and 85% cure rate – will cost approximately US$200 million per year[120]. This will require a focused global programme, with participating countries being given financial, technical and managerial assistance. However, there are some who believe that sufficient funds or personnel will never be available in Africa to support the widespread use of short-course chemotherapy, and that radical short courses of chemotherapy (1

day to 8 weeks) in association with immunotherapy (killed *M. vaccae*) should be evaluated
urgently[121] (Chapter 5, p. 67). Because of
the enormous logistic problems that undoubtedly would accompany primary
isoniazid prophylaxis in Africa, the same
authors also believe that preventive immunotherapy, using killed *M. vaccae*, should be
considered. Evidence so far indicates that
immunotherapy with *M. vaccae* has great
potential for the prevention and treatment of
tuberculosis[122, 123], and this option should
certainly be studied. Given the disastrous
impact that HIV is having on the incidence
and clinical course of tuberculosis in many
developing countries, it is essential that in
the field of scientific and operational research
HIV and tuberculosis control programmes
collaborate as much as possible. In order to
reach as many patients as possible, these
programmes must also be fully integrated
into the primary health care systems. The
task ahead is formidable (Chapter 15b).

REFERENCES

1. WHO (1992) *Weekly epidemiological record*, WHO, Geneva, 6 April.
2. WHO (1991) *Point of Fact*, No. 74, May.
3. Fleming, A.F. (1988) Seroepidemiology of human immunodeficiency viruses in Africa. *Biomed. Pharmacother.*, **42**, 309–20.
4. Goodgame, R.W. (1990) AIDS in Uganda – clinical and social features. *N. Engl. J. Med.*, **323**, 383–9.
5. De Cock, K.M., Barrere, B., Diaby, L. *et al.* (1990) AIDS – the leading cause of adult death in the West African City of Abidjan, Ivory Coast. *Science*, **249**, 793–6.
6. Braun, M.M., Heyward, W.L. and Curran, J.W. (1990) The global epidemiology of HIV infection and AIDS. *Ann. Rev. Microbiol.*, **44**, 555–77.
7. Quinn, T.C., Mann, J.M., Curran, J.W. and Piot, P. (1986) AIDS in Africa: an epidemiologic paradigm. *Science*, **234**, 955–63.
8. Kreiss, J.K. and Castro, K.G. (1990) Special considerations for managing suspected human immunodeficiency virus infection and AIDS in patients from developing countries. *J. Inf. Dis.*, **162**, 955–960.
9. Kochi, A. (1991) The global tuberculosis situation and the new control strategy of the World Health Organisation. *Tubercle*, **72**, 1–6.
10. Murray, C.J.L., Styblo, K. and Rouillon, A. (1990) Tuberculosis in developing countries: burden, intervention and cost. *Bull. Int. Union Tuberc. Lung Dis.*, **65**, 2–20.
11. WHO (1989) Childhood tuberculosis and BCG vaccine. *EPI Update Supplement*, World Health Organization, Geneva.
12. Cauthen, G.M., Pio, A. and ten Dam, H.G. (1988) Annual risk of tuberculous infection. World Health Organization, Geneva WHO/TB/88.154.
13. Sudre, P., ten Dam, G. and Kochi, A. (1992) Tuberculosis: a global overview of the situation today. *Bull. WHO*, **70**, 149–59.
14. East African and British Medical Research Council (1987) A study of the use of maternity and child welfare clinics in case-finding for pulmonary tuberculosis in Kenya. *Tubercle*, **68**, 93–103.
15. Nkhoma, W., Harries, A.D. and Wirima, J.J. (1988) Pulmonary tuberculosis in Malawian adults: why the delay in diagnosis? *Medical Quarterly (J. Med. Assoc. Malawi)*, **5**, 22–3.
16. Styblo, K. (1986) Tuberculosis control and surveillance, in *Recent Advances in Respiratory Medicine* (eds D.C. Flenley and T.L. Petty), Churchill Livingstone, Edinburgh, 77–108.
17. Kleeberg, H.H. and Boshoff, M.S. (1980) A world atlas of initial drug resistance. Report to the Scientific Committee on Bacteriology and Immunology of the IUAT.
18. Fox, W. (1983) Compliance of patients and physicians: experience and lessons from tuberculosis – I. *Br. Med. J.*, **287**, 33–5.
19. Murray, C.J.L., Dejonghe, E., Chum, H.J. *et al.* (1991) Cost-effectiveness of chemotherapy for pulmonary tuberculosis in three sub-Saharan African countries. *Lancet*, **338**, 1305–8.
20. Pitchenik, A.E. and Fischl, M.A. (1983) Disseminated tuberculosis and the acquired immunodeficiency syndrome. *Ann. Intern. Med.*, **97**, 112.
21. Pape, J.W., Liautaud, B., Thomas, F. *et al.* (1983) Characteristics of the acquired immunodeficiency syndrome (AIDS) in Haiti. *N. Engl. J. Med.*, **309**, 945–50.
22. Sunderam, G., McDonald, R.J., Maniatis, T. *et al.* (1986) Tuberculosis as a manifestation of

the acquired immunodeficiency syndrome (AIDS). *J. Am. med. Assoc.* **256**, 362–6.

23. Clumeck, N., Sonnet J., Taelman H. *et al.* (1984) Acquired immunodeficiency syndrome in African patients. *N. Engl. J. Med.*, **310**, 492–7.

24. Lester, F.T., Ayehunie, S. and Debrework, Z. (1988) Acquired immunodeficiency syndrome: seven cases in Addis Ababa (Ethiopia) hospital. *Ethiop. Med. J.*, **26**, 139–47.

25. McLeod, D.T., Latif, A., Neill, P. and Lucas, S. (1988) Pulmonary diseases in AIDS patients in Central Africa. *Am. Rev. Respir. Dis.*, **137**, 119.

26. Reeve, P.A. (1989) HIV infection in patients admitted to a general hospital in Malawi. *Br. Med. J.*, **298**, 1567–8.

27. Wadhawan, D. and Hira, S.K. (1989): Tuberculosis and HIV-1 in medical wards. *Med. J. Zambia*, **24**, 16–18.

28. Gilks, C.F., Brindle, R.J., Otieno, L.S. *et al.* (1990) Extrapulmonary and disseminated tuberculosis in HIV-1-seropositive patients presenting to the acute medical services in Nairobi. *AIDS*, **41**, 981–5.

29. Barr, R.D. (1972) A two-year prospective analysis of emergency admissions to an adult medical unit at the Kenyatta National Hospital, Nairobi. *East Afr. Med. J.*, **49**, 772–82.

30. Turner, P.D. (1962) The pattern of disease as seen by medical admission to the Coast General Hospital in 1960. *East Afr. Med. J.*, **39**, 121–35.

31. Mann, J.M., Snider, D.E., Francis, H. *et al.* (1986) Association between HTLV-III/ LAV infection and tuberculosis in Zaire. *J. Am. Med. Assoc.*, **256**, 346.

32. Standaert, B., Niragira, F., Kadende, P. and Piot, P. (1989) The association of tuberculosis and HIV infection in Burundi. *AIDS Res. Hum. Retroviruses*, **5**, 247–51.

33. Colebunders, R.L., Karahunga, C., Ryder, R. *et al.* (1988) Seroprevalence of HIV-1 antibody among tuberculosis patients in Zaire 1985–1987. XIIth International Congress for Tropical Medicine and Malaria. *Int Congr. Ser.*, **810**, 222.

34. Slutkin, G., Leowski, J. and Mann, J. (1988) Tuberculosis and AIDS. The effects of the AIDS epidemic on the tuberculosis problem and tuberculosis programmes. *Bull. Int. Union Tuberc. Lung Dis.*, **63**, 21–4.

35. Kool, H.E., Bloemkolk, D., Reeve, P.A. and Danner, S.A. (1990) HIV seropositivity and tuberculosis in a large general hospital in Malawi. *Trop. Geogr. Med.*, **42**, 128–32.

36. Lesbordes, J.L., Baquillon, G., Georges, M.C. *et al.* (1988) La tuberculose au cours de l'infection par le virus de l'immunodeficience humaine a Bangui (Republique Centrafricaine). *Med. Trop. (Mars.)*, **48**, 21–5.

37. Simooya, O.O., Maboshe, M.N., Kaoma, R.B. *et al.* (1991) HIV infection in newly diagnosed tuberculosis patients in Ndola, Zambia. *Centr. Afr. J. Med.* **37**, 4–7.

38. Willame, J.C., Nkoko, B., Pauwels, P. *et al.* (1988) Tuberculose et sero-positive anti VIH à Kinshasa, Zaire. *Ann. Soc. Belge Med. Trop.*, **68**, 165–7.

39. Colebunders, R.L., Ryder, R.W., Nzilambi, N. *et al.* (1989) HIV infection in patients with tuberculosis in Kinshasa, Zaire. *Am. Rev. Respir. Dis.*, **139**, 1082–5.

40. Meeran, K. (1989) Prevalence of HIV infection among patients with leprosy and tuberculosis in rural Zambia. *Br.Med.J.*, **298**, 364–5.

41. Mbolidi, C.D., Cathebras, P. and Vohito, M.D. (1988) Parallel increase in the prevalence of pulmonary tuberculosis and infection with HIV in Bangui. *Presse Med.*, **17**, 872–3.

42. Cathebras, P., Vohito, J.A., Yete, M.L. *et al.* (1988) Tuberculose et infection par le virus de l'immunodeficience humaine en Republique Centrafricaine. *Med. Trop. (Mars.)*, **48**, 401–7.

43. Ouattara, S.A., Diallo, D., Meite, M. *et al.* (1988) Epidemiologie des infections par le virus de l'immunodeficience humaine VIH -1 et VIH -2 en Cote d'Ivoire. *Med. Trop. (Mars.)*, **48**, 375–79.

44. Braun, M., Mamadou, T., Damet, G. *et al.* (1989) HIV-1, HIV-2 and tuberculosis in Abidjan, Cote d'Ivoire. V International Conference on AIDS, Montreal, June (abstract MGP24).

45. Nunn, P., Gicheha, C., Hayes, R. *et al.* (1992) Cross-sectional survey of HIV infection among patients with tuberculosis in Nairobi, Kenya. *Tuberc. Lung Dis.*, **73**, 45–51.

46. Malkin, J.E., Prazuck, T., Simmonet, F. *et al.* (1990) Tuberculosis and HIV infection: a longitudinal study in West Africa: Burkina-Faso. VI International Conference on AIDS, San Francisco, June (abstract ThC733).

47. Kelly, P., Burnham, G. and Radford, C. (1990) HIV seropositivity and tuberculosis in

a rural Malawi hospital. *Trans. Roy. Soc. Trop. Med. Hyg.*, **84**, 725–7.

48. Elliott, A.M., Luo, N., Tembo, G. *et al.* (1990) Impact of HIV on tuberculosis in Zambia: a cross-sectional study. *Br. Med. J.*, **301**, 412–15.

49. Mets, T., Ngendahayo, P., Van de Perre, P. and Mutwewingabo, A. (1989) HIV infection and tuberculosis in Central Africa. *N. Engl. J. Med.*, **320**, 542–3.

50. De Cock, K.M., Gnaore, E., Adjorlolo, G. *et al.* (1991) Risk of tuberculosis in patients with HIV-1 and HIV-2 infections in Abidjan, Ivory Coast. *Br. Med. J.*, **301**, 496–9.

51. Mahari, M., Legg, W., Hoston, S. *et al.* (1990) Association of tuberculosis and HIV infection in Zimbabwe. VI International Conference on AIDS, San Francisco, June (abstract ThB494).

52. Mukadi, Y., Perriens, J., Willame, J.C. *et al.* (1990) HIV seroprevalence among new cases of pulmonary tuberculosis stable between 1987 and 1989 in Kinshasa, Zaire. VI International Conference on AIDS, San Francisco, June (abstract FC608).

53. Eriki, P.P., Okwera, A., Aisu, T., *et al.* (1991) The influence of human immunodeficiency virus infection on tuberculosis in Kampala, Uganda. *Am. Rev. Respir. Dis.*, **143**, 185–7.

54. Naucler, A., Albino, P., Da-Silva, A.P. *et al.* (1991) HIV-2 infection in hospitalized patients in Bissau, Guinea-Bissau. *AIDS*, **5**, 301–4.

55. Rwandan HIV Seroprevalence Study Group (1989) Nationwide community-based serological survey of HIV-1 and other human retrovirus infections in a central African country. *Lancet*, **i**, 941–3.

56. Ferebee, S.H. (1970) Controlled chemoprophylaxis trials in tuberculosis: a general review. *Adv. Tuberc. Res.*, **17**, 28–106.

57. Selwyn, P.A., Hartel, D., Lewis, V.A. *et al.* (1989) A prospective study of the risk of tuberculosis among intravenous drug users with human immunodeficiency virus infection. *N. Engl. J. Med.*, **320**, 545–50.

58. Di Perri, G., Cruciani, M., Danzi, M.C. *et al.* (1989) Nosocomial epidemic of active tuberculosis among HIV-infected patients. *Lancet*, **ii**, 1502–4.

59. Daley, C.L., Small, P.M., Schecter, G.F. *et al.* (1992) An outbreak of tuberculosis with accelerated progression among persons infected with the human immunodeficiency virus. *N. Engl. J. Med.*, **326**, 231–5.

60. Wadhawan, D., Hira, S., Mwansa, N. *et al.* (1990). Isoniazid prophylaxis among patients with HIV-1 infection. VI International Conference on AIDS, San Francisco, June (abstract ThB510).

61. Batungwanago, J., Allen, S., Bogaerts, J. *et al.* (1990) Etude prospective du risque de tuberculosis dans une cohort de femmes HIV-seropositives à Kigali, Rwanda. V International Conference on AIDS in Africa, Kinshasa, October (abstract WOD4).

62. Braun, M.M., Badi, N., Ryder, R.W. *et al.* (1991) A retrospective cohort study of the risk of tuberculosis among women of childbearing age with HIV infection in Zaire. *Am. Rev. Respir. Dis.*, **143**, 501–4.

63. Crowe, S.M., Carlin, J.B., Stewart, K.I. *et al.* (1991) Predictive value of CD4 lymphocyte numbers for the development of opportunistic infections and malignancies in HIV-infected persons. *J. Acq. Immun. Def. Syndr.*, **4**, 770–6.

64. Theuer, C.P., Hopewell, P.C., Elias, D. *et al.* (1990). Human immunodeficiency virus infection in tuberculosis patients. *J. Infect. Dis.*, **162**, 8–12.

65. Perronne, C., Ghoubontni, A., Leport, C. *et al.* (1992) Should pulmonary tuberculosis be an AIDS-defining diagnosis in patients infected with HIV? *Tuberc. Lung Dis.*, **73**, 39–44.

66. Mukadi, Y., Perriens, J., Willame, J.C. *et al.* (1990) Short-course antituberculous therapy for pulmonary tuberculosis in HIV-seropositive patients: a prospective controlled study. VI International Conference on AIDS, San Francisco, June (abstract ThB507).

67. Styblo, K. (1988) The potential impact of AIDS on the tuberculosis situation in developed and developing countries. *Bull. Int. Union Tuberc. Lung Dis.*, **63**, 25–8.

68. Styblo, K. (1991) The impact of HIV infection on the global epidemiology of tuberculosis. *Bull. Int. Union Tuberc. Lung Dis.*, **66**, 27–32.

69. Schulzer, M., Fitzgerald, J.M., Enarson, D.A. and Grzybowski, S. (1992) An estimate of the future size of the tuberculosis problem in sub-Saharan Africa resulting from HIV infection. *Tuberc. Lung Dis.*, **73**, 52–8.

70. Pitchenik, A.E., Cole, C., Russell, B.W. *et al.* (1984) Tuberculosis, atypical mycobacteriosis

and the acquired immunodeficiency syndrome among Haitian and non-Haitian patients in South Florida. *Ann. Intern. Med.*, **101**, 641–5.

71. Pape, J.W., and Johnson, W.D. (1988) Epidemiology in the Caribbean. AIDS and HIV infection in the tropics. *Bailliere's Clin. Trop. Med. Commun. Dis.*, **3**, 31–42.

72. Long, R., Scalcini, M., Manfreda, J. *et al.* (1991) Impact of human immunodeficiency virus type 1 on tuberculosis in rural Haiti. *Am. Rev. Respir. Dis.*, **143**, 69–73.

73. Ponce de Leon, R., Ruiz-Palacios, G., Schnieders, B., and Cruz, A. (1988) Characteristics of AIDS in a reference hospital in Mexico City. Proceedings of the IV International Conference on AIDS, Stockholm, June (Abstract 5074).

74. Kritski, A.L., Matida, A., and Galvao-Castro, B. (1989) Tuberculosis and AIDS – Rio De Janeiro, Brazil 1983–1988. Proceedings of the V International Conference on AIDS. Montreal, June (abstract ThBP74).

75. Kritski, A.L., Werneck, E.B., Medeiros, D. *et al.* (1988) Study of association between active pulmonary tuberculosis and human immunodeficiency virus (HIV), at a sanatorium in Rio De Janeiro, Brazil. A prospective study. *Am. Rev. Respir. Dis.*, **137**, 494.

76. Kritski, A.L., Magalhaes, J.C.Q., Werneck, E.B. *et al.* (1989) A study of the association between extrapulmonary tuberculosis (EPTB) and HIV infection, as seen in 13 primary health centres (PHC) in Rio De Janeiro, Brazil. *Am. Rev. Respir. Dis.*, **139**, A185.

77. East African and British Medical Research Council Co-operative Investigation. (1978) Tuberculosis in Kenya. A second national sampling survey of drug resistance and other factors, and a comparison with the prevalence data from the first national sampling survey. *Tubercle*, **59**, 155–77.

78. Kenya/British Medical Research Council Co-operative Investigation (1989) Tuberculosis in Kenya 1984: a third national survey and a comparison with earlier surveys in 1964 and 1974. *Tubercle*, **70**, 5–20.

79. East African and British Medical Research Council Co-operative Investigation (1975) Tuberculosis in Tanzania: a national sampling survey of drug resistance and other factors. *Tubercle*, **56**, 269–94.

80. Tanzanian/British Medical Research Council

collaborative study (1985) Tuberculosis in Tanzania – a national survey of newly notified cases. *Tubercle*, **66**, 161–78.

81. Barnes, P.F., Verdegem, T.D., Vachon, L.A. *et al.* (1988) J.M., Ov. Chest roentgenogram in pulmonary tuberculosis: new data on an old test. *Chest*, **94**, 316–20.

82. Harries, A.D., Thomas, J. and Chugh, K.S. (1985) Malnutrition in African patients with pulmonary tuberculosis. *Hum. Nutr. Clin. Nutr.*, **39C**, 361–3.

83. Scalcini, M., Occenac, R., Manfreda, J. and Long, R. (1991) Pulmonary tuberculosis, human immunodeficiency virus type-1 and malnutrition. *Bull. Int. Union. Tuberc. Lung Dis.*, **66**, 37–41.

84. De Cock, K.M., Selik, R.M., Soro, B., *et al.* (1991) AIDS surveillance in Africa: a reappraisal of case definitions. *Br. Med. J.*, **303**, 1185–8.

85. Chaisson, R.E., Schecter, G.F., Theuer, C.P., *et al.* (1987) Tuberculosis in patients with the acquired immunodeficiency syndrome. *Am. Rev. Respir. Dis.*, **136**, 570–4.

86. Harries, A.D. (1990) Tuberculosis and human immunodeficiency virus infection in developing countries. *Lancet*, **335**, 387–90.

87. Noronha, D., Pallangyo, K.J., Ndosi, B.N. *et al.* (1991) Radiological features of pulmonary tuberculosis in patients infected with human immunodeficiency virus. *East Afr. Med. J.*, **68**, 210–15.

88. White, D.A., and Matthay, R.A. (1989) Non infectious pulmonary complications of infection with the human immunodeficiency virus. *Am. Rev. Respir. Dis.*, **140**, 1763–87.

89. Murray, J.K., and Mills, J. (1990) Pulmonary infectious complications of human immunodeficiency virus infection. *Am. Rev. Respir. Dis.*, **141**, 1356–72; 1582–96.

90. Taelman, H., Kagame, A., Batungwanayo, J. *et al.* (1991) Tuberculosis and HIV infection. *Br. Med. J.*, **302**, 1206.

91. Miller, R.F., Kocjan, G., Buckland, J., *et al.* (1991) Sputum induction for the diagnosis of pulmonary disease in HIV-positive patients. *J. Infect.*, **23**, 5–15.

92. Wilkins, E.G.L and Ivanyi, J. (1990) Potential value of serology for diagnosis of extrapulmonary tuberculosis. *Lancet*, **336**, 641–4.

93. Cegielski, J.P., Ramaiya, K., Lallinger, G.J. *et al.* (1990) I.A., M. Pericardial disease and

human immunodeficiency virus in Dar-es-Salaam, Tanzania. *Lancet*, **335**, 209–12.

94. Nambuya, A., Sewankambo, N., Mugerwa, J. *et al.* (1988). Tuberculous lymphadenitis associated with human immunodeficiency virus (HIV) in Uganda. *J. Clin. Pathol.*, **41**, 93–6.

95. Katzenstein, D.A., Latif, A.S., Grace, S.A. *et al.* (1990) Clinical and laboratory characteristics of HIV-1 infection in Zimbabwe. *J.Acq. Immun. Def. Syndr.*, **3**, 701–7.

96. Voetberg, A., and Lucas, S.B. (1991) Tuberculosis or persistent lymphadenopathy in HIV disease? *Lancet*, **337**, 56–7.

97. Lynn, W., Whyte, M., and Weber, J. (1989) Nocardia, mycobacteria and AIDS. *AIDS*, **3**, 766–7.

98. Shafer, R.W., Goldberg, R., Sierra, M. and Glatt, A.E. (1989) Frequency of *Mycobacterium tuberculosis* bacteraemia in patients with tuberculosis in an area endemic for AIDS. *Am. Rev. Respir. Dis.*, **140**, 1611–13.

99. Long, R., Maycher, B., Scalcini, M. and Manfreda, J. (1991) The chest roentgenogram in pulmonary tuberculosis patients seropositive for human immunodeficiency virus type 1. *Chest*, **99**, 123–7.

100. Levi, G.C., Mendes, W.S., Rodrigues, G.A. *et al.* (1988) Tuberculosis (TB) and acquired immunodeficiency syndrome (AIDS). XIIth International Congress for Tropical Medicine and Malaria. *Int. Congr. Ser.*, **810**, 66.

101. Small, P.M., Schecter, G.F., Goodman, P.C., *et al.* (1991) Treatment of tuberculosis in patients with advanced human immunodeficiency virus infection. *N. Engl. J. Med.*, **324**, 289–94.

102. Kritski, A.L., Silva, R.A., Boechat, N.L. *et al.* (1989) Association between tuberculosis (TB) and AIDS in 135 patients: an overview. *Am. Rev. Respir. Dis.*, **139**, A147.

103. Kibuga, D.K., and Gathua, S. (1990) A study of HIV infection in association with tuberculosis as seen in infectious diseases hospitals (IDH) in Nairobi. VI International Conference on AIDS, San Francisco, June (abstract ThB489).

104. Mann, J.M., Francis, H., Quinn, T.C. *et al.* (1986) HIV seroprevalence among hospital workers in Kinshasa, Zaire. *J. Am. Med. Assoc.*, **256**, 3099–102.

105. WHO (1991) Guidelines for tuberculosis treatment in adults and children in National Tuberculosis Programmes. WHO/TUB/91.161. World Health Organization, Geneva.

106. Gilks, C.F., Brindle, R.J., Otieno, L.S. *et al.* (1990) Life-threatening bacteraemia in HIV-1 seropositive adults admitted to hospital in Nairobi, Kenya. *Lancet*, **336**, 545–9.

107. Perriens, J.H., Colebunders, R.L., Karahunga, C. *et al.* (1991) Increased mortality and tuberculosis treatment failure rate among human immunodeficiency virus (HIV) seropositive compared with HIV seronegative patients with pulmonary tuberculosis treated with 'standard' chemotherapy in Kinshasa, Zaire. *Am. Rev. Respir. Dis.*, **144**, 750–5.

108. Miller, A.B., Fox, W. and Tall, R. (1966) An international co-operative investigation into thiacetazone (thioacetazone) side effects. *Tubercle*, **47**, 33–73.

109. Pearson, C.A. (1978) Thiacetazone toxicity in the treatment of tuberculosis patients in Nigeria. *J. Trop. Med. Hyg.*, **81**, 238–42.

110. Naraqi, S. and Temu, P. (1980) Thiacetazone skin reaction in Papua New Guinea. *Med. J. Aust.*, *i*, 480–1.

111. Nunn, P., Kibuga, D., Gathua, S. *et al.* (1991) Cutaneous hypersensitivity reactions due to thiacetazone in HIV-1 seropositive patients treated for tuberculosis. *Lancet*, **337**, 627–30.

112. Wirima, J.J. and Harries, A.D. (1991) Stevens–Johnson syndrome during anti-tuberculosis chemotherapy in HIV-seropositive patients: report on six cases. *East Afr. Med. J.*, **68**, 64–6.

113. Nunn, P., Porter, J., Githui, W. and Odhiambo, J. (1991) Treating tuberculosis in HIV-positive Africans. *Lancet*, **338**, 1141.

114. Ninane, J., Grymonprez, A., Burtonboy, G. *et al.* (1988) Disseminated BCG in HIV infection. *Arch. Dis. Childh.*, **63**, 1268–9.

115. Colebunders, R.L., Izaley, L., Musampu, M. *et al.* (1988) BCG vaccine abscesses are unrelated to HIV infection. *J. Am. Med. Assoc.*, **259**, 352.

116. Lallemant-Le Coeur, S., Lallemant, M., Cheynier, D. *et al.* (1991) Bacillus Calmette–Guerin immunization in infants born to HIV-1-seropositive mothers. *AIDS*, **5**, 195–9.

117. Von Reyn, C.F., Clements, C.J. and Mann, J.M. (1987) Human immunodeficiency virus infection and routine childhood immunisation. *Lancet*, **ii**, 669–72.

118. Jordan, T.J., Lewit, E.M., Montgomery, R.L.

et al. (1991). Isoniazid as preventive therapy in HIV-infected intravenous drug users. A decision analysis. *J. Am. Med. Assoc.*, **265**, 2987–91.

119. Edwards, D. and Kirkpatrick, C. (1986) The immunology of mycobacterial diseases. *Am. Rev. Respir. Dis.*, **34**, 1062–71.

120. WHO (1992) Tuberculosis control and research strategies for the 1990s: memoran-dum from a WHO meeting. *Bull. WHO*, **70**, 17–21.

121. Stanford, J.L., Grange, J.M. and Pozniak, A. (1991) Is Africa lost? *Lancet*, **338**, 557–8.

122. Grange, J.M. (1990) Immunotherapy of tuberculosis. *Tubercle*, **71**, 237–9.

123. Pozniak, A., Stanford, J.L. and Grange, J.M. (1991) *Mycobacterium vaccae* immunotherapy. *Lancet*, **338**, 1533–44.

ENVIRONMENTAL MYCOBACTERIA

J. Banks

13.1 INTRODUCTION

In addition to *Mycobacterium tuberculosis* and *Mycobacterium bovis*, other species of mycobacteria may cause human disease. Variously referred to as opportunist, non-tuberculous, atypical, mycobacteria other than tuberculosis (MOTT) and environmental mycobacteria, these micro-organisms are ubiquitous in nature and have been isolated from sources including soil, dust, water and milk, and a variety of animals and birds[1–4]. Infection usually occurs in patients with pre-existing chronic lung disease or states of immunodeficiency but rarely may also develop in patients with no obvious predisposing condition. Infection is not transmitted from person to person but is most likely to be acquired from the environment, although the source and portal of entry may differ between individuals.

Environmental mycobacteria that are potentially pathogenic are shown in Table 13.1. Clinicians should be aware of non-pathogenic species that are occasionally isolated from sputum and other clinical specimens, which are rarely of clinical significance. These include *M. gordonae, M. gastri, M. terrae* complex, and *M. flavescens*[5,6].

M. kansasii is the commonest species encountered in Western Europe, Texas and the upper central states of North America[6,7] while the *Mycobacterium avium-intracellulare* complex (MAC) predominates in the south-eastern USA, Western Australia and Japan, where the prevalence of pulmon-

Table 13.1 Major environmental mycobacteria that may cause human disease

Species	Major sites of infection
M. avium \	\ Pulmonary
M. intracellulare } MAC[a]	} Lymph gland
M. scrofulaceum /	/ Disseminated
M. kansasii	Pulmonary
M. xenopi	Pulmonary
M. malmoense	Pulmonary
M. fortuitum	Soft tissues/surgical wounds
M. chelonei	Soft tissues/surgical wounds
M. ulcerans	Skin
M. marinum	Soft tissues/surgical wounds

[a] Also referred to as 'MAIS'.

ary infection caused by the MAC is approximately 10% of that resulting from *M. tuberculosis*[7,8]. Geographical patterns of disease also emerge within the UK. Overall, *M. kansasii* is the commonest species encountered in Britain but infection in London and south-east England is predominantly caused by *M. xenopi*[9]. Of 533 clinically confirmed new cases of environmental mycobacterial infection recorded by the Regional Centre for Tuberculosis Bacteriology, Dulwich, 37% were due to *M. xenopi*, 28% to *M. kansasii*, 20% to the MAC, and 8% to *M. fortuitum* or *M. chelonei*[10]. The emerging problem of disseminated infection caused by the MAC in patients infected with the human immunode-

Clinical Tuberculosis. Edited by P.D.O. Davies. Published in 1994 by Chapman & Hall, London. ISBN 0 412 48630 X

ficiency virus (HIV) is likely to alter the pattern of disease in due course.

Diagnosis depends upon identification of the infecting micro-organism by the bacteriologist. Differential skin testing cannot be relied upon to make a diagnosis because of the non-specificity of mycobacterial antigens, which results in cross-reactivity between different mycobacterial species. Hypersensitivity to purified protein derivative (PPD) from the MAC, for example, can arise as a result of infection with a wide range of mycobacterial species and does not specifically indicate MAC infection[11]. Similarly skin testing using multiple types of PPD does not discriminate between infection caused by *M. tuberculosis* and *M. kansasii*[12], and is no substitute for the isolation and identification of the infecting mycobacterium.

Many sites of infection have been reported, including soft tissue, bone, joint and genitourinary tract, but pulmonary disease, lymphadenitis and disseminated infection are the commonest and most important clinical problems encountered.

13.2 PULMONARY DISEASE

Pulmonary disease most often results from infection with either *M. kansasii*, the MAC, *M. xenopi* or *M. malmoense*, the prevalence varying according to the geographical patterns previously described. Patients may present with an acute or sub-acute illness that is clinically and radiographically identical to that caused by infection with *M. tuberculosis*. Symptoms, which may develop over several weeks, frequently include cough with sputum, haemoptysis and night sweats and the chest radiograph usually shows confluent upper lobe shadows with cavities [13,14]. Although infection may occur in previously healthy individuals, the majority have co-existing lung disease, commonly chronic bronchitis and emphysema, bronchiectasis or pneumoconiosis[13–16]. Not surprisingly, many patients are thought to

have tuberculosis when acid-fast bacilli are seen on sputum smear, and the correct diagnosis is only confirmed several weeks later on the results of culture.

Although the diagnosis is usually straightforward in patients who present with this acute pattern of disease, the diagnosis may be difficult when infection pursues a more chronic insidious course developing over a period of months or even years. In these cases clinical manifestations of weight loss and cachexia, which often accompany respiratory symptoms, may be attributed to co-existent pulmonary disease and not to mycobacterial infection. The chest radiograph can be difficult to interpret, often showing chronic, apparently indolent abnormalities, which may also be attributed to other causes, e.g. post-tuberculous fibrosis. Mycobacteria isolated from the sputum of such patients may be thought to represent colonization of previously damaged lung rather than signifying active infection. Indeed, distinguishing colonization from genuine infection may be difficult. Genuine infection is likely if multiple colonies of the same strain of mycobacteria are repeatedly isolated in the absence of other pathogens from a symptomatic patient whose chest radiograph shows abnormalities consistent with mycobacterial disease[17]. A single isolate from sputum that cannot be repeated is unlikely to be of any significance. Two positive cultures of *M. kansasii*[18] or *M. malmoense*[15] obtained on separate occasions usually signify genuine infection, but three or four isolates of *M. xenopi* or the MAC should be obtained to establish a diagnosis[19,20]. Colonization should not be lightly dismissed, however, since transformation to invasive disease may occur unpredictably, sometimes following years of apparent quiescence[21]. Patients with the MAC in their sputum do not always develop progressive disease but they can do so with a fatal outcome[16], while disease caused by *M. kansasii* has progressed insidiously in some patients over several years in the absence of new symptoms at the time of diagnosis[22]. If doubt exists about the significance of repeated isolates it is probably wise to treat the patient with antimycobacterial drugs.

13.2.1 THE CHEST RADIOGRAPH

Certain radiographic abnormalities may suggest infection with environmental mycobacteria. These include the presence of thin-walled, often unilateral cavities with little surrounding infiltrates or a single well-circumscribed opacity containing multiple lucencies[23–27]. Increased cavitation relative

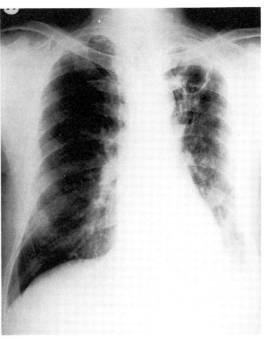

Fig. 13.2 Chest radiograph showing a single cavity in the left apex in a 60-year-old man. *M. malmoense* was isolated from the sputum on repeated occasions.

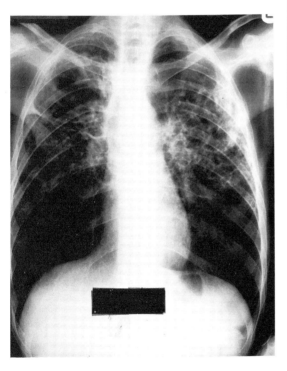

Fig. 13.1 Chest radiograph showing extensive pulmonary disease caused by *M. xenopi* in an elderly male.

to total lung involvement has been emphasized, although in one series[28] cavitating upper lobe infiltrates were present in only 50% of patients. The remainder had patchy

nodular infiltrates without upper lobe predominance and multiple small cavities resembling bronchiectasis. Any of these findings may be seen in tuberculosis, however, and are not pathognomonic of infection with environmental mycobacteria (Figs 13.1 and 13.2).

13.3 DISSEMINATED DISEASE

Prior to the HIV pandemic, disseminated infection with environmental mycobacteria was rare. In a large review series[29] only 30 cases of disseminated infection caused by the MAC and 26 cases of disease caused by *M. kansasii* could be identified from the literature. The dramatic increase in incidence of disseminated infection associated with the acquired immunodeficiency syndrome

(AIDS) has been caused predominantly by the MAC[30–33]. Patients usually have pronounced immunodeficiency and complain of fever with weight loss and general malaise. Gastrointestinal symptoms may predominate[30,34], while pulmonary symptoms are less marked and occur late. Enlarged lymph glands, hepatosplenomegaly and skin lesions are the commonest findings[30,35]. Physical signs in the chest are less common but the chest radiograph is usually abnormal and may show mediastinal lymphadenopathy, pulmonary nodules or patchy alveolar infiltrates[35,36]. Pulmonary cavitation in disseminated infection is uncommon. The diagnosis is usually made by tissue biopsy of lymph nodes, liver, bone marrow or gastrointestinal tract[36]. Infected tissue typically shows poorly formed granulomata teeming with acid-fast bacilli. Bacteraemia is frequently present and serially performed blood cultures may be used to monitor the response to treatment[31].

13.4 OTHER SITES OF INFECTION

Lymphadenitis, usually affecting the cervical glands, occurs not infrequently in children aged between 1 and 5 years. The infecting micro-organisms usually belong to the MAC and the affected glands are usually painless and non-tender[37,38]. There is rarely any accompanying constitutional illness. The diagnosis is made by aspiration or resection of the involved glands. Infection with *M. fortuitum* or *M. chelonei* usually occurs as a skin or soft-tissue infection following penetrating trauma or surgery giving rise to recurrent abscess and fistula formation. Sternotomy wounds have become a particularly common site of infection[39–42]. Inoculation of the skin by *M. marinum* may occur following abrasions acquired in contaminated swimming pools or aquaria[43]. The initial lesion, which is often papular but which may later form a superficial ulcer, is known as the 'swimming pool' or 'fishtank' granuloma. The skin may also be infected by *M. ulcerans*, giving rise to chronic indolent necrotic ulcers known as 'Buruli ulcer', most commonly seen in Central Africa[44]. Although infection of bone, joint and genitourinary tract have been reported, these are rare sites of infection.

13.5 TREATMENT

13.5.1 PULMONARY DISEASE

There is no general agreement about the treatment of pulmonary infection caused by environmental mycobacteria and many different approaches to treatment have been advocated. This lack of consensus reflects the absence of large clinical trials assessing treatment and the subsequent reliance upon results from small, non-comparable retrospective or prospective series for guidance. The variable degrees of pulmonary infection and co-existing lung disease in patients included in these series have usually influenced both treatment and eventual prognosis[45]. Recommendations about treatment have also been hampered by inappropriate comparisons with the treatment of tuberculosis. For example, the use of chemotherapy for the treatment of *M. kansasii* infection was originally questioned because patients remained sputum culture-positive and showed persistent cavities on their chest radiographs after a few months of treatment with isoniazid, para-aminosalicyclic acid (PAS) and streptomycin[46–49]. Since this compared unfavourably with the prompt bacteriological and radiographic response seen in patients with tuberculosis given the same treatment, drug therapy was discouraged in favour of surgical treatment for this condition[50]. The apparent failure of chemotherapy was attributed to drug resistance. Subsequent reports, however, showed that despite poor *in vitro* drug susceptibility, successful treatment was possible in 85% of patients when the duration of chemotherapy was prolonged beyond that normally con-

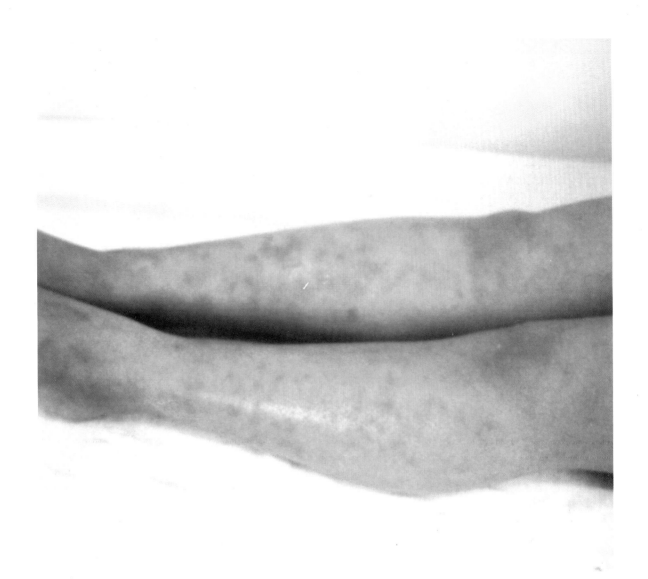

Plate 8 (Chapter 11) **Erythema nodosum in a teenage girl with pulmonary tuberculosis.**

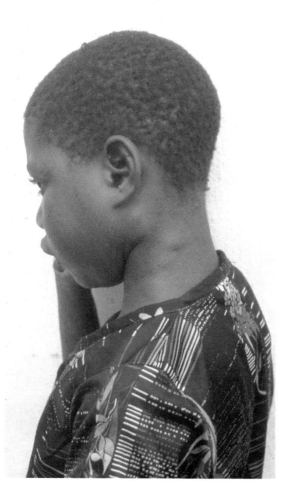

Plate 9 (Chapter 12b) **Extrapulmonary tuberculosis in the pre-AIDS era.**

Plate 10 (Chapter 12b) **Tuberculous cervical lymphadenopathy and tuberculous spondylitis.**

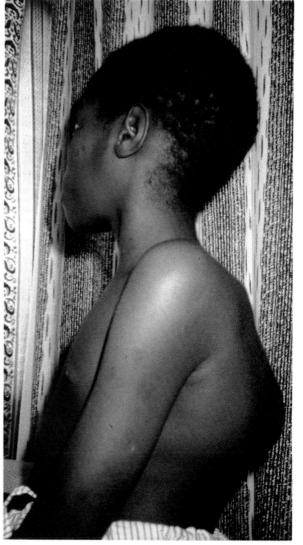

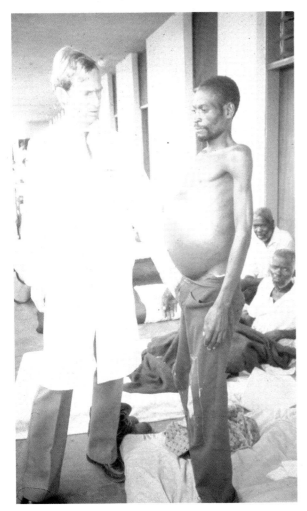

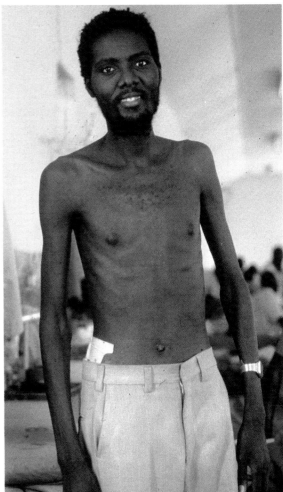

Plate 11 (Chapter 12b) **Tuberculous ascites in a patient on a general medical ward.**

Plate 12 (Chapter 12b) **Malnourished patient with pulmonary tuberulosis.**

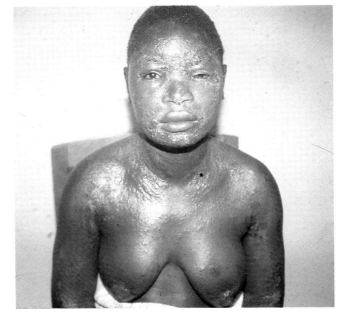

Plate 13 (Chapter 12b) **Cutaneous drug reaction.** HIV-positive patient who developed a severe cutaneous reaction 3 weeks after starting streptomycin, isoniazid and thiacetazone for a tuberculous pleural effusion.

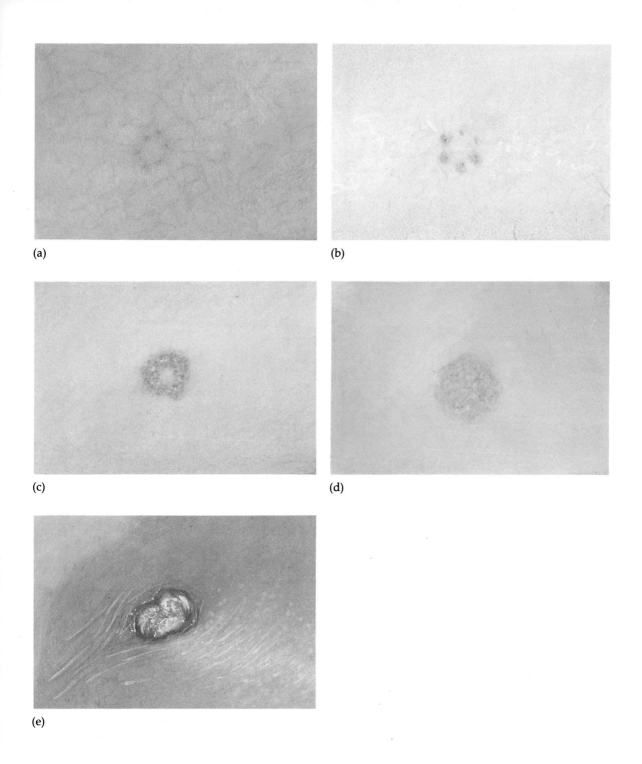

(a)

(b)

(c)

(d)

(e)

Plate 14 (Chapter 15d) **Grades of reaction to the Heaf tuberculin test.** (a) Grade 0; (b) Grade I; (c) Grade II; (d) Grade III; (e) Grade IV. (Artwork by Miss G. Rycroft.)

sidered adequate for tuberculosis[51–53]. Poor *in vitro* drug susceptibility to conventional anti-mycobacterial drugs did not predict treatment failure but indicated a need for prolonging treatment for 18–24 months. Clearly, criteria of *in vitro* drug susceptibility that govern the treatment of infection caused by *M. tuberculosis* do not apply to disease caused by other mycobacterial species.

(a) *Mycobacterium kansasii*

Pulmonary infection caused by *M. kansasii* can be treated using regimens that include rifampicin. Combining rifampicin with ethambutol is particularly effective[13,54]. Nine months of treatment is usually adequate, reflecting the micro-organisms' *in vitro* susceptibility to both drugs. In a recent prospective study[54], treatment failure occurred in only 1 of 158 patients who completed 9 months' treatment with rifampicin and ethambutol and poor compliance with treatment was thought to be a major problem in the single patient who failed to respond. Fifteen patients (9%) subsequently relapsed between 6 and 50 months after completing treatment, but relapse in eight of these was influenced by factors such as lack of compliance with treatment, malnourishment and the development of carcinoma.

(b) MAC

The outcome of treatment for MAC infection is less predictable than for that caused by *M. kansasii*. Poor *in vitro* susceptibility to conventional anti-mycobacterial drugs and failure of chemotherapy in some patients have led to recommendations for surgical treatment whenever possible[55] (Chapter 8c). Good results following surgical treatment for pulmonary MAC infection have been reported, with conversion to sputum culture-negative occurring postoperatively in 93–100% of cases and relapses occurring in only 5%

during prolonged follow-up[55,56]. Results in other series, however, have been less impressive, with 33% of patients ultimately relapsing postoperatively[45]. Surgery may not be feasible in the majority of patients with co-existent lung conditions or those with extensive lung involvement secondary to mycobacterial infection. Medical treatment is the only therapeutic option for the majority of patients.

As with early reports describing chemotherapy in patients with *M. kansasii* infection, chemotherapy for MAC infection may have failed in many cases because treatment was not continued for long enough. In more recent series, successful results were achieved in 60–94% of patients given combinations of rifampicin, ethambutol, isoniazid and streptomycin for at least 18 months[16,57]. *In vitro* drug susceptibility did not predict the eventual clinical response but did correlate in some studies with the time taken to convert to sputum culture-negative[58,59]. Both the initial response to treatment and late relapse following cessation of chemotherapy may be influenced by the severity of co-existing pulmonary disease. Ninety-four percent of patients in one study who were not breathless at the start of treatment responded to rifampicin, isoniazid and ethambutol given for 18 months[57], and only 6% relapsed during follow-up. In another study[60], 91% of patients with moderately advanced cavitating disease responded to treatment with three or more standard antituberculosis drugs compared with only 64% of those with advanced disease given the same treatment. Although treatment with five or six drugs has been recommended[61–63], there have been no comparative studies to show that such multiple regimens are more effective than those comprising fewer drugs.

(c) *Mycobacterium xenopi*

There is little information at present concerning treatment for pulmonary infection caused by *M. xenopi*. Patients treated with combinations of rifampicin, ethambutol and isoniazid usually show clinical improvement and convert to sputum culture-negative while receiving treatment, despite the microorganisms' poor *in vitro* susceptibility to these agents[14,64]. Unfortunately, relapse has occurred in up to 25% of patients following cessation of treatment. Other patients have developed progressive disease while receiving treatment with drugs such as ethionamide and cycloserine, even though these agents were highly effective on *in vitro* testing[14]. Drug toxicity and poor compliance with treatment were thought to contribute to the poor outcome in some patients. Surgical treatment has been effective in controlling the disease in small numbers of patients[65,66] but has been associated with a high rate of postoperative complications and may not be feasible because of co-existing pulmonary conditions.

(d) *Mycobacterium malmoense*

There have been few reports describing the response to treatment of pulmonary infection caused by *M. malmoense*[15,67]. Rifampicin, ethambutol and isoniazid given for 18–24 months was effective in patients in one series, although the rate of relapse could not be determined since follow-up was relatively short[15]. The inclusion of ethambutol in treatment regimens appears to be crucially important since its withdrawal has been followed by *clinical* deterioration in some patients[15].

(e) *Mycobacterium fortuitum*

Pulmonary infection with *M. fortuitum* occurs infrequently and reports on the efficacy of treatment are mostly anecdotal. Successful treatment with ciprofloxacin or ofloxacin has been reported[68,69]. Since single-agent treatment may permit the emergence of quinolone-resistant strains[70], treatment should also include a second drug, such as amikacin, imipenem, doxicycline or a sulphonamide, which have also been effective for this condition.

13.5.2 SUMMARY OF TREATMENT FOR PULMONARY DISEASE

Although effective treatment for pulmonary infection caused by environmental mycobacteria is possible using combinations of standard anti-mycobacterial drugs, success cannot be guaranteed in every case. Rifampicin combined with ethambutol is the treatment of choice for infection caused by *M. kansasii* but new drugs are clearly needed for treating infection caused by the MAC, *M. xenopi* and *M. malmoense*. Agents that have shown promise for treating disseminated MAC infection in patients with AIDS, such as clarithromycin, azithromycin, ciprofloxacin, amikacin and clofazamine[71–73], may also prove to be effective for the treatment of infection localized to the chest. Studies assessing the value of combinations of these drugs in patients with pulmonary infection are clearly needed.

13.5.3 LYMPH GLAND INFECTION

Lymphadenitis caused by infection with the MAC or *M. scrofulaceum* is effectively treated by local resection of the involved glands without the need to resort to chemotherapy[37,38]. Wound infections with *M. fortuitum* or *M. chelonei* should be treated by surgical debridement combined with ciprofloxacin and an amino-glycoside or imipenem[39–42]. Skin lesions caused by *M. marinum* often heal spontaneously, although successful treatment has been reported using co-trimoxazole[74] or tetracycline[75]. Wide surgical excision with skin grafting is the treatment of choice for skin infection caused by *M. ulcerans*[76].

13.6 *IN VITRO* DRUG SENSITIVITY TESTS AND ENVIRONMENTAL MYCOBACTERIA

In contrast to infection caused by *M. tuberculosis*, drug resistance defined by laboratory tests does not correlate with the clinical response to treatment in patients with infection caused by environmental mycobacteria. There are several possible explanations for this discrepancy. *In vitro* minimum inhibitory concentrations (MICs), which predict the clinical response to treatment, are not known for mycobacterial species other than *M. tuberculosis*. It has become customary to classify environmental mycobacteria as being drug- resistant if their MICs exceed those that have been established for drug-sensitive strains of *M. tuberculosis*[77]. This assumes that all mycobacterial species have the same critical MICs as *M. tuberculosis*. This is unlikely, however, considering that the basic mechanisms of drug resistance differ between mycobacterial species. Isoniazid resistance for *M. tuberculosis* usually occurs by a single mutational step and is dependent upon the loss of catalase peroxidase activity[78–80], yet the MAC show natural resistance to isoniazid despite possessing catalase peroxidase activity[62]. It is inappropriate therefore to use MICs established for *M. tuberculosis* as yardsticks to define drug resistance for the MAC. Compared with strains of *M. tuberculosis*, environmental mycobacteria are undoubtedly less sensitive to conventional anti-mycobacterial drugs *in vitro*, but this may simply indicate a need to prolong treatment in order to achieve a successful therapeutic result.

Drug resistance cannot be defined simply by relating *in vitro* MICs to serum drug concentrations since serum levels do not always reflect drug concentrations achieved within tissues or macrophages. For example, concentrations of ethambutol in normal and caseous lung tissue are three- to tenfold higher than plasma levels[81]. Even higher concentrations are achieved within alveolar macrophages[82,83], yet concentrations required to kill phagocytosed bacilli are lower than bactericidal concentrations required in culture medium[84]. Intracellular levels of rifampicin, clarithromycin and ciprofloxacin

are also several-fold higher than their respective serum levels[85]. These high intracellular concentrations coupled with the enhanced bactericidal action of drugs within macrophages may account for the effectiveness of some drugs in treatment despite their poor action in culture medium.

Synergy may account for the effectiveness of some drugs in treatment. Drug combinations *in vitro* have been shown to be more effective than single agents against *M. kansasii*, the MAC, *M. xenopi* and *M. malmoense*[86–92]. The particular efficacy of rifampicin and ethambutol can be explained on theoretical grounds. Rifampicin acts against mycobacteria by inhibiting bacterial DNA-dependent RNA polymerase thereby blocking transcription[93]. Rifampicin-resistant strains of *M. tuberculosis* have a resistant polymerase[94]. In contrast, rifampicin resistance among environmental mycobacteria results from a failure of the drug to penetrate the bacterial cell wall[95]. The RNA polymerase of rifampicin-resistant strains belonging to the MAC is in fact highly sensitive to rifampicin but is protected by the cell wall permeability barrier[96]. Ethambutol even in low concentrations induces morphological changes in the bacterial cell wall *in vitro*[97], probably by interfering with mycolic acid and phospholipid synthesis[97,98]. This action on the cell wall might facilitate access of rifampicin into the cell thus exposing its rifampicin-sensitive polymerase. A similar mechanism operating *in vivo* could explain the effectiveness of these two drugs in treatment.

13.7 SUMMARY

The treatment of infection caused by environmental mycobacteria, in particular the MAC, *M. xenopi* and *M. malmoense*, remains a clinical challenge. Physicians are often left confused about which treatment regimen to use in the face of seemingly conflicting recommendations made in the literature. These issues can only be resolved by conducting large prospective studies assessing and comparing different approaches to treatment. Such studies are currently being conducted and co-ordinated by the British Thoracic Society.

REFERENCES

1. Chapman, J.S. (1971) The ecology of the atypical mycobacteria. *Arch. Environ. Hlth*, **22**, 41–6.
2. Chapman, J.S., Bernard, J.S. and Speight, M. (1965) Isolation of mycobacteria from raw milk. *Am. Rev. Respir. Dis.*, **91**, 351–5.
3. Marks, J. Jenkins, P.A. (1971) The opportunist mycobacteria – a 20 year retrospect. *Postgrad. Med. J., 1971*, **47**, 705–9.
4. McSwiggan, D.A. and Collins, C.H. (1974) The isolation of *M. kansasii* and *M. xenopi* from water systems. *Tubercle*, **55**, 291–7.
5. Runyon, E.H. (1974) Ten mycobacterial pathogens. *Tubercle*, **55**, 235–40.
6. Jenkins, P.A. (1981) Nontuberculous mycobacteria and disease. *Eur. J. Respir. Dis.*, **62**, 69–71.
7. Selkon, J.B. (1969) 'Atypical' mycobacteria: a review. *Tubercle*, **50** (Suppl.), 70–8.
8. Edwards, F.G.B. (1970) Disease caused by 'atypical' (opportunist) mycobacteria: a whole population review. *Tubercle*, **51**, 285–95.
9. Marks, J. and Schwabacher, H. (1965) Infection due to *M. xenopi*. *Br. Med. J.*, **1**, 32–3.
10. Grange, J.M. and Yates, M.D. (1986) Infections caused by opportunist mycobacteria: a review. *J. Roy. Soc. Med.*, **79**, 226–9.
11. Wijsmuller, G. and Erickson, P. (1974) The reaction to PPD–Battey. A new look. *Am. Rev. Respir. Dis.*, **109**, 29–40.
12. Hyde, L. and Hyde, C.l. (1974) Skin testing with multiple PPD antigens in the differential diagnosis of mycobacterial disease. *Chest*, **66**, 108–9.
13. Banks, J., Hunter, A.M., Campbell, I.A. *et al.* (1983). Pulmonary infection with *Mycobacterium kansasii* in Wales, 1970–9: review of treatment and response. *Thorax*, **38**, 271–4.
14. Banks, J., Hunter, A.M., Campbell, I.A. *et al.* (1984) Pulmonary infection with *Mycobacterium xenopi*: a review of treatment and response. *Thorax*, **39**, 376–82.
15. Banks, J. Jenkins, P.A. and Smith, A.P. Pulmonary infection with *Mycobacterium malmoense* – a review of treatment and response. *Tubercle*, **66**, 197–203.
16. Hunter, A.M., Campbell, I.A., Jenkins, P.A. and Smith, A.P. (1981) Treatment of pulmonary infection caused by mycobacteria of the *Mycobacterium avium–intracellulare* complex. *Thorax*, **36**, 326–9.
17. Diagnostic Standards and Classification of Tuberculosis and other Mycobacterial Diseases, 14th edn. (1981). *Am. Rev. Respir. Dis.*, **123**, 343–58.
18. Harris, G.D., Johanson, W.G. Jr and Nicholson, D.P. (1975) Response to chemotherapy of pulmonary infection due to *Mycobacterium kansasii*. *Am. Rev. Respir. Dis.*, **112**, 31–6.
19. Ahn, C.H., Nash, D.R. and Hurst, G.A. (1976) Ventilatory defects in atypical mycobacteriosis, a comparison study with tuberculosis. *Am. Rev. Respir. Dis.*, **113**, 273–9.
20. Yamamoto, M., Ogura, Y., Sudo, K. and Hibino, S. (1967) Diagnostic criteria for disease caused by 'atypical' mycobacteria. *Am. Rev. Respir. Dis.*, **96**, 773–8.
21. Banks, J. (1988) Treatment of pulmonary disease caused by non-tuberculous mycobacteria. MD Thesis, University of Manchester.
22. Francis, P.B., Jay, S.J., Johanson, W.G. Jr (1975) The course of untreated *Mycobacterium kansasii* disease. *Am. Rev. Respir. Dis.*, **111**, 477–87.
23. Cook, P.L., Riddell. R.W. and Simon, G. (1971) Bacteriological and radiographic features of lung infection by opportunist mycobacteria; A review. *Tubercle*, **52**, 232–41.
24. Seibert, C.E and Tabrisky, J. (1969) Radiological features of pulmonary atypical mycobacterial infections. *Br. J. Radiol.*, **42**, 140–4.
25. Anderson, D.H., Grech, P., Townsend, R.H. and Jephcott, A.E. (1975) Pulmonary lesions due to opportunist mycobacteria [review includes 30 cases of *M. kansasii* infections]. *Clin. Radiol.*, **26**, 461–9.
26. Tsukamura, M. (1975) Roentgenographic features of lung disease due to *Mycobacterium intracellulare* (Primary and secondary infection). *Kekkaku*, **50**, 17–30.
27. Zvetina, J.R., Demos, T.C., Maliwan, N., *et al.* (1984) Pulmonary cavitations in *Mycobacterium kansasii*: Distinctions from *M. tuberculosis. Am. J. Radiol.* **143**, 127–30.
28. Albelda, S.M., Kern, J.A., Marinelli, D.L. and Miller, W.T. (1985) Expanding spectrum of pulmonary disease caused by nontuberculous mycobacteria. *Radiology*, **157**, 289–96.

29. Wolinsky, E. (1979) Nontuberculous mycobacteria and associated diseases. *Am. Rev. Respir. Dis.*, **119**, 107–59.

30. Greene, J.B., Siou, G.S., Lewin, S. *et al.* (1982) *Mycobacterium avium-intracellulare*: A cause of disseminated life-threatening infection in homosexuals and drug abusers. *Ann. Intern. Med.*, **97**, 539–46.

31. Wong. B., Edwards, F.F., Kiehn, T.E. *et al.* (1985) Continuous high-grade *Mycobacterium avium-intracellulare* bacteraemia in patients with the acquired immunodeficiency syndrome. *Am. J. Med.*, **78**, 35–40.

32. Fainstein, V., Bolivar, R., Mavlight, G. *et al.* (1982) Disseminated infection due to *Mycobacterium avium-intracellulare* in a homosexual man with Kaposi's sarcoma. *J. Infect. Dis.*, **145**, 586.

33. Small, C.B., Klein, R.S., Friedland, G.H. *et al.* (1983) Community-acquired opportunistic infections and defective cellular immunity in heterosexual drug abusers and homosexual men. *Am. J. Med.*, **74**, 433–41.

34. Zakowski, P., Fligiel, S., Berlin, G.W. and Johnson, B.L. Jr (1982) Disseminated *Mycobacterium avium-intracellulare* infection in homosexual men dying of acquired immunodeticiency. *J. Am. Med. Assoc.*, **248**, 2980–2.

35. Horsburgh, C.R. Jr, Mason, U.G., Farhi, D.C. and Iseman, M.D. (1985) Disseminated infection with *Mycobacterium avium-intracellulare*. A report of 13 cases and a review of the literature. *Medicine*, **64**, 36–48.

36. Marinelli, D.L., Albelda, S.M., Williams, T.M. *et al.* (1986) Nontuberculous mycobacterial infection in AIDS: clinical, pathologic, and radiographic features. *Radiology*, **160**, 77–82.

37. Prissick, F.H. and Masson, A.M. (1956) Cervical lymphadenitis in children caused by chromogenic mycobacteria. *Canad. Med. Assoc. J.*, **75**, 798–803.

38. MacKellar, A. (1976) Diagnosis and management of atypical mycobacterial lymphadenitis in children. *J. Paediatr. Surg.*, **11**, 85–9.

39. Wallace, R.J., Musser, J.M., Hull, S.I. *et al.* (1989) Diversity and sources of rapidly growing mycobacteria associated with infections following cardiac surgery. *J. Infect. Dis.*, **159**, 708–16.

40. Hanson, P., Thomas, J. and Collins, J. (1987) *Mycobacterium chelonei* and abscess formation in soft tissues. *Tubercle*, **68**, 297–9.

41. Wallace, R.J. Jr, Swenson, J.M., Silcox, V.A. *et al.* (1983) Spectrum of disease due to rapidly growing mycobacteria. *Rev. Infect. Dis.*, **5**, 657–79.

42. Rappaport, W., Dunington, G., Norton, L. *et al* (1990). The surgical management of atypical mycobacterial soft-tissue infections. *Surgery*, **108**, 36–9.

43. Greenberg, A.E. and Kupka, E. (1957) Swimming pool injuries, mycobacteria, and tuberculosis like disease. *Publ. Hlth. Rep.*, **72**., 902.

44. Meyers, W.M., Shelly, W.M., Connor, D.H. and Meyers, E.K. (1974) Human *Mycobacterium ulcerans* infections developing at sites of trauma to skin. *J. Trop. Med. Hyg.*, **23**, 91.

45. Rosenzweig, D.Y. (1979) Pulmonary mycobacterial infections due to *Mycobacterium intracellulare-avium* complex. *Chest*, **75**, 115–19.

46. Lester, W., Jr, Botkin, J. and Colton, R. (1958) An analysis of forty-nine cases of pulmonary disease caused by photochromogenic mycobacteria. *Trans.17th Conf.Chemother.Tuberc. V A Armed Forces*, Cleveland, Ohio, pp. 289–97.

47. Jenkins, D.E., Bahar, D., Chofnos, I., Foster, R. *et al.* (1959). The clinical problem of infection with atypical acid-fast bacilli. *Trans. Am. Clin. Climat. Assoc.*, **71**, 21–33.

48. Christianson, L.C. and Dewlett, H.J. (1960) Pulmonary disease in adults associated with unclassified mycobacteria. *Am. J. Med.*, **29**, 980–91.

49. Phillips, S., Larkin, J.C. Jr (1964) Atypical pulmonary tuberculosis caused by unclassified mycobacteria. *Ann. Intern. Med.*, **60**, 401–8.

50. Corpe, R.F., Runyon, E.H. and Lester, W. (1963) Status of disease due to unclassified mycobacteria. A statement of the subcommittee on unclassified mycobacteria of the committee on therapy. *Am. Rev. Respir. Dis.*, **87**, 459–61.

51. Pfuetze, K.H., Vo, L.V., Reimann, A.F. *et al.* (1965) Photochromogenic mycobacterial pulmonary disease. *Am. Rev. Respir. Dis.*, **92**, 470–5.

52. Pfuetze, K.M., Nuchprayoon, C.V., Berg, G.S. and Pamintuan, R. (1966) Present status of open negative cavities due to photochromogenic mycobacteria among co-operative patients. *Am. Rev. Respir. Dis.*, **94**, 467.

53. Lester, W. (1966) Unclassified mycobacterial disease. *Ann. Rev. Med.*, **17**, 351–60.

54. Campbell, I.A. for BTS Research Committee. BTS study of treatment of *M. kansasii* (1993) *Thorax* (Abstract) (in press).

55. Corpe, R.F. (1981) Surgical management of pulmonary disease due to *Mycobacterium avium-intracellulare*. *Rev. Infect. Dis.*, **3**, 1064–7.

56. Moran, J.F., Alexander, L.G., Staub, E.W. *et al.* (1983) Long-term results of pulmonary resection for atypical mycobacterial disease. *Ann. Thoracic Surg.*, **35**, 597–604.

57. Engbaek, H.C., Vergmann, B. and Bentzon, M.W. (1984) A prospective study of lung disease caused by *Mycobacterium avium/ Mycobacterium intracellulare*. *Eur. J. Respir. Dis.*, **65**, 411–18.

58. Etzkorn, E.T., Aldarondo, S., McAllister, C.K. et al. (1986) Medical therapy of *Mycobacterium avium-intracellulare* pulmonary disease. *Am. Rev. Respir. Dis.*, **134**, 442–45.

59. Horsburgh, C.R. Jr, Mason, U.G. III, Heifets, L.B. *et al.* (1987) Response to therapy of pulmonary *Mycobacterium avium-intracellulare* infection correlates with results of *in vitro* susceptibility testing. *Am. Rev. Respir. Dis.*, **135**, 418–21.

60. Tsukamura M., Ichiyama, S. and Takuaya, M. (1989) Superiority of enviomycin or streptomycin over ethambutol in initial treatment of lung disease caused by *Mycobacterium avium* complex. *Chest*, **95**, 1056–8.

61. Yaeger, H. Jr, and Raleigh, J.W. (1973) Pulmonary disease due to *Mycobacterium intracellulare*. *Am. Rev. Respir. Dis.*, **108**, 547–52.

62. Lester, T.W. (1979) Drug-resistant and atypical mycobacterial disease. Bacteriology and treatment. *Arch. Intern. Med.*, **139**, 1399–401.

63. Lester, W., Moulding, T., Fraser, R.I., McClatchy, K. *et al.* (1969) Quintuple drug regimens in the treatment of Battey-type infections. *Trans. 28th Pulm. Dis. Res. Conf. VA Armed Forces*, Cleveland, Ohio, p. 83.

64. Smith, M.J. and Citron, K.M. (1983) Clinical review of pulmonary disease caused by *Mycobacterium xenopi*. *Thorax*, **38**, 373–7.

65. Thibier, R., Vivien, J.N. and Lepeuple, A. (1970) Sept cas de pleuropneumopathie a 'Mycobacterium xenopi, *Rev. Tuberc. Pneumol.*, **34**, 623–5.

66. Parrot, R.G. and Grosset, J.H. (1988) Postsurgical outcome of 57 patients with *Mycobacterium xenopi* pulmonary infection. *Tubercle*, **69**, 47–55.

67. France, A.J., McLeod, D.T., Calder, M.A. and Seaton, A. (1987) *Mycobacterium malmoense* infections in Scotland: an increasing problem. *Thorax*, **42**, 593–5.

68. Burns, D.N., Rohatgi, P.K., Rosenthal, R. *et al.* (1990) Disseminated *Mycobacterium fortuitum* successfully treated with combination therapy including ciprofloxacin. *Am. Rev. Respir. Dis.*, **142**, 468–70.

69. Yew W.W., Kwan, S.Y.L., Wong, P.C. and Lee, J. (1990) Ofloxacin and imipenem in the treatment of *Mycobacterium fortuitum* and *Mycobacterium chelonae* lung infections. *Tubercle*, **71**, 131–3.

70. Wallace, R.J. Jr, Bedsole, G., Sumter, G., *et al.* (1990) Activities of ciprofloxacin and ofloxacin against rapidly growing mycobacteria with demonstration of acquired resistance following single-drug therapy. *Antimicrob. Agents Chemother.*, **34**, 65–70.

71. Young, L.S. *Mycobacterium avium* complex infection. (1988) *J. Infect. Dis.*, **157**, 863–7.

72. Young, L.S., Wiviott, L., Wu M. *et al.* (1991) Azithromycin for treatment of *Mycobacterium avium-intracellulare* complex infection in patients with AIDS. *Lancet*, **338**, 1107–9.

73. Dautzenberg, B., Truffot, C., Legris, S. (1991) Activity of clarithromycin against *Mycobacterium avium* infection in patients with the acquired immune deficiency syndrome. *Am. Rev. Respir. Dis.*, **144**, 564–9.

74. Black, M.M. and Eykyn, S.J. (1977) The successful treatment of tropical fish tank granuloma (*Mycobacterium marinum*) with co-trimoxazole. *Br. J. Dermatol.*, **97**, 689.

75. Izumi, A.K., Hanke, C.W. and Higaki, M. (1977) *Mycobacterium marinum* infections treated with tetracycline. *Arch. Dermatol.*, **113**, 1067.

76. Glynn, P.J. (1972) The use of surgery and local temperature elevation in *Mycobacterium ulcerans* infection. *Aust. NZ J. Surg.*, **41**, 312.

77. Marks, J. (1976) A system for the examination of tubercle bacilli and other mycobacteria. *Tubercle*, **57**, 207–25.

78. Middlebrook, G. (1954) Isoniazid resistance and catalase activity of tubercle bacilli. *Am. Rev. Tuberc.*, **69**, 471–2.

79. Dunbar, F.P., McAllister, E. and Jeffries, M.B. (1959) Catalase and peroxidase activation of isoniazid-susceptible and resistant strains of *Mycobacterium tuberculosis*. *Am. Rev. Tuberc.*, **79**, 669–71.

80. Youatt, J. (1969) A review of the action of isoniazid. *Am. Rev. Respir. Dis.*, **99**, 729–49.

81. Djurovic, V., DeCroix, G. and Daumet, P. (1973) L'ethambutol chez l'homme. Etude

comparative des taux seriques erythrocytaires et pulmonaires. *Nouv. Presse Med.*, **2**, 2815–16.

82. Johnson, J.D., Hand, W.L., Francis, J.B. *et al.* (1980) Antibiotic uptake by alveolar macrophages. *J. Lab. Clin. Med.*, **95**, 429–39.

83. Liss, R.H. (1983) Antimycobacterial activity of ethambutol in human pulmonary mononuclear phagocytes. *Prax. Klin. Pneumol.*, **37**, 485–6.

84. Crowle, A.J., Sbarbaro, J.A., Judson, F.N. and May, M.H. (1985) The effect of ethambutol on tubercle bacilli within cultured human macrophages. *Am. Rev. Respir. Dis.*, **132**, 742–5.

85. Ellner, J.J., Goldberger, M.J. and Parenti, D.M. (1991) *Mycobacterium avium* infection and AIDS: A therapeutic dilemma in rapid evolution. *J. Infect. Dis.*, **163**, 1326–35.

86. Tsang, A.Y., Bentz, R.R., Schork, M.A. and Sodeman, T.M. (1978) Combined vs single drug studies of susceptibilities of *Mycobacterium kansasii* to isoniazid, streptomycin and ethambutol. *Am. J. Clin. Pathol.*, **138**, 816–20.

87. Zimmer, B.L., DeYoung, D.R. and Roberts, G.D. (1982) *In vitro* synergistic activity of ethambutol, isoniazid, kanamycin, rifampicin, and streptomycin against *Mycobacterium avium-intracellulare* complex. *Antimicrob. Agents Chemother.*, **22**, 148–50.

88. Nash, D.R. and Steingrube, V.A. (1982) Selecting drug combinations for treatment of drug-resistant mycobacterial diseases. *J. Clin. Pharmacol.*, **22**, 297–300.

89. Heifets, L.B. (1982) Synergistic effect of rifampicin, streptomycin, ethionamide, and ethambutol on *Mycobacterium intracellulare*. *Am. Rev. Respir. Dis.*, **125**, 43–8.

90. Kuze, F. (1984) Experimental chemotherapy in chronic *Mycobacterium avium-intracellulare* infection of mice. *Am. Rev. Respir. Dis.*, **129**, 453–9.

91. Banks, J. and Jenkins, P.A. (1987) Combined versus single antituberculosis drugs on the *in vitro* sensitivity patterns of non-tuberculous mycobacteria. *Thorax*, **42**, 838–42.

92. Hoffner, S.E., Svenson, S.B. and Kallenium, G. (1987) Synergistic effects of antimycobacterial drug combinations on *Mycobacterium avium* complex determined radiometrically in liquid medium. *Eur. J. Clin. Microbiol.*, **6**, 530–5.

93. Sippel, A. and Hartmann, G. (1968) Mode of action of rifampicins on the RNA polymerase reaction. *Biochim. Biophys. Acta*, **157**, 218–19.

94. Wehrli, W., Knusel, F., Schmid, K. and Staehelin, M. (1968) Interaction of rifamycin with bacterial RNA polymerase. *Proc. Natl. Acad. Sci. USA*, **61**, 667–73.

95. Tsukamura, M. (1972) The pattern of resistance development to rifampicin in *Mycobacterium tuberculosis*. *Tubercle*, **53**, 111–17.

96. Hui, J., Gordon, N. and Kajioka, R. (1977) Permeability barrier to rifampicin in mycobacteria. *Antimicrob. Agents Chemother.*, **11**, 773–9.

97. Kilburn, J.O. and Greenberg, J. (1977) Effect of ethambutol on the viable cell count in *Mycobacterium smegmatis*. *Antimicrob. Agents Chemother.*, **11**, 534–40.

98. Takayama, K., Armstrong, E.L., Kunugi, K.A. and Kilburn, K.O. (1979) Inhibition by ethambutol of mycolic acid transfer into the cell wall of *Mycobacterium smegmatis*. *Antimicrob. Agents Chemother.*, **16**, 240–2.

PREVENTION 14

PREVENTIVE THERAPY FOR TUBERCULOSIS

14a

R.J. O'Brien

14a.1 INTRODUCTION

In both developed and developing countries, a significant proportion of tuberculosis cases arise from the pool of persons with remote infection with *Mycobacterium tuberculosis*. In the USA and other developed countries where tuberculosis rates are low and the majority of cases are in older persons, it is estimated that approximately 90% of tuberculosis cases occur in those infected more than 1 year previously. With nearly 2 billion of the world's population infected with the tubercle bacillus, the potential for continued disease and transmission is enormous.

Among the intervention and control measures that could significantly decrease current tuberculosis morbidity, preventive chemotherapy, i.e. treatment of infected persons to prevent the development of active disease, is of great importance. Even if other well-established tuberculosis control measures were fully available and fully effective, tuberculosis cases would continue to occur well into the future as new cases continued to develop among persons previously infected. A highly effective vaccine would protect only those who were not earlier infected. Aggressive case detection and prompt treatment of infectious cases certainly reduces tuberculosis transmission but does not prevent new cases arising from endogenous reinfection.

With the introduction of isoniazid for the treatment of tuberculosis in 1952, preventive therapy became a possibility. The drug was safe, inexpensive and could be given orally without supervision. After animal studies indicated that the drug was effective as a chemoprophylactic, large-scale preventive therapy, clinical trials demonstrated its efficacy in man. In spite of the theoretical benefit of preventive therapy for tuberculosis and its proven efficacy, this intervention measure has never gained widespread acceptance outside developed countries, particularly in North America. However, several factors appear to have rekindled interest in this intervention method.

The first is the shortening of tuberculosis treatment with 6-month chemotherapy regimens using isoniazid, rifampicin and pyrazinamide ('short-course' chemotherapy or SCC). In a number of SCC studies, drugs were administered twice or three times weekly, either throughout the entire treatment period or following an initial period of daily therapy. The results of these studies suggest that preventive therapy may be similarly shortened and perhaps given intermittently. The second factor is the epidemic of HIV infection resulting in significant increases in tuberculosis in areas where HIV and tuberculosis co-infection is common. It has become apparent that the only presently

Clinical Tuberculosis. Edited by P.D.O. Davies. Published in 1994 by Chapman & Hall, London. ISBN 0 412 48630 X

available intervention method that might reduce the occurrence of HIV-associated tuberculosis is preventive therapy of co-infected persons.

This chapter will review the scientific basis for preventive therapy, detail its limitations and outline recommendations for its use in both developed and developing countries. The focus will be on isoniazid preventive therapy; however, some emphasis will be given to rifampicin-containing regimens that are currently under investigation. Throughout the chapter, the term 'preventive therapy' will be used. Although the word 'chemoprophylaxis' has commonly been used to designate this intervention, the administration of a drug to prevent the progression of latent infection to clinical disease is not truly chemoprophylaxis.

14a.2 SCIENTIFIC BASIS FOR PREVENTIVE THERAPY

14a.2.1 ISONIAZID

Before clinical trials of isoniazid preventive therapy were begun in the USA, its efficacy in guinea-pigs was demonstrated. In a large study conducted by the US Public Health Service, guinea-pigs receiving varying doses of isoniazid were challenged with virulent tubercle bacilli[1]. Those animals receiving a daily dose of at least 5 mg/kg were protected, i.e. survival was comparable with control animals who were not challenged with the bacillus. On the basis of these studies, the dose of 5 mg/kg was chosen for clinical studies in man. These animal studies also demonstrated that infection was partially but incompletely protective against rechallenge by the organism.

The results of a large number of randomized placebo-controlled clinical trials of isoniazid preventive therapy have been summarized by Ferebee[2]. The description of these studies and results are given in Tables 14a.1 and 14a.2. The studies were conducted in seven countries, both deve-

loped and developing, and involved over 100 000 participants at risk of tuberculosis, including children with primary tuberculosis, contacts of active cases, tuberculin skin test convertors, institutionalized patients with mental disease, and persons with inactive tuberculosis. The outcomes measured in these studies included progression of primary tuberculosis, tuberculin conversion in uninfected contacts, prevention of disease in infected persons, and recurrence of disease.

In these studies the effectiveness of preventive therapy, as measured by the decrease in disease among all persons participating in these trials, varied between 25 and 92%. However, when analysis was restricted to persons who were apparently compliant with medication, the protective efficacy appeared to be in the order of 90%. Substantial protection was conferred even if pill-taking was irregular but sustained, suggesting the possibility that intermittent isoniazid preventive therapy may be efficacious.

While the mechanism of preventive therapy is not known, it is assumed that administration of isoniazid results in sterilization of infection and elimination of organisms from infected persons. On the basis of skin test reversions among newly infected persons given isoniazid preventive therapy, this mechanism has been inferred[3].

Studies in Alaska indicated that the maximal effect was achieved by between 6 and 12 months of isoniazid and that there was no advantage to extending treatment beyond 1 year[4] (Fig. 14a.1). Follow-up studies have shown that the duration of protection in areas where the rate of new infection is low is at least 19 years[5], indicating that protection may be life-long. The results of a large placebo-controlled isoniazid preventive therapy study in seven eastern European countries sponsored by the International Union Against Tuberculosis (IUAT) have suggested that treatment for less than 1 year is effective[6]. In this study of infected persons with fibrotic lesions on chest radiograph, 6

Table 14a.1 Summary of results of controlled trials of prescribing isoniazid to prevent manifest tuberculosis

Type of subjects	No.	Outcome	Years of observation	% reduction
Children with primary tuberculosis, USA	2750	Tuberculous complications	10	88
Children with primary tuberculosis, France	2970	Tuberculous complications	3–10	64
Household contacts to old cases, USA	2814	Tuberculous disease	4	54
Household contacts to new cases, USA	27 847	Tuberculous disease	10	60
Household contacts to new cases, Japan	2238	Tuberculous disease	1	30
Household contacts, Kenya	764	Positive bacteriology	3	80
Household contacts, Philippines	327	Abnormal chest radiographs	2	41
Shipboard contacts, Netherlands	261	Tuberculous disease	7	92
Railway workers, Japan	548	Tuberculous disease	6–12	62
Greenland villagers	8801	Tuberculous disease	6	31
Alaskan villagers	6064	Positive bacteriology	6	59
Tunisian villagers, urban residents	15 910	Positive bacteriology	1	25
Mental institutions, USA	25 210	Tuberculous disease	10	62
Alaskan schools	1670	Tuberculous disease	6–10	67

Table 14a.2 Summary of results of controlled trials of prescribing isoniazid to prevent reactivation of previously untreated inactive disease

Source of subjects	No.	Outcome	Years of observation	% reduction
Mental institutions, New York State	513	Active tuberculosis	6	43
Health Departments, USA	1992	Active tuberculosis	5	60
Chest clinic patients, India	317	Positive bacteriology	6	83
Chest clinic patients, Canada	2405	Active tuberculosis	7–13	53
Veterans hospitals, USA	2389	Positive bacteriology	5	59

months of therapy conferred substantial protection against recurrence of disease (Fig. 14a.2). Among those persons with small lesions, 6 months and 12 months of therapy were associated with equivalent protection.

Preliminary results have been reported from a placebo-controlled study of daily isoniazid preventive therapy for 6 months among adults with HIV infection in Zambia[7]. In this trial no tuberculin skin testing was done, and persons were entered after exclusion of clinically active tuberculosis. After approximately 1 year of follow-up, 1% of those receiving isoniazid had developed tuberculosis compared with 14% of those receiving placebo. However, there was no significant difference in mortality at 1 year, and with increased follow-up the pro-

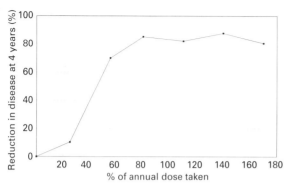

Fig. 14a.1 Alaska village isoniazid preventive therapy studies: reduction in tuberculosis by amount of isoniazid taken. (Adapted from G.W. Comstock and F.H. Ferebee, *Am. Rev. Respir. Dis.*, 1970, **101**, 780–2.

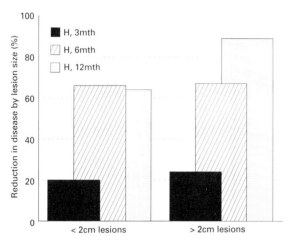

Fig. 14a.2 IUAT trial of isoniazid preventive therapy: reduction in tuberculosis by duration of therapy and lesion size. (Adapted from IUAT Committee on Prophylaxis, *Bull. WHO*, 1982, **60**, 555–64.)

tective efficacy of isoniazid seemed to be lessened. Whether this is due to a failure of isoniazid to eradicate dormant bacilli or to new infection after cessation of preventive therapy is not known. Apparent failure of isoniazid preventive therapy in HIV infection

was noted in a single case report from the USA[8].

14a.2.2 RIFAMPICIN AND OTHER DRUGS

In early studies of rifampicin in a mouse model of disease, Grumbach and Rist showed that rifampicin had greater sterilizing activity than isoniazid[9]. Furthermore, resistance to rifampicin developed more slowly than to isoniazid. More recent studies of the sterilizing properties of rifampicin, isoniazid and pyrazinamide in a mouse model of chronic tuberculosis demonstrated the superiority of rifampicin and rifampicin combined with pyrazinamide[10]. In this study, rifampicin alone for 2 or 3 months and rifampicin plus pyrazinamide for 2 months were more effective than isoniazid alone for 6 months. Moreover, the addition of isoniazid to the rifampicin/pyrazinamide regimen appeared to have an inhibiting effect on sterilizing activity. The only regimen consistently to result in sterilization at the end of the treatment period was the 2-month regimen of rifampicin plus pyrazinamide. Subsequent studies by these investigators suggested pharmacological antagonism between isoniazid and rifampicin leading to lower rifampicin levels and thus reduced efficacy[11]. The significance of these findings in mice for tuberculosis prevention in man is unclear.

In a study by Japanese investigators of another mouse model of chronic infection, employing a streptomycin-dependent strain of tubercle bacilli that had been starved of the antibiotic, the superiority of rifampicin over isoniazid as a sterilizing agent was also demonstrated[12].

Mitchison and co-workers[13,14] have provided evidence for a model of drug action in which isoniazid provides a rapid kill of the largest portion of bacteria, i.e. those that are extracellular and rapidly metabolizing, in the first few days of therapy. However, according to this model, rifampicin and pyrazinamide subsequently provide for the final sterilization of tissue, killing the slowly and/or intermittently metabolizing bacilli, including those within macrophages, the probable site of tubercle bacilli in infected persons without disease. It is likely that the effect of drugs in the sterilizing phase of short-course therapy would be similar to their effect when given as preventive therapy. In Mitchison's model, the effect of pyrazinamide is achieved during the first 8 weeks of therapy, while rifampicin appears to have an important effect throughout the entire course of therapy.

Short-course chemotherapy of less than 6 months has proved to be inadequate for the treatment of bacteriologically confirmed disease[15,16]. However, 2- and 3-month therapy regimens of isoniazid, rifampicin, pyrazinamide and streptomycin were shown to be 86% and 93% effective, respectively, in the treatment of individuals whose chest radiographs indicated active disease but whose sputum smears and cultures were negative for *M. tuberculosis*[17]. Other studies of 6-month short-course therapy have suggested that streptomycin does not contribute greatly to the sterilizing activity of rifampicin and pyrazinamide. However, streptomycin does increase the rate of adverse reactions and is associated with an increase in patient non-compliance[18].

A recent placebo-controlled study of daily preventive therapy among silicotic patients in Hong Kong suggested that the rifampicin alone for 3 months was of comparable efficacy to 3 months of rifampicin plus isoniazid and isoniazid alone for 6 months[19]. Compared with placebo, the reductions in culture-confirmed tuberculosis at 5 years were 63% for 3 months of rifampicin, 48% for 6 months of isoniazid, and 41% for 3 months of rifampicin and isoniazid. The difference among the active regimens was not statistically significant.

The largest published experience with rifampicin preventive therapy involved infected children at high risk of tuberculosis living in Blackburn, England[20]. In this report, the administration of either a 9-month or a 6-month regimen of rifampicin/isoniazid to 339 children was associated with a significant decrease in the incidence of childhood tuberculosis in the community.

Of new antimycobacterial agents, several new compounds related to rifampicin may be highly effective as tuberculosis preventive therapy[21]. Two of these, rifapentine and rifabutin, are of particular interest. Rifapentine is a cyclopentyl rifamycin derivative with a long half-life and good activity against *M. tuberculosis*. In studies in mice, rifapentine administered once weekly appeared as active as daily rifampicin[22]. Rifabutin, a spiro-piperidyl-rifamycin, has recently been approved in the USA for the prophylaxis for *M. avium* complex in severely immuno-compromised persons with HIV infection[23]. Its activity against *M. tuberculosis* is comparable with rifampicin, and its long half-life and high tissue levels suggest that it may be an effective chemoprophylactic drug. Recent studies in an animal model of chronic tuberculosis infection have indicated that these two agents given intermittently may be as effective as daily rifampicin (B. Ji, personal communication). Among the new quinolone antibiotics with antimycobacterial activity, sparfloxacin has been found to have excellent sterilizing activity in mice, comparable with rifampicin and isoniazid[24]. This drug may also be useful for preventive therapy.

Clinical studies of these new drugs that might shed light on their usefulness in preventive therapy are limited. However, placebo-controlled clinical studies of rifabutin in the USA have demonstrated this drug's usefulness in preventing disseminated *M. avium* complex disease in severely immuno-compromised patients with HIV infection[25]. In these studies, which involved over 500 participants, three cases of tuberculosis occurred among those receiving placebo treatment, but none among those receiving the active drug (P. Olliaro, personal communication). Because of this drug's long half-life and high tissue and macrophage levels, it may be an excellent agent for preventive therapy, especially in regimens given intermittently.

14a.3 LIMITATIONS

14a.3.1 TOXICITY

In 1965, when isoniazid was first recommended in the USA for preventive therapy for infected persons at risk of tuberculosis, it was believed to be remarkably free of serious toxicity. In the US Public Health Service studies among tuberculosis contacts, percentages of persons stopping treatment for suspected drug reactions were low and approximately equivalent for the placebo and isoniazid groups[2]. While rates of adverse reactions were more common among both placebo and isoniazid groups in the studies of persons with inactive tuberculosis, no type of reaction appeared to be more common in the isoniazid group. The occurrence of hepatitis was a rare event, not thought to be due to isoniazid.

Reports in the late 1960s suggested that isoniazid caused hepatitis and studies indicated that asymptomatic increase in hepatic transaminases occurred among persons receiving the drug[26]. However, it was not until the occurrence of several deaths from hepatitis among persons receiving isoniazid preventive therapy in the early 1970s that the potential of isoniazid hepatitis was appreciated[27].

The largest and most comprehensive study of isoniazid hepatitis was conducted by the US Public Health Service during 1971–1972[28]. In this survey nearly 14 000 persons receiving isoniazid preventive therapy were monitored for the development of hepatitis. The overall rate of probable isoniazid hepatitis was 1% but was clearly age-related, with no cases occurring among those under 20 years and the highest rate of 2.3% among

those over 50 years. An association of hepatitis was also seen with alcohol consumption, with rates being four times higher among those consuming alcohol daily than among those who did not drink. Rates among males and females were equivalent. Rates were lower among Blacks and higher among Asians compared with rates among Whites. Hepatitis rates were much lower among participants in the IUAT trial, although the same positive association with age was seen[6].

In the US Public Health Service surveillance study, a total of eight deaths from hepatitis occurred among the participants, seven of those among persons living in Baltimore. Several years after completion of the study a review of death certificates showed a marked increase in deaths from cirrhosis during 1972 in Baltimore and surrounding counties, suggesting that a cofactor may have been responsible for the cluster of deaths see in the study[29].

Estimates of hepatitis morbidity and mortality from this study have commonly been used for cost–benefit analyses. Subsequently, recommendations for the USA excluded the low-risk tuberculin reactor over age 35 from preventive therapy and recommended issuance of no more than 1 month's drug supply at a time, together with monthly questioning and education about signs and symptoms of hepatitis. Although isoniazid-associated hepatitis deaths continue to be reported sporadically, it is probable that in many, if not the majority of cases the guidelines for monitoring have not been followed[30]. A more recent analysis of isoniazid-associated hepatitis deaths in the USA found that women may be at increased risk of death and suggested that guidelines on administration of isoniazid preventive therapy for women may require revision[31]. Other reports have suggested that the risk of isoniazid hepatitis may be increased by the administration of the drug to pregnant women in the third trimester and the immediate postpartum period[32] and by the concomitant administration of acetaminophen [33]. There is also evidence from animal studies supporting increased hepatotoxicity by the combination of isoniazid and acetaminophen[34].

Of other effects of isoniazid, the occurrence of peripheral neuritis secondary to isoniazid-induced pyridoxine (vitamin B6) deficiency may be avoided by the administration of supplemental pyridoxine. However, this is recommended only for persons whose diet may be deficient and persons with diseases known to be associated with peripheral neuropathies[35]. Other possible effects of isoniazid, such as effects on mental activity and its carcinogenic potential, have been evaluated carefully, and no serious long-term consequences have been demonstrated[2]. Furthermore, there is no apparent adverse effect on the fetus if a pregnant woman receives isoniazid during pregnancy[36].

Rifampicin is thought to have less hepatotoxic potential than isoniazid but may be more frequently associated with less serious adverse effects, such as nausea and pruritus. In the Hong Kong study of tuberculosis preventive therapy in persons with silicosis, hepatotoxic reactions were noted among those receiving isoniazid but were not reported among those receiving rifampicin alone[19]. Furthermore, no increase in serum alanine aminotransferase was seen among those receiving rifampicin alone, in contrast to those receiving isoniazid.

Pilot studies of rifampicin alone and the combination of rifampicin and pyrazinamide for preventive therapy have been conducted in North America and Europe[37–39]. The results suggest safety and good tolerance of these regimens among both children and adults in Europe[38,39]. However, in the North American studies, hepatotoxic reactions, as well as elevations in hepatic transaminases, were significantly greater among adults allocated to the 2-month rifampicin–pyrazinamide regimen than among those receiving either rifampicin

alone for 4 months or isoniazid for 6 months[37]. On the other hand, excellent tolerability with a 2-month regimen of rifampicin and pyrazinamide given twice weekly to adults with HIV infection in Haiti has been suggested[40].

In general, little is known about the tolerability and toxicity of new drugs that might be used for preventive therapy. An exception, however, is rifabutin, which had an excellent safety profile in placebo-controlled studies of MAC prophylaxis[41]. Surprisingly, although there was a slight increase in arthralgia and myalgia in the active treatment group, no overall difference in adverse effects was seen among those significantly immunosuppressed patients receiving rifabutin. This finding suggests that the drug would also be well tolerated when given to persons who are not ill.

14a.3.2 COMPLIANCE

A major limitation to the effective use of tuberculosis preventive therapy is the requirement that an asymptomatic person takes medication for a relatively long period of time, in most cases to achieve a personal benefit that is marginal. The available studies and surveys indicate that noncompliance with preventive therapy is considerable. In the US Public Health Service isoniazid surveillance study, only 22% of patients collected all 12 monthly supplies of medication[28]. Data compiled by the Division of Tuberculosis Control at the Centers for Disease Control from tuberculosis programmes throughout the USA found that, in 1990, only 63% of persons begun on preventive therapy completed the prescribed course of treatment (D. Brown, personal communication). However, among contacts under the age of 15 years, the highest risk group, 76% completed.

In a study of compliance with isoniazid preventive therapy among Canadian Indians in Saskatchewan, only 5% of persons beginning treatment completed the 12-month course[42]. Education and a short period of directly supervised therapy had a modest but transient effect on compliance. Considering the large number of persons who were lost before beginning preventive therapy, only 2% of possible tuberculosis cases were prevented by this programme. Another study of isoniazid preventive therapy among prisoners in New York City suggested that education significantly improved compliance[43]. Provision of twice-weekly supervised isoniazid preventive therapy for men in a homeless shelter in the USA resulted in a completion rate of only 49%[44]. The authors concluded that this rate would probably be improved only by the availability of short drug regimens.

Other data from the USA indicate that provider compliance with recommendations on preventive therapy has decreased during the past decade, particularly in prescribing isoniazid for persons over the age of 15 years[45]. This phenomenon may be due in part to concerns about isoniazid hepatitis and to ongoing controversy in the USA over the age cut-off for preventive therapy for the low-risk tuberculin reactor[46,47].

It is also expected that compliance would be a limiting factor for the usefulness of this intervention for HIV-infected persons in developing countries. However, recent information from a study of the feasibility of isoniazid preventive therapy at an HIV voluntary testing site in Uganda indicates good compliance for persons who begin preventive therapy[48]. However, the major impediments to the wider use of preventive therapy in this setting are the lack of inexpensive and easily applied methods to identify HIV-infected persons who are also at higher risk of tuberculosis and mechanisms to provide preventive therapy to them safely and efficiently.

14a.3.3 DRUG RESISTANCE

Concern has been expressed about the possibility that isoniazid preventive therapy might induce resistance to isoniazid, particularly if the bacillary population were sufficiently large so that spontaneously resistant mutant bacilli were present. Data on drug resistance from the US Public Health Service studies indicate that among cases of tuberculosis developing among persons in the contact studies, isoniazid resistance was not more common among isoniazid recipients than among placebo recipients[2]. Among persons with inactive disease previously treated with isoniazid, there appeared to be a slight increase in isoniazid-resistant disease among preventive therapy patients.

The efficacy of isoniazid preventive therapy would be expected to be reduced if given to a population in which primary drug resistance to isoniazid is high. In a study of preventive therapy prescribed for 2795 South East Asian refugees in Seattle, isoniazid resistance was seen in seven of the 15 bacteriologically confirmed cases of tuberculosis arising in the 4 years following therapy[49]. Resistant disease was more frequently pulmonary than extrapulmonary and occurred more frequently among compliant persons, suggesting that isoniazid failed because of the existence of infection from isoniazid-resistant organisms rather than from acquired resistance during preventive therapy.

Based on decision analysis, rifampicin has been recommended for preventive therapy for persons infected by isoniazid-resistant organisms[50]. However, there have been no clinical trials of rifampicin preventive therapy for isoniazid-resistant infection, and a least one instance of failure of rifampicin preventive therapy with development of rifampicin resistance has been reported[51]. In the Hong Kong study, rifampicin resistance was not seen among those persons 'failing' the rifampicin alone regimen[19]. None the less, there is justifiable concern about the development of drug resistance when monotherapy is used, especially in persons with HIV infection. This concern stems from the difficulty in diagnosing active tuberculosis in HIV-infected persons, especially in settings where adequate facilities are limited, and the consequent possibility of recommending preventive monotherapy for persons with active disease. Furthermore, the unsupervised use of drugs might also lead to increases in drug-resistant tuberculosis. This consideration applies especially to rifampicin preventive therapy.

14a.3.4 REINFECTION

Another potential limitation to the use of preventive therapy is that it would not prevent disease associated with reinfection after the completion of treatment. While this concern is not of particular relevance in developed countries with very low annual rates of infection, it is an important consideration in countries with high rates. However, even in the latter situation, its use for infected persons with very high risks for disease (e.g. tuberculin reactors with HIV infection, infected children in households with infectious cases) may be indicated. In areas with high rates of tuberculosis infection (e.g. an annual risk of infection of 2% or more), life-long preventive therapy may be reasonable to consider for high-risk persons such as those with HIV infection. In such cases, this intervention would become true primary prophylaxis.

Obviously, widespread implementation of preventive therapy, as has been undertaken in North America, would only be considered in the context of efficient tuberculosis control programmes with effective case finding and high rates of completion of treatment of patients with disease. In such cases, an efficient programme should result in a significant decrease in the rate of infection.

14a.3.5 FEASIBILITY

Perhaps the most significant impediment to implementation of isoniazid preventive therapy is its cost and the requirement of an adequate infrastructure for provision of tuberculosis services. National programmes lacking the resources to provide modern chemotherapy (i.e. short-course therapy) for cases, could not consider a general preventive therapy programme. However, when resources are available for case finding and treatment, preventive therapy of high-risk persons, especially HIV-infected persons and children living in households with infectious patients, should be considered. In the latter instance, chemotherapy and preventive therapy would be given to members in the same household at the same time.

Cost-effectiveness analysis has been applied to the question of duration of isoniazid preventive therapy in the USA[52]. It was determined that the most cost-effective duration was 6 months, at a cost per case prevented of US$7112. These calculations used data on disease risk and expected reduction in disease from the IUAT preventive therapy trial. For persons having a greater risk of disease (e.g. persons with HIV infection), the cost-effectiveness would be much more favourable. In developing countries, preventive therapy is unlikely to be more cost-effective than case treatment of symptomatic persons, except possibly for HIV-infected persons and high-risk children [53].

A number of cost–benefit and cost-effectiveness analyses have been applied to the question of preventive therapy of infected adults with very low risks of tuberculosis and have come to varying conclusions about an appropriate age cut-off[46,47]. However, these analyses have little relevance to developing countries. The feasibility study in Uganda mentioned above is unique, in that it is the only one implemented directly to address the questions of cost, demand and sustainability.

14a.4 RECOMMENDATIONS

Because isoniazid preventive therapy administered daily is the only regimen that has been proven to be efficacious in controlled clinical trials, and because it is inexpensive and well tolerated, this drug is the agent commonly recommended for use in most circumstances. However, the data presented above suggest that tuberculosis preventive therapy employing other drugs with potent sterilizing properties, e.g. rifampicin and pyrazinamide, given together for periods as short as 2 months, may be more effective than single-drug therapy with isoniazid given for a much longer period of time. The studies also suggest that rifampicin alone may be more effective than isoniazid alone even when given for a shorter period of time.

Rifampicin is the only drug other than isoniazid that has been recommended for preventive therapy. Its advantages include its high sterilizing activity, in theory much more effective than isoniazid alone, the low level of adverse effects compared with isoniazid, and the low rate of primary resistance to rifampicin. However, there is a risk of adverse effects (immune reactions) if taken irregularly, its expense precludes its use in developing countries, and the optimal duration for administration of this drug is unknown. There is also the risk of the induction of acquired drug resistance when given to an unsuspected case of tuberculosis.

As intermittent therapy during the continuation (sterilizing) phase of therapy is as effective as daily therapy, the administration of intermittent preventive therapy (i.e. giving drugs twice weekly) would be expected to be as efficacious as daily preventive therapy. Providing for supervised therapy, decreasing drug costs and minimizing drug toxicity are potential advantages to intermittent preventive therapy.

The following combination regimens are being evaluated in clinical trials and may be recommended in the future.

(a) Rifampicin/isoniazid

There is clinical experience with this combination in a 4-month regimen of chemother-apy, and it has been used as preventive therapy in England. The use of more than one drug decreases the risk of acquired drug resistance, and tablets of the combined drugs are available. However, isoniazid hepatotoxicity is not avoided, and rifampicin may actually increase isoniazid hepatotoxicity[54].

(b) Rifampicin/pyrazinamide

As noted above, there is experimental evidence that these two drugs can be given for as short a period as 2 months with good sterilizing effect. This combination avoids the toxic effects of isoniazid and may be as effective for preventive therapy as the three-drug combination with isoniazid. However, this combination is also expensive and may have additive adverse effects as suggested by the results of the pilot studies in North America. A combined tablet is not currently available, and the safety of pyrazinamide in pregnancy has not been demonstrated.

(c) Rifampicin/pyrazinamide/isoniazid

This three-drug combination is currently the most effective combination for treating tuberculosis. A 2-month regimen has been found to be effective in preventing reactivation in patients with culture-negative pulmonary tuberculosis. A combined tablet is available, which makes administration simpler. If given to an unsuspected case of active tuberculosis, drug resistance is unlikely to develop. However, it is expensive, and there is potential additive toxicity from the three different drugs. Again, the safety of pyrazinamide in pregnancy has not been demonstrated.

14a.4.1 INDICATIONS

In countries with adequate resources for tuberculosis control and a well-functioning programme for case finding and treatment, highest priority for isoniazid preventive therapy should be given to persons with a positive tuberculin skin test reaction and any of the risk factors listed below. The appropriate criterion for defining a positive skin-test reaction depends on the likelihood of tuberculous infection and the risk of tuberculosis given infection[55]. For persons with HIV infection, close contacts of infectious cases and those with fibrotic lesions on chest radiograph, a reaction of ≥5 mm to 5 i.u is considered positive (see also Chapter 12a, Fig. 12a.5, p. 233). For other at-risk persons, a reaction of ≥10 mm is positive. For those persons at low risk of tuberculous infection, a reaction ≥15 mm is positive. For persons who have received BCG vaccination, higher cut-off points may be indicated. However, studies in developing countries have suggested that for persons with HIV infection, even in countries where BCG is commonly given, use of the 5 mm cut-off is appropriate[56]. The most important situation where the choice of the cut-off may vary is for young children who are household contacts to infectious cases. The World Health Organization currently recommends the use of a 5 mm cut-off regardless of a history of BCG vaccination (S. Spinaci, personal communication), while other authorities recommend higher cut-off points[57].

(a) Persons with TB/HIV co-infection

The annual risk of tuberculosis in a tuberculin-positive person with HIV infection may be as high as 8% per year[58], and the lifetime risk in a co-infected person may be 50% or more. Thus, the identification of persons with dual infection and the administration of preventive therapy to these persons is of great importance. Tuberculin skin testing is recommended for all persons with HIV infection, and those with PPD-tuberculin reactions of ≥5 mm should be considered for isoniazid preventive therapy after active tuberculosis has been excluded. However, anergy to PPD-tuberculin and to other delayed-type hypersensitivity skin test (DTH)

antigens may occur before signs and symptoms of HIV infection develop. DTH anergy becomes increasingly common as HIV infection progresses, making the diagnosis of tuberculous infection difficult. Anergy testing with two DTH skin-test antigens (*Candida albicans*, mumps or tetanus toxoid) in conjunction with tuberculin testing is now recommended to identify anergic persons at risk of tuberculosis[59]. Recent studies have shown that the risk of tuberculosis in anergic, HIV-infected injecting drug users in New York City approximates the risk of those who are tuberculin positive[60]. Thus, anergic persons with an estimated risk of tuberculous infection of ≥10% should be considered for isoniazid preventive therapy. However, there are no data supporting the routine use of isoniazid preventive therapy without tuberculin testing for persons with HIV infection in developing countries where HIV-associated tuberculosis is common, although this policy has been suggested. Interestingly, a recent cost–benefit analysis applied to injecting drug users in New York City recommends the routine use of isoniazid preventive therapy in selected persons at risk of both HIV and tuberculosis infections without either PPD or HIV testing[61].

(b) Household contacts of infectious cases

Household contacts of infectious (i.e. sputum smear-positive) cases are likely to have been recently infected and have a risk of developing tuberculosis of up to 5% during the 2 years following infection. The risk of disease, and especially for severe disease, for very young children is especially great. Therefore, tuberculin-positive contacts of infectious cases are candidates for preventive therapy[62,63]. In addition, young tuberculin-negative (<5 mm) children who have been in contact with an infectious case within the past 3 months are candidates for preventive therapy until a repeat tuberculin skin test is done 3 months after last contact with the infectious source. If the repeat skin test is positive (≥5 mm), therapy should be continued. If the reaction remains negative, therapy need not be continued unless there is continuing exposure to an infectious source-case. In programmes where skin testing is not available, the World Health Organization recommends isoniazid preventive therapy for all childhood contacts of infectious cases (S. Spinaci, personal communication).

(c) Recent tuberculin convertors

Persons who are being routinely screened for tuberculosis by tuberculin skin testing should be considered for preventive therapy if their skin test converts from negative to positive. An example would be a hospital worker with potential exposure to tuberculosis patients where the risk of tuberculosis given recent infection would be comparable with household contacts of infectious cases. Because of the problem of boosting of PPD reactions, conversion has been defined as an increase in reaction size of 10 mm for persons under age 35 years and of 15 mm for those 35 years and older[64].

(d) Persons with other medical risk factors

A number of medical conditions, in addition to HIV infection, have been reported to increase the risk of active tuberculosis in infected persons. The most important of these conditions and the estimate of risk for disease are given in Table 14a.3 [65]. Persons with these conditions who also have a positive skin test should be considered for preventive therapy. Other medicial risk factors for tuberculosis that have not been quantified include prolonged therapy with adrenocorticosteroids (e.g. the equivalent of at least 15 mg of prednisone daily for over 4 weeks), some haematological and reticuloendothelial diseases that are associated with suppressed cellular immunity (e.g. leukaemia and Hodg-

Table 14a.3 Risk factors for tuberculosis following infection

	Measurement of incidence	
Risk factor	Absolute/1000 person-years	Relative risk
Infection >7 years past	0.7	
Infection<1 year past	10.4	
HIV infection	79	
AIDS		170.3
Fibrotic lesion	2.0–13.6	
Silicosis		30
Immunosuppressive treatment		11.9
Haemodialysis		10–15
Gastrectomy		5
Jejunoileal bypass		27–63
Carcinoma of head or neck		16
Diabetes		2.0–3.6

Adapted from H.L. Rieder *et al.*, *Epidemiol. Rev.*, 1989, **11**, 79–98. Additional references for these data are given in the text.

kin's disease), and other conditions associated with substantial rapid weight loss or chronic undernutrition (e.g. chronic peptic ulcer disease, chronic malabsorption syndromes and chronic alcoholism). Persons injecting illicit drugs may also be at increased risk of tuberculosis even if not infected with HIV[66].

(e) Other indications

In addition, even in the absence of any identified risk factors, persons under 35 years of age in the following high-incidence groups are appropriate candidates for preventive therapy if their skin test is positive [64]. These include foreign-born persons from high-prevalence countries, medically underserved low-income populations, including high-risk racial or ethnic minority populations, residents of facilities for long-term care (e.g. correctional institutions, nursing homes and mental institutions), and the staff of facilities in which an individual with current tuberculosis would pose a risk to large numbers of susceptible persons (e.g. correctional institutions, nursing homes, mental institutions, other health-care facilities, schools and child-care facilities).

14a.4.2 SCREENING PROCEDURES

Before preventive therapy is started it is necessary to exclude bacteriologically positive or radiographically progressive tuberculosis. This is especially important for persons with HIV infection in whom the signs of tuberculosis may be atypical and extrapulmonary disease is common. A history should be taken to determine if medical conditions exist that might contraindicate the use of preventive therapy or mandate closer monitoring of preventive therapy. These include the history of severe adverse drug reactions, acute or active liver disease of any aetiology. Hepatitis B surface-antigen positivity is not a contraindication unless associated with chronic active hepatitis.

Special precautions are indicated for persons over age 35 years, those using alcohol daily and those with hepatic disease, the existence of peripheral neuropathy or of a condition such as diabetes mellitus or alcoholism, which might predispose to the development of neuropathy associated with isoniazid. Although no harmful effects of isoniazid to the fetus have been observed, preventive therapy generally should be delayed until after delivery, except for pregnant women likely to have been recently infected or with high-risk medical conditions, especially HIV infection. The safety of pyrazinamide in pregnancy has not been shown, and therefore this drug should not be used for preventive therapy in pregnant women.

14a.4.3 ADMINISTRATION

Isoniazid is used alone for preventive therapy and given in a single daily dose of 5 mg/kg body weight, not to exceed 300 mg per day. It is advisable to dispense isoniazid in monthly allotments. The minimal duration of treatment is 6 months, but 9 months has been recommended for children [67] and 12 months for those with HIV infection [68]. Persons who have an abnormal radiograph (i.e. stable parenchymal lesions or silicosis) should receive 12 months of therapy. For persons at especially high risk of tuberculosis whose adherence is questionable, supervised preventive therapy may be indicated, with isoniazid given twice weekly at the dose of 15 mg/kg.

The person receiving preventive therapy or a responsible adult in a household with children on preventive therapy should be questioned carefully, either in person or by telephone, at monthly intervals for symptoms or signs consistent with liver damage or other adverse effects. Up to 20% of individuals receiving isoniazid will develop some mild abnormality of liver function tests, which tend to resolve even if isoniazid is continued. Except for persons at increased risk of hepatic injury, routine liver function tests are not recommended; however, they are needed to evaluate signs and symptoms of adverse reactions.

There are occasional situations in which alternative forms of preventive therapy might be desirable. In the situation where there is confidence that the source case has isoniazid-resistant organisms, it appears reasonable to treat child contacts and those adult contacts who appear particularly susceptible to tuberculosis (e.g. immunocompromised hosts) with rifampicin [50]. Some clinicians would add a second drug, such as ethambutol, to which the organism is believed susceptible. The drug(s) should be given in standard therapeutic doses for 6 months; paediatric authorities recommend a 9-month treatment period for children. In situations in which there is less confidence that the infection is due to isoniazid-resistant organisms, isoniazid should be used.

In persons likely to have been infected with isoniazid-resistant organisms (e.g. immigrants and refugees from Asia), including rifampicin with isoniazid for preventive treatment may be considered. In persons likely to have been infected with bacilli resistant to both isoniazid and rifampicin, observation without preventive therapy has usually been recommended, because no other drugs have been evaluated for preventive therapy. However, in persons with an especially high risk of tuberculosis (e.g. persons with HIV infection), preventive therapy should be considered[69]. If the organisms are thought to be susceptible, 6 months of daily ethambutol and pyrazinamide at the usual therapeutic doses are recommended. If infection is due to organisms resistant to ethambutol as well, the combination of pyrazinamide plus a quinolone (ciprofloxacin or ofloxacin) for 6 months is recommended. Careful assessment to exclude active tuberculosis prior to the initiation of preventive therapy is mandatory.

14a.5 SPECIAL CONSIDERATIONS FOR DEVELOPING COUNTRIES

As noted above, there are two situations in which preventive therapy might be considered in a developing country setting. Both assume the establishment of a well-functioning National Tuberculosis Programme (NTP) that is effectively identifying and successfully treating cases. The first priority is for childhood contacts of infectious cases. In this situation, children living in the same household are treated at the same time as the adult index case. Specific guidelines are given above.

The second situation concerns the provision of preventive therapy for persons with HIV infection who are also at risk of tuberculosis. Because voluntary HIV testing is not readily available in many developing countries, opportunities to implement preventive therapy for this indication are limited. However, tuberculosis screening and the provision of preventive therapy should be considered for any site where voluntary HIV testing is available. Feasibility studies of isoniazid preventive therapy are needed to assess the cost, demand for services, sustainability and potential impact of such preventive therapy programmes. In most cases these studies should be conducted by the National AIDS Control Programme in settings where voluntary HIV testing is practised. However, close collaboration with the NTP in these studies and, if successful, in programme implementation, is essential. In addition to capability for HIV testing and counselling, these programmes must be able to screen patients for tuberculosis and refer tuberculosis suspects to appropriate facilities for additional examination and treatment.

REFERENCES

1. Ferebee, S.H. and Palmer, C.E. (1956) Prevention of experimental tuberculosis with isoniazid. *Am. Rev. Tuberc. Pul. Dis.*, **73**, 1–18.
2. Ferebee, S.H. (1969) Controlled chemoprophylaxis trials in tuberculosis. A general review. *Adv. Tuberc. Res.*, **17** 29–106.
3. Houk, V.N., Kent, D.C., Sorensen, K. and Baker, J.H. (1968) The eradication of tuberculosis infection by isoniazid chemoprophylaxis. *Arch. Environ. Hlth*, **16**, 46–50.
4. Comstock, G.W. and Ferebee, S.H. (1970) How much isoniazid is needed for prophylaxis? *Am. Rev. Respir. Dis.*, **101**, 780–2.
5. Comstock, G.M., Baum, C. and Snider, D.E. (1979) Isoniazid prophylaxis among Alaskan Eskimos: a final report of the Bethel isoniazid studies. *Am. Rev. Respir. Dis.*, **119**, 827–30.
6. International Union Against Tuberculosis Committee on Prophylaxis (1982) Efficacy of various durations of isoniazid preventive therapy for tuberculosis: five years of follow-up in the IUAT trial. *Bull. WHO*, **60**, 555–64.
7. Wadhawan, D., Hira, S., Mwansa, N. and Perine, P. (1992) Preventive tuberculosis chemotherapy with isoniazid among persons infected with HIV. Presented at the Eighth International Conference on AIDS, Amsterdam, 19–24 July.
8. Johnson, S.C., Stamm, C.P. and Hicks, C.B. (1990) Tuberculosis psoas muscle abscess

following chemoprophylaxis with isoniazid in a patient with human immunodeficiency virus infection. *Rev. Infect. Dis.*, **12**; 754–6.

9. Grumbach, F. and Rist, N. (1967) Activite antituberculeuse experimentale de la rifampicine, derive de la rifamycine SV. *Rev. Tuberc. Pneumol. (Paris)*, **31**, 749–62.

10. Lecoeur, H.F., Truffot-Pernot, C. and Grosset, J.H. (1989) Experimental short-course preventive therapy of tuberculosis with rifampin and pyrazinamide. *Am. Rev. Respir. Dis.*, **140**, 1189–93.

11. Grosset, J., Truffot-Pernot, C., Lacroix, C. and Ji, B. (1992) Antagonism between isoniazid and the combination pyrazinamide-rifampin against tuberculosis infection in mice. *Antimicrob. Agents Chemother.*, **36**, 548–51.

12. Kondo, E. and Kanai, K. (1988) An experimental model of chemotherapy on dormant tuberculous infection with particular reference to rifampicin. *Jpn J. Med. Sci. Biol.*, **41**, 37–47.

13. Mitchison, D.A. (1985) The action of antituberculosis drugs in short-course chemotherapy. *Tubercle*, **66**, 219–25.

14. Jindani, A., Aber, V.R., Edwards, E.A. and Mitchison, D.A. (1980) The early bactericidal activity of drugs in patients with pulmonary tuberculosis. *Am. Rev. Respir. Dis.*, **121**, 939–47.

15. Singapore Tuberculosis Service/British Medical Research Council (1986) Longterm follow-up of a clinical trial of six-month and four-month regimens of chemotherapy in the treatment of pulmonary tuberculosis. *Am. Rev. Respir. Dis.*, **133**, 779–83.

16. East African/British Medical Research Councils. (1981) Controlled clinical trial of five short-course (4-month) chemotherapy regimens in pulmonary tuberculosis. *Am. Rev. Respir. Dis.*, **123**, 165–70.

17. Hong Kong Chest Service/Tuberculosis Research Center, Madras/British Medical Research Council (1984) A controlled trial of 2-month, 3-month, and 12-month regimens of chemotherapy for sputum-smear-negative pulmonary tuberculosis: results at 60 months. *Am. Rev. Respir. Dis.*, **130**, 23–8.

18. Zierski, M. and Bek, E. (1980) Side-effects of drug regimens used in short-course chemotherapy for pulmonary tuberculosis. A controlled clinical study. *Tubercle*, **61**, 41–9.

19. Hong Kong Chest Service/Tuberculosis Research Centre, Madras/British Medical Research Council (1992) A double-blind placebo-controlled clinical trial of three anti-tuberculosis chemoprophylaxis regimens in patients with silicosis in Hong Kong. *Am. Rev. Respir. Dis.*, **145**, 36–41.

20. Ormerod, L.P. (1987) Reduced incidence of tuberculosis by prophylactic chemotherapy in subjects showing strong reactions to tuberculin testing. *Arch. Dis. Child.*, **62**, 1005–8.

21. Dickinson, J.M. and Mitchison, D.A. (1987) *In vitro* observations on the suitability of new rifamycins for the intermittent chemotherapy of tuberculosis. *Tubercle*, **68**, 183–93.

22. Truffot-Pernot, C., Grosset, J., Bismuth, R. and Lecoeur, H. (1983) Activité de la rifampicine administrée de manière intermittente et de la cyclopentyl rifamycine (ou DL473) sur la tuberculose experimentale de la souris. *Rev. Fr. Mal. Resp.*, **11**, 875–82.

23. O'Brien, R.J., Lyle, M.A., and Snider, D.E. (1987) Rifabutin (ansamycin LM427): a new rifamycin-S derivative for the treatment of mycobacterial diseases. *Rev. Infect. Dis.* **9**, 519–30.

24. Truffot-Pernot, C., Lanlande, V., Ji, B. and Grosset, J.H. (1992) Powerful bactericidal activity of sparfloxacin against *M. tuberculosis* in mice. Presented at 32rd Interscience Conference on Antimicrobial Agents and Chemotherapy, Anaheim, 11–14 October.

25. Gorin, F., Nightingale, S., Wynne, B. *et al.* (1992) Rifabutin monotherapy prevents or delays *Mycobacterium avium* complex (MAC) bacteremia in patients with AIDS. Presented at Eighth International Conference on AIDS, Amsterdam, 19–24 July.

26. Mitchell, J.R., Zimmerman, H.J., Ishak, K.G. *et al.* (1976) Isoniazid liver injury: clinical spectrum, pathology and probable pathogenesis. *Ann. Intern. Med.*, **84**, 181.

27. Garibaldi, R.A., Drusin, R.E., Ferebee, S.H. and Gregg, M.B. (1972) Isoniazid-associated hepatitis. Report of an outbreak. *Am. Rev. Respir. Dis.*, **106**, 357–65.

28. Kopanoff, D.E., Snider, D.E. and Caras, G.J. (1978) Isoniazid-related hepatitis. A US Public Health Service cooperative surveillance study. *Am. Rev. Respir. Dis.*, **117**, 991–1001.

29. Comstock, G.M. (1986) Prevention of tuberculosis among tuberculin reactors: maximizing benefits, minimizing risks. *J. Am. Med. Assoc.*, **256**, 2729–30.

30. Moulding, T.S., Redeker, A.G. and Kanel,

G.C. (1989) Twenty isoniazid-associated deaths in one state. *Am. Rev. Respir. Dis.,* **140,** 700–5.

31. Snider, D.E. and Caras, G.J. (1992) Isoniazid-associated hepatitis deaths: a review of available information. *Am. Rev. Respir. Dis.,* **145,** 494–7.

32. Franks, A.L., Binkin, N.J., Snider, D.E. *et al.* (1989) Isoniazid hepatitis among pregnant and postpartum Hispanic patients. *Publ. Hlth Rep.,* **104,** 151–5.

33. Murphy, R., Sxartz, R. and Watkins, P.B. (1990) Severe acetaminophen toxicity in a patient receiving isoniazid. *Ann. Intern. Med.,* **113,** 799–800.

34. Burk, R.F., Hill, K.E., Hunt, R.W. and Martin, A.E. (1990) Isoniazid potentiation of acetaminophen hepatotoxicity in the rat and 4-methylpyrazole inhibition of it. *Res. Commun. Chem. Path. Pharmacol.,* **69,** 115–18.

35. Snider, D.E. (1980) Pyridoxine supplementation during isoniazid therapy. *Tubercle,* **61,** 191–6.

36. Holdiness, M.R. (1987) Teratology of the antituberculosis drugs. *Early Hum. Develop.,* **15,** 61–74.

37. Geiter, L.J., O'Brien, R.J. and Kopanoff, D.E. (1990) Short-course preventive therapy for tuberculosis. *Am. Rev. Respir Dirs.,* **141** (Part 2), A437.

38. Rusche, A.F., Geiter, L.J., Magdorf, K. *et al.* (1991) Short-course preventive therapy for tuberculosis: a study of rifampin and pyrazinamide regimens in children. *Am. Rev. Respir. Dis.,* **143** (Part 2), A119.

39. Graczyk, J., O'Brien, R.J., Bek, E. *et al.* (1991) Assessment of rifampin-containing regimens for tuberculosis preventive therapy: results of a pilot study in Poland. *Am. Rev. Respir. Dis.,* **143** (Part 2), A119.

40. Clermont, H., Hohnson, M., Coberly, J. *et al.* (1991) Tolerance of short-course TB chemoprophylaxis in HIV-infected individuals. Presented at Seventh International AIDS Conference, Florence, 16–20 June.

41. Sullam, P., Burnside, A., Chew. T. (1992) Safety profile of rifabutin for the prevention of *M. avium* complex (MAC) bacteremia in patients with AIDS. Presented at the Eighth International AIDS Conference, Amsterdam 19–24 July.

42. Wobeser, W., To, T. and Hoeppner, V.H. (1989) The outcome of chemoprophylaxis on tuberculosis prevention in the Canadian Plains Indians. *Clin. Invest. Med.,* **12,** 149–53.

43. Alcabes, P., Vossenas, P., Cohen, R. *et al.* (1989) Compliance with isoniazid prophylaxis in jail. *Am. Rev. Respir. Dis.,* **140,** 1194–7.

44. Nazar-Stewart, V. and Nolan, C.M. (1992) Results of a directly observed intermittent isoniaizd preventive therapy program in a shelter for homeless men. *Am. Rev. Respir. Dis.,* **146,** 57–60.

45. Mehta, J.B., Dutt, A.K., Harvill, L. and Henry, W. (1988) Isoniazid preventive therapy for tuberculosis. Are we losing our enthusiasm? *Chest,* **94,** 138–41.

46. Taylor, W.C., Aronson, M.D. and Delbancho, T.L. (1981) Should young adults with a positive tuberculin test take isoniazid? *Ann. Intern. Med.,* **94,** 808–13.

47. Rose, D.N., Schechter, C.B. and Silver, A.L. (1986) The age threshold for isoniazid chemoprophylaxis. A decision analysis for low-risk tuberculin reactors. *J. Am. Med. Assoc.,* **256,** 2709–13.

48. Aisu, T., Van Praag, E., Raviglione, M.C. *et al.* (1992) Feasibility of preventive chemotherapy for HIV-associated tuberculosis (TB) in Uganda. Presented at the Eighth International Conference on AIDS, Amsterdam 19–24 July.

49. Nolan, C.M., Aitken, M.L., Elarth, A.M. *et al.* (1988) Active tuberculosis after isoniazid chemoprophylaxis of Southeast Asian refugees. *Am. Rev. Respir. Dis.,* **133,** 431–6.

50. Koplan, J.P. and Farer, L.S. (1980) Choice of preventive treatment for isoniazid-resistant tuberculous infection. Use of decision analysis and the Delphi technique. *J. Am. Med. Assoc.,* **244,** 2736–40.

51. Livengood, J.R., Sigler, T.G., Foster, L.R. *et al.* (1985) Isoniazid-resistant tuberculosis. A community outbreak and report of a rifampin prophylaxis failure. *J. Am. Med. Assoc.,* **253,** 2847–49.

52. Snider, D.E, Caras, G.J. and Koplan, J.P. (1986) Preventive therapy with isoniazid. Cost-effectiveness of different durations of therapy. *J. Am. Med. Assoc.,* **255,** 1579–83.

53. Murray, C.J.L. Styblo, K. and Rouillon, A. (1990) Tuberculosis in developing countries: burden, intervention and cost. *Bull. Int. Union. Tuberc. Lung Dis.,* **65,** 6–24.

54. Steele, M.A., Burk, R.F. and DesPrez, R.M. (1991) Toxic hepatitis with isoniazid and rifampin, a meta-analysis. *Chest,* **99,** 465–71.

55. American Thoracic Society/Centers for Disease Control (1990) Diagnostic standards and classification of tuberculosis. *Am. Rev. Respir. Dis.*, **142**, 725–35.

56. Johnson, M.P., Coberly, J.S., Clermont, H.C. *et al.* (1990) Tuberculin skin test reactivity among adults infected with human immunodeficiency virus. *J. Infect. Dis.*, **166**, 194–8.

57. Joint Tuberculosis Committee (1990) Chemotherapy and management of tuberculosis in the United Kingdom: recommendations of the Joint Tuberculosis Committee of the British Thoracic Society. *Thorax*, **45**, 403–8.

58. Selwyn, P.A., Hartel, D., Lewis, V.A. *et al.* (1989) A prospective study of the risk of tuberculosis among intravenous drug users with human immunodeficiency virus infection. *N. Engl. J. Med.*, **320**, 545.

59. Centers for Disease Control (1991) PPD-tuberculin anergy in persons with HIV infection. Guidelines for anergy testing and management of anergic persons at risk of tuberculous infection. *Morbid. Mortal. Weekly Rep.*, **40** (Suppl. RR-5), 27–33.

60. Selwyn, P.A., Sckell, B.M., Alcabes. P. *et al.* (1992) High risk of active tuberculosis in HIV-infected drug users with cutaneous anergy. *J. Am. Med. Assoc.*, **268**, 504–9.

61. Jordon, T.J., Lewit, E.M., Montgomery, R.I. and Reichman, L.B. (1991) Isoniazid as preventive therapy in HIV-infected intravenous drug abusers. A decision analysis. *J. Am. Med. Assoc.*, **265**, 2987–91.

62. American Thoracic Society/Centers for Disease Control (1986) Treatment of tuberculosis and tuberculosis infection in adults and children. *Am. Rev. Respir. Dis.*, **134**, 355–63.

63. International Union Against Tuberculosis and Lung Diseases (1991) Tuberculosis in children – guidelines for diagnosis, prevention and treatment. *Bull. Int. Union Tuberc. Lung Dis.*, **66**, 61–7.

64. Centers for Disease Control (1990) The use of preventive therapy for tuberculous infection in the United States. Recommendations of the Advisory Committee for Elimination of Tuberculosis. *Morbid. Mortal. Weekly Rep.*, **39**(RR-6), 9–12.

65. Rieder, H.L., Cauthen, G.M., Comstock, G.W., and Snider, D.E. (1989) Epidemiology of tuberculosis in the United States. *Epidemiol. Rev.*, **11**, 79–98.

66. Reichman, L.B., Felton, C.P. and Edsall, J.R. (1979) Drug dependence, a possible new risk factor for tuberculosis disease. *Arch. Intern. Med.*, **139**, 337–9.

67. American Academy of Pediatrics (1992) Chemotherapy for tuberculosis in infants and children. *Pediatrics*, **89**, 161–5.

68. Centers for Disease Control (1989) Tuberculosis and human immunodeficiency virus infection: recommendations of the Advisory Committee for the Elimination of Tuberculosis. *Morbid. Mortal. Weekly Rep.*, **38**, 236–8, 243–50.

69. Villarino, M.E., Dooley, S.W., Geiter, L.J. *et al.* (1992) Management of persons exposed to multidrug-resistant tuberculosis. *Morbid. Mortal. Weekly Rep.*, **41**(RR-11), 59–71.

BCG VACCINATION

P.G. Smith

14b.1 INTRODUCTION

Case-finding with effective treatment and mass BCG vaccination have been the central pillars of tuberculosis control activities in most countries. BCG vaccination has been regarded as of special importance in less developed countries where the identification and treatment of cases of tuberculosis has posed considerable logistic problems, because of scanty and poorly financed medical services. In such situations, BCG offered obvious attractions as a means of tuberculosis control, especially among children, where its value is likely to lie mostly in the protection of vaccinated individuals, rather than in reducing the overall level of infection in the community[1]. The vaccine is simple to administer and causes few complications. In freeze-dried form it is stable and relatively easy to store and transport. Furthermore, in some situations, a single injection has been shown to give protection against tuberculosis that lasts for a decade or more. Unfortunately, it has been difficult to predict in which situations this last finding will hold. In placebo-controlled trials, the protection afforded by BCG against tuberculosis has been shown to vary from zero to nearly 80% in studies conducted in different areas of the world. Despite the variable findings in these studies, the evidence in favour of a protective effect was considered to be strong enough in the early 1950s for the World Health Organization to recommend mass vaccination campaigns. These were conducted in many countries. In some BCG was given to persons showing no reaction to tuberculin, as it was not expected that giving the vaccine to those who had already been infected with the tubercle bacillus would confer any protection and, furthermore, there were fears that giving BCG to those already infected might actually increase the incidence of tuberculosis or lead to more virulent disease. Studies coordinated by the WHO indicated that it was safe to give BCG to those already infected and thus in many of the mass vaccination campaigns an attempt was made to vaccinate all children, without prior skin testing. Following the mass campaigns, vaccination coverage has been maintained by immunizing newborn children and/or school children as part of the routine health care system.

Because of the variation in protective efficacy that had been observed in trials of BCG vaccination and because few of these studies had been conducted in less developed countries, where the problem of tuberculosis is now concentrated, the Indian Council for Medical Research, in collaboration with the WHO and the US Centers for Disease Control, set up, in 1968, a large and carefully designed trial in south India. It was hoped that this trial would provide definitive answers regarding the role of BCG in tuberculosis control in less-developed countries. The first results from this trial were presented in 1979[2] and, to the surprise and consternation of most observers, it was reported that BCG had offered no protection at all against

Clinical Tuberculosis. Edited by P.D.O. Davies. Published in 1994 by Chapman & Hall, London. ISBN 0 412 48630 X

tuberculosis – in fact, the incidence of tuberculosis was slightly higher in the vaccinated group than in those given a placebo. It thus seemed possible, if these results were applicable on a widespread basis, that the millions of BCG vaccinations that had been administered in the mass campaigns had been a complete waste of time and money.

There was, naturally, a considerable reluctance to accept this possibility and much thought has been devoted to trying to work out what these results mean in relation to other knowledge of the epidemiology of tuberculosis and of the effects of BCG. In summary, no hypothesis has been formulated that, on the basis of present evidence, provides a wholly satisfactory explanation of the results in the Indian trial and in other controlled trials and definitive answers are likely to come only through further research.

In the mean time, a considerable number of attempts have been made to assess the efficacy of BCG against tuberculosis in different parts of the developing world, using case-control and similar approaches. Such studies are more susceptible to bias than randomized controlled trials and this complicates their interpretation, but they are much quicker and cheaper to conduct and have produced important new information about the heterogeneity of BCG efficacy in parts of the world where the public health importance of tuberculosis is greatest.

In this chapter, the results of the trials that have been conducted to assess BCG efficacy are reviewed and some of the hypotheses that have been advanced to explain the different findings are discussed. The results of recent retrospective evaluations of the efficacy of BCG as used in control programmes are also summarized. The implications of these findings for future BCG policies are assessed, taking into account the complication of the situation by the rapidly growing HIV pandemic.

14b.2 EARLY WORK ON BCG

The observation that persons infected with tuberculosis early in life (as measured by their reaction to tuberculin) were more resistant to tuberculosis than those uninfected, together with similar observations in experimental animals, led Calmette to postulate that an artificial infection with an organism whose virulence has been attenuated may also protect against the disease. By 1921, Calmette and Guerin had developed a vaccine from a strain of *Mycobacterium bovis*, that had been through 231 serial cultures over 13 years and that had lost its pathogenicity in animals. This vaccine (Bacille Calmette–Guerin) was used in Europe in a fairly uncontrolled way in the 1920s, but some results reported by Heimbeck[3,4] suggested that the protective effect against tuberculosis might be considerable. He had offered BCG to student nurses in an Oslo hospital from 1927 onwards. Not all accepted the offer and he was able to show that the incidence of tuberculosis in those who had been given BCG was less than one-quarter of that in those who had refused vaccination. The possibility of bias in this study cannot be excluded as the vaccine had not been administered to the nurses 'at random' in the context of a controlled trial, but the findings offered encouragement to those advocating widespread use of the vaccine. A severe setback came, however, following an accident in Germany in which 251 infants were given vaccine orally and 72 died of tuberculosis, mostly within a few months of administration. Although it was soon established that the vaccine had been accidentally contaminated with a virulent strain of *M. tuberculosis*, the damage to its reputation persisted[5].

It was only in 1935 that the first well-controlled trial was started to evaluate the efficacy of BCG against tuberculosis in humans and, in this study, a 75% protective efficacy was reported[6] – an effect similar in magnitude to that observed in the uncontrolled study of Heimbeck[4]. (A protective

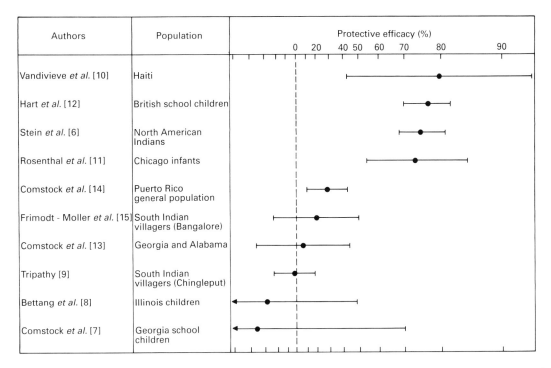

Fig. 14b.1 Protective efficacy of BCG vaccination against tuberculosis measured in randomized controlled trials. (The bars on the efficacy estimates are 95% confidence intervals.)

efficacy of 75% means that 75% of the cases that would have been expected in the vaccinated group, had they not been given the vaccine, were prevented by the vaccination.) However, this unfortunately, was only the beginning of the story and, over the next 20 years, a number of further trials were set up in different parts of the world and the protective efficacy of BCG in different studies varied from zero to 77%.

14b.3 TRIALS OF BCG VACCINATION

Fig. 14b.1 summarizes the results from nine large, controlled trials of BCG vaccination against tuberculosis that were started between 1935 and 1966. Also shown are the results from the largest and most recent trial, conducted in south India (Chingleput), which started in 1968[2]. In all of these trials the division of the population into a vacci-

nated and an unvaccinated group was done using some 'random', or close to random, procedure. In general, an individual was first given a tuberculin test and those showing a 'positive' reaction were excluded from the randomization procedure, though in some trials this was not the case. The diagnosis of tuberculosis in a participant was made without knowledge of whether or not the patient had been given BCG. Thus, the results are free from the biases that may be present in uncontrolled studies.

The protective efficacy of BCG varied from zero in three trials among Georgia[7] and Illinois[8] children and in south Indian villagers (Chingleput)[9] (in all of these the incidence of tuberculosis was slightly higher in the group given BCG than in the unvaccinated group) to over 70% in four other trials: in a low socioeconomic group in Haiti[10], among North American Indians[6], newborn

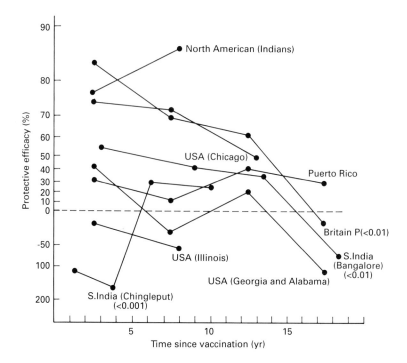

Fig. 14b.2 Changes in protective efficacy of BCG against tuberculosis with time since vaccination, in randomized controlled trials. *P* values refer to changes in efficacy over course of years studied. No *P* value signifies no significant change.

children in Chicago[11] and school children in Britain[12]. Low protective efficacies were seen in the three remaining trials: 6% among the general population of Georgia and Alabama[13]; 29% in Puerto Rico[14]; and 19% among south Indian villages near Bangalore[15]. (The protective efficacies quoted are those based upon the results from the most recent follow-up of the trial population). Some of the variation in the results between different trials may be due to statistical fluctuations caused by the small numbers of cases of tuberculosis observed, but this certainly cannot explain all the variation. For example, we can be reasonably confident that the protective efficacy among North American Indians and British school children was truly above 65% and for south Indian villagers (Chingleput) was below 20%.

Follow-up continued for extended periods in most of the trials. Fig. 14b.2 shows the variation in the protective efficacies with time since vaccination in ten of the trials. In those trials in which a protective effect of BCG was

evident, the effect persisted for over a decade, although there was a tendency for the efficacy to decrease at longer periods after vaccination, which was statistically significant only in the trial among British school children. The curious excess of cases of tuberculosis in the BCG-vaccinated group in the early years of the south Indian (Chingleput) trial is evident in Fig. 14b.2. This phenomenon has not been observed in other trials and may be a chance finding.

14b.4 POSSIBLE EXPLANATIONS FOR THE DIFFERENCES IN RESULTS

Several hypotheses have been put forward in an attempt to explain the variation in the results in the different trials and some of these are reviewed below.

14b.4.1 METHODOLOGICAL BIASES

Deficiencies in the design and conduct of some of the trials may account for some of the variation in the levels of protective efficacy reported[16], but it seems most unlikely that all of the variation is due to differences or biases in the methodologies used. In general, the trials were designed carefully to avoid the biases possible in uncontrolled studies and, in particular, an expert committee of the WHO conducted a rigorous review of the procedures used in the Chingleput trial and agreed that it was of a high scientific standard and that no errors in the conduct of field operations or in data processing could have been serious enough to have invalidated the results[17]. The differences in protective efficacy between trials are more than would be expected on the basis of statistical variation due to sampling errors and thus it must be concluded that the differences are real and satisfactory hypotheses regarding the mechanism of the action of BCG must account for these differences.

14b.4.2 VACCINE STRAINS AND DOSES

Different strains of BCG vary in their ability to protect laboratory animals against tuberculosis. A strain produced by the Tice Laboratory in Chicago in the late 1940s and early 1950s was shown, by a number of workers, to be of reduced potency compared with other vaccines in experimental animals and this may account for the weak or absent protective effect seen in the trials conducted among Georgia and Illinois children and in the general population of Georgia and Alabama, compared with the earlier trial using a Tice vaccine among Chicago infants[18,19]. Willis and Vandiviere noted a close correlation between the protective efficacies of the BCG strains used in trials in North American Indians, the Georgia and Alabama population and in Puerto Rico and the protective efficacies of the same strains in experimental animals[18]. As always, it is difficult to know to what extent it is reasonable to extrapolate from the findings in experimental animals to man.

In three of the trials showing low efficacies, BCG was given by the multiple puncture method[7,8,13] and it is known that this may result in inoculation of a low dose of BCG and this may inhibit multiplication of BCG. The multiple puncture method was also used, however, in the trial among Chicago infants[11], in which a high efficacy was observed. In the trial in Puerto Rico[14] intradermal injection was used and thus a low vaccine dose cannot explain the low efficacy observed in this trial, although there is some evidence that the potency of this strain of BCG may have been low[18].

It seems likely that some of the variation in the results in the trials shown in Fig. 14b.1 was due to differences in vaccine potency and, perhaps, also in dosages administered. This was recognized at the time the Chingleput trial was designed and, for these reasons, it was decided to include two potent vaccine strains (one of which, the Danish strain, had been shown to be highly protective among British school children) and to give each of these in two different doses to different groups of trial participants, using the intradermal method of inoculation. Neither vaccine at either dose showed any evidence of a protective effect, though both strains of BCG protect experimental animals[2]. We must search, therefore, for factors in addition to vaccine strain and dose to explain the different results.

The Chingleput study was the first controlled trial in which freeze-dried vaccines had been used and it was suggested that this may explain the absence of protection. It is noteworthy, however, that Springett and Sutherland[20], when analysing changes in tuberculosis morbidity among school children in Birmingham, England, found that the freeze-dried batches of BCG that had been issued between 1962 and 1968 gave a high protective efficacy, similar to that of the liquid batches that had been issued between 1953 and 1961. Their observations were not made in the context of a controlled trial, but they suggest very strongly that freeze-drying *per se* cannot be incriminated.

14b.4.3 INFECTION WITH ENVIRONMENTAL MYCOBACTERIA

Palmer and Long suggested that the prevalence of sensitization to environmental mycobacteria may modify the protective effect to be expected from BCG[21]. Experiments in animals had shown that infection with certain environmental mycobacteria conferred some protection against a subsequent challenge with *M. tuberculosis* and that giving BCG in addition, before challenge with *M. tuberculosis*, brought the level of protection only up to that conferred by BCG alone [21,22]. Thus, if BCG was given in situations where infection with environmental mycobacteria was common, a reduced protective efficacy might be expected, which might, for example, explain the differences between the results of the trials in Puerto Rico, where environmental mycobacteria are common, and in British school children, in whom there was a low prevalence of infection with such mycobacteria. It was thought that such an explanation might account for some of the variation in the results from the different trials. It seems unlikely, however, that this is the complete explanation. Observations in animals indicate that the protection against tuberculosis afforded by infection with environmental mycobacteria is not as strong as that given by BCG[21]. Thus, while a reduced effect of BCG might be expected if there was infection with environmental mycobacteria, the complete absence of an effect would not be predicted. Calculations by Hart[23] and ten Dam and co-workers[19], suggested that such sensitization alone could not explain the differences in protection observed between the British and American studies. It is noteworthy, also, that in a number of trials, persons with a low-grade response to tuberculin were excluded from the group randomized to receive vaccine or placebo. This will

have effectively excluded many of those with prior infections with environmental mycobacteria. Furthermore, in the trial in Puerto Rico, the protective effect of BCG was found to be essentially the same for persons with no reaction to tuberculin and for those with low-grade reactions[14].

Stanford *et al.*[15] proposed that infection with certain kinds of environmental mycobacteria may directly inhibit the protective effect of BCG and thus the effect of the vaccine would be dictated by the kinds of organisms present in the environment. The evidence in support of this hypotheses is not yet strong and its evaluation must await further studies.

14b.4.4 DIFFERENT STRAINS OF *M. TUBERCULOSIS*

Strains of *M. tuberculosis* isolated from patients in south India are of lower virulence in the guinea-pig than strains from Europe. There is some evidence that this 'south Indian' strain may be of reduced virulence to man also. It is likely that this organism is prevalent also in the area where the Chingleput vaccine trial was conducted, but its distribution in other parts of India and in other countries is incompletely known. The extent to which BCG may protect differently against different strains of tubercle bacilli is unknown, but recent developments in molecular 'fingerprinting' of isolates (Chapter 17c) may facilitate better study of this issue.

The pattern of tuberculosis in the Chingleput trial was markedly different from that seen in other areas of the world, and even from that in the close-by area in Bangalore District, where an earlier trial was conducted. The prevalence of tuberculosis infection was very high, indicating a very infectious organism, but there was an unexpectedly low incidence of bacillary tuberculosis among those recently infected. The incidence of tuberculosis among adults was, however, very high. Few persons were found who did not show some reaction to tuberculin, and indeed, in the initial trial report those with reactions to PPD-S of less than 8 mm were considered together, with no further breakdown. It is possible that some of these persons had already been infected with tuberculosis – perhaps by a strain of low virulence producing a poor tuberculin response – and thus no effect of BCG would be expected (given prior to infection, BCG is thought to stop the haematological spread of an initial infection, but it is not expected that BCG will protect if administered after the initial infection). Such a situation, however, would lead to a reduced efficacy for BCG but would not be expected to eliminate completely any protective effect.

In the British trial the incidence of tuberculosis in those who were tuberculin-'positive' at entry to the trial was initially high but, after a few years, declined to a level below that in the unvaccinated (tuberculin-'negative') group[24]. The high incidence initially was probably due to recently infected persons being included in the group, with disease following soon after infection. In the trials in Puerto Rico, Georgia–Alabama and south India (Chingleput) the incidence of tuberculosis was much higher in persons initially tuberculin-positive than in those initially tuberculin-negative and unvaccinated. This was true for the total duration of the follow-up and the incidence was not especially high just after the start of the trial. Ten Dam and Pio[25] have interpreted these observations as being compatible with disease being of the exogenous reinfection type rather than of the endogenous type. In the trial among North American Indians, both the levels of infection and the rates of disease were very high, suggesting that the disease was not due to exogenous reinfection. It is postulated that in some areas of the world tuberculosis may be largely due to exogenous reinfection: in such areas BCG is likely to be of little use – except perhaps if given at birth

to protect against infant tuberculosis due to the initial infection.

14b.4.5 OTHER FACTORS

The possibility of genetic differences between populations in their response to BCG cannot be excluded and could explain the differences in protection observed. (A common feature of genetic hypotheses, however, is their adaptability!) Certainly work to examine this possibility should be encouraged but it seems an unlikely explanation and should not be given high priority. It seems much more likely that the determining factor is the environment in which people live.

Poor nutritional status has been advanced as a factor that might modify the effect of BCG, but this fails to account for the similarity of the finding among well-nourished British school children and poorly nourished North American Indians[23]. Furthermore, no association between efficacy and thickness of subcutaneous fat was found in the Georgia–Alabama trial[26].

If the initial infection with tuberculosis arose following intense exposure (either through infection with a large number of bacilli or through frequent exposure to an infected person), it is possible that this might overwhelm any protective effect offered by BCG against less intense exposure. Indeed, this may explain why, even in areas where BCG does offer good protection, it does not offer complete protection. It is, of course, almost impossible to determine the size of the infecting dose and it is difficult to measure the frequency of exposure in different areas and, thus, it is not possible to test directly whether this could explain the variation in the effects of BCG in different trials. Indirect evidence that this is not the explanation is provided by continuing studies in Britain, where over a 30-year period there has been a dramatic fall in the incidence of tuberculosis but no apparent decline in the efficacy of BCG[27–29]. It does not follow, of course, that a declining incidence necessarily leads to less intense exposures among those infected, but this study does suggest that the prevalence of tuberculosis is not the major determinant of the effect of BCG.

14b.5 RETROSPECTIVE ASSESSMENT OF BCG EFFICACY IN CONTROL PROGRAMMES

BCG vaccination is compulsory in 64 countries and officially recommended in a further 118. It is in widespread use in almost all less developed countries[30]. Publication of the initial findings from the Chingleput trial[2] caused widespread concern about the role of BCG in tuberculosis control activities. It is important to note, however, that the Chingleput trial provided no information on the effects of BCG in infants or children, as those under 10 years old were not included in the assessment and, in any case, tuberculosis was measured by the incidence of sputum-positive pulmonary tuberculosis and this form of disease is relatively rare in children. As most BCG campaigns in less developed countries have been focused on infants and young children, it might be argued that the controlled trials offered little guidance on the value of these policies. At that time there had been few controlled trials of BCG in developing countries and, for example, none in Latin America or Africa. The prospect of setting up further long-term, large and expensive trials was daunting after the experience in the Chingleput study. It was suggested, however, that it might be possible to assess retrospectively the effect on tuberculosis rates that BCG had had, when given in routine vaccination programmes and in mass vaccination campaigns. Two methods were suggested for doing this. One, the case-control approach[31] involved ascertaining the history of BCG vaccination among cases of tuberculosis and among suitable chosen 'controls', without tuberculosis. Estimates of efficacy could be derived by comparing the proportions of cases and controls vaccinated. The second method, contact studies[32], involved comparing the incidence and prevalence of tuberculosis in vaccinated and unvaccinated child contacts of infectious adult cases of tuberculosis. Both methods were dependent upon obtaining an accurate history of past vaccination, based on vaccination records or, more usually, on the presence or absence of a BCG scar.

The major disadvantage of these approaches was that they were based on comparing the incidence of tuberculosis in those who had, or had not, been vaccinated in routine programmes or campaigns. Thus, unlike the controlled trials, the selection of the vaccinated group was not by randomization and it is possible that those reporting for vaccination may be at higher or lower risk of tuberculosis that those not so reporting, for reasons unrelated to vaccination. For example, those in higher socio-economic groups may be more likely to use health services and are also, independently, at lower risk of tuberculosis. Such a bias would tend to bias towards observing an apparent protective effect of vaccination. By careful design, it is possible to minimize such biases[31], but the possibility of their existence cannot be eliminated completely, and this must be borne in mind when interpreting the results of such studies. Against this disadvantage must be balanced the enormous advantage that such studies are relatively quick, cheap and simple to conduct, and can be undertaken with relatively few resources.

Over the past 5–10 years a comparatively large number of these kinds of study have been published. They have focused mostly on childhood tuberculosis, which brings with it additional diagnostic problems (Chapter 11), and many have been in developing countries and, thus, have been of direct value to national health services in evaluating their past vaccination strategy. Fig. 14b.3 summarizes the findings in most of the published studies. Most of the studies have been of the

Authors	Population	Type of Study	Protective efficacy (%)
Wunsch Filho et al. [33]	Brazil (São Paulo)[a]	C	
Sharma et al. [34]	India (Delhi)[a]	C	
Sirinavin et al. [35]	Thailand (Bangkok)	C	
Chavalittamrong et al. [36]	Thailand (Bangkok)	C	
Jin et al. [37]	Korea (Seoul)	Co	
Miceli et al. [38]	Argentina (Buenos Aires)	C	
Blin et al. [39]	Cameroon (Yaounde)	C	
Tidjani et al. [40]	Togo (Lomé)	Co	
Packe et al. [41]	England (Birmingham Asians)	C	
Young et al. [42]	Canada (Manitoba Indians)	C	
Padungchan et al. [43]	Thailand (Bangkok)	Co	
Houston et al. [44]	Canada (Treaty Indians)	C	
Rodrigues et al. [45]	England (Asians)	C	
Murtagh [46]	Papua New Guinea	C	
Myint et al. [47]	Burma (Rangoon)	C	
Putrali et al. [48]	Indonesia (Jakarta)	C	
Smith [49]	Sri Lanka (Colombo)	C	
Shapiro et al. [50]	Colombia (Cali)	C	
Ponnighaus et al. [51]	Malawi (Rural)	P	

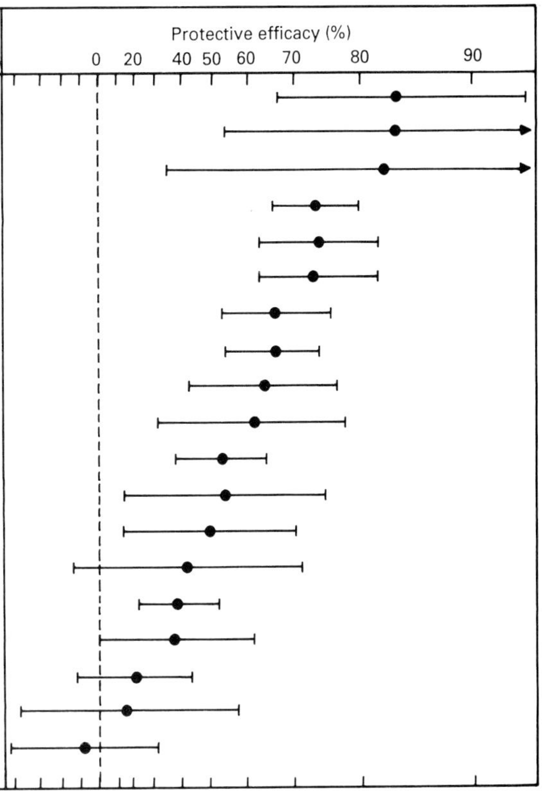

[a] Tuberculous meningitis ●

C, case-control; Co, contact study; P, prospective study.

Fig. 14b.3 Protective efficacy of BCG vaccination against tuberculosis, as assessed in case-control, contact and cohort studies, in developing countries or in disadvantaged communities. (The bars on the efficacy estimates are 95% confidence intervals.)

case-control type, but also included are three contact studies[37,40,43] and one cohort study[51] conducted in the special context of a large longitudinal study of leprosy and tuberculosis in Malawi. There are several striking features of these results. Firstly, the range of variation in the estimates of protective efficacy is as great as that seen in the controlled trials, spanning zero to 80% protection. Secondly, in most though not all of the studies, the estimated efficacy is significantly different from zero, with over half of the studies reporting a protective efficacy in the range of 40–70%. Thirdly, in those studies that were confined to cases of tuberculous meningitis, or in those where this subset of patients was examined separately, the protective effects appeared to be higher, indicating that either there was more diagnostic uncertainty for some other forms of tuberculosis (which would tend to bias the estimate of efficacy towards zero), or that the protection against meningitis was indeed strongest.

Of special interest among the studies summarized in Fig. 14b.3 are two that were conducted in England among children of Asian (Indian subcontinent) ethnic origin. As the overall incidence of tuberculosis has declined in England, some health authorities have stopped the routine vaccination of school children (at age 13 years) and instead have targeted BCG vaccination at infants at relatively high risk of infection, a group that includes Asian infants. The two studies conducted among children with tuberculosis in this group reported 49%[45] and 64%[41] protection associated with vaccination in the first year of life. These findings provide some evidence against the view that genetic factors may explain the results of the Chingleput trial.

The finding of little protection in Malawi contrasts with the relatively high efficacies reported in Togo and Cameroon and further studies in Africa would be useful. It is of interest that though BCG was reported not to protect against tuberculosis in the Malawi study, the vaccine appeared to have offered substantial protection against leprosy[51].

Although the studies summarized in Fig. 14b.3 have not yet led to unifying hypotheses to explain the variation in efficacy, they have enabled a number of national tuberculosis control programmes to ascertain the usefulness of BCG vaccination in their local situation. In general, BCG appears to have offered some protection against tuberculosis, though not everywhere, and variably from place to place. Certainly the overall evidence would seem to be strong enough to encourage the continuance of BCG vaccination to infants and young children. This is in line with the conclusion reached by ten Dam and Hitze [52], who reviewed the evidence on newborn and young child vaccination, before the series of studies in Fig. 14b.3 were available.

14b.6 BCG AND HIV INFECTION

The profound impact that HIV infection has had, and will have, on tuberculosis is reviewed elsewhere in this volume (Chapter 12). For BCG vaccination, as for other aspects of the disease, the full import of the infection is still not known. There are two main concerns. Firstly, is it safe to give BCG to someone whose immune system might be compromised by HIV? Secondly, even if BCG protects against tuberculosis in the absence of HIV, will it continue to so do in HIV-infected individuals? There are limited data available on the first of these questions but few on the second.

In 1986, the WHO recommended that, in countries where tuberculosis in children was still a significant problem, BCG should continue to be given according to standard schedules to children with asymptomatic HIV infection, but should not be given to individuals with clinical AIDS[53]. In countries where the risk of tuberculosis in children is low, BCG vaccination of HIV-infected infants is not recommended.

The occurrence of adverse effects associated with BCG vaccination in those with HIV infection or AIDS has been documented mostly in case reports, which makes quantitation of the risks difficult. However, some population-based studies have been reported. Lalleant-Le Coeur *et al.*[54] followed-up 64 infants of HIV-infected mothers and 130 control babies and found no significant differences in complication rates of BCG in the two groups, or in the children who were later proven to have been perinatally infected, though fewer children in this last group showed tuberculin skin test conversion. A study of the children of 209 seropositive mothers and 213 seronegative mothers in Rwanda reported similar findings[55].

As discussed above, our knowledge of the efficacy of BCG against tuberculosis, in the absence of HIV infection, is patchy. Whether or not BCG is less effective in HIV-infected individuals is not known. There is evidence that the conversion to a positive tuberculin skin test following BCG vaccination is less common among those HIV-infected, which may suggest lower likely efficacy, but it is unclear if the BCG-induced tuberculin response bears any relationship to protection. One of the striking findings in the trial among British school children was that the protection conferred by BCG vaccination was as good among those who showed little or no response to tuberculin after vaccination as among those who showed a strong response[56].

14b.7 PRIORITIES FOR RESEARCH

Immunity to tuberculosis is clearly complicated (Chapter 5, p. 55). Advances in immunology may provide clues for the variations in BCG efficacy seen in different communities. Similarly, this variation must be telling us something important about the epidemiology and immunology of tuberculosis. Following the publication of the first results of the Chingleput trial, an expert group met and laid out an agenda for research to try to explain the variable findings in different BCG trials[17]. In the decade that has passed since that group reported, it is not clear that we are significantly closer to having an answer. Much of our knowledge of the epidemiology of tuberculosis is based on studies that were conducted in the now developed countries and it is possible that extrapolation of these findings to developing countries is not straightforward. We know relatively little about the epidemiology of tuberculosis in those areas of the world where the problem is now concentrated. Large-scale longitudinal studies of the epidemiology of tuberculosis in developing countries must be a priority for the future, especially in view of the likely impact of HIV infection. Better knowledge of the epidemiology of tuberculosis is likely to provide further important clues to the reasons for BCG's variable value.

The case-control and contact studies reviewed above have shown that rapid assessments of efficacy are possible, and even if this does not tell us the reason for the variation it does provide vital information to national disease control programmes on the effectiveness of BCG as an intervention measure in a local context. Adaptation of these methods to assess whether BCG offers pro-

tection against tuberculosis among those HIV-infected must also be on the research agenda.

In most developing countries BCG is given shortly after birth. It is generally considered that vaccination at this age is unlikely to give life-long protection against tuberculosis and that revaccination is necessary at school age. The value of such revaccination has never been assessed. There is one controlled trial of this question under way in Malawi[51], but further evaluation is necessary, possibly using case-control or similar approaches, in situations where revaccination has been part of the routine vaccination programme.

In developed countries, where tuberculosis is now a much reduced problem, it may be necessary to adapt BCG policies to changing circumstances. For example, it has been estimated that in 1950, in England and Wales, it was necessary to vaccinate 67 school children with BCG to prevent one notified case of tuberculosis, whereas in 1989, 3600 vaccinations were necessary to prevent one case and, in 1999, the number necessary will be 9300[57]. Clearly the time will come when it will no longer be cost-effective to continue the mass BCG vaccination strategy. However, the possible impact of HIV infection on trends in tuberculosis add an additional element of uncertainty to the projection of a continuing decline in tuberculosis rates.

Because of the equivocal results of a protective effect in the controlled trials conducted in the USA, that country has been one of the very few countries not to have instituted a routine BCG vaccination policy. The emergence of strains of tuberculosis that are multi-drug resistant may lead to a reassessment of vaccination policies in high-risk groups. For example, BCG vaccination is not currently recommended for health care workers in the USA, but a recent evaluation of tuberculosis control strategies in this group suggested that it would only be necessary for the efficacy of BCG to be around 13% for routine vaccination to be a more effective strategy than annual screening with a tuberculin test and chemoprophylaxis for those found to be infected[58].

It is to be hoped that in the longer term a vaccine against tuberculosis will be developed that will give more consistent protection against tuberculosis in different geographical areas than BCG. Such a vaccine may be rather distant, however, and, in the mean time, the weight of the evidence suggests that in much of the world BCG is an effective and cheap method of providing individual protection against tuberculosis.

REFERENCES

1. Styblo, K. and Meijer, J. (1976) Impact of BCG vaccination programmes in children and young adults on the tuberculosis problem. *Tubercle*, **57**, 17–43.
2. Tuberculosis Prevention Trial (1979) Trial of BCG vaccines in south India for tuberculosis prevention: first report. *Bull. WHO*, **7**, 819–27.
3. Heimbeck, J. (1928) Immunity to tuberculosis. *Arch. Intern. Med.*, **41**, 336–42.
4. Heimbeck, J. (1948) BCG vaccination of nurses. *Tubercle*, **28**, 84–8.
5. Wilson, G.S. (1967) Faulty production: use of wrong culture, in *The Hazards of Immunization*, London, Athlone Press, pp. 66–74.
6. Stein, S.C. and Aronson, J.D. (1953) The occurrence of pulmonary lesions in BCG vaccinated and unvaccinated persons. *Am. Rev. Tuberc. Pulmon. Dis.*, **68**, 695–712.
7. Comstock, G.W. and Webster, R.G. (1969) Tuberculosis studies in Muscogee County, Georgia. VII. A twenty-year evaluation of BCG vaccination in a school population. *Am. Rev. Respir. Dis.*, **100**, 839–45.
8. Bettag, O.L., Kaluzny, A.A., Morse, D. and Radney, D.B. (1964) BCG study at a state school for mentally retarded. *Dis. Chest*, **45**, 503–07.
9. Tripathy, S.P. (1986) Fifteen year follow-up of the Indian BCG prevention trial, in *Tuberculosis and Respiratory Diseases*. Papers presented at the plenary sessions of the XXVth World Conference of the International Union against Tuberculosis, Singapore 4–7 November 1986. Professional Postgraduate Services, pp. 69–72.
10. Vandiviere, H.M., Dworski, M., Melvin, I.G.

et al. (1973) Efficacy of Bacillus Calmette–Guerin and isoniazid-resistant Bacillus Calmette–Guerin with and without isoniazid chemoprophylaxis from day of vaccination. II. Field trial in man. *Am. Rev. Respir. Dis.*, **108**, 301–13.
11. Rosenthal, S.R., Loewinsohn, E., Graham, M.L. et al, (1961) BCG vaccination against tuberculosis in Chicago. A twenty-year study statistically analyzed. *Pediatrics*, **28**, 622–41.
12. Hart, P.D. and Sutherland, I. (1977) BCG and vole bacillus vaccines in the prevention of tuberculosis in adolescence and early adult life. *Br. Med. J.*, **2**, 293–5.
13. Comstock, G.W., Woolpert, S.F. and Livesay, V.T. (1976) Tuberculosis studies in Muscogee County, Georgia. Twenty-year evaluation of a community trial of BCG vaccination. *Publ. Hlth Rep.*, **91**, 276–80.
14. Comstock, G.W., Livesay, V.T. and Woolpert, S.F. (1974) Evaluation of BCG vaccination among Puerto Rican children. *Am. J. Publ. Hlth*, **64**, 283–91.
15. Frimodt-Moller, J., Acharyulu, G.S. and Kesava Pillai, K. (1973) Observations on the protective effect of BCG in a South Indian rural population: fourth report. *Bull. Int. Union. Tuberc.*, **48**, 40–9.
16. Clemens, J.D., Chuong, J.J. and Feinstein, A.R. (1983) The BCG controversy: a methodological and statistical appraisal. *J. Am. Med. Assoc.*, **249**, 2362–9.
17. World Health Organization (1980b) Vaccination against tuberculosis: report of an ICMR/WHO Scientific Group. *WHO Techn. Rep. Ser.*. No. 651.
18. Willis, M.S. and Vandiviere, M.R. (1961) The heterogeneity of BCG. *Am. Rev. Respir. Dis.*, **84**, 288–90.
19. ten Dam, H.G., Toman, K., Hitze, K.L. and Guld, J. (1976) Present knowledge of immunisation against tuberculosis. *Bull. WHO*, **54**, 255–69.
20. Springett, V.H. and Sutherland, I. (1970) Comparison of the efficacy of liquid and freeze-dried strains of BCG vaccine in preventing tuberculosis. *Brit. Med. J.*, **4**, 148–50.
21. Palmer, C.E. and Long, M.W. (1966) Effects of infection with atypical mycobacteria on BCG vaccination and tuberculosis. *Am. Rev. Respir. Dis.*, **94**, 553–68.
22. Youmans, G.P., Parlett, R.C. and Youmans,

A.S. (1961) The significance of the response of mice to immunization with viable unclassified mycobacteria. *Am. Rev. Respir. Dis.*, **83**, 903–5.

23. Hart, P.D. (1967) Efficacy and applicability of mass BCG vaccination in tuberculosis control. *Br. Med. J.*, **1**, 587–92.

24. Medical Research Council (1972) BCG and vole bacillus vaccines in the prevention of tuberculosis in adolescence and early adult life. *Bull. WHO*, **46**, 371–85.

25. ten Dam, H.G. and Pio, A. (1982) Pathogenesis of tuberculosis and effectiveness of BCG vaccination. *Tubercle*, **63**, 225–33.

26. Comstock, G.W. and Palmer, C.E. (1966) Long- term results of BCG vaccination in the Southern United States. *Am. Rev. Respir. Dis.*, **93**, 171–83.

27. British Thoracic and Tuberculosis Association (1975) Present effectiveness of BCG vaccination in England and Wales. *Tubercle*, **56**, 129–37.

28. British Thoracic Association (1980) Effectiveness of BCG vaccination in Great Britain in 1978. *Br. J. Dis. Chest*, **74**, 215–27.

29. Sutherland, I. and Springett, V.H. (1987) Effectiveness of BCG vaccination in England and Wales in 1983. *Tubercle*, **68**, 81–92.

30. World Health Organization (1980a) BCG Vaccination Policies. *WHO Techni. Rep. Ser.*, No. 652.

31. Smith, P.G. (1982) Retrospective assessment of the effectiveness of BCG vaccination against tuberculosis using the case-control method. *Tubercle*, **62**, 23–35.

32. ten Dam, H.G. (1987) Contact studies on the effectiveness of BCG vaccination in childhood, in *Tuberculosis and Respiratory Diseases*. Papers presented at the plenary sessions of the XXVIth World Conference of the International Union against Tuberculosis, Singapore, 4–7 November 1986. Professional Postgraduate Services, pp. 80–3.

33. Wunsch Filho, V., de Castilho, E.A., Rodrigues, L.C. and Huttly, S.R.A. (1990) Effectiveness of BCG vaccination against tuberculous meningitis: a case-control study in Sao Paulo, Brazil. *Bull. WHO*, **68**, 69–74.

34. Sharma, R.S., Srivastava, D.K., Singh, A.A. *et al.* (1989) Epidemiological evaluation of BCG vaccine efficacy in Delhi – 1989. *J. Commun. Dis. (India)*, **21**, 200–6.

35. Sirinavin, S., Chotpitayasunondh, T., Suwanjutha, S. *et al.* (1991) Protective efficacy of neonatal Bacillus Calmette–Guerin vaccination against tuberculosis. *Pediat. Infect. Dis. J.*, **10**, 359–65.

36. Chavalittamrong, B., Chearskul, S. and Tuchinda, M. (1986) Protective value of BCG vaccination in children in Bangkok, Thailand. *Pediat. Pulmonol.*, 2,202–5.

37. Jin, B.W., Hong, Y.P. and Kim, S.J. (1989) A contact study to evaluate the BCG vaccination programme in Seoul. *Tubercle*, **70**, 241–8.

38. Miceli, I., de Kantor, I.N., Colaiacovo, D. *et al.* (1988) Evaluation of the effectiveness of BCG vaccination using the case-control method in Buenos Aires, Argentina. *Int. J. Epidemiol.*, **17**, 629–34.

39. Blin, P., Delolme, H.G., Heyraud, J.D *et al.* (1986) Evaluation of the protective effect of BCG vaccination by a case-control study in Yaounde, Cameroon. *Tubercle*, **67**, 283–8.

40. Tidjani, O., Amedome, A. and ten Dam, H.G. (1986) The protective effect of BCG vaccination of the newborn against childhood tuberculosis in an African community. *Tubercle*, **67**, 269–81.

41. Packe, G.E. and Innes, J.A. (1988) Protective effect of BCG in infant Asians: a case-control study. *Arch. Dis. Childh.*, **63**, 277–81.

42. Kue Young, T. and Hershfield, E.S. (1986) A case-control study to evaluate the effectiveness of mass neonatal BCG vaccination among Canadian Indians. *Am. J. Pub. Hlth*, **76**, 783–6.

43. Padungchan, S., Konjanart, S., Kasiratta, S. *et al.* (1986) The effectiveness of BCG vaccination of the newborn against childhood tuberculosis in Bangkok. *Bul. WHO*, **64**, 247–58.

44. Houston, S., Fanning, A., Soskolne, C.L. and Fraser, N. (1990) The effectiveness of Bacillus Calmette–Guerin (BCG) vaccination against tuberculosis. *Am. J. Epidemiol.*, **131**, 340–48.

45. Rodrigues, L.C., Gill, O.N. and Smith, P.G. (1991) BCG vaccination in the first year of life protects children of Indian sub-continent ethnic origin against tuberculosis in England. *J. Epidemiol. Comm. Hlth*, **45**, 78–80.

46. Murtagh, K. (1980) Efficacy of BCG. *Lancet*, **1**, 423.

47. Myint, T.T., Win, H., Aye, H.H. and Kwaw-Mint, T.O. (1987) Case-control study on evaluation of BCG vaccination of newborn in Rangoon, Burma. *Ann. Trop. Paediatr.*, **7**, 159–66.

48. Putrali, J., Sutrisna, B., Rahayoe, N. and Gunardi, A.S. (1983) A case-control study of effectiveness of BCG vaccination in children in Jakarta, Indonesia. Proceedings of the Eastern Regional Tuberculosis Conference of IUAT, Jakarta, Indonesia, pp. 194–200.

49. Smith, P.G. (1987) Evaluating interventions against tropical diseases. *Int. J. Epidemiol.*, **16**, 159–66.

50. Shapiro, C., Cook, N., Evans, D. *et al.* (1985) A case-control study of BCG and childhood tuberculosis in Cali, Colombia. *Int. J. Epidemiol.*, **14**, 441–6.

51. Ponnighaus, J.M., Fine, P.E.M., Sterne, J.A.C. *et al.* (1992) Efficacy of BCG vaccine against leprosy and tuberculosis in northern Malawi. *Lancet*, **339**, 636–9.

52. ten Dam, H.G. and Hitze, K.L. (1980) Does BCG vaccination protect the newborn and young infants? *Bull. WHO*, **58**, 37–41.

53. World Health Organization (1987) Expanded programme on immunization. Joint WHO/UNICEF statement on immunization and AIDS. *Weekly Epidemiol. Rec.*, **62**, 53–4.

54. Lallemant-Le Coeur, S., Lallemant, M., Cheynier, D. *et al.* (1991) Bacillus Calmette–Guerin immunization in infants born to HIV-1-seropositive mothers. *AIDS*, **5**, 195–9.

55. Msellati, P., Dabis, F., Lepage, P., *et al.* (1991) BCG vaccination and pediatric HIV infection – Rwanda, 1988–1990. *Morbid. Mortal. Weekly Rep.*, **40**, 833–6.

56. D'Arcy Hart, P., Sutherland, I. and Thomas, J. (1967) The immunity conferred by effective BCG and vole bacillus vaccines, in relation to individual variations in induced tuberculin sensitivity and to technical variations in the vaccines. *Tubercle*, **48**, 201–10.

57. Sutherland, I. and Springett, V.H. (1989) The effects of the scheme for BCG vaccination of schoolchildren in England and Wales and the consequences of discontinuing the scheme at various dates. *J. Epidemiol. Comm. Hlth*, **43**, 15–24.

58. Greenberg, P.D., Lax, K.G. and Schechter, C.B. (1991) Tuberculosis in house staff. A decision analysis comparing the tuberculin screening strategy with the BCG vaccination strategy. *Am. Rev. Respir. Dis.*, **143**, 490–5.

CONTROL 15

CONTROL OF TUBERCULOSIS IN LOW-PREVALENCE COUNTRIES

A.G. Leitch

15a.1 INTRODUCTION

In the low-prevalence countries the most powerful weapons for control of tuberculosis are **case-finding** and **treatment**[1,2]. As the rate of fall of notification of tuberculosis in developed countries begins to slow down, stop or even reverse, as in the USA[3–6], special high-risk groups with a continuing or increasingly high disease frequency begin to exert an ever-growing influence on notification rates[4,7–11]. The need for identification and monitoring of these high-risk groups and intervention with specific programmes for control of tuberculosis is well recognized. This need occurs against a recent background of generally diminishing tuberculosis notifications, declining public health concern and reduction in provision of tuberculosis services[10–14]. In addition, the medical profession has less experience of tuberculosis – 'the fading away of the old soldier' effect[13]; in Holland a family doctor will see only one case of tuberculosis every 4 years and a chest physician only 4 cases per year[9].

The diagrammatic representation of the origin of cases of tuberculosis in the USA in 1983 (Fig. 15a.1)[15], however much one may debate the illustrative population figures, points to the possible interventions available for control of tuberculosis. Tuberculin non-reactors (group A in Fig. 15a.1) could be offered a high degree of protection utilizing BCG immunization[15–17] (Chapter 14b,

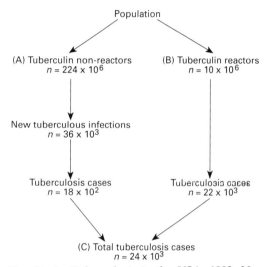

Fig. 15a.1 Tuberculosis in the USA, 1983. New cases may arise either from the small pool of recently infected individuals or from reactivation disease occurring in the much larger pool of positive skin test reactors.

p. 297); in low-prevalence countries this approach has either not been used or, where still used on a population-wide basis, is now coming to the end of its useful life[18–20] with a predictable but tolerable small increase in childhood tuberculosis in those countries where it has been discontinued[21–24]. Tuberculin reactors (group B in Fig. 15a.1) can theoretically be prevented from developing disease by isoniazid chemoprophylaxis

Clinical Tuberculosis. Edited by P.D.O. Davies. Published in 1994 by Chapman & Hall, London. ISBN 0 412 48630 X

Table 15a.1 Mode of detection of smear-positive tuberculosis cases in Kolin, Czechoslovakia, 1961–1969, and the Netherlands, 1951–1967

Country or area	Period of observation	No. of smear +ve cases	Percentage of smear +ve cases discovered by			
			Symptoms	Chest clinic	Mass radiog.	Other
Kolin	1961–1969	193	45	21	25	9
Netherlands	1951–1955	6027	58	12	14	15
	1956–1961	3823	57	15	13	14
	1962–1967	2460	54	17	15	13

[15,24,25]. (Chapter 14a, p. 280) The balancing of the benefits of chemoprophylaxis against the costs, of which hepatitis is the most expensive[26], is a continuing source of debate[25,27–29] and not all of the indications for chemoprophylaxis are crystal clear. The tuberculosis cases (group C in Fig. 15a.1), whether they are due to new infection or reactivation, are the focus of attention for the tuberculosis service. As case-finding moves from the population at large to well-defined high-risk groups, so the contributions of **BCG immunization** and **chemoprophylaxis** become more clearly defined.

15a.2 CASE-FINDING

Mass screening of the population by radiological examination of the chest, although identifying cases of tuberculosis, makes no substantial impact on the number of new cases arising in that population. The evidence for this observation is derived principally from studies in Kolin, Czechoslovakia[30,31], where 95% of the population over 14 years old had chest radiography at 3-year intervals between 1960 and 1972. All identified cases were treated. The number of infectious cases did not differ significantly from year to year between 1960 and 1972, i.e. despite repeated 'cleaning-up' of the population by radiographic detection of disease and treatment, new cases of infectious disease continued to develop in the period between the screening radiographs. The methods of discovery of infectious cases in Czechoslovakia and in the Netherlands where screening by mass miniature radiography was also carried out[32] are shown in Table 15a.1. In both countries then, as now[9], the most common method of discovery was presentation with symptoms. Smaller numbers were detected at chest clinics (e.g. contacts, recent convertors and those with fibrotic lesions) and by mass radiography. Case-finding in the general population most frequently results therefore from radiological and sputum examination of patients presenting with symptoms.

Although mass radiography is not indicated as a case-finding method in the population at large, a clear case exists for radiological and other methods of screening of selected populations and these are outlined below.

15a.2.1 HIGH-YIELD GROUPS

(a) Symptoms group

This consists of patients who have symptoms suggestive of tuberculosis, for example, patients presenting with a productive cough that fails to respond to treatment. Commonly, patients may tolerate a productive cough for weeks or months before seeking medical advice. They may then have several courses of antibiotics extending to weeks or months before they are referred for radiological examination of the chest or a chest clinic opinion. Waiting lists for radiological examination or clinic appointments may further prolong the period the undiagnosed (and often infectious) tuberculosis patient spends in the community before the diagnosis is considered and made. In the Netherlands the mean 'patient plus doctor delay' is reported to be as much as 4 months[9]. Continuing education of the public and practitioners is needed. An open access chest radiology service to which general practitioners can immediately refer their patients may obviate some of the delay[33].

(b) Contacts

It is most important following notification of a case of tuberculosis that appropriate contact procedures be initiated with a view to identifying other cases of tuberculosis. If the first notified or index case is one of primary tuberculosis, then a source case is being sought; if the index case has smear-positive post-primary or reactivation tuberculosis then, although a source case may still be sought, the concern is that other contacts may have been infected by the index case. In most reports, 10–14% of all notifications have been detected by contact screening[34–39], contacts being some ten to 60 times more likely to have the disease than the general population[4,7]. In other reports contact procedures have been less rewarding[40–43]. It is clear that the procedures to be adopted may vary from region to region depending on the local prevalence of tuberculosis, particularly smear-positive tuberculosis, and the ethnic make-up of the population[43]. Departures from standard contact tracing procedures[44–46], are not recommended but much unnecessary screening can be avoided if a rational approach is adopted[47].

Close contacts are defined as household contacts, i.e. living under the same roof as the index case, but other contacts, e.g. those sharing a confined working area with the index case, may equally qualify for the same

description – some interpretative sense is required in the use of this term. All other contacts are **casual**.

The basic tools of contact tracing are tuberculin skin testing and chest radiography. In the USA the Mantoux test with 5TU is used[25] whereas in the UK, where the national BCG programme complicates the interpretation of skin tests, the Heaf test is preferred. BCG-vaccinated individuals and individuals with atypical mycobacterial infection usually have Heaf grade 1 or 2 skin test and those infected with TB grade 3 or 4 skin test results[48] (Chapter 15d, p. 346). In other countries of Europe the Mantoux test is given with PPD RT 23, 2TU.

Where the index case is primary, close contacts should be tuberculin-tested and those with positive tuberculin tests (Mantoux > 5 mm; Heaf test grade 2–4 without and grade 3–4 with previous BCG) should have chest radiography performed. Some detective work may be necessary, employing the 'stone in the pond principle' (screen the inner circle before moving to the outer rings)[49]. Identified cases will be investigated and treated and **their** contacts (who may differ) also screened. Chemoprophylaxis should be recommended for those judged to have been infected by the source case[44,45]. School outbreaks due to infectious disease in a teacher demonstrate the principles of screening in this situation[50,51], although the ageing grandparent, procedures 'invading' the respiratory tract[52] or public service employees[53] may be equally potent sources of infection.

The majority of notified cases of tuberculosis in low-prevalence countries have post-primary or reactivation disease. Where the index case has smear-positive pulmonary disease, initial screening is by skin testing of close and casual contacts. Contacts with negative or weakly positive skin tests (Mantoux < 5 mm; Heaf test grade 0 or 1 without and grade 0–2 with previous BCG) should be retested after 6–8 weeks to exclude the possibility of recent primary infection. Those converting to positive skin tests (Mantoux ≥ 10 mm; Heaf test grade 2–4 without and grade 3–4 with previous BCG) should have chest radiography, those with positive radiographs being investigated and treated and those with negative radiographs receiving chemoprophylaxis. In the UK it is recommended that skin-test-negative contacts under the age of 35 years be immunized with BCG[44] although this may now only be of proven value in Asians[54]. Contacts with positive initial tuberculin tests (Mantoux ≥ 5 mm; Heaf test grade 2–4 without and grade 3–4 with previous BCG) should have chest radiography. Positive radiographs qualify the patient for investigation and treatment. The management of contacts of smear-positive index cases who have positive tuberculin tests and negative initial chest radiographs may be by:

1. Chemoprophylaxis[25,45], possibly restricted to those under 16 years of age[44].
2. Radiological follow-up.

Radiological follow-up for tuberculin-positive contacts of smear-positive index cases has been recommended for a duration of 1 year extending to 2 years for contacts of Asian cases[44]. Most cases detected radiologically among contacts are diagnosed within 6 months [47,55] and extending follow-up beyond this time may be unproductive as well as uneconomic. Audit of the productivity of local procedures will help to determine the policy locally appropriate[47].

Screening of contacts of smear-negative pulmonary disease should be restricted to close contacts who require only initial chest radiography. If chemoprophylaxis is to be offered to all tuberculin-positive contacts of smear-negative pulmonary cases or, as recommended by the British Thoracic Society [44], only to those under 16 years of age, then their skin test status must also be determined. Similarly, the skin test status of contacts of Asian smear-negative pulmonary cases must

be determined for they qualify for BCG immunization if skin-test-negative and aged less than 35 years and for chemoprophylaxis if tuberculin-positive[54,56].

Screening of contacts of patients with extrapulmonary tuberculosis is unproductive[38] and need not be performed except where a recent primary infection is suspected as with pleural effusion, meningitis or erythema nodosum in children. Any tuberculosis screening service, whether organized and run by consultants in public health medicine or chest physicians, is dependent on health visitors or their nursing equivalent who ensure that contact tracing is followed through and that defaulters are encouraged by every possible means to attend for screening. Efficient record-keeping and regular review of contact and case records are essential[33].

(c) Lodging houses, prisons and mental institutions

Tuberculosis is more common in the population variously referred to as the homeless, 'down-and-outs', lodging house or hostel dwellers among whom alcohol and drug abuse are often commonplace[57–63] (Chapter 10, p. 193). The advent of HIV infection among intravenous drug abusers in this population has led to an increase in tuberculous disease in this group[64–66] (Chapter 12a; p. 228) and focused attention on the marked deficiencies in public health services offered to them[14,67]. These individuals are notoriously unreliable, frequently moving address and usually hostile to and suspicious of the attentions of the health services.

In an ideal world the tuberculin skin test and radiological status of each of these individuals would be known and updated as required. Where appropriate, chemoprophylaxis would be prescribed[25] and services would be available to ensure that it was taken. Reality is different, in New York at least; even when hospitalized with active tuberculosis and started on treatment, 89% of the patient population were lost to follow-up and a very significant minority were re-admitted within 12 months with active tuber-culosis, to be discharged and lost to follow-up yet again[65].

Attitudes to screening for tuberculosis among this population will depend largely on the scale of tuberculous and HIV infection and disease among them. Where this is perceived to be a problem, skin-testing pro-grammes with supervised chemoprophylaxis for skin-test-positive individuals should be offered[45]. At the very least the threshold of suspicion for active tuberculous disease in individuals should be set low with early bacteriological and radiological investigation followed by supervised treatment of dis-ease[68]. Contact screening, known to be very productive in this situation[62,63] should be pursued rigorously. The provision of a health service for this group and the education of their carers are important for success. Staff working with this population should be protected by BCG immunization or annual tuberculin testing with chemoprophy-laxis for convertors. In either case they should be educated to present early for radiographic examination if they develop symptoms.

The increasing prevalence of HIV infection has focused attention on the possible conse-quences to the prison service of incarcerating individuals with dual tuberculous and HIV infection who are predisposed to the risk of developing active tuberculosis with all the attendant risks of transmission of infection to other inmates and staff[69]. This problem has not so far been actively addressed in the UK where radiological screening of prison popu-lations ceased (because it was unproductive) some years ago. In the USA clear guidelines for the control and prevention of tuberculosis in correctional institutions have been given [70] based on annual tuberculin testing for inmates and staff with chemoprophylaxis/ radiological investigation where appropriate.

These recommendations have not been universally implemented[71]. Clearly, a low threshold of suspicion and for detection of disease in this population is desirable with contact screening if and when a case is diagnosed.

Residential facilities other than hostels and prisons, such as homes for the mentally ill or handicapped, are also potential sites for spread of tuberculous infection and disease. Radiological screening of such establish-ments in the UK ceased many years ago as it had latterly proved unproductive perhaps reflecting a decrease in tuberculous infection (and therefore risk of reactivation disease) in these patients. There appear to have been no untoward consequences of abandoning such screening; the occasional identified case leads to prompt and usually unproductive contact screening, which is nevertheless reassuring to all concerned. Were significant problems with tuberculosis to develop locally in such a population then a programme of skin testing and intervention might be necessary.

(d) Immigrants and ethnic group distinctions

New immigrants from high-prevalence countries, most commonly Asians, may import active tuberculosis to their new low-prevalence home; more commonly, they develop disease reactivation within 5 years of their arrival[72–76]. Tuberculosis in this high-risk group is a component but by no means the only or principal component in the higher incidence of tuberculous disease in ethnic minorities in the USA; in comparison with Whites, tuberculosis is four times more common in Hispanics, five times more common in American Indians, six times in Blacks and 11 times in Asians and Pacific Islanders[77–82]. In the UK and Canada tuberculosis is at least 15 times more common in Asian immigrants and in Germany nine times more common in immigrants than in the general population[4, 7, 83] (Chapter 11, p. 191).

Ideally, immigrants should have had radiography in their country of origin. At the port of arrival they should be seen by a medical officer who obtains relevant details (chest radiograph, BCG status, skin-test status, previous disease or treatment) where possible, including the address of intended settlement. These details may not be reliable and chest radiography carried out at the port of arrival is to be preferred. These details can then be forwarded to the relevant health service officer in the appropriate district. Complementary local initiatives for identifying new immigrants may be employed, such as regular scrutiny of family doctor lists with referral of any new immigrant names to the tuberculosis service for follow-up by a health visitor. Immigrants should be contacted as soon as possible after arrival as they are highly mobile (Chapter 10, p. 203)

A visit by a tuberculosis health visitor allows organization of Heaf (or Mantoux) testing either at a clinic or at home. An interpreter service is often helpful. In the UK those with negative tuberculin reactions aged less than 35 years are referred for BCG vaccination[54]. Those with positive tuberculin reactions (Mantoux $\geq$ 10 mm; Heaf test grade 2–4 without and grade 3–4 with previous BCG) are offered chest radiography and those aged less than 35 years are offered chemoprophylaxis[44].

Childhood tuberculosis in children of Asian parents in the UK is 25 times more common among those born abroad and 15 times more common among those born in the UK than in native white children[84]. BCG vaccination should therefore be given at birth in those born in the UK and as soon as possible after arrival in the country to those born abroad who are tuberculin-negative.

The medical and allied professions need to continue to be aware of the high incidence of tuberculosis in immigrants.

(e) The elderly in nursing homes

The elderly are at risk not only of endogenous reactivation of tuberculosis but possibly also of exogenous reinfection, particularly in nursing homes[85]. Outbreaks of tuberculosis among the elderly in nursing homes have been reported from Arkansas, USA[86] and subsequent studies of such chronic care populations have shown as much as a 5% rate of tuberculin skin-test conversion in elderly residents[87,88] with the development of significant disease in those not given chemoprophylaxis with isoniazid[88].

Given the permanence, in most circumstances, of a move to long-term residential care, often somewhat removed from medical, radiological and other investigative services, it would make sense to determine, at the time of admission, either tuberculin skin-test status or recent/current radiological status or both[89,90]. Skin testing should be performed using the two-step method to identify reactors whose reaction has waned with time[88] (Chapter 15d, p. 348).

Studies in nursing home residents in Liverpool, UK[91] have not, so far, confirmed the findings from Arkansas, but this should not detract from the need for a high level of suspicion among carers for the possibility of tuberculosis in their charges. Where skin test or radiological status are known to be positive for previous tuberculous infection then nursing home residents developing 'bronchitis or pneumonia' should be examined for clinical manifestations of tuberculosis and have sputum examined microbiologically for tuberculosis.

15a.2.2 HIGH-RISK GROUPS

(a) Doctors, dentists, nurses and other clinical practitioners

Tuberculosis still occurs among hospital doctors[92,93] and is most commonly acquired during training[94,95]. Many of these doctors will have evaded screening[96,97] and some may transmit the disease to their patients[98].

In the UK, members of the medical, dental and nursing professions as well as others regularly working with patients and medical laboratory technicians[99–101] are subjected to pre-employment health screening and tuberculin testing (unless there is a history of previous BCG supported by a scar). Tuberculin-negative individuals are immunized with BCG. Strongly positive tuberculin reactors are referred for chest radiographic examination[44], although in the absence of symptoms this may be unnecessary[102]. In countries where BCG vaccination programmes are not routinely employed, such as the USA, annual tuberculin skin testing may be used for those who are initially tuberculin-negative, with chemoprophylaxis being offered to those who are initially tuberculin-positive and to those who subsequently convert their skin-test status. Booster reactions need to be identified and separated from true skin-test conversions[103,104]. It has been suggested that BCG vaccination may be preferable to a tuberculin skin-testing programme[105].

(b) Teachers and others working with children

The important consideration with regard to school teachers and others working with children is the detection of active pulmonary tuberculosis by medical examination and investigation of those about whom there is any suspicion after the pre-employment health questionnaire[44].

15a.3 BCG VACCINATION

BCG vaccination is considered in Chapter 14a. For control purposes, as discussed above, the administration of BCG to school children in the UK (and other countries) may be discontinued in the next few years[44]. Other categories of individuals currently offered tuberculin testing and BCG vaccination if negative are health service employees and some contacts of cases of tuberculosis [44]. Tuberculin-negative children and neonates in Asian (and other high-risk ethnic group) families should also be vaccinated[54]. BCG vaccination may be an alternative to annual tuberculin testing of health service employees in the USA[105].

15a.4 CHEMOPROPHYLAXIS

Chemoprophylaxis is also considered in Chapter 14a. Secondary chemoprophylaxis with isoniazid 300 mg daily (5 mg/kg for children up to a maximum of 300 mg daily) for 1 year (for alternatives see Chapter 14a) is recommended in the following situations [44,45]:

1. *Tuberculin positive contacts of cases of tuberculosis*, including recent skin-test convertors who have no evidence of disease. Radiological follow-up of tuberculin-positive adults is preferred in the UK.
2. *Tuberculin skin-test reactors with an abnormal chest radiograph* suggestive of inactive tuberculous disease, who are bacteriologically negative and have not previously been treated, may qualify for chemoprophylaxis, which reduces the incidence of disease[106,107] although large numbers have to be treated to prevent one case[27].
3. *Positive skin-test reactors with special clinical conditions*[25,45]

Mantoux ≥ 5 mm	HIV-seropositive patients
Mantoux ≥ 10 mm	Silicosis
	Gastrectomy
	Jejuno-ileal bypass
	Malnutrition
	Chronic renal failure

Diabetes mellitus
Corticosteroid therapy
Immunosuppressive treatment
Haematological malignancy
Intravenous drug abusers

4. *Healthy positive skin-test reactors aged < 35 years* with Mantoux test ≥ 15 mm. This group would qualify for chemoprophylaxis in the UK.

With chemoprophylaxis, as with chemotherapy for tuberculosis, success can only be measured in treatments completed. Problems with patient compliance are commonplace and a number of strategies designed to improve compliance have been described [108].

15a.5 ORGANIZATION OF TUBERCULOSIS SERVICES

Control of tuberculosis in low-prevalence countries is critically dependent on efficient and effective monitoring and surveillance of disease. Notification systems already exist, with cases notified locally or regionally being passed to a National Tuberculosis Register where annual statistics can be collated [4,13,44,109]. Not all cases are notified [110, 111]. Separate notifications by microbiologists and pathologists of positive specimens may uncover and remedy clinical lapses in practice[110]. Data on standard notification forms are not adequate to provide effective surveillance of population risk groups and it has been suggested[10] that the minimum information supplied for each case should include: age, sex, nationality, ethnic status (including year of immigration), bacteriological status and site of disease. Disease initially notified as tuberculous and subsequently found to be due to an environmental mycobacterium should be denotified.

Each district or region should appoint a chest physician and/or consultant in public health medicine with responsibility for pro-viding the tuberculosis service[33]. Adequate medical, nursing and clerical staff[112] should be available to ensure that necessary contact tracing and screening is performed and that interventions such as BCG vaccination, chemoprophylaxis, radiological follow-up and chemotherapy itself are not only implemented but also, where necessary, supervised to ensure compliance[106]. The extreme consequences of deficiencies in such services have been described in New York [14,64,113]. Organization of the service for BCG immunization of immigrant neonates is best carried out by the consultant in public health medicine but chest and family physicians also have a role to play in identifying tuberculin-negative immigrant children who qualify for BCG vaccination.

Adequate surveillance of tuberculosis in low-prevalence countries should permit the identification and targeting of services on high-risk groups whether they constitute 40%[4] or 80%[7] of all tuberculosis notifications. It is only by developing, applying and maintaining such services that the aim of 'eradication of tuberculosis' will seem nearer rather than further away[114].

REFERENCES

1. Styblo, K. (1991) Epidemiology of tuberculosis. *Royal Netherlands Tuberculosis Association, Selected Papers*, **24**, 1–115.
2. Styblo, K. and Enarson, D.A. (1991) Epidemiology of tuberculosis in HIV prevalent countries. *Royal Netherlands Tuberculosis Association, Selected Papers*, **24**, 116–36.
3. Davies, P.D.O. (1989) The slowing of the decline in tuberculosis notifications and HIV infection. *Respir. Med.*, **83**, 321–2.
4. Schilling, W. (1990) Epidemiology and surveillance of tuberculosis in the German Democratic Republic. *Bull IUATLD*, **65**, 2–3, 40–2.
5. Murray, J.F. (1989) The white plague: down and out or up and coming? *Am. Rev. Respir. Dis.*, **140**, 1788–95.
6. Bloch, A.B., Rieder, H.L., Kelly, G.D. *et al.*

(1989). The epidemiology of tuberculosis in the United States. Implications for diagnosis and treatment. *Clin. Chest. Med.*, **10**, 297–313.

7. Enarson, D.A., Fanning, E.A. and Allen, E.A. (1990) Case finding in the elimination phase of tuberculosis: high-risk groups in epidemiology and clinical practice. *Bull. Int. Union Tuberc. Lung Dis.*, **65**, 2–3, 73–4.

8. Styblo, K. (1990) The elimination of tuberculosis in the Netherlands. *Bull. Int. Union Tuberc. Lung Dis.*, **65**, 2–3, 49–55.

9. Veen, J. (1990) Methods of tuberculosis case-finding in the Netherlands. *Bull. Int. Union Tuberc. Lung Dis.*, **65**, 2–3, 67–9.

10. Rieder, H.L. (1992) Misbehaviour of a dying epidemic: a call for less speculation and better surveillance. *Tuberc. Lung Dis.*, **73**, 181–3.

11. Sbarbaro, J. (1990) 'Elimination': of tuberculosis or tuberculosis control programmes. *Bull. Int. Union Tuberc. Lung Dis.*, **65**, 2–3, 47–8.

12. Leff, D.R. and Leff, A.R. (1989) Tuberculosis control policies in major metropolitan health departments in the United States. *Am. Rev. Respir. Dis.*, **139**, 1350–5.

13. Broekmans, J.F. (1990) Maintenance of a tuberculosis programme in the elimination phase. *Bull. Int. Union Tuberc. Lung Dis.*, **65**, 2–3, 92–3.

14. Reichman, L.B. (1991) The U-shaped curve of concern. *Am. Rev. Respir. Dis.*, **144**, 741–2.

15. Research Committee of the British Thoracic Association (1980) Effectiveness of BCG vaccination in Great Britain in 1978. *Br. J. Dis. Chest*, **74**, 215–27.

16. Sutherland, I. and Springett, V.H. (1987) Effectiveness of BCG vaccination in England and Wales in 1983. *Tubercle*, **68**, 81–92.

17. Capewell, S., France, A., Uzel, N. and Leitch, A.G. (1986) The current value of tuberculin testing and BCG vaccination in schoolchildren. *Br. J. Dis. Chest*, **80**, 254–64.

18. Sutherland, I. and Springett, V.H. (1989) The effects of the scheme for the BCG vaccination of schoolchildren in England and Wales and the consequences of discontinuing the scheme at various dates. *J. Epidemiol. Comm. Hlth*, **43**, 15–24.

19. Conway, S.P. (1990) BCG vaccination in schoolchildren. *Br. Med. J.*, **301**, 1059–60.

20. Joseph, C.A., Watson, J.M. and Fern, K.J. (1992) BCG immunisation in England and Wales: a survey of policy and practice in schoolchildren and neonates. *Br. Med. J.*, **305**, 495–8.

21. Romanus, V. (1990) Experience in Sweden 15 years after stopping general BCG vaccination at birth. *Bull. Int. Union*, **65**, 2–3, 32–5.

22. Trnka, L., Dankova, D., Machova, A. *et al.* (1990) Project on discontinuation of BCG in newborns in Czechoslovakia. *Bull. Int. Union Tuberc. Lung Dis.*, **65**, 2–3, 36–7.

23. Romanus, V., Svensson, A. and Hallander, H.O. (1992) The impact of changing BCG coverage on tuberculosis incidence in Swedish-born children between 1969 and 1989. *Tubercle Lung Dis.*, **73**, 150–61.

24. Centers for Disease Control. (1989) A strategic plan for the elimination of tuberculosis in the United States. *Morbid. Mortal. Weekly Rep.*, **38** (Suppl. S-3).

25. Bass, J.B. (1990) Tuberculin test, preventive therapy and elimination of tuberculosis. *Am. Rev. Respir. Dis.*, **141**, 812–13.

26. Kopanoff, D.E., Snider, D.E. and Caras, G.J. (1978) Isoniazid-related hepatitis. A US Public Health Service Co-operative Surveillance Study. *Am. Rev. Respir. Dis.*, **117**, 991–1001.

27. Leading Article (1981) Chemoprophylaxis for tuberculosis. *Tubercle*, **62**, 69–72.

28. Taylor, W.C., Aronson, M.D. and Delbanco, T.L. (1981) Should young adults with a positive tuberculin test take isoniazid? *Ann. Intern. Med.*, **94**, 808–13.

29. Jordan, T.J., Lewitt, E.M. and Reichman, L.B. (1991) Isoniazid preventive therapy for tuberculosis. Decision analysis concerning ethnicity and gender. *Am. Rev. Respir. Dis.*, **144**, 1357–60.

30. Styblo, K., Dankova, D., Drapela, J. *et al.* (1967) Epidemiological and clinical study of tuberculosis in the district of Kolin, Czechoslovakia. *Bull. WHO*, **37**, 819–74.

31. Krivinka, R., Drapela, J., Dankova, D. *et al.* (1974) Epidemiological and clinical study of tuberculosis in the district of Kolin, Czechoslovakia. Second Report (1965–1972). *Bull. WHO*, **51**, 59–69.

32. Meijer, J., Banneti, G.D., Kubik, A. and Styblo, K. (1971) Identification of sources of infection. *Bull. Int Union Tuberc. Lung Dis.* **45**, 5–12.

33. Leitch, A.G. (1987) Setting up and running a local tuberculosis service. *Br. J. Dis. Chest*, **87**, 6–13.

34. Payne, C.R. (1978) Surveillance of tuberculosis contacts? Experience at Ealing Chest Clinic. *Tubercle*, **59**, 179–84.

35. British Thoracic Association (1978) A study of a standardised contact procedure in tuberculosis. *Tubercle*, **59**, 245–59.

36. Rose, C.E., Zerbe, G.O., Lantz, S.O. and Bailey, W.C. (1979) Establishing priority during investigation of tuberculosis contacts. *Am. Rev. Respir. Dis.*, **119**, 603–9.

37. American Thoracic Society (1983) Control of tuberculosis. *Am. Rev. Respir. Dis.*, **128**, 336–42.

38. Capewell, S. and Leitch, A.G. (1984) The value of contact procedures for tuberculosis in Edinburgh. *Br. J. Dis. Chest*, **78**, 317–29.

39. Management of contacts of tuberculosis (1990) *Drug Ther. Bull.*, **28**, 21–2.

40. Spencer-Jones, J. (1982) A tuberculosis outbreak in Deal, Kent. *Lancet*, **1**, 1060–1.

41. Spencer-Jones, J. (1983) Tuberculosis case-finding in coastal South-East Kent 1977–1981. *Lancet*, **i**, 232–3.

42. Esmonde, T.F.G. and Petheram, I.S. (1991) Audit of tuberculosis contact tracing procedures in S. Gwent. *Resp. Med.*, **85**, 421–4.

43. Hussain, S.F., Watura, R., Cashman, B. *et al.* (1992) Audit of a tuberculosis contact tracing clinic. *Br. Med. J.*, **304**, 1213–15.

44. Sub-Committee of the Joint Tuberculosis Committee of the British Thoracic Society (1990) Control and prevention of tuberculosis in Britain: an updated code of practice. *Br. Med. J.*, **300**, 995–9.

45. Centers for Disease Control (1990) Screening for tuberculosis and tuberculous infections in high risk populations and the use of preventive therapy for tuberculous infection in the United States. *Morbid. Mortal. Weekly Rep.*, **39**, RR-8.

46. American Thoracic Society (1992) Control of tuberculosis in the United States. *Am. Rev. Respir. Dis.*, **146**, 1623–33.

47. Leitch, A.G. (1992) Rationalising tuberculosis contact tracing in low-prevalence areas. *Respir. Med.*, **86**, 371–3.

48. Rathus, E.M. (1956) The Heaf multiple puncture test compared with the Mantoux test in epidemiological surveys. *Med. J. Aust.*, **1**, 696–8.

49. Veen, J. (1991) Tuberculosis in a low prevalence country: a wolf in sheep's clothing. *Bull. Int. Union Tuberc. Lung. Dis.*, **66**, 203–5.

50. Wales, J.M., Buchan, A.R., Cookson, J.B. *et al.* (1985) Tuberculosis in a primary school: the Uppingham outbreak. *Br. Med. J.*, **291**, 1039–40.

51. Frew, A.J., Mayon-White, R.T. and Benson, M.K. (1987) An outbreak of tuberculosis in an Oxfordshire school. *Br. J. Dis. Chest*, **81**, 293–5.

52. Catanzaro, A. Nosocomial tuberculosis. *Am. Rev. Respir. Dis.*, **125**, 559–62.

53. Rao, V.R., Joanes, R.F., Kilbane, P. and Galbraith, N.S. (1980) Outbreak of tuberculosis after minimal exposure to infection. *Br. Med. J.*, **281**, 187–9.

54. Ormerod, L.P. (1990) Tuberculosis screening and prevention in new immigrants 1983–1988. *Resp. Med.*, **84**, 269–71.

55. Selby, C.D., Allen, M.B. and Leitch, A.G. (1989) Optimal duration of radiological follow-up for tuberculosis contacts. *Resp. Med.*, **83**, 353–5.

56. Ormerod, L.P. (1987) Reduced incidence of paediatric tuberculosis following prophylactic chemotherapy in strongly tuberculin positive children. *Arch. Dis. Childh.*, **62**, 1005–8.

57. Patel, K.R. (1985) Pulmonary tuberculosis in residents of lodging houses, night shelters and common hostels in Glasgow: a five-year prospective study. *Br. J. Dis. Chest*, **79**, 60–6.

58. Capewell, S., France, A., Anderson, M. and Leitch, A.G. (1986) The diagnosis and management of tuberculosis in common hostel dwellers. *Tubercle*, **67**, 125–31.

59. Barry, M.A., Wall, C., Shirley, L. *et al.* (1986) Tuberculosis screening in Boston's homeless shelters. *Publ. Hlth Rep.*, **101**, 487–94.

60. Wosornu, D., Macintyre, D. and Watt, B. (1990) An outbreak of isoniazid resistant tuberculosis in Glasgow 1981–1988. *Resp. Med.*, **84**, 361–4.

61. Friedman, L.N., Sullivan, G.M., Bevilaqua, R.P. and Loscos, R. (1987) Tuberculosis screening in alcoholics and drug addicts. *Am. Rev. Respir. Dis.* **136**, 1188–92.

62. Anon. (1990) Tuberculosis among residents of shelters for the homeless, Ohio 1990. *Morbid. Mortal. Weekly Rep.*, **40**, 869–77.

63. Nolan, C.M., Elarth, A.M., Bass, H., *et al.* (1991). An outbreak of tuberculosis in a shelter for homeless men. *Am. Rev. Respir. Dis.*, **143**, 257–61.

64. Selwyn, P.A., Hartel, D., Lewis, V.A., *et al.*

(1989) A prospective study of the risk of tuberculosis among intravenous drug users with human immunodeficiency virus infection. *N. Engl. J. Med.*, **320**, 545–50.

65. Brudney, K. and Dobkin, J., (1991) Resurgent tuberculosis in New York City. Human immunodeficiency virus, homelessness and the decline of tuberculosis control programs. *Am. Rev. Respir. Dis.*, **144**, 745–9.

66. Daley, C.L., Small, P.M., Schecter, G.F. *et al.* (1992) An outbreak of tuberculosis with accelerated progression among persons infected with the human immunodeficiency virus. *N. Engl. J. Med.*, **326**, 231–5.

67. Sbarbaro, J. (1987) To seek, find and yet fail. *Am. Rev. Respir. Dis.*, **136**, 1072–3.

68. Schieffelbein, C.W. and Snider, D.E. (1988) Tuberculosis control among the homeless population. *Arch. Intern. Med.*, **148**, 1843–6.

69. Darbyshire, J. (1989) Tuberculosis in prisons. Possible links with HIV infection. *Br. Med. J.*, **299**, 874.

70. Centers for Disease Control (1989) Prevention and control of tuberculosis in correctional institutions: recommendations of the Advisory Committee for Elimination of Tuberculosis. *Morbid. Mortal. Weekly Rep.*, **38**, 313–25.

71. Snider, D.E. and Hutton, M.D. (1989) Tuberculosis in correctional institutions. *J. Am. Med. Assoc.*, **261**, 436–7.

72. British Thoracic and Tuberculosis Association (1975) Tuberculosis among immigrants related to length of residence in England and Wales. *Br. Med. J.*, **3**, 698–9.

73. Nolan, C.M. and Elarth, A.M. (1988) Tuberculosis in a cohort of South-East Asian refugees. A five-year surveillance study. *Am. Rev. Respir. Dis.*, **137**, 805–9.

74. Tala, E. (1989) Migration, ethnic minorities and tuberculosis. *Eur. Resp. J.*, **2**, 492–3.

75. Enarson, D.A., Wang, J.S. and Grzybowski, S. (1990) Case-finding in the elimination phase of tuberculosis: tuberculosis in displaced people. *Bull. Int. Union Tuberc. Lung. Dis.*, **65**, 2–3, 71–2.

76. Wang, J.S., Allen, E.A., Enarson, D.A. and Grzybowski, S. (1991) Tuberculosis in recent Asian immigrants in British Columbia, Canada: 1982–1985. *Tubercle*, **72**, 277–83.

77. Leads from MMWR (1987) Tuberculosis among Hispanics – United States, 1985. *J. Am. Med. Assoc.*, **258**, 1583.

78. Leads from MMWR (1987) Tuberculosis in Blacks, United States. *J. Am. Med. Assoc.*, **257**, 2407–8.

79. Leads from MMWR (1987) Tuberculosis among Asians/Pacific Islanders – United States 1985. *J. Am. Med. Assoc.*, **258**, 181–2.

80. Rieder, H.L., Cauthen, G.M. Kelly, G.D., *et al.* (1989) Tuberculosis in the United States. *J. Am. Med. Assoc.*, **262**, 385–9.

81. Snider, D.E., Salinas, L. and Kelly, G.D. (1989) Tuberculosis: an increasing problem among minorities in the United States. *Publ. Hlth Rep.*, **104**, 646–53.

82. Rieder, H.L., Cauthen, G.M., Comstock, G.W. and Snider, D.E. (1989) Epidemiology of tuberculosis in the United States. *Epidemiol Rev.*, **11**, 79–98.

83. Medical Research Council, (1986) The geographical distribution of tuberculosis notifications in a national survey of England and Wales in 1983. *Tubercle*, **67**, 163–78.

84. Medical Research Council Tuberculosis and Chest Diseases Unit (1988) Tuberculosis in children: a national survey of notifications in England and Wales in 1983. *Arch. Dis. Childh.*, **63**, 266–76.

85. Leading article (1983) Tuberculosis in old age. *Tubercle*, **64**, 69–71.

86. Stead, W.W. (1981) Tuberculosis among elderly persons: an outbreak in a nursing home. *Ann. Intern. Med.*, **94**, 606–10.

87. Welty, C., Burstin, S., Muspratt, S. and Tager, I.B. (1985) Epidemiology of tuberculous infection in a chronic care population. *Am. Rev. Respir. Dis.*, **132**, 133–6.

88. Stead, W.W., Lofgren, J.P., Warren, E. and Thomas, C. (1985) Tuberculosis as an endemic and nosocomial infection among the elderly in nursing homes. *N. Engl. J. Med.*, **312**, 1483–7.

89. Stead, W.W. (1989) Special problems in tuberculosis. Tuberculosis in the elderly and in residents of nursing homes, correctional facilities, long-term care hospitals, mental hospitals, shelters for the homeless and jails. *Clin. Chest Med.*, **10**, 397–405.

90. Stead, W.W. and Dutt, A.K. (1991) Tuberculosis in elderly persons. *Ann. Rev. Med.*, **42**, 267–76.

91. Davies, P.D.O., Nisar, M., Williams, C.S.D. and Ashby, D. (1992) Risk of tuberculosis

infection in residential houses for the elderly. *Thorax*, **47**, 228P.

92. Festenstein, F. (1984) Tuberculosis in hospital doctors. *Br. Med. J.*, **289**, 1327–8.

93. Belfield, P.W., Arnold, A.G., Williams, S.E. *et al.* (1984) Recent experiences of tuberculosis in junior hospital doctors in Leeds and Bradford. *Br. J. Dis. Chest*, **78**, 313–16.

94. Geiseler, P.J., Nelson, K.E., Crispen, R.G. and Moses, V.K. (1986) Tuberculosis in physicians: a continuing problem. *Am. Rev. Respir. Dis.*, **133**, 773–8.

95. Malasky, C., Jordan, T., Potielski, F. and Rachman, L.B. (1990) Occupational tuberculous infections among physicians in training. *Am. Rev. Respir. Dis.*, **142**, 505–7.

96. Geiseler, P.J., Nelson, K.E. and Crispen, R.G. (1987) Tuberculosis in physicians. Compliance with preventive measures. *Am. Rev. Respir. Dis.*, **135**, 3–9.

97. Clague, J.E., Fields, P., Graham, D.R. and Davies, P.D.O. (1991) Screening for tuberculosis: current problems and attitudes of hospital workers. *Tubercle*, **721**, 265–7.

98. Stewart, C.J. (1976) Tuberculous infection in a paediatric department. *Br. Med. J.*, **1**, 30–2.

99. Harrington, J.M. and Shannon, H.S. (1976) Incidence of tuberculosis, hepatitis, brucellosis and shigellosis in British medical laboratory workers. *Br. Med. J.*, **1**, 759–62.

100. Capewell, S., Leaker, A.R. and Leitch, A.G. (1988) Tuberculosis in health service staff – is it a problem? *Tubercle*, **69**, 113–18.

101. Goldman, K.P. (1988) Tuberculosis in hospital doctors. *Tubercle*, **69**, 237–40.

102. Gottridge, J., Meyer, R., Schwartz, N.S. and Lesser, R.S. (1989) The non-utility of chest roentgenographic examination in asymptomatic patients with positive tuberculin test results. *Arch. Intern. Med.*, **149**, 1660–2.

103. Thompson, N.J., Glassroth, J.L., Snider, D.E. and Farer, L.S. (1979) The booster phenomenon in serial tuberculin testing. *Am. Rev. Respir. Dis.*, **119**, 587–97.

104. Bass, J.B. and Serio, R.A. (1981) The use of repeat skin tests to eliminate the booster phenomenon in serial tuberculin testing. *Am. Rev. Respir. Dis.*, **123**, 394–6.

105. Greenberg, P.D., Lax, K.G. and Schecter, C.B. (1991) Tuberculosis in house staff. A decision analysis comparing the tuberculin screening strategy with the BCG vaccination. *Am. Rev. Respir. Dis.*, **143**, 490–95.

106. International Union Against Tuberculosis Committee on Prophylaxis. (1982) Efficacy of various durations of isoniazid preventive therapy for tuberculosis: 5 years of follow-up. *Bull. WHO*, **60**, 555–64.

107. Comstock, G.W. (1983) New data on preventive treatment with isoniazid. *Ann. Intern. Med.*, **98**, 663–5.

108. Cuneo, W. and Snider, D.E. (1989) Enhancing patient compliance with tuberculosis therapy. *Clin. Chest Med.*, **10**, 375–80.

109. Aoki, M. (1990) Tuberculosis surveillance system in Japan. *Bull. Int. Union Tuberc. Lung Dis.*, **65**, 2–3, 44–7.

110. Bradley, B.L, Kerr, K.M, Leitch, A.D. and Lamb, D. (1988) Notification of tuberculosis: can the pathologist help? *Br. Med. J.*, **297**, 595.

111. King, K., Cock, H., Sheldon, C.D. *et al.* (1992) Notification of tuberculosis: how many cases are never reported? *Thorax*, **47**, 1015–18.

112. Joint Tuberculosis Committee (1988) *Nursing Service for Tuberculosis.* British Thoracic Society, London Newsletter No. 3.

113. Glassroth, J.L. (1992) Tuberculosis in the United States: looking for a silver lining among the clouds. *Am. Rev. Respir. Dis.*, **146**, 278–9.

114. Horne, N.W. (1983) Eradication of tuberculosis in Europe – so near and yet so far. *Eur J. Resp. Dis.*, **64** (Suppl. 126), 169–73.

TUBERCULOSIS CONTROL IN HIGH-PREVALENCE COUNTRIES

15b

Petra Graf

15b.1 THE EXTENT OF THE PROBLEM

Tuberculosis has declined in industrialized countries during the past decades, but it still represents a major health problem in developing countries. There are two basic factors influencing the difference of tuberculosis control between high- and low-prevalence countries; the prevalence of tuberculosis infection and disease within the communities, and the different socio-economic conditions.

If we talk about tuberculosis control in high-prevalence countries, we can synonymously talk about tuberculosis control in developing countries. Only a few of the problems that make proper tuberculosis control in developing countries such an extraordinary challenge can be mentioned here: poor overall health status of the population in developing countries; poor economies; poor infrastructure; bad roads; heavy rainy seasons, which make vast areas inaccessible for months; remote areas, inaccessible by car; the problem of nomads, migrants and refugees, and civil war. This list is far from being comprehensive. Not all of these aspects are specific for developing countries alone, but one has to face these problems when planning health intervention strategies in developing countries.

Table 15b.1 shows clearly that the tuberculosis problem is mainly a problem of the developing world. Out of approximately 8

Table 15b.1 The global toll of tuberculosis

Region	No. infected (000)	New cases (000)	Deaths (000)
Africa	171 000	1398	656
Americas	117 000	564	220
E Mediterranean	52 000	594	163
SE Asia	426 000	2480	932
W Pacific	574 000	2557	894
Industrialized countries	382 000	409	42
Total	1 722 000	8002	2907

Source: First Programme Report (1989–1990) and Future Plan (1991–1995), World Health Organization, Document WHO/TB/91.159.

million new cases per year, only 5% occur in industrialized countries and out of approximately 3 million deaths reported in tuberculosis cases per year, only 1.5% occur in industrialized countries. In other words, 95% of the cases are to be found in developing countries and more than 98% of related deaths occur in developing countries[1].

The causative agent of tuberculosis in developing countries is mainly *Mycobacterium tuberculosis* complex (*M. tuberculosis* and *M. africanum*); in areas where cattle holding is common one may still find *M. bovis*, but all these are equally responsive to modern chemotherapy.

Table 15b.2 shows the current average

Clinical Tuberculosis. Edited by P.D.O. Davies. Published in 1994 by Chapman & Hall, London. ISBN 0 412 48630 X

Table 15b.2 Epidemiological pattern of tuberculosis

Country/areas	Annual risk (%)		
	Current level of ARI	Declining trend of ARI	Availability of health resources
I Industrial countries	0.1–0.01	>10	Excellent
II Middle-income countries in Latin America, W Asia	0.5–1.5	5–10	Good
III Middle-income countries E/SE Asia	1.0–2.5	<5	Good
IV Sub-Saharan Africa, Indian subcontinent	1.0–2.5	0–3	Poor

ARI, annual risk of infection.
Souce: First Programme Report (1989–1990) and Future Plan (1991–1995), World Health Organization, Document WHO/TB/91.159.

levels of annual risk of infection with the tubercle bacillus in various regions. The annual tuberculosis infection rate, or incidence of infection, can be derived from tuberculin-test results in a representative sample of non-BCG-vaccinated children. The annual risk of infection is an approximation of the annual incidence of infection in a population. High-prevalence countries are countries with an annual risk of infection of 1% or more.

In some middle-income countries (Table 15b.2, II), tuberculosis has declined. In other middle-income developing countries (Table 15b.2, III), the decline is slow and tuberculosis still remains a major public health problem. In the majority of low-income, developing countries (Table 15b.2, IV), almost no decline has been observed and the absolute number of cases is probably increasing[1].

So which population group in high-prevalence countries is the major source of infection? Some 1.3 million cases and 40 000 deaths per annum occur in children under 15 years. This group also represents 10–20% of new cases, but only a very small proportion of smear-positive cases[2]. In Tanzania, a high-prevalence developing country, which forms a particular focus for this chapter (see pp. 335–338), only 2.1% of all smear-positive cases are younger than 15 years[3]. Therefore children do not play a major role as a source of infection.

It is the adult smear-positive case (index case) who spreads the disease within the community. Such a smear-positive case may arise from endogenous reactivation of an existing infection, from exogenous infection, or from reinfection.

In developing countries tuberculosis is not limited to certain high-risk groups, although one may find more cases in the poorer communities and in HIV-seropositive patients (see also Chapter 12). In other words, in developing countries the greatest incidence and mortality is concentrated in the economically most productive group of the population (15–59 years). More than 80% of the tuberculosis toll in the developing world falls in this age group[1]. Moreover, with the emergence of HIV epidemics, which affect also mainly the 15–59 year age group, one can assume that the extent of the problem in many developing countries, above all in sub-Saharan Africa, is likely to increase in the next decade.

What would happen in high-prevalence countries if no intervention methods were applied? In the absence of chemotherapy 50% of cases would die within 5 years, 30% would recover spontaneously and 20% would remain sputum-positive and continue to spread the disease[4]. Therefore there is a medical and ethical obligation to plan adequate intervention measures in order to get tuberculosis under control.

15b.2 THE PRINCIPLES OF TUBERCULOSIS CONTROL

In principle there are four methods for prevention of tuberculosis:

- Improvement of socio-economic conditions.
- Chemoprophylaxis.
- Vaccination.
- Case-finding and treatment[5].

Improvement of socioeconomic conditions is the measure that has the most profound effect on reducing the disease load, as tuberculosis is intimately associated with poverty and deprivation[5]. The major part of the decrease in the incidence of the disease in developed countries occurred long before effective therapy and vaccinations were available[6]. Unfortunately for many countries, socioeconomic development is a very complex and long-term solution.

Chemoprophylaxis and vaccination (Chapter 14) are expected to protect the individual, but not to have an immediate impact on transmission[5]. BCG vaccination in children provides a certain degree of protection against serious forms of the disease, such as miliary tuberculosis and tuberculosis meningitis, therefore BCG vaccination should be included in the Expanded Programme on Immunization in developing countries (Chapter 14b, p. 297). Chemoprophylaxis for infected contacts, especially children, since they have a high risk of developing the disease, is recommended to protect these individuals.

A *quick* reduction in the risk of transmission can be achieved by giving effective treatment to all smear-positive cases found in the community in order to make them non-infectious, taking into account that a single smear-positive case infects approximately 10–14 people in a year[7]. Consequently, the principles for tuberculosis control in high-prevalence areas are:

- To cure the individual and, by doing so, restore their quality of life (work capacity: socio-economic position, individual health and welfare).
- To decrease the risk of tuberculosis infection in the community, preferably to an extent where tuberculosis will no longer present a public health problem. This will improve the economic and social conditions of the respective community as a whole.

One has to make sure that a sufficiently high proportion of those patients put on treatment do complete it. Therefore, in Tanzania the more specified policy in the National TB Leprosy Programme is to aim at a cure ratio of 85% of all smear-positive cases put on short-course chemotherapy, which is also the WHO policy[8], in order to cure the individual and to reduce transmission in the community.

15b.3 CASE-FINDING

A case of tuberculosis for control purposes in high-prevalence countries is defined as 'an individual, discharging TB bacilli, especially if the bacilli in the sputum smear can be seen by direct smear microscopy'.[9]

Bacteriologically unconfirmed cases, such as pulmonary tuberculosis (PTB) smear-negative cases and extra pulmonary cases should, of course, also be treated, but must be notified separately[9]. For field purposes pulmonary TB should be suspected when a patient presents with:

- Persistent cough for more than 3 weeks, usually productive (with sputum), sometimes bloodstained.
- Loss of body weight, night sweats, fever.
- Chest pain.

The symptoms of extrapulmonary TB depend on the organs involved (see Chapter 7) and the diagnosis is sometimes not easy to make due to limited facilities in developing countries.

The diagnosis of pulmonary tuberculosis is based on bacteriological examination of sputum smears. Smear-positive cases are diagnosed by direct smear microscopy only [10,11].

The role of microscopy is crucial in developing countries.

- It is the diagnostic tool for smear-positive cases before starting treatment.
- It is also the essential tool for monitoring treatment in smear-positive cases after the end of the intensive phase of short- course chemotherapy, during the continuation phase and at the end of treatment.

Pulmonary smear-negative cases should preferably be diagnosed by chest radiography with the assessment of a competent medical officer.

Radiological diagnosis of tuberculosis is unreliable, because other lung diseases can imitate the picture of PTB. Smear-negative disease may present with an uncharacteristic radiographic pattern, especially when associated with HIV-infection[9]. The costs of radiographic examinations are high and therefore very often not affordable for all cases of tuberculosis in developing countries.

Of course radiographs can be helpful in clinical work, especially for diagnosis of tuberculosis in children (where sputum is frequently negative), in miliary tuberculosis, in pulmonary smear-negative and in extrapulmonary tuberculosis.

The tuberculin test has a limited value in clinical work, especially in high-prevalence countries like Tanzania, where approximately 50% of the adult population is infected with the tubercle bacillus. But in children, the presence of a history of contact, together with a positive tuberculin test, is likely to reflect recent infection and therefore a high risk of developing disease[12,16].

Case-finding in high-prevalence countries' control programmes is in principle passive, which means that patients with symptoms present themselves to health facilities and are then examined. The promotion of awareness in the community and within medical staff

may increase the yield of new tuberculosis cases. The only exception to passive case-finding is the active tracing of contacts of a smear-positive index case, such as household contacts, especially children[12].

15b.4 TREATMENT

When cases are identified as tuberculosis cases they should be handled with adequate and effective treatment. In industrialized countries costs do not play a major role in deciding which treatment regimen to choose. In developing countries limited resources force health officials very often to apply affordable treatment, which may not always be optimal treatment.

Short-course chemotherapy, preferably for all smear-positive cases, containing at least three effective drugs in the intensive phase and preferably two different drugs in the follow-up phase, in order to prevent resistance, should be the treatment of choice in a well-structured programme.

'Short course' means that the duration of treatment should be 8 months or less in order to maintain an acceptable level of compliance on the part of the patient (Chapter 8). The intensive phase should usually last 2–3 months, a time period during which up to 90% of the smear-positive cases turn to sputum smear-negativity.

In poor resource countries the intermittent application of rifampicin unsupervised in the continuation phase has to be very carefully considered. The risk that the drug, even in a combined tablet, may be diverted and sold unsupervised is high.

In Tanzania, fortunately levels of resistance to antituberculosis drugs are low (see Table 15b.3). There are several reasons for this. Firstly, Tanzania is poor. Therefore, for decades antituberculosis drugs were only available through the National Programme; they were not sold on the private market. Secondly, the drugs given through the National Tuberculosis Programme were

Table 15b.3 Drug resistance pattern in Tanzania for new smear-positive cases (1991)

Drug	% resistance
H	8
R	3
S	<1
E	3
HR	<1
HRS	0
HRSE	1
HS	1
HE	0
RS/RE/SE	0

H, isoniazid; R, rifampicin; S, streptomycin; E, ethambutol.

strictly supervised, daily in the initial phase of 2 months, monthly in the continuation phase of 6 months. Since almost 90% of the smear-positive cases converted to smear-negative after the intensive phase (month 2 or 3 of treatment), the chance of developing resistance was very low.

Nowadays antituberculosis drugs are available on the private market and are imported by voluntary agencies outside the National Programme as well. The partial loss of control over the distribution of these drugs will, in the future, probably make effective treatment more difficult in Tanzania as resistance is likely to emerge.

It is desirable that in the future even more effective drug combinations will be available, with a shorter duration of treatment. This would enable control programmes to cure patients in a shorter time period. Therefore it would be possible to cope better with the increasing case load in many places and eventually to overcome the tuberculosis problem more rapidly.

PTB smear-negative cases in Tanzania, as in many other African countries, are treated differently from smear-positive cases. Currently they still receive a 12-month SThH regimen (2SThH/10ThH), but hopefully this regimen can be changed soon. This is because of limited funds and lack of facilities

for proper supervision for a rifampicin-containing component.

In the rural areas of Tanzania, and in many other developing countries, smear-positive patients have to be hospitalized for the intensive 2-month phase, not because they are so sick, but simply because there is no other way to ensure regular daily drug intake in areas where a patient has to walk 20 or 30 km to get to health care.

Table 15b.4 Short-course chemotherapy (SCC) regimen currently used within the NTLP, Tanzania

	Initial phase (2/12)	Continuation phase (6/12)
SCC for sputum smear +ves	S H R Z	Th H or E H
Non-rifampicin regimen for sputum smear −ves	S Th H	Th H or E H

S, streptomycin; H, isoniazid; R, rifampicin; Z, pyrazinamide; Th, thiacetazone; E, ethambutol.

Table 15b.4 shows the treatment regimen currently used in the National Tuberculosis and Leprosy Programme in Tanzania. This regimen is about to be changed. In the wake of the HIV endemic the programme will gradually abandon streptomycin injections, because of the risk of transmitting other infections to the tuberculosis patients, such as hepatitis or HIV[13]. Basic hygiene cannot always be guaranteed in countries where only limited resources are available, means for sterilization sometimes are poor and safe disposal of used needles is not always guaranteed.

Another argument for stopping injection in tuberculosis patients is to reduce the workload of an already overstrained staff by replacing time-consuming and work-

Table 15b.5 Cost of essential antituberculosis drugs[a]

Drugs	Dosage/form	Packaging (no. per box)	Price ($ US)[b]
Isoniazid	Tablets 100 mg	1000	3.95
	300 mg	1000	11.07
Rifampicin	Tablets 150 mg	100	4.83
	(or capsules) 300 mg	100	9.87
Pyrazinamide	Tablets 500 mg	100	4.30
Isoniazid + rifampicin	Tablets 100 + 150 mg	100	5.8
	150 + 300 mg	100	10.2
Isoniazid + rifampicin + pyrazinamide	Tablets 50 + 120 + 300 mg	1000	115[c]
Isoniazid + thiacetazone	Tablets 100 + 50 mg	1000	5.19
	300 + 150 mg	1000	11.34
Streptomycin (sulphate)	Ampoules (powder) 1 g	50	13.57
Water for injection	Ampoules 5 ml	50	1.65
Ethambutol	Tablets 400 mg	500	11.90

Source: Chaulet *et al.* (1992), *Review of the International Children's Centre*, No. 196–7.
[a] Based on the UNICEF 1991 price list.
[b] The FOB price (free on board) of orders through UNICEF may be calculated by adding 4–6% to the price listed above.
[c] This is a special price for international organizations aiding National Tuberculosis Programmes. It includes the FOB price and the cost of air transportation.

intensive injections by tablets[3]. Moreover, the programme is looking for additional long-term financial support in order to be able to use other, unfortunately more expensive, drugs instead of the cheap thiacetazone in the follow-up phase. This is to avoid the serious adverse effects such as Stevens–Johnson syndrome, which thiacetazone causes in HIV-positive tuberculosis patients (Chapter 12b)[14]. The same is planned for PTB smear-negative patients, at least for the known HIV-positive patients.

Since costs are always a key factor in health-intervention strategies, Table 15b.5 gives an overview of the present costs of TB drugs used in control programmes in high-prevalence countries.

As a rule-of-thumb one can keep in mind that one short-course chemotherapy treatment with 2 months' SHRZ and 6 months' ThH costs approximately 40 US$ (at 1991 prices). Other costs such as expenses for admission and staff salaries are not included in that figure.

15b.5 OTHER ASPECTS OF TUBERCULOSIS CONTROL

15b.5.1 MONITORING AND EVALUATION

A proper monitoring and evaluation system, based on a meticulous recording and reporting system is of utmost importance in order to assess the effectiveness of both the treatment given and the particular programme's and staff's performance.

The Tanzanian recording and reporting system developed by the International Union Against Tuberculosis and Lung Disease under the guidance of Dr K. Styblo is now serving as a model for many National Tuberculosis Programmes. The reporting system is based mainly on two reports, which are compiled at district level, for each respective district four times a year. They are the district quarterly report on case-finding and the district quarterly report on treatment results in smear-positive patients. The basic information made available is drawn from the **district register**, which, being an individual case register, contains all relevant patient information on the cases enrolled for treatment:

- Name
- Home address, treatment unit
- Sex
- Age
- Disease classification (PTB-positive, PTB-negative, EP)
- Category (new pulmonary disease, relapse, transferred in, treatment after default, others – e.g. failures)

The district register also contains all relevant information on outcome of treatment:

- Smear results (at 0, 2, 5 and 8 months for an 8-month short-course regimen).
- Cured (confirmed by sputum smear microscopy).
- Treatment completed (last available smear negative, but no final smear result obtained).
- Died (from any cause whatsoever).
- Bacteriological positive (failure).
- Defaulted (out of control).
- Transferred out (from one region to another while being on treatment).

The district register contains all information needed to compile the two essential types of reports.

For epidemiological purposes the **quarterly reports on case-finding** are used (Fig. 15b.1) and compiled at central level for all districts. These reports enable information on trends in disease to be obtained (e.g. increased overall case load, newly detected smear-positive cases) but only as an indication of the incidence of disease, as not all cases will be detected. Such data are useful for planning staff needs, drug supplies and so on.

Trends in relation to a change in age or sex distribution or changes in sputum smear-positivity results can also be observed by data recording on these forms. Fig. 15b.2 illustrates the shift to the younger age groups in the National Tuberculosis Programme in Tanzania in the wake of the HIV endemic.

The other source of information is the **quarterly report on results of treatment**, also compiled at district level. This report is a cohort report. The cohort is the number of patients enrolled in a respective quarter, observed for the whole treatment period (8 months) for outcome of treatment (Fig. 15b.3).

This report, compiled at central level, enables programme managers to evaluate by cohort analysis – among many other subjects – the effectiveness of the programme as such, of the treatment applied and of the staff's performance.

15b.5.2 HEALTH EDUCATION

Health education of the individual patient is an essential tool to improve compliance. It has to be explained how the patient can avoid spreading the disease, how to identify other persons with symptoms in the household, why drugs must be taken regularly and why all of the drugs given must be taken until treatment is completed.

Health education of the community, at village level or through mass media at national level, has to explain what tuberculosis is, what the symptoms of the disease are, how it is spread, how it can be cured and that it is indeed curable.

Another important element of a good tuberculosis-control programme is continuous **systematic supervision** at all levels, from central (government) level down to the dispensary. All aspects of the programme have to be supervised, such as proper diagnosis, which means also supervision of staff, including that of the microscopy centres, and quality control. Supervision of proper case-holding, including individual patient care and overall treatment compliance, has to be assured throughout the year.

Supervision of recording and reporting at all levels is crucial, as well as supervision of managerial and administrative aspects, such as drug supplies and proper use of funds.

Ministry of Health
National Tuberculosis/Leprosy Programme

Quarterly report on new cases and relapses of tuberculosis

Patients registered during

☐ quarter of 19

Name of DTLC _____

Date of completion of this form : _____

Signature : _____

Name of district :

_____

District no : _____ __

Block 1

PULMONARY TUBERCULOSIS					SMEAR-NEGATIVE (3)		EXTRA-PULMONARY TUBERCULOSIS (4)		TOTAL (5)		
SMEAR-POSITIVE											
NEW CASES (1)			Relapses (2)								
Males	Females	Total	M	F	M	F	M	F	Males	Females	Total

NEW SMEAR-POSITIVE CASES : from Column (1) above

Block 2

Age-group (years)														TOTAL		
0-14		15-24		25-34		35-44		45-54		55-64		65 or more				
M	F	M	F	M	F	M	F	M	F	M	F	M	F	Males	Females	Total

Explanations on how to fill in the form

District Register Number ⇥ identification number of the district

Quarters : 1st quarter ⇥ January, February, March
 2nd quarter ⇥ April, May, June
 3rd quarter ⇥ July, August, September
 4th quarter ⇥ October, November, December

Block 1 : NEW CASES AND RELAPSES OF TUBERCULOSIS registered during _____ quarter of (year) _____

Fill in the quarter and the year.

Column (1) : NEW SMEAR-POSITIVE CASES ⇥ patients with pulmonary tuberculosis, sputum smear-positive, who have never received antituberculosis treatment.

Column (2) : SMEAR-POSITIVE RELAPSES ⇥ patients with pulmonary tuberculosis, sputum smear-positive, who have been declared cured but have now got the disease again.

Column (3) : SMEAR-NEGATIVE CASES ⇥ patients with pulmonary tuberculosis, having a negative sputum for AFB, in whom the diagnosis of tuberculosis was made by means other than sputum microscopy.

Column (4) : EXTRA-PULMONARY TUBERCULOSIS ⇥ patients with tuberculosis of organs other than the lungs

Column (5) : TOTAL Males — Add **all male** patients in columns 1 + 2 + 3 + 4
 Females — Add **all female** patients in columns 1 + 2 + 3 + 4
 Total — Add **all patients** (males + females) in columns 1 + 2 + 3 + 4.

Block 2 : NEW SMEAR-POSITIVE CASES : from Column (1) above

In this block enter the patients (already recorded in Block 1, column (1)) according to their sex and age group. If the exact age of a patient, at the time of his registration, is unknown, it should be estimated to the nearest 5 years, e.g. 15, 20, 25, etc.

Fig. 15b.1 Quarterly report of new cases of tuberculosis.

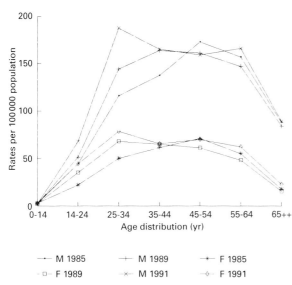

--- M 1985   --- M 1989   --- F 1985
--- F 1989   --- M 1991   --- F 1991

Fig. 15b.2 Age and sex distribution in the National Tuberculosis and Leprosy Programme in Tanzania.

15b.5.3 TRAINING

Training and refresher courses contribute largely to the success of a programme, because they are helpful to maintain quality and enthusiasm within an already established programme.

A systematic plan of training, based on the actual needs should be established, which takes into consideration activities in previous years, and looks ahead for at least 1–2 years.

15b.6 STARTING A TUBERCULOSIS CONTROL PROGRAMME IN A HIGH-PREVALENCE COUNTRY

Whenever possible such a control programme should be designed as a National Programme. It should be permanent, organized on a country-wide basis (serving rural and urban areas equally), be a well-balanced component of the country's health programme, integrated into the community health structure, meet the public demand, and be accessible, available and convenient for the consumer rather than for those providing the services[15].

Firstly, the commitment of the central government is crucial. Unless government authorities are aware of the need to start such a programme, success cannot be achieved. The government has to commit itself to create the necessary structures, including a central unit for the programme, and to make necessary staff available[11]. Another prerequisite is a plan of action. The plan should clearly enumerate the main targets and the actions planned to achieve them. Figure 15b.4 shows how such a programme can be structured.

Before a National Programme for tuberculosis is started, a regular drug supply, including sufficient stock, has to be assured to mid term. Stock replenishment, half-yearly at central level and at least quarterly at regional level, is essential since, in developing countries, weak infrastructure, poor logistics or long rainy seasons sometimes make it impossible to react quickly to drug shortages.

Staff must be recruited and trained **before** the practical work starts. Adequate training for all categories of health personnel should be available. Basic information on the National Tuberculosis Programmes should be added to the curricula of medical, paramedical and nursing schools[15].

Continuous evaluation based on a simple but comprehensive recording and reporting system should be established from the beginning, which should provide information for future planning. A sufficient number of diagnostic (microscopy) centres have to be established, and supervised through a quality control system for laboratories.

Of course, funding of the essential aspects of the programme should be guaranteed for a sufficient time period (5–10 years). As a rule, treatment for tuberculosis should be free in developing countries.

The introduction of a tuberculosis control programme should be stepwise. It is recommended, that a start be made in a pilot area in order to identify the specific problems faced.

REPORT ON THE RESULTS OF TREATMENT OF SMEAR-POSITIVE PULMONARY TUBERCULOSIS PATIENTS REGISTERED 15-18 MONTHS EARLIER

Name of district : _____   District no : _____   Patients registered during   Date of completion of this form : _____

Name of DTLC : _____   ☐ quarter of 19   _____ 19

Signature : _____

Total No of smear-positive patients registered during the above quarter	Regimen	(1) Cured (smear-negative)	(2) Treatment completed (no smear-results)	(3) Died	(4) Failure (smear-positive)	(5) Defaulted	(6) Transferred to another district	Total number evaluated (sum of columns 1 to 6)
M	1. New Cases							
	1.1 short-course							
F	1.2 standard							
	1.3 Total							
T*	2. Retreatment							
	2.1 relapses							
	2.2 others (failure cases)							
	2.3 Total							

* Of those, _____ (number) were excluded from evaluation of chemotherapy for the following reasons : _____

Fig. 15b.3 Quarterly report on the results of treatment.

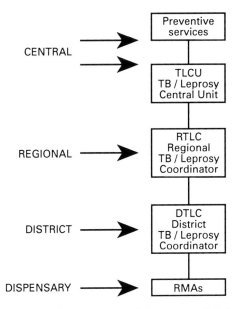

Fig. 15b.4 The structure of the National Tuberculosis and Leprosy Programme in Tanzania (RMA = Rural Medical Assistant).

Later, according to the resources available, the programme can be expanded gradually.

From the experience in Tanzania it is known that other areas, having heard of success in a region where the programme is already functioning fully, are ready to join the activities of a National Tuberculosis Programme.

15b.7 COST-EFFECTIVENESS OF TUBERCULOSIS WORK IN HIGH-PREVALENCE COUNTRIES

The greatest burden of tuberculosis incidence and mortality is concentrated in adults (age 15–59 years). These are the parents, workers and leaders of society. Therefore it is very important to make government officials, and donors to such programmes, aware that establishing a tuberculosis control programme means that they are supporting one of the most cost-effective health interventions available[16]. Systematic tuberculosis chemotherapy (and BCG vaccination) in countries

with a high risk of infection are some of the most cost-effective health interventions available.

An analysis of the National Programme in Tanzania has shown that to treat smear-positive tuberculosis cases costs less than US$230 per death averted. Cost per discounted year of life saved is 1–2 US$ [16]. Cost-effectiveness for HIV-positive patients with smear-positive tuberculosis depends on the survival time of patients after treatment and the indirect benefits of treatment.

In terms of direct benefits, treating HIV-positive patients is much more expensive than treating HIV-seronegative patients. However, HIV-positive, smear-positive patients will also transmit the disease. If HIV-positive, smear-positive patients transmit almost as much tuberculosis as HIV-negative patients, then short-course chemotherapy should also be cost-effective[16]. It is an ethical obligation to treat all tuberculosis patients regardless of their HIV status.

15b.8 THE TANZANIA EXPERIENCE

Tanzania, an East African country situated bordering the Indian Ocean between Kenya in the north and Malawi/Mozambique in the south, has very limited resources (Table 15b.6). Nevertheless, Tanzania has a well-

Table 15b.6 Basic data on Tanzania

Population	~24 million
Area	881 289 km²
Proportion of rural population	82%
GNP	~200 US$
Birth rate	46 (1988)
(per 1000 population)	
Death rate	15 (1988)
(per 1000 population)	
Infant mortality	116 (1988)
(per 1000 live births)	
Life expectancy	~50 years

Table 15b.7   Synopsis: Tuberculosis 1983–1991, mainland Tanzania

	1983	1984	1985	1986	1987	1988	1989	1990	1991
Newly detected cases	11 782	12 089	14 089	15 453	16 920	18 234	19 262	22 249	25 210
Smear +ve PTB	6651	7523	8207	8561	9279	9918	10 479	11 396	11 898
Case detection rate per 100 000	34.1	37.3	39.6	40.2	42.3	44.0	44.0	47.8	48.5
Cohort reported cure rate (%) in SCC	43%	49%	61%	67%	72%	74%	77%	79%	Not yet
AFB +ve patients put on SCC	799	2745	4936	5919	7171	8155	9320	9742	—
% of all AFB +ve	12%	36%	60%	69%	77%	82%	87%	86%	—

PTB, pulmonary tuberculosis; SCC, short-course chemotherapy; AFB, acid-fast bacilli.

functioning Tuberculosis National Programme, established in 1977 as the 'National Tuberculosis and Leprosy Programme' (NTLP), Tanzania – the first combined Leprosy–Tuberculosis programme of its kind in the world. It has functioned successfully, without major breakdowns, for almost 15 years, and one may wonder as to what is the secret of its success.

Firstly, the country, despite its poor resources, has had political stability for many years. It also has a well-established health infrastructure from central to district, and down to dispensary level, although sometimes the well-designed structures cannot be filled with active workers due to limited availability of resources (Fig. 15b.4). The NTLP is fully integrated in this existing health system, no extra structures have been created. Only specialized staff have been made available within the existing system.

These two factors also contributed largely to the success of other programmes, for example in Malawi[17].

The typical problems of developing countries remain: bad roads, heavy rainy seasons, poor communication systems. These are, among others, the daily problems that have had to be faced while running the National Programme. From the beginning, however, the programme had the full committment and reliable support of the government. Now almost all staff are Tanzanians, salaries for them being paid by the government. A continuous, uninterrupted drug supply, including supply of a reasonable stock, by the overseas donors has guaranteed that patients searching for treatment really do get treatment, which unfortunately is not the rule in many other existing programmes.

Reliable means of transport (cars, motorbikes), are one of the biggest cost factors besides drugs, and have been made available by donors.

The programme has served as a model for many other countries. The unique recording and reporting system designed by IUATLD under the guidance of Dr K. Styblo[18,19] is used nowadays – with slight variations only – in many National Tuberculosis Programmes and represents the WHO recommended recording and reporting system.

The combination of programmes for two diseases, tuberculosis and leprosy, has also contributed to the success, the donors from both sides assisting each other. Moreover, combining forces has contributed to making the programmes more cost-effective (one member of staff specialized for two diseases, one vehicle serving several purposes etc.).

Table 15b.8 Treatment results: tuberculosis smear positives, NTLP first half 1990

Cured	79%
Treatment completed	3%
Died	8%
Failure (remained +ve)	1%
Out of control	4%
Transferred out	5%
Total	100%

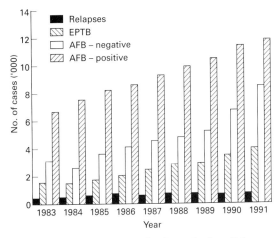

Fig. 15b.5 New cases of tuberculosis, all forms, reported in the National Programme in Tanzania, 1983–1991. (EPTB denotes extrapulmonary disease; AFB = acid-fast bacilli.)

The results are displayed in Tables 15b.7 and 15b.8 and in Fig. 15b.5.

Why did the NTLP Tanzania not reach the goal of an 85% cure rate? Firstly, 8% of all patients died during treatment, not all of tuberculosis, but many also of other causes. A considerable proportion died from AIDS, after converting to sputum smear-negativity.

A 1% failure rate of cases who could not be cured by treatment is acceptable. Another 5% were transferred to another region, again a proportion that cannot be influenced by the programme as such. Another 4% defaulted (out of control), which is a fairly low propor-

tion, even in developed countries. Three per cent of the patients completed treatment without having cure confirmed by a final smear, either because they could not produce sputum or because they did not attend for a final smear examination. This is also an acceptable proportion.

Therefore only 79% of all smear-positive cases were cured. If one assumes that most of the patients in the 'treatment completed' group are cured as well, and if one accepts that those who died are no longer a source of infection, 90% of the positive patients enrolled for treatment are eradicated as a source of infection. Also if up to 50% of those 'transferred out' and 'out of control' are cured, it can be concluded that the 1991 results for short-course chemotherapy in smear-positive patients are very favourable.

Of course the programme also has problems and its quality varies from region to region depending on the motivation of the persons involved. Preliminary results of an ongoing WHO study in Tanzania reveal that some 30–40% of our tuberculosis patients are HIV-positive. The current close association of the two endemics in Tanzania and other developing countries leaves many open questions. Although the response to chemotherapy in HIV/TB-positive patients is generally good, the management of the individual patients has to be adjusted to the new conditions (Chapter 12b).

Drugs that cause serious adverse effects in HIV/TB positive cases should be replaced by better tolerated drugs[20] in order to maintain the 'good reputation' of such programmes. Emphasis should be put on proper diagnosis. Overdiagnosis in HIV/TB-positive cases is common. Is a 'wasting child' a TB case, a malnourished child, or an HIV-infected one? These are questions that require certain skills on the part of the staff involved in tuberculosis diagnosis, to be answered. The proportion of deaths in tuberculosis patients will increase. The prognosis of cure of tuberculosis is good for TB in HIV-positive patients, but poor with regard to other HIV-related diseases. In addition, the compliance of TB/HIV-positive cases may differ from the ordinary tuberculosis patients. There will be problems in handling confidentiality while registering patients. Counselling of known HIV-positive subjects may be a new burden for the tuberculosis programme. The list could be continued with subjects like chemoprophylaxis for HIV-positive patients and BCG in HIV-positive patients.

Overall costs for tuberculosis programmes may rise due to increased case load and probably more frequent need for hospitalization in HIV/TB patients, especially when they present with full-blown AIDS.

The biggest problem now is the increasing figures in tuberculosis case detection, which put a tremendous strain on the programme, especially in the urban areas, where patients from the rural areas search for help. The overall increase can be attributed partly to improved reporting and diagnosing, partly to the influx of immigrants from neighbouring countries, attracted by the quality of the programme, but definitely the HIV endemic in the country contributes most to the steady increase. HIV infection is the highest risk factor so far identified, which increases the risk of latent infection with tuberculosis progressing to an active form of disease by reducing the cell-mediated immunity[21,22].

Moreover, recent studies reveal that HIV-seropositive cases may be infected more quickly and more heavily, resulting in development of the disease sooner than in HIV-seronegative patients[23]. The only way to cope with this increased case load, which can be identified with workload, is to reduce the sources of infection. In turn, this means keeping the cure ratio high. This can be achieved by increasing the staff and space for the patients, especially in the overstrained urban areas, and by intensified health education activities. These activities should make people aware of the further existing possibi-lity and necessity of cure for tuberculosis. In addition, treatment regimens have to be adjusted to the new conditions we are facing in the wake of the HIV pandemic. Lastly, a close co-operation with National Aids Programmes is desirable, since we are sharing a considerable proportion of patients.

The future will show whether measures presently available are sufficient to maintain the standard of the ongoing programmes or whether other, completely new intervention strategies have to be applied.

REFERENCES

1. World Health Organization (1991) First Programme Report (1989–1990) and Future Plan (1991–1995). WHO document WHO/TB 91.159.
2. Chaulet, P., Grangaud, J.P., Mazount, M.S. *et al.* (1992) *Childhood Tuberculosis Still With Us.* . . . International Children's Centre, Paris, (*Children in the Tropics*, No. 196–197).
3. National Tuberculosis and Leprosy Programme, Tanzania (1991) Annual Report.
4. Grzybowski, S. (1991) Natural history of tuberculosis. *Bull. Int. Union Tuberc. Lung Dis.,* **66**, 193–4.
5. Rodrigues, L.C. and Smith, P.G. (1990) Tuberculosis in developing countries and methods for its control. *Trans. Roy. Soc. Trop. Med. Hyg.,* **84**, 739–44.
6. McKeown, T. (1979) *The Role of Medicine: Dream, Mirage or Nemesis?* Basil Blackwell, Oxford.
7. Murray, C.J.L., Styblo, K. and Rouillon, A. (1990) Tuberculosis in developing countries: burden, intervention and cost. *Bull. Int. Union Tuberc. Lung Dis.,* **65**, 6–24.
8. Kochi, A. (1991) The global tuberculosis situation and the new control strategy of the World Health Organization (Leading article). *Tubercle,* **72**, 1–6.
9. International Union Against Tuberculosis and Lung Disease (1991) *Tuberculosis Guide for High Prevalence Countries,* 2nd edn, Misereor/IUATLD, Aachen/Paris.
10. Chum, H.J. *Manual of the National Tuberculosis/Leprosy Programme in Tanzania,* 2nd edn, TB/Leprosy Control Unit, Ministry of Health, Tanzania.
11. Enarson, D.A. (1991) Principles of IUATLD

collaborative tuberculosis programmes. *Bull. Int. Union Tuber. Lung Dis.*, **66**, 195–200.

12. Styblo, K. (1991) The epidemiology of tuberculosis in children. *TSRU/IUAT Progress Report*, **1**, 175–83.

13. Hu, D.J., Kane, M.A. and Heymann, D.L. (1991). Transmission of HIV, hepatitis B virus, and other bloodborne pathogens in health care settings: a review of risk factors and guidelines for prevention. *Bull. WHO*, **69**(5), 623–30.

14. Nunn, P., Kibuga, D. Gathua, S. *et al.* (1991) Cutaneous hypersensitivity reactions due to thiacetazone in HIV-1 seropositive patients treated for tuberculosis. *Lancet*, **377**, 627–30.

15. Shears, P. (1988) Tuberculosis Programmes in Developing Countries, 2nd edn, Oxfam, 274 Banbury Road, Oxford.

16. Murray, C.J.L., DeJonghe, E., Chum, H.J. *et al.* (1991) Cost effectiveness of chemotherapy for pulmonary tuberculosis in three sub-Saharan African countries. *Lancet*, **338**, 1305–8.

17. Nuyangulu, D.S., Nkhoma, W.N. and Salaniponi, F.M.L. (1990/91) Factors contributing to a successful Tuberculosis Control Programme in Malawi. *Bull. Int. Union Tuberc. Lung Dis.* 1990/1991; **66**(Suppl.), 45–6.

18. Styblo, K. (1986) Tuberculosis control and surveillance, in *Recent Advances in Respiratory Medicine* (D.C. Flenley and T.C. Petty), Churchill Livingstone, Edinburgh, **41**, 77–105.

19. Styblo, K. (1989) Overview and epidemiological assessment of the current global TB situation with an emphasis on control in developing countries. *Rev. Inf. Dis.*, **II**(Suppl. 2), 339–46.

20. Narain, J.P., Raviglione, M.C. and Kochi, A. (1992) HIV-associated tuberculosis in developing countries. Epidemiology and strategies for prevention. World Health Organization, Document WHO/TB/92.166.

21. Rieder, H.L., Cauthen, G.W., Bloch, A.B. *et al.* (1989) Tuberculosis and acquired immunodeficiency syndrom – Florida. *Arch. Intern. Med.*, **149**, 1268–73

22. De Cock, K.M., Gnaore, E., Adjorlolo, G. *et al.* (1991) Risk of tuberculois patients with HIV-1 and HIV-2 infections in Abidjan, Ivory Coast. *Br. Med. J.*, **302**, 496–9.

23. Daley, C.L., Small, P.M. and Schecter, G.F. (1992) An outbreak of tuberculosis with accelerated progression among persons infected with the Human Immundeficiency Virus. *N. Engl. J. Med.*, **326**, 231–5.

Ceridwen S.D. Williams

The advances in treatment of tuberculosis, have led to the steady decline in the disease, but we cannot afford to be complacent, for tuberculosis is not a disease of the past.

The mainstay of the tuberculosis service is the contribution made by the tuberculosis visitors. Theirs is an integral part of the local tuberculosis service by controlling the spread of tuberculosis in contact tracing. The nurses performing such work must therefore be competent to undertake the care of these patients. They must have sufficient authority and personality to be able to sustain the patient in his or her return to health. Lack of knowledge and indifference by health workers evokes mistrust in patients and could possibly lead to non-compliance with treatment, resulting in advancement of the disease and spread of infection within their families and among other contacts.

15c.1 NATIONAL ORGANIZATION

England and Wales is divided into approximately 200 local authority areas, each of which has a Consultant in Communicable Disease Control (CCDC) responsible for the control of infection in his or her area. The CCDC receives all notification forms for patients notified in that area and is responsible for alerting the relevant health service personnel to provide measures for control for any outbreak of a notifiable disease that may occur.

In the case of tuberculosis this will involve providing the tuberculosis visitor for that area with enough detail about the notified patient to enable the visitor to see the patient, to establish a relationship with the patient and to draw up a list of contacts. It is therefore vital that each authority area has a sufficient number of trained visitors to enable comprehensive coverage of all patients notified, who are resident in that area. In practice this means at least one full-time visitor for each 50–100 patients, but more visitors may be needed depending on the social and residential circumstances of the area.

If a patient is not notified the disease control services may never become aware of the patient and the disease may spread. Recent evidence from London suggests that up to one-third of patients may not be notified[1].

15c.2 THE ROLE OF THE TUBERCULOSIS VISITOR

The tuberculosis visitor has six main functions:

1. To visit all newly notified tuberculosis patients.
2. To help run an efficient contact screening clinic.
3. To provide a BCG vaccination service.
4. To screen immigrants.
5. To screen tuberculin-test-positive school children.

Clinical Tuberculosis. Edited by P.D.O. Davies. Published in 1994 by Chapman & Hall, London. ISBN 0 412 48630 X

6. To educate other health workers and be used as a resource of information on tuberculosis.

15c.2.1 VISITING THE NEWLY NOTIFIED TUBERCULOSIS PATIENT

When a case of tuberculosis is notified, the health worker responsible for tuberculosis in the community visits the index case in hospital or at home with the primary objective of identifying all contacts at risk and arranging for them to be screened at their nearest chest clinic. Sometimes it is necessary to contact trace outside a particular health authority's area, in this case liaison with other health authorities is undertaken.

The tuberculosis visitor works to the guidelines issued by the Joint Tuberculosis Committee of the British Thoracic Society for the control and prevention of tuberculosis[2].

It is normal practice to screen all close contacts (i.e. household contacts) of all patients with tuberculosis. For patients with smear-positive pulmonary disease, the contact tracing may be extended to include casual contacts (i.e. relatives, schools and play groups, places of work, prisons, nursing homes etc.). Where the index case is a child the search is for the possible source of infection and it may be necessary to extend tracing beyond close contacts to include casual contacts. The principal of the stone in the pond, tracing contact 'ripples' outwards is a useful guide[3].

Once a list of contacts is obtained, each contact is visited and given a clinic appointment card providing details of the time and date they are required to attend clinic. It is important to recognize the need for visiting each contact. Counselling and advising relatives and casual contacts allays any fears they may have and enables them to ask questions. Such measures help to ensure co-operation from contacts.

Adequate explanation and stress on the importance of attending for screening is essential. The majority of all tuberculosis cases are now nursed in the community and so it is essential to form a good relationship with both the patient and their family. The tuberculosis visitor becomes the link between the patient and the physician undertaking the screening of contacts. The physical and mental well-being of that patient is the concern of the nurse responsible for the patient, ensuring compliance with treatment and reporting any problems to the physician undertaking care of the patient. The patients should always be given the name and contact telephone number of their tuberculosis visitor and encouraged to telephone if they encounter any problems. These visits are always documented on a tuberculosis visitor card, which is kept on each patient.

15c.2.2 CONTACT-SCREENING CLINIC

The object of running an efficient contact-screening clinic is to allow detection of disease in contacts of tuberculosis patients. The tuberculosis visitor prepares a contact sheet for each contact. The sheet has on it the name of the index case, the nature of the disease and bacteriological details. The name, age, sex, address, the relationship to the index case and the BCG status is documented on the contact sheet, together with the name and address of the GP. It is also used to record the dates and results of the tuberculin skin test and chest radiographs carried out at the contact clinic. The outcome of the contact procedure is recorded, namely, follow-up examinations, chest radiographs, BCG, prophylactic treatment or discharge.

In Liverpool it is policy to perform tuberculin skin tests on all contacts up to the age of 35 years and a chest radiograph on all contacts. Heaf tests are performed by the tuberculosis visitor, either in the patient's home or in the contact clinic, and read 7 days later. Tuberculin test-negative contacts are re-tested 6 weeks after the last contact to allow time for tuberculin conversion and if still negative are offered BCG. They are given a further appointment 6 weeks later to review the BCG site and discharged.

Chemoprophylaxis is given to children under 5 who are close contacts of smear-positive adult patients with tuberculosis irrespective of their tuberculin state; they can be given BCG after completion of chemoprophylaxis.

Chemoprophylaxis may also be given to contacts with strongly positive Heaf tests with no radiological evidence of disease. The responsibility of counselling and visiting this group of contact patients lies with the tuberculosis visitor (Chapter 15a, p. 315).

The presence of the tuberculosis visitor when clinics are held ensures continuity of care, not only with the patient but also with the contacts of that patient and almost certainly helps with the co-operation of all concerned and reduces the non-attendance rate in the clinics as defaulters can be visited and a further appointment arranged. The tuberculosis visitor has the opportunity to discuss any problems that may require further action with the physician, and whether these concern a patient or contacts.

15c.2.3 PROVISION OF BCG VACCINATION SERVICE

The clinic also provides a BCG vaccination service not only for contacts of tuberculosis patients, but for other selected groups (i.e. children who have missed BCG at school, immigrant children and overseas travellers).

As well as providing a service for the control of infection, the tuberculosis visitors' role is also one of prevention. This is where measures are taken to identify 'at risk' groups and offer BCG vaccination to all tuberculin-negative patients. NHS staff in regular contact with tuberculosis patients, laboratory staff and others who are handling tuberculosis material are considered to be a 'high-risk' group. Suitable pre-employment screening is

recommended; normally a Heaf test and chest radiography. Relevant past history concerning tuberculosis or previous BCG vaccination should be documented.

BCG vaccination is also offered to some neonates, especially those born to Asian (Indian subcontinent) parents and also babies who are close contacts to a patient with pulmonary disease.

15c.2.4 SCREENING OF IMMIGRANTS

Because the incidence of tuberculosis is high among some immigrant groups, especially those coming from countries where tuberculosis is common (e.g. Indian subcontinent, Vietnam, Hong Kong) it is necessary to screen all immigrants coming into the UK (Chapter 10, p. 203).

Screening of immigrants is aimed at identifying patients who are active and infectious; individuals who show evidence of infection (tuberculin test-positive) without having actual disease and who may require chemoprophylaxis, and also identifying non-infected individuals who may require BCG vaccination.

Immigrants, which should also include the student population, are usually referred by the medical officer at the port of entry to the UK (usually Heathrow airport) to the relevant CCDC. An address of intended settlement is obtained. These people are a highly mobile group and it is necessary to try to contact them as soon as possible following their arrival in this country. On occasions this has become a problem and some have been lost to contact. To ensure that a high percentage of immigrants continue to be screened it is suggested that all health workers and general practitioners, and occupational health services in universities and colleges, are made aware of the problem and can, if necessary, refer individuals to the local contact clinics.

The immigrants are screened utilizing the

contact clinic facilities and provision should be made for interpreters to be present.

15c.2.5 SCREENING TUBERCULIN TEST-POSITIVE SCHOOL CHILDREN

The health department recommends that BCG vaccination should be offered routinely in schools to children aged 10–14 years. This programme has been shown to be effective in preventing tuberculosis (Chapter 14b, p. 297). A number of school children present with tuberculin-positive skin tests on pre-BCG testing. These children are referred to the contact clinic for chest radiography. Previously all children with a grade II reaction with previous BCG history were referred for chest radiography. It is now considered unnecessary to refer these children unless they are immigrants from an area with a high prevalence of tuberculosis.

All children with grade III and grade IV reactions are referred to the contact clinic for chest radiography and given 3 months' prophylactic treatment. It is also recommended now that grade IV reactors are contact-traced, usually to include all household contacts.

15c.2.6 EDUCATION

To ensure that the highest possible standards are provided by the community nursing service it is reasonable to suggest that education by specialist nurses is vital. Tuberculosis is still very much present in the community and the fear is now that the increase in the number of people with immunodeficiency, as a result of HIV infection, will cause an increase in tuberculosis.

Published information about tuberculosis, suitable for the general public, is virtually non-existent and the way forward must be to press for better information, more publicity of the facts about tuberculosis and an increase in specialist training.

REFERENCES

1. Sheldon, C.D., King, K., Cock, H. *et al.* (1992). Notification of tuberculosis: how many cases are never reported? *Thorax*, **47**, 1015–18.
2. Subcommittee of the Joint Tuberculosis Committee of the British Thoracic Society (1990) Control and prevention of tuberculosis in Britain: an updated code of practice. *Br. Med. J.*, **300**, 995–9.
3. Veen, J. (1991) Tuberculosis in a low-prevalence country: a wolf in sheep's clothing. *Bull. Int. Union Tuberc. Long Dis.*, **66**, 203–5.

P.D.O. Davies and A.G. Leitch

It is perhaps a measure of the lack of scientific research into tuberculosis that we still employ a method of demonstrating infection by *Mycobacterium tuberculosis* discovered by Koch[1]. One hundred years later the tuberculin test, the only reliable method of determining infection by *M. tuberculosis* is to measure a bump on the arm, a method that remains substantially less than 100% sensitive and specific. Correct interpretation of the tuberculin skin test requires understanding of the antigen used, the immunological basis for the reaction, the methods and techniques of measuring the various tests and the epidemiological and clinical setting in which the test takes place. The immunological basis of the test is discussed in Chapter 5.

15d.1 TUBERCULIN

Infection with *M. tuberculosis* produces sensitivity to antigenic components of the organism called 'tuberculins'. Three tuberculins are commonly available, Old Tuberculin (OT) and the Purified Protein Derivatives (PPD-S and PPD-RT23). The first is available only for multipuncture devices; the latter two can be used either for intradermal injection (the Mantoux test) or with multiple puncture devices (e.g. Heaf test). PPD-S has been adopted as the International Standard for PPD of mammalian tuberculin[2].

Dilutions of PPD-S are prepared and marketed in many countries, including the UK, as follows:

for Heaf test only:

Undiluted PPD	100 000 TU in 1 ml

for Mantoux testing:

1 in 100	1000 TU in 1 ml
1 in 1000	100 TU in 1 ml
1 in 10 000	10 TU in 1 ml

In the USA and other countries where 5TU (0.1 g/0.1 ml of PPD-S) is the standard dose administered by the Mantoux test, dilutions of one-fifth and fifty times the standard dose are available.

Tuberculoprotein, when diluted, may be adsorbed in varying amounts on to glass or plastic. To avoid decreasing potency, tuberculin should not be transferred from one container to another, the skin test being given as soon as the syringe is filled. Problems with adsorption of tuberculin to glass may be resolved by the addition of small quantities of the detergent Tween 80 to the solution. Tuberculin should be kept away from strong light.

15d.2 THE MULTIPLE-PUNCTURE TEST

The most commonly used multiple-puncture device was developed by Heaf[3]. The six-pronged device is used to inject undiluted PPD or OT smeared on the skin, into the epidermis. Most devices can be adjusted to

Clinical Tuberculosis. Edited by P.D.O. Davies. Published in 1994 by Chapman & Hall, London. ISBN 0 412 48630 X

Table 15d.1   Factors that may reduce response to tuberculin

Relating to subject	*Relating to testing*
Infections	Tuberculin
Viral (measles, mumps, chickenpox), HIV	Chemical denaturation
Bacterial (including overwhelming tuberculosis)	Adsorption
Fungal	Wrong dilution
Live virus vaccination	Improper storage
Metabolic disease (renal failure)	Administration
Depleted nutrition	Too little injected
Leukaemias and lymphomas	Wrong site
Sarcoidosis	Subdermal
Drugs (immunosuppressives and steroids)	Readings
Age (newborn and elderly)	Inexperienced reader
Trauma (burns, surgery)	Bias
	Error in recording

allow 1 mm penetration for babies, or 2 mm for children and adults. The skin is first cleaned with alcohol and the tuberculin solution smeared over an area of about 2 cm². The head of the Heaf device is then placed on the tuberculin-smeared skin and the prongs 'fired' into the skin by pressing firmly downwards.

The reaction can be read at any time between 3 and 10 days, as follows (Plate 14)

Grade 0	less than four discrete papules.
Grade I	at least four discrete papules.
Grade II	a coalescent papular reaction forming a ring of induration.
Grade III	an area of induration up to 10 mm diameter.
Grade IV	an area of induration greater than 10 mm diameter or vesiculation of a grade III reaction.

For sterilization the device should be immersed in spirit for at least a minute and then held over a flame until the spirit has been burned off. Recently theoretical concerns over the transmission of viruses such as hepatitis or HIV has lead to the use of disposable magnetic heads for Heaf testing with resultant increase in cost[4]. Disposable multipronged devices such as the Tine test are more convenient and cheaper than disposable heads, but are not currently recommended because of variable impregnation of the prongs, which has given false results[5].

15d.3 THE INTRADERMAL (MANTOUX) TEST

The intradermal injection of a known amount of PPD is the most reliable means currently available of detecting the immunological response resulting from infection with *M. tuberculosis*. A dose of 0.1 ml of PPD solution is injected into the volar surface of the forearm. The tuberculin should be injected just beneath the surface of the skin, with the needle bevel upward. A discrete bleb or wheal up to 10 mm in diameter should be produced. If it is not, the test should be repeated at a different site, since the solution will have been injected subdermally.

The site of injection should be marked or noted so that when the test is read 48–72 h later the reader has a clear idea of where to expect a reaction. The basis of the reading is the presence or absence of induration, which should be determined by inspection and palpation. The area of hyperaemia or flare is irrelevant. The diameter of induration should be measured transversely to the long axis of the forearm and recorded in millimetres.

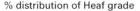

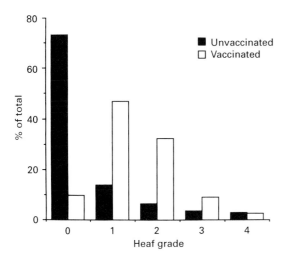

% distribution of Heaf grade

Fig. 15d.1 Histogram showing percentage of reactions by Heaf grade in groups of children before and after receiving BCG vaccination.

When performing a Mantoux test as an aid to diagnosis, the lowest dilution may be given first (i.e. 1 TU) to avoid severe (sometimes systemic) hypersensitivity reactions. If no reaction is present after 24 h the next dilution (10 TU) should be given. For the elderly or patients who may be immunocompromised the strongest dilution (100 TU) may be used if 10 (TU) gives no reaction (Table 15d.1).

15d.4 INTERPRETATION OF THE TUBERCULIN TEST

In persons with a reactive tuberculin test the major confounding factor is infection with resultant hypersensitivity to mycobacteria other than *M. tuberculosis*. Standard tuberculin testing of a population of school children, unlikely to have been infected by *M. tuberculosis*, gives a distribution of Heaf test grades as shown in Fig. 15d.1[6]. Only 6% had strongly positive grade III or IV reactions. While it is possible that these strongly positive reactions represent the tail of the skewed

distribution of uninfected persons, it is also possible that those with grade III or IV reactions represent children infected with an environmental organism or with *M. tuberculosis*. The majority of BCG-unvaccinated children have grade 0 or I Heaf test reactions, whereas the majority of BCG-vaccinated children have weakly positive grade I or II Heaf test reactions (Fig. 15d.1). In practice it is necessary to presume that grades III and IV Heaf test reactions represent infection with *M. tuberculosis*, whether or not BCG has been given. It should, however, be borne in mind that a small proportion of these individuals, whether or not they have had BCG, may not have been infected with *M. tuberculosis*. As yet, there is no means of distinguishing which individuals with strongly positive Heaf test reactions fall into the 'false-positive' and which into the genuinely infected group.

In a similar manner, a Mantoux test reaction of 15 or more millimetres' induration to 10 TU PPD is presumed to represent infection with *M. tuberculosis*. The threshold or cut-off point in millimetres' induration taken to represent infection with *M. tuberculosis* may be varied in different clinical situations.

Different countries may have different criteria for the cut-off point separating positive from negative tests. Also, within any country, classification of a result as positive may differ for different clinical groups. Guidelines from the American Thoracic Society [7,8] classify cut-off points as follows (to 5 TU tuberculin PPD):

A reaction of ≥ 5 mm in: (i) HIV-infected persons or persons with risk factors for HIV of unknown HIV status; (ii) persons who have had close recent contact with infectious tuberculosis cases; (iii) persons with chest radiographs consistent with old healed tuberculosis.

A reaction of ≥ 10 mm is classified as positive in persons who do not have the above risk factors but who include: (i) foreign-born persons from high prevalence countries; (ii) intravenous drug users;

(iii) socially deprived or ethnic minority groups; (iv) residents of long-term care facilities; (v) persons with medical conditions that have been reported to increase the risk of tuberculosis (Table 15d.1); (vi) other high-risk populations.

A reaction of $\geq$ 15 mm is classified as positive in all other persons. In HIV-infected individuals tuberculin reactivity is uncommon when CD4 counts fall below 350/mm^3 and is not seen when below 200/mm^3[9].

15d.5 USE OF THE TUBERCULIN SKIN TEST

Multiple puncture tests such as the Heaf test are useful when screening groups of asymptomatic persons who have been exposed to a case of tuberculosis. Those with grade III or IV Heaf tests are considered to have been infected by *M. tuberculosis* and action taken accordingly.

A Grade II Heaf-test reaction should be considered to indicate infection in the BCG-unvaccinated but is more likely to be due to vaccination in those who have previously received BCG.

The Mantoux test may be used as a screening test in groups of people or as a diagnostic aid. Those with larger reactions are at greater risk of having or of developing disease[10]. A positive test in the presence of symptoms, signs or radiological changes consistent with tuberculosis points strongly towards a diagnosis of tuberculosis. A negative test does not exclude infection or disease (see Table 15d.1).

15d.6 THE BOOSTER PHENOMENON

Delayed hypersensitivity to tuberculin, as represented by a positive tuberculin skin test, once established by infection or BCG, may gradually wane over the years, resulting in reversion to skin test negativity.

The antigenic stimulus of a single tuberculin test may boost or recall hypersensitivity, resulting in an increase in the size of the reaction to a subsequent test. This may cause an apparent conversion from a negative to a positive test, which may be interpreted as representing recent infection. This is termed the booster phenomenon. It may occur at any age, but because age is associated with waning of the hypersensitivity reaction, boosting tends to be a phenomenon of older age groups, particularly over 55 years[11,12].

The booster phenomenon can be to some extent excluded, by performing a two-stage tuberculin test with an interval of 1 week between tests[13]. However, in cases where there has been recent contact with infection it may be impossible to separate true skin test conversion from the booster phenomenon.

It should be borne in mind that hypersensitivity to tuberculin testing may also vary in time even for an individual[14]. Care is always required in the interpretation of tuberculin skin-test findings.

REFERENCES

1. Koch, R. (1891) Weitre Mitteslienger wlier ein Heilmittel gegen Tuberculose. *Dtsch. Med. Wiseln*, **17**, 101–2.
2. Seibert S.B. and Glenn J.T. (1941) Tuberculin puncture protein derivative: preparation and analysis of a large quantity for standard. *Am. Rev. Tuberc.*, **44**, 9–25.
3. Heaf, F. (1951) The multiple puncture tuberculin test. *Lancet*, **21**, 151–3.
4. *Immunization Against Infectious Disease*, 1992 edn, HMSO, London, pp. 84–5.
5. Lunn, J.A. (1980) Reason for variable response to Tine test. *Br. Med. J.*, **280**, 223.
6. Rathus, E.M. (1956) The Heaf multiple puncture test compared with the Mantoux tests in epidemiological surveys. *Med. J. Aust.*, **1**, 696–8.
7. Comstock, G.W. (1975) Frost revisited: the modern epidemiology of tuberculosis. *Am. J. Epidemiol.*, **101**, 363–82.
8. Bass, J.B. (1990) Tuberculin test, preventative therapy and elimination of tuberculosis. *Am. Rev. Respir. Dis.*, **141**, 812–13.
9. Graham, N.M.H., Nelson, K.E., Solomon, L. *et al.* (1992) Prevalence of tuberculin positivity

and skin test anergy in HIV-1 sero-positive and sero-negative intravenous drug users. *J. Am. Med. Assoc.*, **267**, 369–73.

10. Comstock, G.W., Livesay, V.T. and Woolpert, S.F. (1974) The prognosis of a positive tuberculin reaction in childhood and adolescence. *Am. J. Epidemiol.*, **99**, 131–8.

11. Cauthen, G.M. and Snider, D.E. (1986) Delayed tuberculin boosting in the older population. *Am. Rev. Respir. Dis.*, **134**, 857–8.

12. Thompson, N.J., Glassroth, J.L., Snider, D.E. and Farer, L.S. (1979) The booster phenomenon in serial tuberculin testing. *Am. Rev. Respir. Dis.*, **119**, 587–97.

13. Bass, J.B. and Serio, R.A. (1981) The use of repeat skin tests to eliminate the booster phenomenon in serial tuberculin skin testing. *Am. Rev. Respir. Dis.*, **123**, 394–6.

14. Felten, M.K. and Van Der Merwe, C.A. (1989) Random variation in tuberculin sensitivity in schoolchildren. *Am. Rev. Respir. Dis.*, **140**, 1001–6.

E. Anne Fanning

16.1 INTRODUCTION

Mycobacterium bovis (*M. bovis*), a close relative of *Mycobacterium tuberculosis* (*M. tuberculosis*) is a pathogen of humans, cattle and most other animal species[1]. The magnitude of its impact on human health has been debated since Robert Koch described the tubercle bacillus as the cause of tuberculosis in 1882[2]. His initial denial of the existence of different strains of the tubercle bacillus as well as the difficulties of early researchers in differentiating *M. tuberculosis* from *M. bovis* are better understood as today's researchers elucidate the high degree of DNA homology between the strains[3]. Theobald Smith in 1898 showed cultural differences between human and bovine tuberculosis[4]. Koch, having accepted the existence of strain variance, doubted the transmission of the bovine strain to man and the human strain to animals[5]. Koch may have influenced Calmette in the latter's choice of *M. bovis* over *M. tuberculosis* for the development of a vaccine[1]. For the first 40 years of this century, the risk to human health of tuberculous meat and milk and the need for legislated control of animal tuberculosis was debated. The story has recently been chronicled by Pritchard[5], Rosenkrantz[6] and Miller[7]. A misconception, that the only significant route of human inflection with *M. bovis* was via ingestion, placed far too much reliance on pasteurization as the optimal mode of protecting human health from exposure to 'bovine' tuberculosis, at a time when animal tuberculosis control was unpopular[2].

Past descriptions of human morbidity and mortality due to *M. bovis*, both pulmonary and extrapulmonary, demonstrate its pathogenicity and epidemiology and lay to rest any question of its host specificity. *M. bovis* can be transmitted from animal to animal, to humans, between humans and back to animals[8]. Infection occurs by inhalation and ingestion and regardless of the route of infection, may cause life-threatening disease. At the turn of the century, approximately 10% of human tuberculosis cases were attributed to the 'bovine' tubercle bacillus[9]. Differentiation of *M. bovis* from *M. tuberculosis* was initially defined by culture characteristics. Biochemical testing is labour intensive and not routine in many laboratories despite the clinical significance of the predictable resistance of *M. bovis* to pyrazinamide (Z)[10].

Although the present prevalence of *M. bovis* in the developed world is low, its extent in the developing world is unknown, but can reasonably be expected to be greater due to the lack of control programmes in domestic animals. The impact of *M. bovis* on the current resurgence of world wide tuberculosis will not be known until a tool for rapid inexpensive differentiation between *M. bovis* and *M. tuberculosis* has been designed.

Clinical Tuberculosis. Edited by P.D.O. Davies. Published in 1994 by Chapman & Hall, London. ISBN 0 412 48630 X

16.2 MYCOBACTERIOLOGICAL DIFFERENTIATION

In 1868, Villermin demonstrated the inter-species transmission of 'bovine' tuberculosis when tuberculous tissue from cattle, injected into rabbits, resulted in tuberculous lesions [11]. Smith[4], in his description of strain differences for 'bovine', 'human' and 'avian' tubercle bacilli, regretted the animal nomenclature used to differentiate the organisms. Cobbett[12] described the relative pathogenicity of *M. bovis* for most animal species but noted the modifying effect of route of administration. *M. bovis* was more frequent than *M. tuberculosis* in all species except monkeys and dogs.

The 'bovine' bacillus was called *M. tuberculosis* (variant bovis) until the term *M. bovis* was officially accepted in 1970[13]. Both organisms are acid-fast and temperature-dependent (25°C–42°C). The eugonic cultural behaviour of *M. tuberculosis* is not invariable and tests of pathogenicity for laboratory animals are impractical. Hence, many authors have resorted to epidemiological studies of rural and urban tuberculosis to estimate the impact of bovine tuberculosis[8]. In 1956, niacin production by *M. tuberculosis* became the standard tool to differentiate it from *M. bovis*[14]. Subsequently, sensitivity to thiophene-2-carboxylic acid hydrazide (TCH), preference for pyruvate, failure to reduce nitrate, lower oxygen preference, and resistance to pyrazinamide[10] were added to the biochemical tests for *M. bovis*[1]. Although the inhibition of *M. bovis* by glycerol was recognized at the turn of the century[4], both Lowenstein Jensen and Marks media, in most laboratories, contain amounts of glycerol that may inhibit the growth of *M. bovis*. Although most strains of *M. bovis* do not produce amidase and are resistant to pyrazinamide[10], there are some sensitive strains that are referred to as *M. africanum*[15]. *M. africanum* strain I is nitrate-negative and strain II is nitrate-positive.

According to the numeric taxonomy of Wayne[16], *M. africanum*, *M. bovis* and *M. bovis*-BCG and *M. tuberculosis* do not have enough differences to justify classification as separate species. African strains show phenotypic clustering according to their geographic origin, resembling either *M. bovis* or *M. tuberculosis* rather than an intermediate[17]. No proof of strain mutation over time in one host or during transmission from one host to the next has been identified. *M. bovis* BCG has become a therapeutic tool in the treatment of transitional cell carcinoma of the bladder and as such its differentiation from others in the *M. tuberculosis* complex is of clinical importance.

A series of biochemical and cultural tests allow the organisms of the *M. tuberculosis* complex to be differentiated (Table 16.1). The similarity of *M. bovis*, *M. bovis* BCG, *M. tuberculosis*, *M. africanum* and *M. microti* (the vole bacillus) is now confirmed by DNA studies, which demonstrate greater than 95% homology in the DNA of the various strains[18]. High-performance liquid chromatography of mycobacterial mycolic acids cannot differentiate strains in the complex except *M. bovis* BCG[19]. Techniques for other strain differentiation are being developed.

Commercial probes, which identify the *M. tuberculosis* complex do not differentiate strains within the complex, but allow early differentiation from 'atypical' mycobacteria. Rapid radiometric detection of growth on BACTEC (Beckton Dickinson Diagnostic Instrument Systems, Sparks, Maryland) can be probed when the growth index is greater than 100. The fact that BACTEC media does not contain glycerol should increase the yield of *M. bovis*. Upon visualization of an acid-fast organism, application of the probe confirming the presence of *M. tuberculosis* complex and defines the need to treat.

Ellner[20] believes that further differentiation of *M. tuberculosis* complex is unnecessary because of the infrequent isolation of *M. bovis*. Heifits, on the other hand, points out

Table 16.1 Laboratory differentiation of *M. bovis* from other *M. tuberculosis* complex organisms

	Thiphene-2-carboxylic acid hydrazide 5 mg/l	Reduction of nitrate	Oxygen preference	Pyrazin-amide	Cycloserine	Niacin
M. tuberculosis (classical)	R	+	A	S	S	+
M. tuberculosis (Asian)	S	+	A	S	S	
M. bovis	S	−	M	R	S	−
M. tuberculosis						
Africanum I	S	−	M	S	S	+
Africanum II	S	+	M	S	S	+
M. bovis (BCG)	S	−	A	R	R	−
M. microti	S	−		S		+

R, resistant; S, sensitive; A, aerophilic; M, micro-aerophilic.

the need to continue to carry out biochemical testing in order to differentiate various strains of *M. tuberculosis complex*[21]. As seen in Table 16.1, predictable resistance of the *M. bovis* and *M. bovis* BCG organisms to pyrazinamide is one critical reason for continuing to carry out biochemical testing.

The digestion of mycobacterial DNA from culture by restriction enzymes gives different patterns for the tuberculosis complex strains[22]. A repetitive sequence of amino acids, highly conserved in the DNA of mycobacteria belonging to the *M. tuberculosis* complex has proved a useful tool in differentiating members of the complex[23]. This sequence, IS6110, has 10–20 copies in *M. tuberculosis* and *M. microti* but only one to three copies in *M. bovis* and *M. bovis* BCG[23]. The fingerprinting of organisms has been used as an epidemiological tool and will pave the way to a better understanding of the relatedness of *M. bovis* and *M. tuberculosis* and the relationship of *M. africanum* and *M. microti* to both[24]. The use of polymerase chain reaction to amplify DNA sequences when modified by ligation mediation, which amplifies flanking sequence to the insertion sequence, provides a shorter simpler method to differentiate *M. bovis* and *M. tuberculosis* fingerprints[25,26]. Fig. 16.1 illustrates a fingerprint after BamH1 digestion and hybridization with an IS6110 probe. The differ-

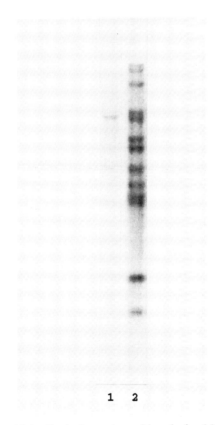

1   2

Fig. 16.1 Typical number of bands for *M. bovis* and *M. tuberculosis* after BamH1 digestion and hybridization with an IS6110 probe. Lanes 1 and 2 contain DNA from *M. bovis* and *M. tuberculosis* respectively. (Courtesy D. Kunimoto, University of Alberta, Canada.)

ences in number of bands between *M. bovis* (lane 1) and *M. tuberculosis* (lane 2) is evident.

16.3 *M. BOVIS* IN CATTLE

The origin of *M. bovis* infection in animals is lost in antiquity. Some believe the prohibition against eating or sacrificing animals with a 'wen' and 'scurvy' in Leviticus 22:22 is a reference to tuberculous animals and a recognition of risk to human health[1]. Early nomads were the first to domesticate cattle. When Europeans arrived in America, no cattle were apparent but the bison served the same purpose for meso-Americans. The origins of the cattle industry in North and South America, and probably the origins of bovine tuberculosis, began with the importation of longhorned Spanish cattle to the West Indies and Mexico.

In the USA in the nineteenth century, tuberculosis was so prevalent that it was considered to be more destructive than all other animal diseases put together. It was estimated that 25–50% of animals were infected with tuberculosis[27]. At that time, both in Europe and North America, tuberculosis was the most common cause of death in man.

16.3.1 PATHOGENESIS

The pathogenesis of tuberculosis in cattle is similar to that in man[27]. The principal route of infection is aerogenous, that is, by coughed droplets containing the organism. The aerolized droplets are subsequently inhaled by close contacts. However, as in man, infection can occur by ingestion, congenitally, sexually or by inoculation.

Cattle and other ruminants eructate rumen gases once per minute. This creates an aerosol in the oral cavity and around the head. In 1941, White reported that calves fed infected milk demonstrated lung lesions much more frequently than mesenteric lesions[28]. Possibly by eructation or after ingestion of infected milk and subsequent absorption and hematogenous transport,

tubercle bacilli reach the lungs. The number of bacilli necessary to infect by ingestion has been widely debated. The Royal Commission on Tuberculosis reported in 1911 that much larger numbers of organisms were required to produce infection by the gastrointestinal route than by the aerosol route[29].

Tuberculous disease in cattle is a slow, wasting illness, which, at post-mortem examination, gives evidence of destruction of organs. By the time it is clinically evident in cattle, it is usually fatal[30]. The primary lesion in the lungs of cattle usually appears in the dorsal areas in a subpleural location and is accompanied by enlargement of bronchial lymph nodes (Fig. 16.2). It is reported in the veterinary literature that primary lesions seldom heal spontaneously but either progress slowly in the lungs or disseminate widely[29]. The distribution of lesions in cattle is 80–90% pulmonary. Less frequently, liver, kidney and spleen are involved. Mastitis is rare, occurring in about 2% of all tuberculous cattle[31]. When the primary infection is in the lungs, the initial symptom complex includes cough, weight loss, dyspnoea and diminished milk production. The organism is shed in coughed secretion, milk, faeces, urine or via uterine discharge. Eradication schemes rely on the detection and removal of infected animals before disease is transmissible.

The interval between infection and symptomatic transmissible disease, as in man, may be years. Before effective bovine tuberculosis control was instituted, the older the animal at slaughter, the greater the likelihood of finding tuberculous lesions. The disease is more common in dairy cattle because they are crowded indoors and mustered daily for milking, whereas beef cattle are sacrificed as yearlings for meat and are usually kept outside.

16.3.2 ANIMAL TUBERCULOSIS CONTROL

Controversy over the best means of tuberculosis control has waged since Koch's era[5].

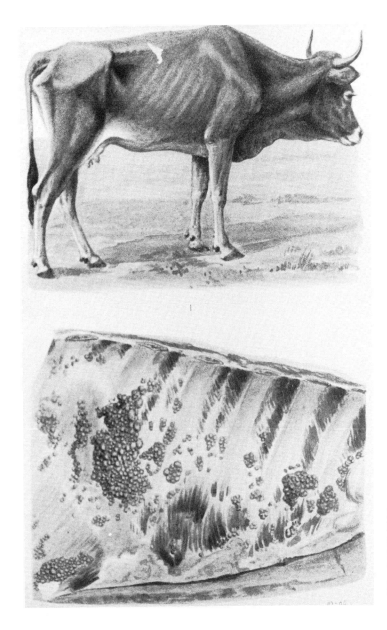

Fig. 16.2 Enlarged subpleural lymph nodes in a cow (Reproduced from A. Calmette, *Tubercle Bacillus Infection and Tuberculosis in Man and Animals*, published by Williams and Wilkins, Baltimore, 1923.)

Animal eradication schemes were originally claimed unnecessary with the establishment of milk pasteurization and meat inspection.

The first legislative attempt to control the sale of cow's milk in Britain failed in 1885[29]. Although *M. bovis* was found in dust, manure and even meat, and although only 2% of tuberculous cattle had mastitis, the pooling of milk for transportation resulted in 9% of samples being positive for the tubercle bacillus. The heating of milk to 185°C to kill *M. bovis* was described in 1899[32]. In the 1920s and 1930s, the frequency of isolation of tubercle bacilli from milk samples ranged from 5 to 12%. The high rate of bovine tuberculosis in childhood and the high rate of extrapulmonary tuberculosis due to *M. bovis* was attributed to drinking unpasteurized milk[33]. On the other hand, the rates of tuberculosis in man in Sweden were demonstrated to be lower in communities with higher rates of cattle tuberculosis. Sjögren attributed this fact to the likelihood that long-term protection against adult infection was conferred by bovine infection in childhood[34].

The tuberculin skin test was developed by using protein from killed *M. tuberculosis* culture originally intended by Robert Koch for treatment of tuberculosis. It induced a skin reaction in tuberculous animals and was first widely used by Bang in 1899[32]. In North America skin testing became routine from 1917 onward. Although human health was the initial reason for animal tuberculosis control, it was soon recognized that the best commercial interests of the cattle industry were served by good tuberculosis control[5]. Legislation for control was approved in the USA in 1917, by which time 95% of herds were tuberculosis-free. By 1940, 99.5% of herds were tuberculosis-free (i.e. all animals in a herd negative on two successive annual tuberculin skin tests). Because the first test is believed to suppress the second test result, animals were to have no tests in the preceding 60 days. In addition, any movement in or out of the herd was to be recorded.

Tuberculosis surveillance and control measures for cattle in high-prevalence areas usually employ area-wide tuberculin skin testing of herds and slaughter of test-positive (infected) animals. When rates are low (less than 0.5% of infected animals), primary surveillance is usually provided by meat inspection. The finding of a tuberculous animal is followed by trace-back investigation of the herd of origin. All cattle, exports and imports, are tuberculin tested. However, if rates of tuberculosis rise or an epidemic occurs, area-herd testing is reinstituted. False-negatives tests are seen in cattle with advanced disease and false-positives in those

with *M. avium* infection. The double comparative cervical test is one in which the response size to the *M. avium* and *M. bovis* antigens differentiates the two infections.

Recent developments in the measurement of immune reactivity of cattle include a battery of tests designed by Frank Griffin of New Zealand, under the title BTB testing[35]. A combination of serological response to *M. bovis* and *M. avium* antigen by ELISA technique, lymphocyte blast transformation with the two antigens, and the identification of serum components associated with inflammation, places the animal on a grid ranging from no infection through infection with no disease to progressive disease. This differentiation attempts to identify animals infected but without disease to allow the non-diseased animals to be quarantined rather than slaughtered. However, as in man, the range of serological and cellular response to antigen spans a wide spectrum, making it difficult to distinguish absolutely between mycobacterial infection and disease.

Other control methods to avoid slaughter of infected animals have included attempts to treat with the antituberculosis agents streptomycin, para-aminosalicylic acid, isoniazid and more recently ethambutol and rifampicin[30]. The problems with treatment include a lack of standardization of treatment dose and duration, record-keeping, prohibitive cost and the difficulty of sorting infected from diseased animals. Similarly, attempts to immunize cattle with BGG and vole vaccines created problems of differentiating those naturally infected and those infected by vaccination. Isoniazid has shown to be protective against the spread of disease in cattle herds[27], however there is general consensus that attempts to treat tuberculous cattle or provide prophylaxis to those infected, perpetuate the disease instead of eradicating it. Critical to the success of any eradication programme is the availability of financial compensation to the farmer. International trade now depends on certification of tuberculosis-free status, most effectively achieved through herd slaughter programmes.

The status of bovine tuberculosis in the world today is summarized in Table 16.2 as extracted from the Pan American Health Organization Zoonoses Centre report for 1991[36]. From 1988 data, it is estimated that of 440 million head of cattle, 1% or 7 million are infected. An asterisk* marks countries with a test and slaughter programme. Epidemiological traceback and contact-herd testing is an essential component of tuberculosis control in cattle[36].

16.4 *M. BOVIS* IN OTHER ANIMALS

A.S. Griffith's early work with animals demonstrated that most species developed tuberculosis disease after intravenous introduction of *M. bovis* (e.g. monkeys, goats, sheep, pigs, horses, dogs, cats and fowl) but the major reservoir of *M. bovis* disease has been in cattle[5].

In the wilds of North America, occasional reports of *M. bovis* isolation are so rare as to suggest that unless animals are herded, the disease is not a significant problem[37]. However, in Britain, *M. bovis* is endemic in the badger (*Meles meles*) population and in New Zealand in the brush-tailed possum (*Trichosurus vulpecula*)[38]. In northern Australia, water buffalo (*Bubalus bubalis*) and feral pigs (*Sus scrofa*) are infected with *M. bovis*. In Canada, bison (*Bison bison*) of Wood Buffalo National Park, are identified as a reservoir of tuberculosis in the wild. The infection was introduced in 1922 with the relocation of a sick herd. The issue of eradication of the herd is still being debated[39]. However, there has been no evidence of transmission to other species[37].

Taking their lead from the prehistoric nomads of Europe and Asia, farmers of Western Europe, New Zealand and North America, have recently turned to the farming of wild animals, especially cervidae (deer and elk) for commerce. In addition to the appeal of wild animal meat for its low fat content, animal parts have some value as medicinals in the Orient. Still a neophyte industry, the first reports of deer farming in New Zealand appeared in 1970. By 1989, there were reported to be 4250 deer farms and 247 under quarantine for tuberculosis. The first instance of tuberculosis diagnosed in the UK occurred in 1985 in red deer imports from Hungary. Nineteen subsequent reports had been recorded by 1991. In Denmark, by 1987, seven reports of tuberculosis infected herds had been received and importation was banned[38].

Tuberculosis control in New Zealand, by the BTB differential method, quarantines infected herds and only requires the slaughter of diseased animals. Only infection-free herds are allowed foreign trade. Recently, in Canada, the infected herd depopulation policy for cattle was applied to an outbreak of tuberculosis in elk (*Cervus elaphus*). In the USA, bovine tuberculosis in captive cervideus became an important issue in 1991. By the end of the year, ten herds of cervidae, in eight states, had been identified as containing diseased animals. Control in the USA is hampered by lack of federal authority to govern tuberculous cervidae[40]. Lesions in cervidae appear to be more purulent[40] than those described in cattle. The reason for this species susceptibility has not been elucidated.

The risk to human health of animal tuberculosis was recognized in an outbreak of tuberculosis in herded elk in Alberta, Canada, 1990[41]. By mid 1993, 15 of the province's 109 elk herds were identified with disease and had been destroyed. Of a total of 564 persons identified as contacts, 110 had positive skin tests. Ten animal workers had tuberculin conversion from negative to positive. In addition one veterinarian who treated the index animal was found to be sputum culture-positive for *M. bovis*, in the absence of symptoms or radiographic abnormality. The

Table 16.2   The status of bovine tuberculosis world wide, 1988

(++/+++)	(+)	(−)
AFRICA		
Algeria*, Angola*, Burundi, Cameroon*, Central African Rep. Chad, Congo, Malawi*, Mali, Rwanda*, Senegal, South Africa*, Sudan, Tunisia*, Zaire*, Zambia*	Burkina Faso, Cape Verde, Ivory Coast*, Egypt*, Ethiopia, Gambia, Ghana, Guinea-Bissau, Libya*, Madagascar, Mauritania*, Mauritius*, Mozambique*, Niger, Nigeria*, Tanzania*, Togo*, Uganda	Gabon, Equatorial Guinea, Liberia, Namibia*, Seychelles*, Sierra Leone*, Zimbabwe*
63 037 000[a]	88 497 000[a]	8 133 000[a]
EUROPE		
Ireland, USSR	Albany, Austria, Bulgaria, France, GFR, GDR, Greece, Italy, Malta, Poland, Portugal, Romania, Spain, Great Britain, Yugoslavia	Belgium, Denmark, Czechoslovakia, Hungary, Finland, Luxembourg, The Netherlands, Sweden, Switzerland
	All countries have programmes or conduct control	
126 173 000[a]	96 766 000[a]	22 353 000[a]
ASIA		
Kampuchea, Kuwait*	Bangladesh*, Burma*, India*, Iran*, Korea*, Japan*, Nepal*, Pakistan*, Syria, Turkey*	Cyprus*, Hong Kong*, Israel*, Malaysia*, Philippines*, Singapore, Sri Lanka, United Arab Emirates
1 976 000[a]	227 445 000[a]	2 743 000[a]
THE AMERICAS		
Argentina, Bolivia, Brazil, Chile, Dominican Republic, El Salvador, Guatemala, Nicaragua, Venezuela	Anguilla, Barbados, Bahamas, Belize, Canada, Costa Rica, Cuba, Jamaica, Panama, Paraguay, St Lucia, St Kitt's, Surinam, USA, Uruguay	Ecuador, Haiti, Mexico
OCEANIA		
New Zealand*	Australia*	
8 062 000[a]	23 500 000[a]	

(++/+++) High occurrence.
(+) Exceptional occurrence.
(−) Not recorded.
* Programmes or control activities.
[a] Estimated bovine population.
Adapted from Isabel N. de Kantor, La TB bovina en Argentina, *Bol. Inf. COLABAT*, 1991, **7** (2), 23.

Table 16.3 Literature estimates of frequency of *M. bovis* isolation in human tuberculosis

Year	Country	Reference	Frequency of M. bovis (%)	
			PTB (%)	EPTB (%)
1937	England	42	1.7	8–50
	Scotland	42	5.2	29–71
	Denmark	42	4.8	
1943	South Africa	42	Rare	Rare
1943–1945	UK	52		15
1944	England ⎰ Scotland ⎱	46	2.2	
1950–1960	Denmark	52	17/177	
1957	Germany	46	19	58.6
1954–1968	USA (Mayo Clinic)	51	0.3	
1956	India	46	Rare	
1969–1983	Liverpool	47	2.9	
1974	Germany	53	15	
1980	Canada	50	0.3	
1078–1981	Argentina	44	1.1	
1983	Peru	44	4.45	
1964–1970	Canada (Ontario)	49	0.5	
1979–1981	USA	43	0.04–0.07	
1977–1989	Argentina	45	2.7	
1977–1987	South-East England	48	1.2	
1980–1991	San Diego (USA)	56	3.0	

PTB, pulmonary tuberculosis, EPTB, extrapulmonary tuberculosis.

highest reactor rate was found in persons who worked in a tanning factory and who had been born outside Canada. The highest conversion rate occurred in renderers, most of whom were born in Canada and had no history of previous exposure to tuberculosis. Two veterinary inspectors and two laboratory workers showed conversion of their skin tests during follow-up. Forty-six received prophylaxis with isoniazid and none has developed signs of active tuberculosis.

16.5 *M. BOVIS* INFECTION IN MAN

In man, *M. bovis* is most efficiently and frequently acquired by the aerosol route. However, the pooling of *M. bovis* infected milk for urban distribution was believed to be the reason for high rates of *M. bovis* disease in children, before pasteurization. Because the differentiation of *M. bovis* from *M. tuberculosis* in the early years of the twentieth century was **not** routinely made in the laboratory, estimates of the frequency of *M. bovis* disease in man are of uncertain reliability.

16.5.1 CLINICAL PRESENTATION

Five to eight weeks after ingestion of *M. bovis*, fever, sore throat, tonsillar and cervical lymphadenopathy may occur. Vague stomach ache and enlargement of mesenteric nodes with or without erythema nodosum and phelectenular conjunctivitis have been reported. After inhalation, a flu-like syndrome with dry cough may occur. Progression to active disease may result in sputum production, fatigue, chest pain or late symptoms at an extrapulmonary site. Table 16.3 [42–53] summarizes reports of frequency of

M. bovis isolates from humans with tuberculosis. Only infrequently are details of method of differentiation of *M. bovis* from *M. tuberculosis* provided. In 1939, a review of 'bovine' tuberculosis[42] in man from several European countries, Australia, Japan, the USA and Canada reported *M. bovis* was isolated from 0 to 13.5% of all human cases. Sweden and Greece reported no *M. bovis*. Germany, Australia and the USA reported 13.5, 12.1 and 11.7%, respectively. Extrapulmonary tuberculosis was more often due to the 'bovine' tubercle bacillus. In Britain, cervical lymph node disease was of 'bovine' aetiology in 50%, skin tuberculosis 40%, bone and joint tuberculosis 19.5–30%, genitourinary 17–31% and meningeal 24–29%. During the years covered by the review, it was estimated that 2–10% of milk contained the 'bovine' bacillus in the same countries. The severity of the disease in the early decades of this century can be understood from the estimate of 25–30% mortality from extrapulmonary tuberculosis and 1–2% for pulmonary disease due to *M. bovis*[27]. It is believed by some that the early downward trend of tuberculosis rates, before the availability of antituberculosis drugs, can be attributed to animal tuberculosis control and pasteurization.

16.5.2 OCCURRENCE

The frequency of *M. bovis* has declined with time and tended to be higher in extrapulmonary isolates. More recent reports from the USA are exceedingly low (0.04–0.07%)[43]. From Latin America, Peru reported *M. bovis* in 4.5%[44] and Argentina 1.1[44] to 2.7%[45] in the 1980s. In India, low rates of *M. bovis* isolation are attributed to the tradition of boiling milk before ingestion[46]. In Liverpool, England, the 2.9% rate of *M. bovis* isolation was associated with extrapulmonary disease and not with foreign birth[47]. In south-east England, the 1.2% *M. bovis* isolates tended to be from Southern Europeans and 43% had pulmonary lesions[48]. In

Ontario, Canada, between 1964 and 1970, 31 cases of *M. bovis* were identified among 629 isolates (5%), of whom 42% had pulmonary disease, 58% were foreign born and all were over the age of 40 years[49]. In non-pulmonary tuberculosis reported in Canada in the 1970s, 0.3% were due to *M. bovis*[50]. From the Mayo Clinic[51] during 14 years ending in 1968, six *M. bovis* isolates accounted for 0.3% of all tuberculosis complex isolates and 17% had pulmonary lesions. In Denmark, from 1959 to 1963, with 2% *M. bovis* isolates, 58% had pulmonary lesions[52]. From Queensland and South Australia, 77 and 80% respectively of *M. bovis* isolates were from pulmonary lesions. Most persons with *M. bovis* isolates in Australia had a history of animal contact[54,55]. Recent communications from laboratories in Massachusetts, Portugal, New Delhi, Japan and Korea, each receiving 15 000 to 200 000 specimens annually, indicate that no *M. bovis* isolates were identified. In an excellent review paper published in 1993, Danker *et al.*[56] reported 73 *M. bovis* isolates between 1980 and 1991, accounting for 3% of all cases of tuberculosis in San Diego County, California (which borders Mexico). The sites of disease were predominantly extrapulmonary in children and 50% pulmonary in adults, and 80% of those affected were of Hispanic origin.

The frequency of *M. bovis* isolation today is somewhat difficult to determine because not all laboratories differentiate organisms in the *M. tuberculosis* complex. However, in Alberta, Canada, one *M. bovis* was isolated in the years 1982–1989, compared with 1467 isolates of *M. tuberculosis*[56]. In the Provincial Laboratory of Alberta, primary isolation was undertaken in Marks media, one vial with glycerol content (0.641%), one without glycerol and one with pyruvate (0.239%). BACTEC (glycerol-free) media was introduced in 1985. In the years 1979–1981, 10, 27 and 20 *M. bovis* isolates, respectively, were reported in the USA, accounting for 0.04, 0.07 and 0.05% of human isolates[43].

In several recent publications[41,45,53, 54,57] the risk of *M. bovis* to animal workers, farmers, meat packers, veterinarians, renderers and zoo keepers has been pointed out. There is potential risk of organisms being disseminated by the cough of a diseased animal or by aerosolization of organisms from contaminated tissue during clean-up with power hoses[41,57].

When humans are exposed to an *M. bovis* aerosol, it is reasonable to assume that they will be infected and that the primary infection will occur in the lungs with the greatest likelihood of reactivation in the respiratory site and occasional dissemination to distant sites. When humans ingest *M. bovis*, the primary infection is more likely to occur in mesenteric nodes and reactivation may be at an abdominal site or site of distant haematogenous spread.

Since *M. bovis* is so closely related to *M. tuberculosis* (greater than 95% DNA homology) and since it is most efficiently transmitted by the respiratory route, it is difficult to understand why *M. bovis* isolation is so infrequent in man, and when it occurs in man, it is so rarely reported to be transmitted from person to person. Magnus[54] showed that there was a significantly lower risk of tuberculosis reactivation in persons presumed (because of their rural Danish origins) infected by *M. bovis* and a slightly lower rate of calcification seen on radiography in those presumed infected by *M. bovis*[58]. These conclusions, which seem to suggest lower pathogenicity, depend on the broad assumption that rural persons were more likely to have been infected by *M. bovis* than *M. tuberculosis*.

Currently in developed countries, the presentation of *M. bovis* disease tends to be at an extrapulmonary site, in persons over 40 years of age and born in a country with uncertain bovine tuberculosis control. The following case is illustrative:

A 76-year-old East Indian woman, who had lived most of her adult life in East

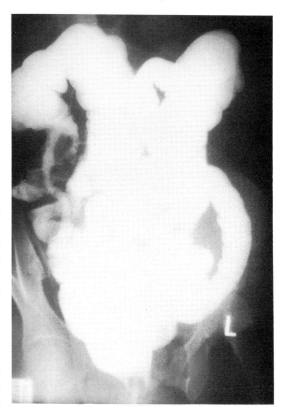

Fig. 16.3 'String sign' from a barium enema examination was caused by narrowing of the terminal ileum due to tuberculous ileitis. Stool cultures were positive for *M. bovis*.

Africa, immigrated to Canada at the age of 74. She presented with obstructive bowel symptoms and a 'string sign' of narrowing of the terminal ileum on barium examination of the colon (Fig. 16.3). The terminal ileum was resected and showed the histological patterns of granulomata in all layers. She was treated with corticosteroids. Two months postoperatively, cervical lymph node enlargement led to further investigation. *M. bovis* was cultured from lymph node, stool and sputum. She responded to treatment with isoniazid, rifampicin and ethambutol.

It is appropriate to treat *M. bovis* with four antituberculosis drugs until a sensitivity pattern is known. Once *M. bovis* is confirmed, resistance to pyrazinamide should be assumed. Hence, when *M. bovis* is suspected, isoniazid, rifampicin, ethambutol and streptomycin would be an optimal combination. Because 90% of *M. bovis* isolates are sensitive to isoniazid[55], prophylaxis is appropriate for household equivalent contacts of smear-positive pulmonary *M. bovis* disease in animals or man.

16.6 SUMMARY

M. bovis has a genome that is greater than 95% homologous with *M. tuberculosis*. A battery of biochemical tests is required to differentiate the two. It is a significant pathogen for cattle, cervidae and other species, including humans. Transmission is most efficient by inhaled aerosol particles containing the organism but the primary infection may be by ingestion. Where bovine tuberculosis control is effective, human isolates are rare. Its frequency in developing countries is unknown because laboratory differentiation is infrequently carried out. Because of predictable resistance to pyrazinamide, better estimates of its frequency would be useful. This will not be possible until a cheap rapid method of differentiation has been designed. DNA fingerprinting holds promise for the future (Chapter 17c).

16.7 CONCLUSIONS

1. There is a need to maintain awareness of *M. bovis* as a pathogen.
2. *M. bovis* is transmitted most efficiently by respiratory aerosol between animals and between animals and man.
3. The similarity of *M. bovis* to *M. tuberculosis* is so close that DNA homology is greater than 95%.
4. Differentiation requires costly biochemical testing.
5. The organism is predictably resistant to pyrazinamide.

6. The likelihood is that standard antituberculosis therapy is adequate to cure.
7. Although isoniazid prophylaxis has not been tested, it is likely to be protective in those infected before disease is active.
8. There is an ongoing need to test susceptible animal populations and to slaughter infected herds.
9. It is essential to maintain surveillance in animal workers, at pre-employment and periodically, in areas where the disease is endemic in animal herds.

ACKNOWLEDGEMENTS

Appreciation is due to the following for their assistance with information about animal tuberculosis and its control: Dr C.O. Thoen, Dr M. Essey, Dr Nick Nation, Dr Stacy Tassaro.

REFERENCES

1. Collins, C.H. and Grange, J.M. (1983) A review: the bovine tubercle bacillus. *J. Appl. Bacteriol.*, **55**, 13–29.
2. Francis, J. (1959) The work of the British Royal Commission on Tuberculosis, 1901–1911. *Tubercle*, **40**, 124–32.
3. McFadden, J., Kunze, Z. and Seechurn, P. (1990) DNA probes for detection and identification, in *Molecular Biology of the Mycobacteria* (ed. J. McFadden), Surrey University Press, London, 139–72.
4. Smith, T. (1898) A comparative study of bovine tubercle bacilli and human bacilli from sputum. *J. Exp. Med.*, **3**, 451–511.
5. Pritchard, D.G. (1988) A century of bovine tuberculosis 1888–1988: conquest and controversy. *J. Comp. Pathol*, **99**, 357–99.
6. Rosenkrantz, G.B. (1985) The trouble with bovine tuberculosis. *Bull. Hist. Med.*, **59**, 155–75.
7. Miller, E.B. (1989) Tuberculous cattle problem in the United States to 1917. *Hist. Med. Vet.*, **14**, 1–64.
8. Sigurdsson, J. (1945) *Studies on the Risk of Infection with Bovine Tuberculosis to the Rural Population*, Ejnar Munksgaard, Copenhagan.
9. Adami, J.G. (1899) On the significance of bovine tuberculosis and its eradication and

prevention in Canada. *Phil. Med. J.*, **41**, 1277–84.

10. Konno, K., Feldmann, F.M. and McDermott, W. (1967) Pyrazinamide susceptibility and amidase activity of tubercle bacilli. *Am. Rev. Respir. Dis.*, **95**, 461–9.

11. Grange, J.M. and Bishop, P.J. (1982) 'Über tuberkulose': A tribute to Robert Koch's discovery of the tubercle bacillus, 1882. *Tubercle*, **63**, 3–17.

12. Cobbett, L. (1970) *The Causes of Tuberculosis*, Cambridge University Press, Cambridge.

13. Karlson, A.G. and Lessel, E.F. (1970) *Mycobacterium bovis*. nom. nov. *Int. J. Sys. Bacteriol.*, **20**, 273–82.

14. Konno, K. (1956) New chemical method to differentiate human-type tubercle bacilli from other mycobacteria. *Science*, **124**, 985.

15. Collins, C.H. and Yates, M.D. (1982) Subdivision of *Mycobacterium tuberculosis* into five variants for epidemiological purposes: methods and nomaclature. *J. Hyg. (Camb.)*, **81**, 235–42.

16. Wayne, L.G. (1981) Numerical taxonomy and cooperative studies: role and limits. *Rev. Infect. Dis.*, **31**, 822–6.

17. David, H.L., Jahan, M.T., Jumin, A. *et al.* (1978). Numerical taxonomy analysis of *Mycobacterium africanum*. *Int. J. Syst. Bacteriol.*, **28**, 467–72.

18. Imaeda, T. (1985) Deoxyribonucleic acid relatedness among selected strains of *Mycobacterium tuberculosis*, *Mycobacterium bovis*, *Mycobacterium bovis*, BCG, *Mycobacterium microti* and *Mycobacterium africanum*. *Int. J. Syst. Bacteriol.*, **35**, 147–50.

19. Floyd, M.M., Silcox, V.A., Jones, W.D., *et al.* (1992). Separation of *Mycobacterium tuberculosis* and *Mycobacterium bovis* by using high-performance liquid chromatography of mycolic acids. *J. Clin. Micro.*, **30**, 1327–30.

20. Ellner, P.D., Kiehn, T.E., Cammarata, R. *et al.* (1988) Rapid detection and identification of pathogenic mycobacteria by combining radiometric and nucleic acid probe methods. *J. Clin. Microbiol.*, **26**, 1349–52.

21. Helfets, L. (1989) Gen-Probe test should not be considered final in *Mycobacterium tuberculosis* identification (Letter). *J. Clin. Microbiol.*, **27**, 299.

22. Collins, D.M. and Delisle, G.W. (1985) DNA restriction endonuclease analysis of *Mycobacterium bovis* and other members of the tuberculosis complex. *J. Clin. Microbiol.*, **21**, 562–4.

23. Cave, M.D., Eisenach, K.D., McDermott, P.F. *et al.* (1991) IS6110: conservation of sequence in the *Mycobacterium tuberculosis* complex andits utilization in DNA fingerprinting. *Mol. Cell. Probe*, **15**, 73–80.

24. van Embden, J.D.A., van Soolingen, D., Small, P. and Hermans, P.W.M. (1992) Genetic markers for the epidemiology of tuberculosis. *Res. Microbiol.* **143**, 385–91.

25. Palittapongampim, P., Chomyc, S. Fanning, A. and Kunimoto, K. (1993) DNA fingerprinting of *Mycobacterium tuberculosis* isolates by ligation-mediated polymerase chain reaction. *Nucleic Acids Res.*, **21**, 761–2.

26. Mazurek, G.H., Cave, M.D., Eisenach, K.D. *et al.* (1991) Chromosomal DNA fingerprinting patterns with IS6110 as strain-specific markers for epidemiologic study of tuberculosis. *J. Clin. Microbiol.*, **29**, 2030–3.

27. Myers, J.A. and Steele, J.H. (1969) *Bovine Tuberculosis Control in Man and Animals*, Warren H. Green, St Louis.

28. White, E.G. and Minett, F.C. (1941) The pathogenesis of tuberculosis in the calf. *Br. J. Tuberc.*, **35**, 69–87.

29. Francis, J. (1958) *Tuberculosis in Animals and Man. A Study in Comparative Pathology*, Cassell, London.

30. Kleeberg, H.H. (1975) Tuberculosis and other mycobacterioses, in *Diseases Transmitted from Animals to Man* (eds W.T. Hubbert, W.F. McCulloch and P.R. Schnurrenberger), 6th edn, Charles C. Thomas, Springfield, Ill. pp. 303–60.

31. Calmette, A. (1923) *Tubercle Bacillus Infection and Tuberculosis in Man and Animals* (trans. W.B. Soper and G.H. Smith), Williams and Wilkins, Baltimore, Med.

32. Bang, B. (1899) *La Lutte contre la tuberculose animals por la prophlaxie* (reprinted in *Selected Works*, 1932), Oxford University Press, London, pp. 366–410.

33. Griffith, A.S. (1937) Bovine tuberculosis in man. *Tubercle*, **18**, 528–43.

34. Sjogren, I. and Sutherland, I. (1974) Studies of tuberculosis in man in relation to infection in cattle. *Tubercle*, **56**, 113–27.

35. Deer Medical Research Laboratory (1987) *Blood TB Testing (BTB): an Aid to Deer Tuberculosis Diagnosis and Management*, New Zealand.

36. Pan American Zoonoses Center (1991) *Current*

Status of Bovine Tuberculosis in Latin America and the Caribbean, Veterinary Public Health Program, PAO, Martinez.

37. Tessaro, S.V. (1989) Zoonotic aspects of *Brucella abortus* and *Mycobacterium bovis* with special consideration of the reservoir of brucellosis and tuberculosis in bison in and around Wood Buffalo National Park. Appendix 3, in Agriculture Canada's Submission to the Northern Diseased Bison Investment Panel, 17 Nov.

38. Clifton-Hadley, R.S. and Wildsmith, J.W. (1991) Tuberculosis in deer: a review. *Vet. Rec.*, **129**, 5–12.

39. Tessaro, S.V. (1986) The existing and potential importance of brucellosis and tuberculosis in Canadian wildlife: a review. *Can. Vet. J.*, **271**, 119–24.

40. Essey, M.A., Fanning, A., Saari, D. and Payeur, J. (1991) Bovine tuberculosis in cervidae; human health concerns. Presented to Committee on Public Health Environmental Quality, United States Animal Health Association, San Diego.

41. Fanning, A. and Edwards, S. (1991) *Mycobacterium bovis* infection in human beings in contact with elk (*Cervus elaphus*) in Alberta, Canada. *Lancet*, **338**, 1253–5.

42. Price, R.M. (1939) The Bovine tubercle bacillus in human tuberculosis. *Am. J. Med. Sci.*, **197**, 411–27.

43. Kent, P.T. and Kubica, G.P. (1985) *Public Health Mycobacteriology: A Guide for the Level III Laboratory*, Centers for Disease Control, Atlanta, p. 124.

44. Acra, P.N. and Szyfus, B. (1987) Zoonotic Tuberculosis, in *Zoonoses and Communicable Diseases Common to Man and Animals*, 2nd edn, Pan American Health Organization, Washington, DC, pp. 181–92.

45. Sequeira de Latini, M.D., Latini, O.A., Lopez, M. and Cecconi, J.O. (1990) *Tuberculosis Bovina en Seres Humanos Periodo 1977–89*, (Laboratorio del Instituto Nacional de Epidemiologia 'Emilio Coni' Casilla de Correo, Santa Fe, Argentina), *Rev. Argent. Torax*, **51**, 13–16.

46. Food and Agriculture Organization of the United Nations (1962) *Milk Hygiene: Hygiene in Milk Production, Processing and Distribution*, World Health Organization, Geneva.

47. Wilkins, E.G.L., Griffiths, R.J. and Roberts, C. (1986) Bovine variants of *Mycobacterium tuberculosis* isolated in Liverpool during the period 1969 to 1983: an epidemiologic survey. *Quart. J. Med.*, **59**, 627–35.

48. Yates, M.D. and Grange, J.M. (1988) Incidence and nature of human tuberculosis due to bovine tubercle bacilli in South-East England: 1977–1987. *Epidemiol. Infect.* **101**(2), 225–9.

49. Wigle, W.D., Ashley, M.J., Killough, E.M. *et al.* (1972) Bovine tuberculosis in humans in Ontario. The epidemiologic features of 31 active cases occurring between 1964 and 1970. *Am. Rev. Respir. Dis.*, **106**, 528–34.

50. Enarson, D.A., Ashley, M.J., Grzybowski, S. *et al.* (1980) Non-respiratory tuberculosis in Canada. *Am. J. Epidemiol.*, **112**, 341–51.

51. Karlson, A.G. and Carr, D.T. (1970) Tuberculosis caused by *Mycobacterium bovis*. *Ann. Intern. Med.*, **701**, 979–83.

52. Magnus, K. (1966) Epidemiologic basis of tuberculosis eradication, 3. Risk of pulmonary tuberculosis after human and bovine infection. *Bull. WHO*, **35**, 483–508.

53. Meissner, G. and Schroder, K.H. (1974) Bovine tuberculosis in man and cattle. *Bull. Int. Union Tuberc.*, **49**, 145–8.

54. Robinson, P., Morris, D. and Antic, R. (1988) *Mycobacterium bovis* as an occupational hazard in abattoir workers. *Aust. NZ J. Med.*, **18**, 701–3.

55. Georghious, P., Patel, A.M. and Konstantinos, A. (1989) *Mycobacterium bovis* as an occupational hazard in abattoir workers. *Aust. NZ J. Med.*, **19**, 409–10.

56. Danker, W.M., Waecker, N.J., Essey, M.A. *et al.* (1993) *Mycobacterium bovis* infections in San Diego: a clinicoepidemiologic study of 73 patients and a historical review of a forgotten pathogen. *Medicine*, **72**, 11–37.

57. Kanic, G., Fanning, A., Mah, H. and Chomyc, S. (1991) Nontuberculous mycobacterial isolates: distribution of species in Alberta. ATS International Conference, Anaheim, CA, May 1991 (Abstract no. 2122).

58. Dalovisio, J.R., Stetter, M. and Mikota-Wells, S. (1992) Rhinoceros' Rhinorrhea: cause of an airborne *Mycobacterium bovis* outbreak in zoo keepers. *Clin. Inf. Dis.*, **15**, 598–600.

59. Magnus, K. (1967) Epidemiological basis of tuberculosis eradication. 5: frequency of pulmonary calcification after human and bovine infection. *Bull. WHO*, **36**, 703–18.

RECENT ADVANCES IN DIAGNOSTIC TECHNIQUES

17

THE SERODIAGNOSIS OF TUBERCULOSIS

E.G.L. Wilkins

17a.1 INTRODUCTION

Despite the large amount of attention currently being focused on AIDS, tuberculosis unassociated with HIV infection still accounts for greater morbidity and mortality. Methods of diagnosis have changed little in 50 years and most laboratories still rely on Ziehl-Neelsen microscopy for rapid diagnosis. The inherent advantages of serology together with the need for an alternative rapid test to microscopy, which is insensitive, has led to the evaluation of many assays. Early tests were bedevilled by poor specificity, but the advent of purified and recombinant antigens, monoclonal antibodies and gel separation techniques has done much to overcome this. Most work has been carried out in smear-positive pulmonary tuberculosis, where the 38 kDa antigen is immunodominant and a sensitivity of over 80% and specificity of 97% can be achieved with several immunoassays. Future emphasis needs to be placed on extrapulmonary, smear-negative pulmonary and childhood tuberculosis. The fact that no single immunoassay has yet emerged as a routine laboratory test underscores the problem of poor sensitivity in paucibacilliary disease. This chapter reviews the present state and discusses the future role of serodiagnosis in tuberculosis.

Diagnostic methods for tuberculosis have altered little since Neelsen described his modified Ziehl stain in 1883 and Jensen his modified Lowenstein medium in 1955[1]. Yet, microscopy is insensitive and culture prohibitively slow. Using rhodamine-auramine fluorescent staining, microscopy is positive in only 60% of confirmed sputum culture-positive cases. Even with contemporary systems such as radiometric (BACTEC)[2] and biphasic (Roche Septi-Chek)[3] culture, which improve the speed of mycobacterial recovery, deferral of treatment to await results (2–4 weeks in smear-negative cases) is impractical. Alternative rapid diagnostic tests to Ziehl-Neelsen and rhodamine-auramine microscopy are therefore needed. One approach is to develop increasingly sensitive methods to detect the causative bacilli or their products. Such techniques include amplification of a defined region of DNA from a few starting copies – the polymerase chain reaction (PCR)[4], immunoassays for detecting antigen, and gas liquid chromotography and mass spectrometry for detecting specific mycobacterial lipids[5]. Of these, PCR is being evaluated most intensely and appears to hold the greatest promise. A number of problems have arisen, as with any new test, which are being addressed but are not yet completely solved (see p. 381)[6].

Another means of achieving the diagnosis is to use the specific humoral or cellular response of the host to infer the presence of disease. Mycobacteria are rich in antigens that stimulate the production of antibodies

Clinical Tuberculosis. Edited by P.D.O. Davies. Published in 1994 by Chapman & Hall, London. ISBN 0 412 48630 X

and serology is simple and readily applicable as a rapid diagnostic test. It also bypasses the need for a specimen from the site of disease, which may not always be obtainable, as in patients with deep-seated infection and children. The major problem is specificity. First tried in 1898[7], antibody responses to preparations of *Mycobacterium tuberculosis* (including purified protein derivative, PPD) or *M. bovis* (including the BCG strain) contain complex antigens (e.g. sonicates, filtrates) that are poorly specific, presumably due to sensitization by cross-reacting antigens of environmental mycobacteria or BCG. Recent studies using enzyme-linked immunosorbent assay (ELISA) methodology have confirmed this in adult smear-positive pulmonary tuberculosis[8], primary disease in children[9,10] and atypical mycobacterial infections[11]. The advent of purified antigens, monoclonal antibodies (MABs) and gel separation techniques have overcome many of the problems relating to specificity.

Test sensitivity depends upon the technique used. The introduction of ELISA, which does not require sophisticated instrumentation or use expensive reagents, generated new interest in the serodiagnosis of tuberculosis. This article reviews the present state of serodiagnosis of tuberculosis with emphasis on ELISA-based methodology using semi-purified and purified fractions of mycobacterial antigens and explores the future development and role for such tests.

17a.2 SEROLOGICAL TECHNIQUES

ELISA, based upon covering a 96-well microtitre plate (solid-phase) with antigen, reacting this with test sera, and developing with an enzyme-labelled anti-human Ig conjugate, is the simplest and most commonly used assay[12]. Enzyme conjugates have superseded isotope labels because of longer shelf-life, safety and ease of use. The major problem with this technique is the necessity to predilute the test serum (1:100 – 1:500) to

counter non-specific binding of human immunoglobulins to plastic, thus reducing the sensitivity of the assay. Also, even purified antigens contain multiple and potentially cross-reactive epitopes, which interfere with the specificity of the test.

Another method is to measure antibody response to individual epitopes by competitive inhibition of the binding of monoclonal antibodies (solid-phase antibody competition test – SACT)[13]. Using microtitre plates coated with crude mycobacterial extract, the binding of MAB is inhibited if epitope-specific antibody is present in the patient's serum. The advantages of this method are that it allows the testing of sera at low (1:5) dilutions without background interference, resulting in higher sensitivity than ELISA, and it bypasses the requirements for purified antigens. One disadvantage is that radio-isotope or enzyme labelling of MABs may interfere with their epitope-specific binding sites, reducing sensitivity and/or specificity. To circumvent this, a modified assay has been developed where unlabelled mouse MAB is used at a limiting high dilution followed by development with an anti-mouse Ig-enzyme conjugate (SACT-SE)[14]. This method is also easy to standardize for screening new MABs. It is, however, somewhat more complex than the standard ELISA.

A general problem with microtitre plates is variability of protein absorption between different batches of plates and between the wells of the same plate, with perimeter wells absorbing more protein than those in the centre[15]. Also, for the interpretation of results an automated ELISA reader is essential, which is not always accessible. Because of these difficulties, dot immunoassays have been developed[16]. This involves sensitizing nitrocellulose strips with the antigen, reacting with test sera, and developing with an enzyme-labelled anti-human Ig conjugate. Strips are then read by visual comparison to standard dots or by densitometry. It is easier to perform and suitable for use in developing countries although results are generally less satisfactory than ELISA tests using the same antigen.

Immunoblotting uses the capacity of gel electrophoresis to separate the component antigens of *M. tuberculosis* so that the level of serum antibodies to multiple, individually resolved antigens can be determined. Protein bands are separated with sodium dodecyl sulphate polyacrylamide gel electrophoresis (SDS-PAGE), transferred to nitrocellulose, reacted with test sera and then developed with a labelled anti-human Ig conjugate. Although too complex as a routine diagnostic test and only identifying linear epitopes, this technique has enabled investigators to identify novel antigens specifically recognized by tuberculous sera[17–20]. MABs against these molecules, or purified antigens, can then be evaluated as potential serodiagnostic tests.

Mention should be made of agglutination-based tests[21] since they are particularly adaptable to field use and therefore would be ideal for tuberculosis serodiagnosis. The method involves antigen coating red cells or inert particles and is excellent for detecting IgM antibody but not IgG, which is the major humoral response in tuberculosis. It is therefore of limited use.

17a.3 ANTIGENS

The ideal antigen for serodiagnosis would show species specificity and strong immunogenicity. Several semi-purified antigens have been produced by chemical or immunological methods[22,23] and evaluated in serodiagnosis. These have been predominantly protein – antigens 5 and 6[23–28], plasma membrane antigen[29,30] and A60 antigen[31–34] – or glycolipid in nature – mannophosphoinositides[35], diacyl trehaloses (DAT_1 and DAT_2)[36], phenolglycolipid (PGL-Tb 1)[37,38], lipoarabinomannan (LAM)[39], sulphatides (SL-I and SL-IV)[40] and polar lipids (C1-C4)[36,41]. The most extensively studied has been protein 5, an affinity-purified antigen of complex composition but known to include arabinomannan and arabinogalactan[23]. The highly immunodominant 38kDa antigen is also contained in antigen 5, which probably explains the relative success of this antigen in serodiagnosis. Antigen 6 is less purified and therefore less satisfactory and equates with the unseparated antigen 85 complex from *M. bovis* BCG[27]. The A60 antigen contains, in addition to protein, both free and bound lipids and polysaccharides and represents the main thermostable component of PPD[34]. Lipoarabinomannan (LAM) is a lipopolysaccharide found in all mycobacteria; the exact nature of plasma membrane antigen is unclear. All these antigens contain numerous non-specific and cross-reactive epitopes, which reduce specificity and they have been superseded by more purified fractions. (Chapter 5, p. 58).

Several distinct protein antigens, which, with a few exceptions, are restricted to *M. tuberculosis*, *M. bovis*, BCG and *M. africanum*, or shared minimally with atypical mycobacteria, have been identified by MABs (mainly murine) and/or immunoblotting. These have molecular masses of 10 kDa, 12 kDa, 14 kDa, 19 kDa, 20 KDa, 23 kDa, 24 kDa, 28 kDa, 30/31 kDa, 33 kDa, 35 kDa, 38 kDa, 45 KDa, 47 kDa, 58/60 kDa, 65 kDa, 70 kDa and 85 kDa [17,20,42–44].

The 14 kDa is a prominent antigen with at least four different epitopes defined by MABs[45]. It is related to the alpha crystallin family of low molecular weight heat-shock proteins[46]. Selectively raised antibody titres to the antigen or the TB68 MAB epitope have been found in primary tuberculosis and contacts of infectious cases[17,46], suggesting that the antigen is particularly immunogenic in the early stages of *M. tuberculosis* infection. The 19 kDa secreted antigen is immunodominant and has limited cross-reactivity with atypical mycobacteria. It has been found to be useful in the diagnosis of smear-negative pulmonary disease[47] and to be negatively correlated with cavitation[48]. The 23 kDa antigen has been identified as the non-secreted superoxide dismutase enzyme but is not a prominent antigen on immunoblotting[49].

The 30/31 kDa antigens are secreted fibronectin-binding proteins that correspond to antigens 85B and 85A (P32) of *M.bovis* BCG[50,51]. Fibronectin may be important to allow the mycobacteria to avoid detection by the immune system or to facilitate interaction with host cells. These antigens are important targets for the human antibody response and have been successfully used as serodiagnostic tests in smear-positive pulmonary tuberculosis[52]. The 35 kDa antigen has been cloned in *Escherichia coli* and is broadly represented among slow-growing mycobacteria; it has not been evaluated as a diagnostic test[53]. The 38 kDa antigen is a phosphate transport protein (PstS) containing seven MAB-defined epitopes specific for *M. tuberculosis*[54]. It is B-cell immunodominant in mice, guinea pigs and man and is secreted *in vivo*, eliciting an early antibody response in mouse and man[55,56]. It has been the most useful single antigen in serodiagnosis in multibacilliary pulmonary tuberculosis[48] and the TB72 MAB epitope has also proved a precise test for extrapulmonary and paucibacilliary pulmonary disease[57]. The 45 kDa antigen has similarly been examined as a serodiagnostic test and is discriminatory in multibacilliary pulmonary but not smear-negative disease[20].

The 47 kDa antigen represents the elongation factor (EF-Tu) protein, a multifunctional conserved protein present in many species [58]. Preliminary data with convalescent sera from tuberculous patients suggest that there is a specific response. The 65 kDa (hsp65) and 71 kDa (hsp70) antigens belong to a family of heat-shock proteins with broadly conserved structure between prokaryocytes and eukaryocytes[59]. Their ubiquity in microorganisms and presence in man would lead one to predict that they would be poor diagnostic antigens. This is certainly true for hsp65 but raised antibody titres to hsp70 have been found in patients with pulmonary and extrapulmonary disease and appear to be associated with late-stage fibrosis[60].

17a.4 RESULTS IN PATIENTS

The ZN stain has a specificity of over 99% and an overall sensitivity of approximately 55% in pulmonary tuberculosis. It is cheap, simple, rapid, uses standard reagents with long shelf lives, and is applied successfully in a developing country context. To be of benefit, a serodiagnostic test must improve upon these test characteristics or complement them. It is unlikely that any test will displace the ZN as the initial screen but it is certain that one or more 'secondary' rapid tests will soon become routine on smear-negative samples. Serology must, therefore, be compared with and compete with other rapid diagnostic tests being developed and should be specifically examined in the area where it is most likely to make a substantial contribution. This is where specimen collection is difficult (e.g. childhood tuberculosis), where disease involves inaccessible sites (e.g. cerebral, pericardial, gastrointestinal, or bone tuberculosis), or where fibrosis is prominent and bacilliary discharge rare (e.g. tuberculous lung fibrosis and constrictive pericarditis). Its use in diagnosis and monitoring should also be evaluated in HIV patients, where early distinction of *M. tuberculosis* from *M. avium-intracellulare* is essential and where sputum microscopy has been found to be less sensitive.

Although important for validation of a rapid diagnostic test, there is little merit in an assay that can only identify smear-positive pulmonary tuberculosis. Unfortunately, the vast bulk of published work on tuberculosis serology solely addresses this group and therefore bears little relevance or application to clinical practice. Only more recently have patients with smear-negative pulmonary, extrapulmonary and childhood tuberculosis

Table 17a.1 Serology results in pulmonary tuberculosis (mainly smear-positive)

Antigen preparations	Sensitivity	Specificity	References
Crude			
Sonicates/filtrates	74 (49–100)	96 (86–100)	[16,23,61]
PPD	69 (32–86)	90 (79–100)	[8,23]
Semi-purified			
Antigen 5	72 (49–87)	97 (92–100)	[23,25,26,27]
A60 antigen	88 (68–96)	91 (87–100)	(31,32,33)
Glycolipids	64 (45–98)	97 (92–99)	[35,37,38,40,41]
Plasma membrane	89 (75–93)	96 (92–97)	[29,30]
LAM	56 (40–81)	94 (92–100)	[39,47,48]
Purified			
kDa 30/31 (85B)	67 (57–75)	99 (98–100)	[50,51,52,62,63]
kDa 71 (hsp70)	82	91	[60]
kDa 45	54	83	[20]
kDa 38	70 (53–83)	97 (93–100)	[18,47,48]
kDa 14	71 (71–72)	85 (74–98)	[47,48]
kDa 19	62 (61–63)	94 (91–98)	[47,48]
MAB epitope-directed			
TB72	74 (63–85)	98 (97–100)	[13,14,17,48,57,64]
TB23	61 (46–76)	99 (98–100)	[13,17,48,57,64]
TB68	36 (21–54)	99 (98–100)	[13,17,48,57,64]
TB78	44 (24–53)	99 (98–100)	[13,17,48,64]

been studied more intensively. It is also important for a diagnostic test to be able to discriminate tuberculosis from diseases that mimic it (e.g. sarcoidosis) and not just from healthy controls. Use of the latter often artificially raises the sensitivity and specificity of an immunoassay. Too often, the details of the cases and controls is given scant mention with emphasis being placed on the new immunoassay. This usually leads to promising early results giving way to later findings of non-specificity. Hence the characteristics of any new immunoassay should be confirmed in another laboratory, in different patient groups, and in areas of low and high tuberculous endemicity.

17a.4.1 SMEAR-POSITIVE PULMONARY TUBERCULOSIS

With the advent of semi-purified and purified antigens and MAB-based epitope-specific immunoassays there has been a slight but noticeable improvement in the test characteristics of immunoassays (Table 17a.1)[23]. It must be realized that there are significant limitations when trying to compare several of these studies. It is impossible to choose the same level of specificity for comparison and thus reports of unexpected higher sensitivity with crude or semi-purified antigens are usually associated with lowered specificity. Also, some investigators examined only smear-positive disease where the humoral response is recognized to be strong, whereas others included significant numbers of smear-negative patients but did not segregate results accordingly or failed to state the smear status of their patients. Lastly, many studies incorporated only healthy controls whereas others correctly used patients with conditions simulating tuberculosis and therefore provided a sterner examination of the assay. Hence, there is a limit to the inference that can be drawn from these comparisons.

Despite these drawbacks, one conclusion can be reached. Whichever test method is used (ELISA, SACT or immunoblotting) and whichever preparation chosen (antigen 5, purified 38 kDa, or TB72-MAB epitope-binding), the 38 kDa antigen is immunodominant in smear-positive pulmonary tuberculosis where a sensitivity of up to 85% can be achieved with a specificity of 97%[18,47,48]. The overriding immunodominance of this antigen is apparent from the fact that sera negative for 38 kDa antibodies are rarely positive for other epitope-specific antibodies[57]. In addition, in those initially antibody-negative, 38 kDa-directed antibodies are usually the first to appear in the first month after commencing treatment[56]. High titres have been linked with recurrent and extensive radiographic disease and a poor prognosis[48]. Levels fall with continued therapy and their reappearance or a marked rise in titre, usually indicates non-compliance[48]. Given the availability of ZN microscopy and its exceedingly high specificity (>99%), the indications for seeking serological testing in a smear-positive patient are restricted to when there is a possibility of an atypical mycobacterial infection, such as *M. avium-intracellulare* infection superimposed on old healed tuberculosis, or in HIV infection where both infections are equally common. Furthermore, monitoring of antibody levels may be useful in predicting recurrence and likely non-compliance.

17a.4.2 SMEAR-NEGATIVE PULMONARY TUBERCULOSIS

Because of the weak humoral response in paucibacilliary disease, very little has been published on this group, especially where crude or semi-purified antigens have been used. In evaluating the serological response to mannophosphoinositide glycolipids in an ELISA assay[35], Mehta and Khuller found a test sensitivity and specificity of 71% and 94% respectively, which was significantly improved upon in the same assay using PPD (54% and 84%). Sada and colleagues, using purified LAM in its native acylated state in an ELISA format, reported a sensitivity of 82% with specificity of 92% in patients with miliary disease[39]. However, in the same patient group using purified 30 kD antigen, the authors found a sensitivity of only 22%[52].

Bothamley and co-workers have identified the 19 kDa antigen as having the best test characteristics of all the purified antigens in smear-negative pulmonary disease (sensitivity 60%; specificity 95%)[47,48]. However, the immunodominant epitope is not that bound by TB23, which only has a 14% sensitivity. Purified 38 kDa antigen is insensitive (15%) in detecting smear-negative disease[47], although using the anti-38 kDa directed MAB TB72 in a sandwich modification of the SACT test, a sensitivity of 70% was achieved (97% specificity)[57]. This modification avoids any potential interference of the conjugate with the epitope-specific binding sites, allowing the use of a much higher dilution of MAB, which may be the reason for the increased sensitivity. Further research is required to confirm the promising SACT-SE results and to examine whether any other MABs directed towards the 38 kDa antigen are useful in serodiagnosis. Future effort should be focused on patients, such as those with smear-negative disease, who have paucibacilliary infection.

17A.4.3 EXTRAPULMONARY TUBERCULOSIS

Using crude antigens and a specificity above 95%, ELISA sensitivity has generally been very poor. This has improved with semi-purified antigen extracts (plasma-membrane 40%[29], LAM 50%[39] A60 antigen 52%[32]) and MAB-based competition assays (SACT) using radioisotope conjugates (34–40%) [17,65], although only 14% of patients with pleural tuberculosis were picked up with an ELISA using 30kD antigen[52]. Occasional reports of exceptional results using crude or semi-purified antigens have been encouraging (if surprising) but remain unsubstantiated[21,28,66]. In all these studies, however, only small numbers of patients have been involved with varying types of extrapulmonary disease. A larger study using SACT-SE gave more promising results[57]. Overall, out of 64 patients with extrapulmonary disease, over 70% had antibodies above the cut-off value giving 97.6% specificity. This was unrelated to site of disease. This is an important development if substantiated and supports the use of the SACT-SE format for detecting low-level antibodies in paucibacilliary disease.

17a.4.4 PRIMARY TUBERCULOSIS AND TUBERCULOSIS IN CHILDREN

Serodiagnosis using crude and semi-purified antigens has been less successful in children than it has in adults[9,10,67], although a report from Argentina using antigen 5 is encouraging[24] with a sensitivity of 86% and specificity of 100%. In this study, 90% of children suffered pulmonary disease and all cases were confirmed by culture: this suggests that the cases studied may represent the more severe end of the spectrum of childhood tuberculosis where seropositivity is more likely. In support of this, Bothamley and colleagues using SACT found 44% of children with microbiologically or histologically proven tuberculosis had positive titres (specificity 95%) compared with only 14% of those with mediastinal lymphadenitis and presumptive (smear-negative) tuberculosis[17]. This was, however, using a combination of five probes, which would not be appropriate for clinical use. Titres were much lower than in adults with tuberculosis although there was a weak association with the TB68 probe, which is directed towards the 14 kDa antigen lending support to the hypothesis that this antigen is important in the early stages of infection[68].

The specific B-cell response after exposure in contacts to wild *M. tuberculosis* or to BCG after immunization has been studied by several investigators[68–71]. No significant antibody response of either IgG or IgM class has been found using 30/31 kDa or to *M. bovis* 65 kDa heat-shock protein[70,71]. This suggests that the level of humoral response after low-level mycobacterial exposure is weak and more sensitive assays need to be developed. Given the difficulty of corroborating the diagnosis in children, a serological test, if one could be developed, would have excellent application.

17a.4.5 LOCAL ANTIBODY PRODUCTION

Antibodies have been looked for and detected in CSF, pleural fluid[72,73] and bronchial washings[74], but only CSF detection holds any diagnostic promise[75–77]. Antibodies to crude or semi-purified extracts of *M. tuberculosis* are found in the CSF in 24–44%[4,75,77,78], a slight improvement on ZN microscopy. Using four purified antigens (14 kDa, 19 kDa, 38 kDa and LAM), this sensitivity could be improved to 61% (77% for culture-positive) while maintaining 100% specificity[79]. Interestingly, the antibody repertoire was quite distinct from that seen in pulmonary or other forms of extrapulmonary tuberculosis in that the 14 kDa antigen and LAM were immunodominant. With the development of PCR technology, however, the place of local antibody detection in diagnosis is probably limited.

17a.4.6 MONITORING OF DISEASE PROGRESSION

Antibody titres in tuberculous patients rise after commencing treatment before falling towards normal[17, 64, 80]. This has generally been ascribed to the release of antigens from killed tubercle bacilli. It has been suggested that, in a seronegative patient, repeat serology after 2 weeks of empirical therapy could be used as a diagnostic test[17]. However, this requires further evaluation. Examining the individual antibody specificities during treatment, those to the 38 kDa antigen appear at 2–4 weeks, followed by a later rise of titres to the 65 kDa/TB78 epitope at 1–4 months[56]. The reappearance of antibody after then, or a marked rise in its level, usually indicates non-compliance[12,48]. Specific and non-specific IgG response may persist for many years after adequate treatment[81]. Allowance for this must be made when interpreting serological results or assessing the discriminative performance of a new immunoassay. Persistent antibody is most likely in recently treated patients who had severe disease and least likely in patients with self-healed remote tuberculosis. Despite this drawback, serology can still be clinically useful in the diagnosis of tuberculosis with the caveat that patients with treated disease should be excluded from the control group.

17a.4.7 IMPACT OF SEROLOGY ON MANAGEMENT OF TUBERCULOSIS

In a large study of extrapulmonary tuberculosis carried out using the SACT-SE assay, the time from admission to diagnosis and treatment was recorded, as well as any invasive procedures to try to establish the diagnosis[57]. Of 55 patients (40 extrapulmonary, 42 smear-negative) whose tuberculosis was not diagnosed for 7 days or longer and 30 patients (27 extrapulmonary, 21 smear-negative) whose tuberculosis was not diagnosed for 14 days or longer, 76% and 77% would have been identifed by the SACT-SE assay carried out on admission. This serological test, which can be performed in a working day, would have obviated the need for 72% and 87%, respectively, of the biopsies carried out to try to establish the diagnosis of tuberculosis in these groups. Fifteen patients were identified in this prospective study who were started on therapy for tuberculosis but later found to have other disorders: only two

were SACT-SE antibody-positive. Overall specificity was 97.6%. It is important that studies gauge the impact of whatever test is being evaluated on the management of patients. Taken to its conclusion, this will mean examining the cost savings accrued by a candidate test over conventional methodology including estimates of savings in terms of hospital stay, overall investigation, patient inconvenience etc.

17a.4.8 SEROLOGY IN PATIENTS WITH CONCOMITANT HIV INFECTION

The humoral response to the tubercle bacillus is still under investigation in HIV infection. With steady evolution of HIV towards AIDS, there is a progressive dwindling in cell-mediated T-helper cell derived function and parallel decline of recall to skin-test antigens. Recent papers addressing the question of humoral response to tubercle antigens in HIV have come up with differing results. Farber and colleagues found antibodies to the 31 kDa antigen in seven out of eight patients with AIDS and ascribed their findings to an anamnestic response to a recall antigen[82]. Another patient was described with AIDS who developed a rise in circulating antimycobacterial titres coinciding with development of tuberculosis[83]. Similar findings have recently been reported by Berlie and co-workers using SL-IV and PGL-Tb1 glycolipid antigens[84]. By contrast, Barrera and colleagues described decreasing humoral responsiveness to PPD antigen with falling CD4 counts[8]. The individual humoral repertoire to particular antigens has yet to be investigated in tuberculous HIV patients as has prospective investigation of antibody-positive and negative populations. As with other infections complicating HIV, it may be possible to predict persons likely to suffer reactivation and protect them accordingly with preventive therapy. With the recognition of multi-drug-resistant strains[85], this takes on added significance. (Chapter 9, p. 172).

17a.5 ANTIGEN DETECTION

Advances have been made in the development of diagnostic tests for the detection of mycobacterial antigens in biological fluids although the advent and enhanced sensitivity of PCR has overshadowed this progress. Diagnostic sensitivity of ZN and rhodamine-auramine staining in this group is only 10–25% but with nearly complete specificity. Published methods for detecting antigen have included sandwich[75,86] and inhibition [87] ELISAs, latex-particle agglutination [88] and reverse-passive haemagglutination [89]. With few exceptions the antibodies used have been polyclonal, raised against crude antigens, often BCG. The exceptions are where antigen 5 has been used in an inhibition ELISA and an MAB (ML34) binding to LAM has been used for sensitizing sheep red cells[87,89]. Assays have been used for detecting antigen in sputum[90], bronchial lavage fluid[74], serum[29], urine[91], ascites, pleural fluid[92], and cerebrospinal fluid (CSF)[86,88,89,93,94]. Results on sputum (sensitivity 60%, specificity 91%), pleural fluid (80% and 38%), bronchoalveolar fluid (67% and 85%) and serum (45% and 100%) reflect the difficulty of detecting antigen in very cellular samples, but those on CSF (sensitivity 75%, specificity 98%) have been encouraging[86,88,89,93,94]. Free mycobacterial antigen at a concentration of 3–20 ng/ml can be detected[74,86,87,90,94].

More recently, Wadee and co-workers have developed a sandwich ELISA using rabbit polyclonal antibody directed against a sonicate extract of *M. tuberculosis* to capture antigen and purified human anti-*M. tuberculosis* antibody conjugated with horseradish peroxidase to reveal it[95]. This immunoassay was evaluated on 253 cerebrospinal, 200 pleural and 117 peritoneal fluid samples. Sensitivity was 100% with specificities ranging from 95% for meningeal to 97% for peritoneal and pleural disease. Analysis of the clinical samples by SDS-PAGE and immunoblotting indicated that the human revealing antibody detects a mycobacterial antigen of 43 kDa. This is probably the same as the 45 kDa antigen recognized on immunoblots using tuberculosis sera and SDS-PAGE separated *M. tuberculosis* antigens[21]. This study indicates the diagnostic potential of antigen detection and the need to evaluate more specific antibodies in antigen assays.

17a.6 CONCLUSIONS AND FUTURE DEVELOPMENTS

At present, the pendulum has swung towards highly sensitive methods to detect *M. tuberculosis* or its products, principally PCR. However, the inherent advantages of simplicity, relative cheapness and potential for speedy automation, together with the need for a rapid diagnostic test for diagnosing tubercle in children and at inaccessible sites, justifies the further development and evaluation of candidate serology assays. Future emphasis must be placed on these defined patient groups with paucibacilliary tuberculosis where a diagnostic test is urgently needed, and in devising appropriate methodology for laboratories in developing countries. The demonstration of antibodies to a single species-specific and immunodominant epitope represents a fundamental advance over the crude antigen-based tests of the past. The more recent finding that many patients with paucibacilliary disease have low levels of epitope-specific antibody to the 38 kDa antigen using SACT-SE is encouraging and needs substantiating. Several new MABs and purified antigens have been identified and their diagnostic potential needs to be assessed. Once the known or predicted amino-acid sequence of a major protein is published, series of small peptides can be synthesized and then probed with MABs or tuberculous sera to identify potential immunodominant epitopes that could be used in serological tests. This will hopefully lead to highly specific assays without any cross-reacting peptide sequences. If an *M. tuberculosis* species-specific strongly immunogenic antigen (or MAB identified epitope) was discovered that demonstrated excellent (>90%) sensitivity with complete specificity in appropriate clinical groups, the pendulum would swing back in favour of serodiagnosis.

REFERENCES

1. Grange, J.M. (1983) The mycobacteria, in *Topley and Wilson's Principles of Bacteriology, Virology and Immunology* (eds G. Wilson, M. Ashley and M.T. Parker), 7th edn, vol. 2, Edward Arnold, London, pp. 60–93.

2. Kirihara, J.M., Hillier, S.L. and Coyl, M.B. (1985) Improved detection times for *Mycobacterium avium* complex and *Mycobacterium tuberculosis* with the BACTEC radiometric system. *J. Clin. Microbiol.*, **22**, 841–5.

3. Isenberg, H.D., D'Amato, F.R.D., Heifets, L. *et al.* (1991) Collaborative feasibility study of a biphasic system (Roche Septi-Chek AFB) for rapid detection and isolation of mycobacteria. *J. Clin. Microbiol.*, **29**, 1719–22.

4. Shankar, P., Manjunath, N., Mohan, K.K. *et al.* (1991) Rapid diagnosis of tuberculous meningitis by polymerase chain reaction. *Lancet*, **337**, 5–7.

5. French, G.L, Chan, C.Y., Cheung, S.W., *et al.* (1987) Diagnosis of tuberculous meningitis by detection of tuberculostearic acid. *Lancet*, **ii**, 117–19.

6. Stoker, N.G. (1990) The polymerase chain reaction and infectious diseases: hopes and realities. *Trans. Roy. Soc. Trop. Med. Hyg.*, **84**, 755–6.

7. Arloing, S. (1898) Agglutination du bacille de la tuberculose vraie. *C R Acad. Sci.*, **126**, 1398–400.

8. Barrera, L., de Kantor, I., Rittaco, I. *et al.* (1992) Humoral response to *Mycobacterium tuberculosis* in patients with human immunodeficiency virus. *Tuberc. Lung Dis.*, **73**, 187–91.

9. Barrera, L., Miceli, I., Rittaco, V. *et al.* (1989) Detection of circulating antibodies to purified protein derivative by enzyme-linked immunosorbent assay: its potential for the rapid diagnosis of tuberculosis. *Pediatr. Infect. Dis. J.*, **8**, 763–7.

10. Srivastava, V.K., Uppal, S.S., Laisram, N. *et al.* (1987) Soluble antigen fluorescent antibody (SAFA) test is not useful in childhood tuberculosis. *Eur. J. Respir. Dis.*, **71**, 292–4.

11. Amando, H., Mizoguchi, K., Tsukamura, M. *et al.* (1989) Enzyme-linked immunosorbent assay for the differential diagnosis of pulmonary tuberculosis and pulmonary diseases due to *Mycobacterium avium-intracellulare* complex. *Jpn J. Med.*, **28**, 196–201.

12. Ivanyi, J. (1993) Serological test for the diagnosis of tuberculosis and leprosy. *Proceedings from the Sixth International Congress on Rapid Methods and Automation* in *Microbiology and Immunology* (eds A. Vaheri, R.C. Tilton and A. Balows), Helsinki, pp. 267–77.

13. Hewitt, J., Coates, A.R.M., Mitchison, D.A. and Ivanyi, J. (1982) The use of murine monoclonal antibodies without purification of antigen in the serodiagnosis of tuberculosis. *J. Immunol. Meth.*, **55**, 205–11.

14. Wilkins, E.G.L., Bothamley, G. and Jackett, P. (1991) A rapid, simple enzyme-linked immuno-sorbent assay to measure antibody to individual epitopes in the serodiagnosis of tuberculosis. *Eur. J. Clin. Microbiol. Infect. Dis.*, **10**, 559–63.

15. Shakarachi, I.C., Sever, J.L., Lee, Y.I. *et al.* (1984) Evaluation of various microtiter plates with measles, toxoplasma and gammaglobulin antigens in enzyme-linked immunosorbent assay. *J. Clin. Microbiol.*, **19**, 89–94.

16. Van Vooren, J.P., Turneer, M., Yernault, J.C. *et al.* (1988) A multidot immunobinding assay for the serodiagnosis of tuberculosis. *J. Immunol. Methods*, **113**, 45–9.

17. Bothamley, G., Udani, P., Rudd, R. *et al.* (1988) Humoral response to defined epitopes of tubercle bacilli in adult pulmonary and child tuberculosis. *Eur. J. Clin. Microbiol. Infect. Dis.*, **7**, 639–45.

18. Espitia, C., Cervera, I., Gonzalea, R. and Mancilla, R. (1989) A 38-kD *Mycobacterium tuberculosis* antigen associated with infection. Its isolation and serological evaluation. *Clin. Exp. Immunol.*, **77**, 373–7.

19. Patarroyo, M.E., Parra, C.A., Pinilla, C. *et al.* (1986) Immunogenic synthetic peptides against mycobacteria of potential immuno-diagnostic and immunoprophylactic value. *Leprosy Rev.*, **57**(Suppl. 2), 163–8.

20. Coates, A.R., Nicolai, H., Pallen, M.J. *et al.* (1989) The 45 kilodalton molecule of *Mycobac-*

terium tuberculosis identified by immunoblotting and monoclonal antibodies as antigenic in patients with tuberculosis. *Br. J. Exp. Pathol.*, **70**, 215–25.

21. Reggiardo, Z. and Vazquez, E. (1981) Comparison of enzyme-linked immunosorbent assay and hemagglutination test using mycobacterial lipids. *J. Clin. Microbiol.*, **13**, 1007–9.

22. Ivanyi, J., Bothamley, G.H. and Jackett, P.S. (1988) Immunodiagnostic assays for tuberculosis and leprosy. *Br. Med. Bull.*, **44**, 635–49.

23. Daniel, T.M. and Debanne, S.M. (1987) The serodiagnosis of tuberculosis and other mycobacterial diseases by enzyme-linked immunosorbent assay. *Am. Rev. Respir. Dis.*, **135**, 1137–51.

24. Alde, S.L., Pinasco, H.M., Pelosi, F.R., *et al.* (1989) Evaluation of an enzyme-linked immunosorbent assay (ELISA) using an IgG antibody to *Mycobacterium tuberculosis* antigen 5 in the diagnosis of active tuberculosis in children. *Am. Rev. Respir. Dis.*, **139**, 748–51.

25. Bengamin, R.G. and Daniel, T.M. (1982) Serodiagnosis of tuberculosis using the enzyme-linked immunosorbent assay (ELISA) of antibody to *Mycobacterium tuberculosis* antigen. *Am. Rev. Resp. Dis.*, **126**, 1013–16

26. Ma, Y., Wang, Y.M. and Daniel, T.M. (1986) Enzyme-linked immunosorbent assay using *Mycobacterium tuberculosis* Antigen 5 for the diagnosis of pulmonary tuberculosis in China. *Am. Rev. Respir. Dis.*, **134**, 1273–5.

27. Benjamin, R.G., Debanne, S.M., Ma, Y. and Daniel, T.M. (1984) Evaluation of mycobacterial antigens in an enzyme linked immunosorbent assay (ELISA) for the serodiagnosis of tuberculosis. *J. Med. Microbiol.*, **18**, 309–18.

28. Stroebel, A.B., Daniel, T.M., Lau, J.H.K. *et al.* (1982) Serological diagnosis of bone and joint tuberculosis by an enzyme-linked immunosorbent assay. *J. Infect. Dis.*, **146**, 280–3.

29. Krambovitis, E., Harris, M. and Hughes, D.T.D. (1986) Improved serodiagnosis of tuberculosis using two assay test. *J. Clin. Pathol.*, **39**, 779–85.

30. Krambovitis, E. (1986) Detection of antibodies to *Mycobacterium tuberculosis* plasma membrane antigen by enzyme-linked immunosorbent assay. *J. Med. Microbiol.*, **21**, 257–64.

31. Charpin, D., Herbault, H., Gevaudan, M.J. *et al.* (1990). Value of ELISA using A60 antigen in the diagnosis of active pulmonary tuberculosis. *Am. Rev. Respir. Dis.*, **142**, 380–4.

32. Zatla, F. and Petithory, J.C. (1989) L'ELISA avec l'antigen A60 dans le diagnostic de la tuberculose. *Techn. Biol.*, **5**, 220–5.

33. Raheman, S.F., Wagner, S., Mauch, H. *et al.* (1988) Evaluation of a dual-antigen ELISA test for the serodiagnosis of tuberculosis. *Bull. WHO*, **66**, 203–9.

34. Cocito, C.G. (1991) Properties of the mycobacterial antigen complex 60 and its applications to the diagnosis and prognosis of tuberculosis. *Chest*, **100**, 1687–92.

35. Mehta, P.K. and Khuller, G.K. (1988) Serodiagnostic potentialities of enzyme-linked immunosorbent assay (ELISA) using mannophosphoinositides of *Mycobacterium tuberculosis* $H_{37}R_v$. *Med. Microbiol. Immunol.*, **177**, 285–92.

36. Ridell, M., Wallerstrom, G., Minnikin, D.E. *et al.* (1992) A comparative serological study of antigenic glycolipids from *Mycobacterium tuberculosis*. *Tuberc. Lung Dis.*, **73**, 101–5.

37. Casabona, N.M., Fuente, T.G., Arce, L.A. *et al.* (1989) Evaluation of a phenolglycolipid antigen (PGL-Tb1) from *M. tuberculosis* in the serodiagnosis of tuberculosis: comparison with PPD antigen. *Acta Leprol.*, **7**(Suppl. 1), 89–93.

38. Torgal-Garcia, J., Papa, F. and David, H.L. (1989) Immunological response to homologous and heterologous phenolic glycolipid antigens in tuberculosis and leprosy. *Acta Leprol*, **7**(Suppl. 1), 102–6.

39. Sada, E., Brennan, P.J., Herrera, T. and Torres, M. (1990) Evaluation of lipoarabinomannan for the serological diagnosis of tuberculosis. *J. Clin. Microbiol.*, **28**, 2587–90.

40. Casabona, N.M., Fuente, T.G., Papa, F. *et al.* (1992) Time course of anti-SL-IV immunoglobulin G antibodies in patients with tuberculosis and tuberculosis-associated AIDS. *J. Clin. Microbiol.*, **30**, 1089–93.

41. Reggiardo, Z., Aber, V.R., Mitchinson, D.A. and Devi, S. (1981) Hemagglutination tests for tuberculosis with mycobacterial glycolipid antigens. *Am. Rev. Respir. Dis.*, **124**, 21–5.

42. Engers, H.D. and Workshop participants. (1986) Results of a World Health Organisation sponsored workshop to characterize antigens recognized by mycobacteria-specific monoclonal antibodies. *Infect. Immun.*, **51**, 718–20.

43. Khanolkar-Young, S., Kolk, A.H.J., Andersen, A.B. *et al.* (1992) Results of the third immunology of leprosy/immunology of tuber-

culosis antimycobacterial monoclonal antibody workshop. *Infect. Immun.*, **60**, 3925–7.

44. Ljungqvist, L., Worsaae, A. and Heron, I. (1988) Antibody responses against *Mycobacterium tuberculosis* in 11 strains of inbred mice: novel monoclonal antibody specificities generated by fusions, using spleens from BALB.B10 and CBA/J mice. *Infect. Immun.*, **56**, 1994–8.

45. Verbon, A., Hartsekerl, R.A., Moreno, C. and Kolk, A.H.J. (1992) Characterisation of B cell epitopes on the 16K antigen of *Mycobacterium tuberculosis*. *Clin. Exp. Immunol.*, **89**, 395–401.

46. Verbon, A., Hartsekerl, R.A., Schiutema, A., et al., (1992) The 14 000-molecular-weight antigen of *Mycobacterium tuberculosis* is related to the alpha-crystallin family of low-molecular-weight heat shock proteins. *J. Bacteriol.*, **174**, 1352–9.

47. Jackett, P.S., Bothamley, G.H., Batra, H.V. et al. (1988) Specificity of antibodies to immunodominant mycobacterial antigens in pulmonary tuberculosis. *J. Clin. Microbiol.*, **26**, 2313–18.

48. Bothamley, G.H. Rudd R., Festenstein F. and Ivanyi J. (1992) Clinical value of the measurement of *Mycobacterium tuberculosis* specific antibody in pulmonary tuberculosis. *Thorax*, **47**, 270–5.

49. Zhang, Y., Lathigra R., Garbe T. et al. (1991) Genetic analysis of superoxide dismutase, the 23 kDa antigen of *Mycobacterium tuberculosis*. *Mol. Microbiol.*, **5**, 381–91.

50. Espitia, C., Sciutto, E., Bottasso, O. et al. (1992), High antibody levels to the mycobacterial fibronectin-binding antigen of 30–31 kD in tuberculosis and lepromatous leprosy. *Clin. Exp. Immunol.*, **87**, 362–7.

51. Van Vooren, J.P., Drowart, A., de Cock, M. et al. (1991) Humoral response of tuberculous patients against the three components of the *Mycobacterium bovis* BCG 85 complex separated by isoelectric focusing. *J. Clin. Microbiol.*, **29**, 2348–50.

52. Sada, E., Ferguson, L.E. and Daniel, T.M. (1990) An ELISA for the serodiagnosis of tuberculosis using a 30 000-Da native antigen of *Mycobacterium tuberculosis*. *J. Infect. Dis.*, **162**, 928–31.

53. Rumschlag, H.S., Yakrus, M.A., Cohen, M.L. et al. (1990) Immunologic characterisation of a 35-kilodalton recombinant antigen of *Mycobacterium tuberculosis*. *J. Clin. Microbiol.*, **28**, 591–5.

54. Andersen, A.B. and Hansen, E.B. (1989) Structure and mapping of antigenic domains of protein antigen b, a 38 000-molecular-weight protein of *Mycobacterium tuberculosis*. *Infect. Immun.*, **57**, 2481–8.

55. Verbon, A., Kuijper, S., Jansen, H.M. et al. (1992) Antibodies against secreted and non-secreted antigens in mice after infection with live *Mycobacterium tuberculosis*. *Scand J. Immunol.*, **36**, 371–84.

56. Bothamley, G., Rudd, R., Festenstein, F. et al. (1990) Antibody levels to *M. tuberculosis* during treatment of smear-positive tuberculosis. *Am. Rev. Respir. Dis.*, **141**, A805.

57. Wilkins, E.G.L. and Ivanyi, J. (1990) Potential value of serology for diagnosing extrapulmonary tuberculosis. *Lancet*, **336**, 641–4.

58. Carlin, N.J., Lofdahl, S. and Magnusson, M. (1992) Monoclonal antibodies specific for elongation factor Tu and complete nucleoside sequence of the tuf gene in *Mycobacterium tuberculosis*. *Infect. Immun.*, **60**, 3136–142.

59. Young, D., Lathigra, R., Hendrix, R. et al. (1988) Stress proteins are immune targets in leprosy and tuberculosis. *Proc. Natl Acad Sci USA*, **85**, 4267–70.

60. Elsaghier, A.A.F., Wilkins, E.G.L., Mehrotra, P.K. et al. (1991) Elevated antibody levels to stress protein hsp70 in smear-negative tuberculosis. *Immun. Infect. Dis.*, **1**, 323–8.

61. Levy, H., Feldman, C., Wadee, A.A. and Rabson, A.R. (1988) Differentiation of sarcoidosis from tuberculosis using an enzyme-linked immunosorbent assay for the detection of antibodies against *Mycobacterium tuberculosis*. *Chest*, **94**, 1254–55.

62. McDonough, J.A., Sada, E., Sippola, A.A. et al. (1992) Microplate and dot immunoassays for the serodiagnosis of tuberculosis. *J. Lab. Clin. Med.*, **120**, 318–22.

63. Van Vooren, J.P., Drowart, A., Bruyn, J. et al. (1992) Humoral responses against the 85A and 85B antigens of *Mycobacterium bovis* BCG in patients with leprosy and tuberculosis. *J. Clin. Microbiol.*, **30**, 1608–10.

64. Hoeppner, V.H., Jackett, P.S., Beck, J.S. et al. (1987) Appraisal of the monoclonal-based competition test for the serology of tuberculosis in Indonesia. *Serodiagn. Immunother.*, **1**, 69–97.

65. Ivanyi, J., Krambovitis, E. and Keen, M. (1983) Evaluation of a monoclonal antibody (TB72) based serological test for tuberculosis. *Clin. Exp. Immunol.*, **54**, 337–45.

66. Chawla, T.C., Sharma, A., Kiran, U. *et al.* (1986) Serodiagnosis of intestinal tuberculosis by enzyme immunoassay and soluble antigen fluorescent antibody tests using a saline extracted antigen. *Tubercle*, **67**, 55–60.

67. Rosen, E.U. (1990) The diagnostic value of an enzyme-linked immune sorbent assay using adsorbed mycobacterial sonicates in children. *Tubercle*, **71**, 127–30.

68. Bothamley, G.H., Beck, J.S., Potts, R.C. *et al.* (1992) Specificity of antibodies and tuberculin response after occupational exposure to tuberculosis. *J. Infect. Dis.*, **166**, 182–5.

69. Das, S., Cheng, S.H., Lowrie, D.B. *et al.* (1992) The pattern of mycobacterial antigen recognition in sera from Mantoux-negative individuals is essentially unaffected by Bacille-Calmette-Guerin (BCG) vaccination in either South India or London. *Clin. Exp. Immunol.*, **89**, 402–6.

70. Daniel, T.M., McDonough, J.A. and Huebner, R.E. (1991) Absence of IgG or IgM antibody response to *Mycobacterium tuberculosis* 30 000-Da antigen to primary tuberculous infection. *J. Infect. Dis*, **164**, 821.

71. Drowart, A., Selleslaghs, J., Yernault, J.C. *et al.* (1992). The humoral immune response after BCG vaccination: an immunoblotting study using two purified antigens. *Tuberc. Lung Dis.*, **73**, 137–40.

72. Levy, H., Wayne, L.G., Anderson, B.E. *et al.* (1990). Antimycobacterial antibody levels in pleural fluid as reflection of passive diffusion from serum. *Chest*, **97**, 1144–7.

73. Murate, T., Mizoguchi, K., Amano, H. *et al.* (1990) Antipurified-protein-derivative antibody in tuberculous pleural effusions. *Chest*, **97**, 670–3.

74. Raja, A. Baughman, R.B., and Daniel, T.M. (1988) The detection by immunoassay of antibody to mycobacterial antigens and mycobacterial antigens in bronchoalveolar lavage fluid from patients with tuberculosis and control subjects. *Chest*, **94**, 133–7.

75. Watt, G., Zaraspe, G., Bautista, S. and Laughlin, L.W. (1988) Rapid diagnosis of tuberculous meningitis by using an enzyme-linked immunosorbent assay to detect mycobacterial antigen and antibody in cerebrospinal fluid. *J. Infect. Dis.*, **158**, 681–6.

76. Kalish, S.B., Radin, R.C., Levitz, D. *et al* (1983). The enzyme-linked immunosorbent assay method for IgG antibody to purified protein derivative in cerebrospinal fluid of patients with tuberculous meningitis. *Ann. Intern. Med.* **99**, 630–33.

77. Coovadia, Y.M., Dawood, A., Ellis, M.E. *et al* (1986). Evaluation of adenosine deaminase activity and antibody to *Mycobacterium tuberculosis* antigen 5 in cerebrospinal fluid and the radioactive bromide partition test for the early diagnosis of tuberculous meningitis. *Arch. Dis. Childh.*, **61**, 428–35.

78. Ashtekar, M.D., Dhalla, A.S., Mazarello, T.B.M.S. and Samuel, A.M. (1987) A study of *Mycobacterium tuberculosis* antigen and antibody in cerebrospinal fluid and blood in tuberculous meningitis. *Clin. Immunol. Immunopathol.*, **45**, 29–34.

79. Chandramuki, A., Bothamley, G.H., Brennan, P.J. and Ivanyi, J. (1989) Levels of antibody to defined antigens of *Mycobacterium tuberculosis* in tuberculous meningitis. *J. Clin. Microbiol.*, **27**, 821–5.

80. Drowart, A., Huygen, K., de Bruyn, J. *et al.* (1991) Antibody level to whole culture filtrate antigens and to purified P32 during treatment of smear-positive tuberculosis. *Chest*, **100**, 685–7.

81. Wilkins, E.G.L. and Ivanyi, J. (1990) Can the SACT-SE (ELISA) really detect active tuberculosis? *Lancet*, **336**, 1516.

82. Farber, C.M., Yernault, J.C., Legros, F. *et al.* (1990). Detection of anti-P32 mycobacterial IgG antibodies in patients with AIDS. *J. Infect. Dis.*, **162**, 279–80.

83. Van Vooren, J.P., Farber, C.M., Motte, S. *et al.* (1988). Assay of specific antibody response to mycobacterial antigen for the diagnosis of a pleural effusion in a patient with AIDS. *Tubercle*, **69**, 303–5.

84. Berlie, H.C., Petit, J.C. and David, H.L. (1991) Use of the SL-IV and PGL-Tb1 glycolipid antigens in ELISA for the diagnosis of tuberculosis in AIDS patients. *Int. J. Med. Microbiol.*, **275**, 351–7.

85. Pearson, M.L., Jereb, J.A., Frieden, T.R. *et al.* (1992) Nosocomial transmission of multidrug-resistant *Mycobacterium tuberculosis*. *Ann. Intern. Med.*, **117**, 191–6.

86. Kadival, G.V., Samuel, A.M., Marazelo, T.B.M. and Chaparas, S.D. (1987) Radioimmunoassay for detecting *Mycobacterium tuberculosis* antigen in cerebrospinal fluids of

patients with tuberculous meningitis. *J. Infect. Dis.*, **155**, 608–11.

87. Radhakrishnan, V.V. and Mathai, A. (1991) Detection of *Mycobacterium tuberculosis* antigen 5 in cerebrospinal fluid by inhibition ELISA and its diagnostic potential in tuberculous meningitis *J. Infect. Dis.*, **163**, 650–2.

88. Krambovitis, E., McIllmurray, M.B., Luck, P.E. *et al.* (1984) Rapid diagnosis of tuberculous meningitis by latex particle agglutination. *Lancet*, **ii**, 1229–31.

89. Chandramuki, A., Allen, P.R.J., Keen, M. and Ivanyi, J. (1985) Detection of mycobacterial antigen and antibodies in the cerebrospinal fluid of patients with tuberculous meningitis. *J. Med. Microbiol.*, **20**, 239–47.

90. Yanez, M.A., Coppola, M.P., Russo, D.A., *et al.* (1986) Determination of mycobacterial antigens in sputum by enzyme immunoassay. *J. Clin. Microbiol.*, **23**, 822–5.

91. Singh, N.B., Choudhary, A. and Bhatnagar, S. (1991) Detection of *M. leprae*-specific antigens with dot-ELISA in urine and nasal samples from leprosy patients. *Int. J. Lepr. Mycobact. Dis.*, **59**, 398–404.

92. Dhand, R., Ganguly, N.K., Vaishnavi, C. *et al.* (1988). False-positive reactions with enzyme-linked immunosorbent assay of *Mycobacterium tuberculosis* antigens in pleural fluid. *J. Med. Microbiol.*, **26**, 241–3.

93. Sada, E., Ruiz-Palacios, G.M., Lopez-Vidal, Y., Ponce de Leon, S. (1983) Detection of mycobacterial antigens in cerebrospinal fluid of patients with tuberculous meningitis by enzyme-linked immunosorbent assay. *Lancet*, **ii**, 651–2.

94. Kadival, G.V., Mazarelo, T.B.M. and Chaparas, S.D. (1986) Sensitivity and specificity of enzyme-linked immunosorbent assay in the detection of antigen in tuberculous meningitis cerebrospinal fluids. *J. Clin. Microbiol.*, **23**, 901–4.

95. Wadee, A.A., Boting, L and Reddy, S.G. (1990) Antigen capture assay for detection of a 43-kilodalton *Mycobacterium tuberculosis* antigen. *J. Clin. Microbiol.*, **28**, 2786–91.

POLYMERASE CHAIN REACTION 17b

R.J. Shaw

17b.1 INTRODUCTION

Two aspects of the diagnosis of tuberculosis continue to pose major problems for the clinician. First, if a patient does not have smear-positive pulmonary disease, a clinician may have to wait many weeks for the results of sputum culture, and in a proportion of cases of active disease an organism may never be identified. This problem is compounded in cases of non-pulmonary tuberculosis where invasive procedures may be required to obtain samples from cases suspected of harbouring infection in inaccessible locations such as the spine or abdomen. Secondly, even when identified, lengthy culture may be required to discriminate *M. tuberculosis* from other mycobacteria. This problem is particularly prominent in patients concurrently infected with the human immunodeficiency virus. Finally, the clinical scientist who is interested to understand why infection by *M. tuberculosis* only progresses to clinical disease in a proportion of cases, has in the past been hampered by the inability to identify infected but clinically healthy individuals. The scientist has had to rely on the secondary phenomenon of increased host immunity, based on a positive Heaf or Tine test. On theoretical grounds, these problems should be answered by taking advantage of the high sensitivity and specifity of identifying mycobacteria by amplifying specific DNA sequences using the polymerase chain reaction (PCR). Two mycobacterial sequences have served as targets for amplification. These are the mycobacteria-specific DNA sequences IS6110, also termed IS986[1–5], which is present as repeats within the genome, and the gene encoding the 65 kDa heat shock protein which is expressed as an antigen in many mycobacteria (65 kDa Ag DNA)[6].

17b.2 THE POLYMERASE CHAIN REACTION IN DIAGNOSIS

The polymerase chain reaction has found widespread application in many areas of science and medicine. Perhaps the best recognized is the DNA fingerprinting used in forensic medicine. The principle stages of applying PCR to a diagnostic problem are:

1. Identify within the organism of interest a sequence of DNA within the genome, which is unique to the organism in question.
2. Design and build two small pieces of DNA (primers), which are complementary to opposite ends to the two different strands of this DNA.
3. Perform a PCR reaction (Fig. 17b.1). In this reaction the native DNA is heated so that the strands separate. As cooling occurs, the primers bind to their regions of complementarity. An enzyme Taq polymerase re-builds the DNA in the region between the primers. At the end of one cycle, the region of DNA between the primers has

Clinical Tuberculosis. Edited by P.D.O. Davies. Published in 1994 by Chapman & Hall, London. ISBN 0 412 48630 X

Double stranded target DNA

DNA denatured

Two DNA targets
available for PCR

PCR
amplification
cycle

Primers bind to target DNA

Double stranded
DNA duplicated

Taq polymerase
rebuilds DNA

Fig. 17b.1 PCR amplification.

been duplicated. This process can then be repeated with doubling of the numbers of target sequences of DNA with each cycle, such that after ten cycles there is 1000-fold more target DNA, after 20 cycles 10^6-fold and 30 cycles 10^9-fold more specific target DNA sequence.

4. The amplified product is placed in a well on a gel and molecules are then separated according to size by electrophoresis. A band of amplified DNA can be visualized by staining with ethidium bromide (Fig. 17b.2). The size of the amplified piece of DNA can be found by comparison with markers of known size. Since the DNA sequence, and thus the number of base pairs between the regions where the primers bind is known, the size of the amplified product can be predicted, and this prediction confirmed on the electrophoresis gel.

5. Under some circumstances it is important to obtain further confirmation of the identity of the amplified product in order to obtain greater sensitivity. The amplified DNA in the gel is transferred by blotting onto a nylon membrane and then probed using a radio-labelled sequence of DNA complementary to the central region of the target DNA sequence. This will only bind if the correct piece of DNA has been amplified. Recently, other detection

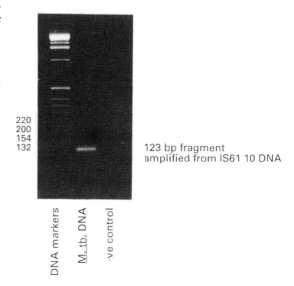

220
200
154
132

123 bp fragment
amplified from IS61 10 DNA

DNA markers

M. tb. DNA

-ve control

Fig. 17b.2 A 123-base pair amplification product from IS6110 DNA of *M. tuberculosis* compared with markers of known size.

systems using non-radioactive techniques have been developed. The primers can be labelled with digoxigenin and the presence of amplified product detected by chemiluminescence[7].

17b.3 SOURCES OF FALSE-POSITIVE RESULTS WITH PCR

PCR is a sensitive technique for detecting a particular sequence of DNA. The identification of the target sequence of DNA does not imply organism viability. It might be possible to identify a DNA sequence specific for *M. tuberculosis* in samples where culture results were negative either because the organism was present in too few numbers to grow in culture or because host defences had rendered the mycobacteria unable to grow. PCR may in the future be used to resolve the argument of whether *M. tuberculosis* organisms are present in a non-viable state in lungs or tissues of patients exposed to tuberculosis or who have previously had treatment for tuberculosis.

The identification of a specific DNA sequence by PCR does not imply that the DNA from the remainder of the organism is present. This may not be relevant in the case of *M. tuberculosis*, but at least in theory it may be possible to identify the DNA of antibiotic-resistant genes in plasmids that are passed between organisms.

A more common cause of false-positive results is contamination of samples by product from previous PCR experiments[8,9]. PCR can identify less than 100 copies of a DNA sequence and amplify these to 10^9 copies. It is very easy during a series a complex laboratory manipulations for microscopic quantities of amplified product to contaminate equipment and later be passed into new samples before amplification, resulting in false-positive results. A number of steps can be taken to avoid this problem. In all experiments, negative controls must be included. In these controls, all manipulations and reagents are used with the exception that the target DNA is omitted. All laboratory equipment must be cleaned regularly and evidence of contamination sought by means of the wipe test[10]. A recent advance is the Cetus 'carry over' kit. Using this system the PCR amplification generates DNA containing UTP in place of TTP found in native DNA. Thus, all amplified products contain UTP, while target DNA contains TTP. Before amplification, the reaction mixture is sub-

jected to enzymic digestion of all molecules containing UTP, but sparing TTP-containing molecules. By this means, DNA amplified from previous reactions cannot become target DNA for subsequent reactions.

17b.4 SOURCES OF FALSE-NEGATIVE RESULTS WITH PCR

False-negative results may occur either because the sample did not contain any *M. tuberculosis* DNA despite being obtained from a patient with tuberculosis. Alternatively, a technical error may occur. To overcome any technical errors causing false-negative results, positive control samples containing *M. tuberculosis* DNA are included. Eisenach *et al.*[11] have constructed a plasmid, which they use in their PCR amplification of the *M. tuberculosis* IS6110 DNA sequence. When amplified, this plasmid produces a 600-base-pair product using the same primers as those for the target sequence. The 600-base-pair product can easily be discriminated from the 123-base-pair product derived from amplification of the native *M. tuberculosis* DNA. In their studies, they have added the control plasmid to all samples. The presence of an amplified product of the 600-base-pair size confirmed that the DNA-extraction procedures were adequate. Other techniques to remove potential inhibitors such as centrifugation through sucrose have been suggested[12].

17b.5 PCR USING THE IS6110 DNA SEQUENCE AS A TARGET

Bacterial chromosomes and plasmids commonly contain insertion sequences of DNA. A number of copies of these sequences may be inserted at varying points in the chromosome. The insertion sequence (IS) 6110 has been identified, sequenced and found to be present up to 16 times in *M. tuberculosis* DNA[1,4,5]. IS6110 is 1361 base pairs long, and contains 28 base-pair imperfect repeats at its extremities, with three mismatches and 3 base-pair direct repeats. The central section exhibits no heterogeneity. A 123 base-pair fragment of this sequence was shown to be present in *M. tuberculosis, M. bovis* and one strain of *M. simiae*[2]. No product was detected with DNA from 28 strains of *M. avium* complex, *M. cheloni* and *M. gordonae*. Others have also confirmed that the IS6110 sequence is specific for the small family of *M. tuberculosis*-like organisms[5].

A number of assessments have been made of the use of PCR amplification of IS6110 DNA in the confirmation of a diagnosis of clinical tuberculosis. Eisenach *et al.*[11] examined 162 sputum samples. IS6110 DNA was amplified in samples from 50 of 51 bacteriologically confirmed cases. IS6110 DNA was found in only 1 of 42 specimens from patients with non-tuberculous mycobacterial disease and all 26 specimens from patients without mycobacterial infection were negative. This study used only 25 cycles of PCR amplification, which may have reduced the sensitivity of the test. Indeed, IS6110 DNA was not identified in at least 40 samples obtained from patients with a clinical diagnosis of tuberculosis in this study. Using 40 cycles and amplification for either IS6110 DNA or the DNA of the gene encodng the 65 kDa antigen, Brisson-Noel *et al.*[13] examined 514 specimens of various body fluids. They found a 97% correlation between PCR findings and bacteriological or clinical data. This study had six false-negatives and three false-positive results. Our studies used 35 cycles of PCR and examined 90 sputum and bronchoscopy samples[14]. IS6110 DNA was detected in six of six samples of patients with active disease, 15 of 18 patients with past tuberculosis, five of nine contacts and five of 54 patients with other lung disease. We speculate that this high number of positive results in those without active disease reflects a greater sensitivity obtained using more cycles and the high prevalence of TB in our urban community. Other body fluids, which are less likely to be a natural reservoir of organisms, may be more useful in pathological conditions, as material in which to identify *M. tuberculosis* DNA. When pleural fluid from patients with tuberculous pleural effusion was examined using 50 cycles of amplification, IS6110 DNA was identified in nine patients, whereas organisms were cultured from the fluid in only three patients[15]. We have examined peripheral blood and found a surprisingly high rate of positive results[16]. IS6110 was identified in the buffy coat not only in the patients with active disease but also in samples from contacts and a proportion of elderly patients with other lung disease, but not in blood samples from young normal volunteers, who were selected on the basis of no exposure to tuberculosis. These data suggest that it may be important to quantify the amount of IS6110 DNA in order to obtain a closer correlation with the clinical picture.

17b.6 PCR USING THE 65kDa GENE AS TARGET

Historically the 65kDa antigen gene was the first candidate as a target DNA sequence for PCR amplification. Hance *et al.*[17] developed a method suitable for clinical application. They amplified a 383 base-pair DNA fragment using primers that bound to DNA of all mycobacteria. The amplified fragment was then hybridized to species-specific oligonucleotide probes. When applied to a small number of clinical samples, the results using this methodology gave a good correlation with the microbiological diagnosis[18].

Amplification of 65kDa antigen gene DNA is less sensitive than IS6110 DNA detection since there is only one copy per organism. There is also a risk of a loss of specificity since all mycobacteria contain this gene and species identification depends on the extent of binding of the probe to the species-specific regions within the amplified segment. These theoretical considerations were confirmed in our study examining respiratory samples from patients with a variety of diseases[14]. When visualization of the DNA by simple ethidium bromide staining versus the additional complexity of probing was compared, there was no benefit using the additional step in the case of IS6110 identification, whereas both sensitivity and specificity were lost if this was omitted in the case of 65kDa Ag gene identification. Similarly, mycobacterial DNA was identified using PCR amplification of 65kDa antigen DNA in 15 of 43 samples from patients with diagnoses other than tuberculosis. By contrast, IS6110 DNA was amplified from only six of 56 samples from this patient group.

17b.7 PCR USING MPB 64 GENE AS TARGET

MPB 64 is an immunogenic protein that has been cloned and characterized from *M. bovis*[19]. MPB 64 is believed to be specific for the *M. tuberculosis* complex[19–21]. PCR amplification of MPB64 DNA has been used to identify *M. tuberculosis* in CSF[22]. Of 20 cases of highly probable tuberculous meningitis on clinical grounds, 15 had MPB64 DNA in the CSF, whereas CSF culture was positive in only four of these cases. Among the 51 controls, there were initially thought to be six positive PCR results, but these were negative on subsequent re-checking. This study highlighted the difficulty in correlating positive PCR results with confirmed clinical tuberculosis, when the test used as a 'gold standard', namely identification of the organism in CSF, is often negative in active clinical infection.

17b.8 OTHER DNA SEQUENCES USED AS TARGETS FOR PCR AMPLIFICATION

A number of other sequences have been used as targets for amplification. De Wit *et al.*[23] have identified another DNA sequence, which is specific for *M. tuberculosis* and is present in multiple copies within the genome. PCR amplification of a 336 base-pair fragment of this sequence was able to identify *M. tuberculsosis* in clinical samples. Hermans *et al.*[24] identified another sequence specific for *M. tuberculosis* complex strains. A 158 base-pair fragment of this sequence was amplified from a range of clinical samples from patients with tuberculosis. Patel *et al.*[25] also identified a sequence of DNA that could be amplified from all mycobacterial species. A region of this was more specific for strains of *M. tuberculosis*. This target has been used in a clinical study of 96 samples of which 74 were positive by PCR and culture, eight were negative by both assessments, and 14 were negative by culture but positive by PCR[26]. Del Portillo *et al.*[27] have also cloned and sequenced a region of DNA specific for *M. tuberculosis*. They amplified a 396 base-pair piece from this region, which was used to identify the organism in clinical samples. Ralphs *et al.*[28] have utilized a 1.5 kb EcoR1-BamH1 restriction fragment from *M. tuberculosis*, which hybridized specifically to *M. tuberculosis* as a target for PCR.

More recently, Altamirano *et al.*[29] cloned a 959 base-pair sequence that is specific for *M. tuberculosis*. PCR identification of this sequence in 200 sputum specimens of which 44 were culture-positive for *M. tuberculosis*, 50 for mycobacteria other than *M. tuberculosis* and 106 of which were culture-negative, gave a sensitivity of 98% and a specificity of 100%. However, the exact clinical characteristics of the patients from whom the samples were collected was not stated.

17b.9 DETECTION OF MYCOBACTERIA BY AMPLIFICATION OF RIBOSOMAL RNA SEQUENCES

Ribosomal RNA (rRNA) is present in large copy numbers in cells and the sequence is characteristic for nearly every organism. Furthermore, there are stretches of highly conserved sequences and regions of considerable variability[30]. These features suggest that PCR amplification of rRNA may offer a suitable target sequence for the identification of mycobacteria. The presence of defined regions of great variability in sequence may offer a tool to assist with epidemiology. Boddinghaus *et al.*[31] have used primers to regions of rRNA to detect fewer than ten mycobacteria, and suggest that the choice of primer can identify the different types of mycobacteria. Probes to such regions of rRNA are available commercially (The Gen-Probe Corp., San Diego, California, USA)[32,33].

17b.10 TARGET DNA SEQUENCES FOR MYCOBACTERIA OTHER THAN *M. TUBERCULOSIS*

Many other mycobacteria contain insertion sequences that may be specific for these different organisms. IS1081 is present in both *M. bovis* and *M. tuberculosis*, but there are six copies in *M. bovis*[34]. IS900 is present in *M. paratuberculosis* and PCR amplification has been used to diagnose infection in cattle[35]. IS1096 is a 2275 base-pair DNA sequence unique to *M. smegmatis*[36]. The presence of insertion sequences may be related to pathogenicity. IS901 is an insertion sequence found in pathogenic strains of *M. avium-intracellulare* but which is absent from *M. avium* complex isolates from HIV-infected individuals[37]. Other sequences may be useful in discriminating between closely related organisms. PCR amplification of the sequence encoding the MPB70 antigen has been used to identify *M. bovis*[38].

17b.11 COMBINED PCR WITH BACTEC OR CULTURE

Taking into account the expense and technical difficulty, it is unlikely that it will be possible to screen large numbers of clinical samples in a routine bacteriology laboratory using PCR amplification. An alternative approach is to use regular or BACTEC culture and once positive growth has been identified, DNA can be amplified and the organism identified using PCR[39,40]. This combination can detect 83% of *M. tuberculosis* culture-positive specimens within 18 days[41].

17b.12 PCR TO IDENTIFY DRUG-RESISTANT *M. TUBERCULOSIS*

The recent association of defects in the mycobacterial katG gene, which encodes both catalase and peroxidase, with isoniazid resitance[42], offers a DNA marker of drug resistance. This DNA sequence may serve as a target for PCR amplification allowing early detection of isoniazid resistance.

17b.13 PCR FOR MYCOBACTERIAL DNA IN SARCOIDOSIS

PCR for mycobacterial DNA in sarcoidosis offers a new approach to resolving the debate over a possible mycobacterial aetiology for sarcoidosis[43]. In a very thorough study Bocart *et al.*[44] found no evidence of IS6110 DNA in extracts from granulomatous lesions from patients with sarcoidosis. To look for evidence of other mycobacteria, granulomatous tissue or bronchoalveolar lavage cells were examined for the presence of DNA encoding the 65 kDa antigen. Great sensitivity was obtained by using up to 100 cycles of PCR and by using a reamplification protocol with nested primers[45]. Under these conditions one set of amplification cycles are performed using the first set of primers. This is followed by a further set of amplification cycles using a second set of primers, which bind to the target sequence of DNA inside the binding sights of the first set of primers. This allows for greater sensitivity and specificity. Bocart *et al.*[44] found DNA of mycobacterial origin in 32 of 84 patients and 34 of 77 controls using this technique. Sequencing of the amplified DNA failed to find any one organism common to all cases of sarcoidosis.

These results conflict with those of Sabour et al.[46] who found IS6110 DNA in samples obtained at bronchoscopy from half the patients with sarcoidosis. This latter study, however, was performed in London and the results may reflect the high prevalence of tuberculosis and exposure to *M. tuberculosis* in this urban community. The possibility of sarcoidosis and tuberculosis coexisting has recently been reviewed[47].

17b.14 FUTURE DEVELOPMENTS

The PCR technology is in its infancy. It is likely that technical developments will allow improved quantification and reduce the risk of contamination giving false-positive results. This may improve the ability of this technique to discriminate between the patients who have been infected in the past by *M. tuberculosis* and those who have clinically active disease. In most infected individuals, disease is prevented by the host immune response. However, in many infected individuals the organisms may remain viable and capable of causing disease at a later date, if host immunity is decreased[48]. The sensitivity of the PCR technique may now for the first time be able to identify these individuals who are infected but do not have active disease, and allow us to ask questions about the relationship between the continued presence of organisms and host immunity.

REFERENCES

1. Eisenach, K.D., Crawford, J.T. and Bates, J.H. (1988) Repetitive DNA sequences as probes for *Mycobacterium tuberculosis*. *J. Clin. Microbiol.*, **26**, 2240–5.
2. Eisenach, K.D., Cave, M.D., Bates, J.H. and Crawford, J.T. (1990) Polymerase chain reaction amplification of a repetitive DNA sequence specific for *Mycobacterium tuberculosis*. *J. Infect. Dis.*, **161**, 977–81.
3. Patel, R.J., Freis, W.U., Piessens, W.F. and Wirth, D.F. (1990) Sequence amplification by polymerase chain reaction of a cloned DNA fragment for identification of *Mycobacterium tuberculosis*. *J. Clin. Microbiol.*, **28**, 513–18.
4. Thierry D., Cave, M.D., Eisenach, K.D. *et al.* (1990) IS6110, an IS-like element of *Mycobacteria tuberculosis* complex. *Nucleic Acid Res.*, **18**, 188–9.
5. Thierry, D., Brisson-Noel, A., Vincent-Levy-Frebault, V. *et al.* (1990) Characterization of a *Mycobacterium tuberculosis* insertion sequence, IS6110, and its application in diagnosis. *J. Clin. Microbiol.*, **28**, 2668–73.
6. Shinnick, T.M. (1987) The 65-kilodalton antigen of *Mycobacterium tuberculosis*. *J. Bacteriol.*, **169**, 1080–8.
7. Fiss, E.H., Chehab, F.F., and Brooks, G.F. (1992) DNA amplification and reverse dot blot hybridization for detection and identification of mycobacteria to the species level in the clinical laboratory. *J. Clin. Microbiol.*, **30**, 1220–4.
8. Kwok, S. and Higuchi, R. (1989) Avoiding false positives with PCR. *Nature*, **339**, 237–8.
9. Porter-Jordan, K. and Garret, C.T. (1990) Source of contamination in polymerase chain reaction assay. *Lancet*, **335**, 1220.
10. Cone, R.W., Hobson, A.C., Huang, M.-L.W. and Fairfax, M.R. (1990) Polymerase chain reaction decontamination: the wipe test. *Lancet*, **ii**, 686 7.
11. Eisenach, K.D., Sifford, M.D., Cave, D. *et al.* (1991) Detection of *Mycobacterium tuberculosis* in sputum samples using a polymerase chain reaction. *Am. Rev. Respir. Dis.*, **144**, 1160–3.
12. Victor, T., du Toit, R. and van Helden, P.D. (1991) Purification of sputum samples through sucrose improves detection of *Mycobacterium tuberculosis* by polymerase chain reaction *J. Clin. Microbiol.*, **30**, 1514–17.
13. Brisson-Noel, A., Aznar, C., Chureau, C. *et al.* (1991) Diagnosis of tuberculosis by DNA amplification in clinical practice evaluation. *Lancet*, **338**, 364–6.
14. Walker, D., Taylor, I., Mitchell, D.M. and Shaw, R.J. (1992) Comparison of polymerase chain reaction (PCR) amplificaton of two mycobacterial DNA sequences IS6110 and the 65kD antigen gene, in the diagnosis of tuberculosis. *Thorax*, **47**, 690–4.
15. de Lassence, A., Lecossier, D., Pierre, C. *et al.* Detection of mycobacterial DNA in pleural fluid from patients with tuberculous pleurisy by means of the polymerase chain reaction comparison of two protocols. *Thorax*, **47**, 265–9.
16. Shaw, R.J., Taylor, I.K., Walker, D. and

Mitchell, D.M. (1992) Assessment of PCR amplification of IS6110 DNA in blood as a diagnostic test for tuberculosis. *Thorax*, **47**, 876 (Abstract).

17. Hance, A.J, Grandchamp, P.B., Levy-Frebault, V. *et al.* (1989) Detection and identification of mycobacteria by amplification of mycobacterial DNA. *Mol. Microbiol.*, **3**, 843–9.

18. Brisson-Noel, A., Gicquel, B., Lecossier, D. *et al.* (1989) Rapid diagnosis of tuberculosis by amplification of mycobacterial DNA in clinical samples. *Lancet*, **ii**, 1069–71.

19. Yamaguchi, R., Matsuo, K., Yamazaki, A. *et al.* (1989) Cloning and characterisation of the gene for immunogenic protein MPB64 by *Mycobacterium bovis* BCG. *Infect. Immun.*, **57**, 283–8.

20. Harboe, M., Nagai, S., Patarrogo, M.E. *et al.* (1986) Properties of proteins MPB64, MPB70 and MPB80 or *Mycobacterium bovis* BCG. *Infect. Immun.*, **52**, 293–302.

21. Shankar, P. Manjunath, N., Lakshmi, R. *et al.* (1990) Identification of *Mycobacterium tuberculosis* by polymerase chain reaction. *Lancet*, **335**, 423.

22. Shankar, P., Manjunath, N., Mohan, K.K. *et al.* (1991) Rapid diagnosis of tuberculous meningitis by polymerase chain reaction. *Lancet*, **337**, 5–7.

23. De Wit, D., Steyn, L., Shoemaker, S. and Sogin, M. (1990) Direct detection of *Mycobacterium tuberculosis* in clinical specimens by DNA amplification. *J. Clin. Microbiol.*, **28**, 2437–41.

24. Hermans, P.W., Schuitema, A.R., Van-Soolingen, D. *et al.* (1990) Specific detection of mycobacteria tuberculosis complex strains by polymerase chain reaction. *J. Clin. Microbiol.*, **28**, 1204–13.

25. Patel, R.J., Fries, J.W.U., Piessens, W.F. and Wirth, D.F. (1990) Sequence analysis and amplification by polymerase chain reaction of a cloned DNA fragment for identification of *Mycobacterium tuberculosis*. *J. Clin. Microbiol.*, **28**, 513–18.

26. Sritnaran, V. and Barker, R.H. Jr (1991) A simple method for diagnosing *M. tuberculosis* infection in clinical samples using PCR. *Mol. Cell Probes*, **5**, 385–95.

27. Del Portillo, P., Murillo, L.A. and Patarroyo, M.E. (1991) Amplification of a species-specific DNA fragment of *Mycobacterium tuberculosis* and its possible use in diagnosis. *J. Clin. Microbiol.*, **29**, 2163–8.

28. Ralphs, N.T., Garret, S., Morse, R. *et al.* (1991) A DNA primer/probe system for the rapid and sensitive detection of *Mycobacterium tuberculosis*-complex pathogens. *J. Appl. Bacteriol.*, **70**, 221–6.

29. Altamirano, M., Kelly, M.T., Wong, A. *et al.* (1992) Characterization of a DNA probe for detection of *Mycobacterium tuberculosis* complex in clinical samples by polymerase chain reaction. *J. Clin. Microbiol.*, **30**, 2173–76.

30. Woese, C.R. (1987) Bacterial evolution. *Microbiol. Rev.*, **51**, 221–71.

31. Boddinghaus, B., Rogall, T., Flohr, T. *et al.* (1990) Detection and identification of mycobacteria by amplification of rRNA. *J. Clin. Microbiol.*, **28**, 751–9.

32. Kiehn, T.E. and Edwards, F.F. (1987) Rapid identification using a specific DNA probe of *Mycobacterium avium* complex from patients with acquired immunodeficiency syndrome. *J. Clin. Microbiol.*, **25**, 1551–2.

33. Drake, T.A., Hindler, J.A., Berlin, O.G. and Bruckner, D.A. (1987) Rapid identification of *Mycobacterium avium* complex in culture using DNA probes. *J. Clin. Microbiol.*, **25**, 1442–5.

34. Collins, D.M. and Stephens, D.M. (1991) Identification of an insertion sequence, IS1081, in *Mycobacterium bovis*. *FEMS Microbiol. Lett.*, **67**, 11–15.

35. van der Giessen, J.W.B., Haring, R.M., Vauclare, E. *et al.* Evaluation of the abilities of three diagnostic tests based on polymerase chain reaction to detect *Mycobacterium paratuberculosis* in cattle: application in control program. *J. Clin. Microbiol.*, **30**, 216–19.

36. Cirillo, J.D., Barletta, R.G., Bloom, B.R. and Jacobs, W.R. Jr (1991) A novel transposon trap for mycobacteria: isolation and characterization of IS1096. *J. Bacteriol.*, **173**(24), 7772–80.

37. Kunze, Z.M., Wall, S., Appelberg, R. *et al.* IS901, a new member of a widespread class of atypical insertion sequences, is associated with pathogenicity in *Mycobacterium avium*. *Mol. Microbiol.*, **5**(9), 2265–72.

38. Cousins, D.V., Wilton, S.D., Francis, B.R. and Gow, B.L. Use of polymerase chain reaction for rapid diagnosis of tuberculosis. *J. Clin. Microbiol.*, **30**(1), 255–8.

39. Ellner, P.D., Kiehn, T.E., Cammarata, R. and Hosmer, M. (1988). Rapid detection and identification of pathogenic mycobacteria by com-

bining radiometric and nucleic acid probe methods. *J. Clin. Microbiol.*, **26**, 1349–52.

40. Body, B.A., Warren, N.G., Spicer, A. *et al.* (1990) Use of Gen-Probe and BACTEC for rapid isolation and identification of myco-bacteria. Correlation of probe results with growth index. *Am. J. Clin. Pathol.*, **93**, 415–20.

41. Peterson, E.M., Lu, R., Floyd, C. *et al.* Direct identification of *Mycobacterium tuberculosis*, *Mycobacterium avium*, and *Mycobacterium intra-cellulare* from amplified primary cultures in BACTEC media using DNA probes. *J. Clin. Microbiol.*, **27**, 1543–47.

42. Zhang, Y., Heym, B., Allen, B. *et al.* (1992). The catalase-peroxidase gene and isoniazid resistance of *Mycobacterium tuberculosis*. *Nature*, **358**, 591–3.

43. Joyce-Brady, M. (1992) Tastes Great, Less Fillings: The debate about mycobacteria and sarcoidosis. *Am. Rev. Respir. Dis.*, **145**, 986–7.

44. Bocart, D., Lecossier, D., De Lassence, A. *et al.* (1992). A search for mycobacterial DNA in granulomatous tissues from patients with sarcoidosis using the polymerase chain reaction. *Am. Rev. Respir. Dis.*, **145**, 1142–8.

45. Pierre, C., Lecossier, D., Boussougant, Y. *et al.* (1991). Use of a reamplification protocol improves sensitivity of detection of *Myco-bacteria* tuberculosis in clinical samples by amplification of DNA. *J. Clin. Microbiol.*, **29**, 712–17.

46. Saboor, S.A., Johnson, N.M. and McFadden, J. (1992) Detection of mycobacterial DNA in sarcoidosis and tuberculosis with polymerase chain reaction. *Lancet*, **339**, 1012–15.

47. Case Records of the Massachusetts General Hospital (1990) Case 24–1990. *N. Engl. J. Med.*, **322**, 1728–38.

48. Snider, D. (1989) Reviews of infectious dis-eases (Editorial). **11** (Suppl. 2)., S336–338.

DNA FINGERPRINTING: A POWERFUL NEW TOOL FOR THE STUDY OF TUBERCULOSIS

P. Godfrey-Faussett

The past decades have seen an escalation in our understanding of the molecular basis of life. New technologies are being used for the diagnosis of many old diseases, including tuberculosis, as discussed in the previous section. The study of the molecular genetics of the mycobacteria has been a new arrival in the research laboratory[1] but already tools are emerging with which to clarify questions about the epidemiology and pathogenesis of tuberculosis that were previously obscure. The development and application of one such method, DNA fingerprinting, will be the focus of this chapter.

17c.1 DIFFERENTIATION OF ISOLATES FROM *M. TUBERCULOSIS* COMPLEX

The distinction between the two major species within the *Mycobacterium tuberculosis* complex (*M. tuberculosis* and *M. bovis*) was originally necessary for public health considerations rather than taxonomic certainties. The similarities between these two species are greater than between individual isolates of other distinct mycobacterial species. None the less, it has proved possible to distinguish these two on the basis of their cultural and biochemical requirements and by their colonial morphology. Similarly, broad distinctions have been drawn between isolates of *M. tuberculosis* from India and Africa. Observations on colonial morphology have been supported by differences in virulence in guinea-pigs and by patterns of susceptibility to different mycobacteriophages[2].

Although phage typing distinguishes more groups[3], increasing numbers of phages are required to increase discrimination, and the standardization and repeatability of phage stocks becomes a problem. Serological methods for typing, which have proved the mainstay of classification for many other bacteria, have not been found to be useful with *M. tuberculosis*[4], because of the rather limited variation in antigens on the waxy cell wall and the tendency for spontaneous clumping of mycobacterial cell suspensions. On the other hand, analysis of mycolic acid components of the cell wall by high-performance liquid chromatography can distinguish different mycobacterial species[5] and may also differentiate between some isolates within the *M. tuberculosis* complex. However the equipment and expertise required are expensive and not widely available (Chapter 17a, p. 367).

Our understanding of the chain of transmission of tuberculosis has been discussed earlier. Following primary infection with tubercle bacilli, a proportion of people deve-

Clinical Tuberculosis. Edited by P.D.O. Davies. Published in 1994 by Chapman & Hall, London. ISBN 0 412 48630 X

lop tuberculosis quite soon but in a substantial majority the initial challenge is overcome without symptoms and the bacilli then lie dormant. Post-primary tuberculosis can then result either from endogenous reactivation of the original infection following a waning of immunity or from a further exogenous infection. The relative contribution of the two mechanisms is not known because the clinical result is identical and most isolates of *M. tuberculosis* could not be distinguished from each other (Chapter 5, p. 60).

Molecular techniques that are able to differentiate between isolates of *M. tuberculosis* will therefore help to answer not only fundamental questions about the pathogenesis of tuberculosis but also more pragmatic ones about clusters of infection and likely routes of transmission. The changes that HIV has produced in susceptibility to infection[6], risk of reactivation[7] and possibly chance of transmission[8] makes this an opportune time to address these issues.

17c.2 REPETITIVE SEQUENCES IN EUKARYOTES AND PROKARYOTES

Repeated DNA sequences have been recognized in eukaryotes since the 1960s[9] and in prokaryotes since the 1970s[10]. Within the bacterial genome there may be repeated genes of known function, such as those encoding ribosomal RNA subunits[11]; noncoding repetitive DNA, such as the repetitive extragenic palindromic sequence, which may occupy up to 1% of the total genome of *Escherichia coli*[12], and transposable elements, comprising insertion sequences and transposons. Insertion sequences are able to transpose to different sites on bacterial plasmids or chromosomes and in doing so frequently generate extra copies of themselves. Transposons are more complex sequences, often including a gene for antibiotic resistance or some other phenotypic variant along with the gene necessary for transposition. The factors governing the regulation of transposition are largely unknown, although increased copy numbers of elements coding for antibiotic resistance have been documented in bacteria cultivated in low concentrations of that antibiotic[13]. Similarly the function of these elements, particularly the more vestigial insertion sequences, remains conjectural[14]. Whether they serve a biological role for their host or merely continue to exist solely through their ability to replicate, they are proving useful as markers for particular strains both for diagnosis and epidemiology.

17c.3 FINGERPRINTING WITH IS6110

Repetitive sequences with variable locations in the genome have been used for a range of applications in both eukaryotes and prokaryotes from forensic pathology among humans[15], through diagnosis of malaria[16] to ecology of yeasts[17]. Repeated sequences were first recognized in *M. tuberculosis* in 1988[18,19]. One of these, identified with a gene probe from a *Mycobacterium fotuitum* plasmid[20], was shown to be an insertion element coding for a transposase of the IS3 family[21]. It was labelled IS986 but in fact is essentially the same element as IS6110, which had been described earlier the same year[22]. It is found in multiple copies (usually between one and twenty) in almost all isolates of *M. tuberculosis* so far studied and is also present in smaller numbers (usually one to five copies) in all isolates of *M. bovis*. BCG has either a single copy or two copies depending on the origin of the batch of vaccine[23]. With the exception of BCG, in which the position of the element(s) is fixed[24], the insertion sequences are scattered throughout the genome with considerable polymorphism between isolates.

Like virtually all bacteria, *M. tuberculosis* has a single circular chromosome. Following digestion with a restriction endonuclease, which will only cut the DNA at a specific motif, fragments of varying size will be generated. Because they are charged, these

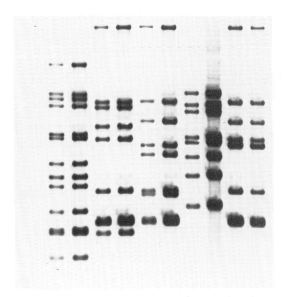

Fig. 17c.1   An example of DNA fingerprints from five isolates of *M. tuberculosis* from patients in central London. Each isolate has been subcultured both on solid and in liquid medium. The number and position of the bands varies from lane to lane. The are no differences in the patterns of isolates grown on solid or in liquid medium.

fragments can be separated by electrophoresis through an agarose gel and then transferred to a nylon membrane. A short piece of DNA complementary to the insertion element, labelled with horseradish peroxidase (Amersham, UK ECL gene detection system) is used as a probe. This will bind to the fragments of DNA on the membrane that contain the insertion element, and will then catalyse the oxidation of luminol, which generates light that can be detected by exposing photographic film to the membrane in an X-ray cassette to produce an autophotograph. This system avoids the safety and storage problems of radioactive probes, although the same result can be obtained with a radiolabelled probe. The resulting DNA fingerprint will consist of a variable number of bands at varying positions along a 'lane' of the photograph (Fig. 17c.1).

A consensus has recently been achieved between various groups using this technique to standardize the methodology in order to facilitate comparisons between different laboratories. The restriction endonuclease used is *Pvu*II, the probe is a specified fragment of IS*6110* and the same internal markers should be used by all groups.

17c.4 VALIDATION OF FINGERPRINTING

Fingerprinting studies in areas of both high and low endemicity have shown that there is much heterogeneity between clinical isolates of *M. tuberculosis*[25–27]. In general each clinical isolate has been shown to have a distinct banding pattern unless a group of isolates have arisen from a common source. In a study of about 50 strains, largely from the Netherlands, two groups of isolates were found with identical fingerprints[28]. One was a set of nine strains cultured from a cluster of patients thought to have been infected from a common source. The other group came from three patients, in whom subsequent investigation suggested a common source of infection was likely. Since then there have been several reports of outbreaks of tuberculosis in Europe[29] and the USA[6] in which fingerprints from patients within the clusters were identical while those from unrelated patients were all distinct.

In Central and East Africa, transmission of tuberculosis is more common, making clusters more difficult to identify. However, most isolates still have unique fingerprints although there is less heterogeneity[25,26]. Amongst 119 isolates from Malawi and Kenya, 71 had unique fingerprints while in 48 the pattern matched one or more other isolate. Of these 48, 32 were multiple isolates from the same individuals, and so would be expected to be identical. Of the remaining 16 strains, eight came from a rather close community of women in one particular district of Nairobi where it is possible that person-to-person spread was occurring. There was no obvious epidemiological link between the patients from whom the last eight isolates originated.

It may seem a paradox to use patterns generated by the position of insertion elements within the genome as an epidemiological marker. The only gene encoded on the insertion element is for the enzyme responsible for moving the element around the chromosome. The range of diversity seen in the number and positions of the elements in different strains attests to the efficacy of this transposition mechanism. However the rate of transposition appears to be sufficiently slow to use fingerprinting for such studies. Hermans and his colleagues[28] showed that neither repeated subculture nor passage through guinea-pigs altered the fingerprint pattern and in the few patients with relapsed tuberculosis in whom the original isolate had been stored, the recurrent strain has usually been identical to the stored one[30]. In one patient from Kenya, the recurrent strain differed from the original. The fingerprints of the two isolates were completely different, which would suggest that reinfection with a new strain had occurred rather than a transposition event within the original population of bacilli[31]. Similarly in most of the sequential isolates that have been studied, transposition has rarely occurred, although the numbers are rather small.

The finding that multiple isolates from the same individual are generally identical also suggests that in a particular infection the bacilli responsible are all of one strain. Further larger studies are required to confirm this point but it raises new questions about the pathogenesis of tuberculosis. Tuberculous infection follows inhalation of droplet nuclei containing a few bacilli in each. If the infector was only carrying one type of *M. tuberculosis*, the bacilli would all be of the same type and when, years later, they reawoke and broke through the infectee's immunity, multiple isolates would all be expected to be identical irrespective of how many of the original droplet nuclei had been

successful in establishing a dormant infection. If, however, we consider the situation in an endemic area, it is probable that many individuals have inhaled droplets from several different infectors. The data are consistent with the idea that only one of these is able to establish infection or that when reactivation occurs only one strain flourishes. Does the first encounter with *M. tuberculosis* generate a sufficient immune response to kill subsequent bacilli before infection is established? Presumably not, because exogenous reinfection in people who are known to be already infected (on the basis of a past history of tuberculosis or a positive tuberculin skin test) is well recognized to be able to lead to active disease.

17c.5 IDENTICAL FINGERPRINTS

DNA fingerprinting therefore provides a method for typing isolates of *M. tuberculosis* that seems well suited for research into the epidemiology and pathogenesis of tuberculosis. The patterns produced from an individual with tuberculosis are consistent, stable and heterogeneous. Isolates that share the same pattern are likely to have a common origin. The method is therefore appropriate for determining possible routes of transmission of disease and for tracking a particular isolate of interest, for example one that is resistant to standard antituberculosis drugs. However, there are important limitations to its use in surveillance. In order to identify clusters that were not suspected, it will be necessary to type isolates and compare fingerprints of each one with each other. As the size of the population grows, the number of comparisons rises rapidly and will require suitable pattern-recognition software and databases. Furthermore, most infections with *M. tuberculosis* lead either to latent infection or to progressive primary disease, which is frequently associated with negative cultures, so many instances of transmission will not be documented. The increased susceptibility of people infected with HIV to progressive disease following recent infection[6] may allow fingerprinting to be particularly useful in this context.

Another use for fingerprinting is for the detection of laboratory contamination, as illustrated by the following case history.

An HIV-infected man was admitted to hospital for investigation of a curious skin lesion. A biopsy revealed non-specific abnormalities and fungal cultures were negative. Treatment with topical antifungal ointment was given and over the next weeks the lesion improved. Several weeks later the cultures from the biopsy grew *M. tuberculosis*. In view of the resolving problem no further action was taken. The patient died shortly thereafter and at autopsy acid-fast bacilli were seen in the bowel wall. No mycobacteria could be cultured. Initially it was thought that the patient may have had a novel presentation of tuberculosis in association with HIV infection. However, a more likely explanation was provided by fingerprinting the isolate from the skin biopsy and also the only other isolate of *M. tuberculosis* that had grown from the samples processed in the mycobacteriology laboratory on the same day. Both isolates shared an identical pattern although the second patient, who had pulmonary tuberculosis, had no connection with the first patient and had never been treated in the same clinic. The most likely explanation is that during the processing of the two samples, live bacilli from one had been transferred to the other.

Similarly in studies of the effect of chemotherapeutic regimens on tuberculosis in Hong Kong, it was noted that in a few patients who had completed treatment satisfactorily and were symptomatically well, a single sputum sample grew *M. tuberculosis*. Comparison of the isolates from those patients with more typical relapsed disease with multiple positive cultures and symptoms showed that they were identical, confirming relapse whereas the 'isolated positive cultures' had distinct fingerprints from the original stored culture[32]. It is probable that these 'relapses' were due to laboratory contamination but differences in the fingerprints of original and recurrent isolates could also be due to reinfection rather than relapse being the cause of the recurrence. Among five HIV-seropositive Kenyan patients with recurrence of tuberculosis after satisfactory treatment and for whom the original isolate had been stored, one was found to have a new isolate at the time of recurrence while the other four still had the original strain[31]. To determine the contribution of reinfection and relapse to recurrence, large numbers of isolates will need to be stored prospectively and matched with subsequent cultures from the same individual.

17c.6 SIMILAR FINGERPRINTS

It is relatively straightforward to check whether fingerprint patterns from different strains of *M. tuberculosis* are identical or not; however, it may also be possible to use the similarity between non-identical isolates for epidemiological purposes. The factors that govern transposition and its mechanism are not known. In other model systems, when transposition occurs there is often a duplication of the insertion elements. The pressure to reduce the number of copies is less certain, although if the insertion disrupts other mycobacterial genes it may confer a selective disadvantage on that strain, which will then become extinct. It is of note that while *M. tuberculosis* functions effectively with 20 or more copies of IS*6110*, the number found in *M. bovis* is much fewer. Transposition will not be a random process and there are known to be particular sites at which integration is more likely[24]. If transposition was a truly random event it would be possible to compute the phylogenetic distance between any two isolates. None the less, it is a reasonable assumption that isolates that have more similar fingerprints evolved from a common ancestor more recently than those with less similar patterns.

The relatedness of different isolates of *M. tuberculosis* can be defined by a similarity coefficient between the fingerprints of the strains. Similarity coefficients (S_{AB}) can be calculated by the formula S_{AB} = [number of bands shared between A and B]/[(number of bands in A) + (number of bands in B) − (number of bands shared between A and B)]. This is a simplification of the formula used by Schmid and colleagues[33] and ignores differences in intensity of hybridization. Since *Pvu*II cuts at one end of the insertion sequence, there will only be a single copy of the target on a given restriction fragment. Assuming that different restriction fragments can be distinguished on the gel, each band should be an all or none signal. Identical isolates have an S_{AB} value of 1.0 whereas isolates with no bands in common have a value of 0.0.

A dendrogram can then be constructed from the matrix of S_{AB} values of any group of isolates. If transposition was a random event, the dendrogram could be transformed to a phylogenetic tree since D (a measure of phylogenetic distance) = -1n S_{AB}.

Whereas identity is easy to establish, the definition of a cluster of related isolates based on S_{AB} values or a dendrogram is arbitrary. Furthermore, the difficulties alluded to above in developing software for pattern recognition and storage are compounded when every band in every fingerprint has to be compared to define the dendrogram. If fingerprints of the same isolate, run on different gels, are compared between different autophotographs both visually and using a flatbed scanner and software designed to define the molecular weights of fragments, such as Gelreader Version 1.0 (public domain software from the National Center for Super-

computing Applications, University of Illinois at Urbana-Champaign), the variability between the molecular weights calculated by the computer for the same band on different gels is greater than that between different bands on the same gel. For small numbers of isolates (less than 30) it is possible to calculate S_{AB} values and construct a tree by visual inspection; however, the number of comparisons makes this method impractical for larger samples.

Despite these technical problems, there are early suggestions that fingerprint patterns from Africa are distinct from those from Europe[26] and that within Britain, indigenous tuberculosis differs from that imported from the Indian subcontinent[29]. Assuming that the size of the database continues to expand and that the problems of image analysis, storage and retrieval are unravelled, it may become possible to define the region of origin of a particular *M. tuberculosis* isolate. This would allow a clear definition of whether cases of post-primary tuberculosis had arisen by reactivation of endogenous infection or reinfection from a new source. There is now good evidence both for increased susceptibility of patients with HIV infection to new infection with accelerated disease progression[6] and also for increased risk of reactivation for those already latently infected with *M. tuberculosis*[7]. The relative contribution of the two mechanisms will differ according to the proportion of the population already infected with each pathogen and the risk of transmission of *M. tuberculosis* in a given setting. There are implications for public health. If reactivation remains the principal pathogenetic mechanism, chemoprophylaxis with a defined course of isoniazid or some other antituberculosis drug or drugs remains a valid approach. If, on the other hand, most disease is due to reinfection, prophylaxis will have to be life-long or other measures will be required to reduce the risk of acquiring disease.

The ability to define groups of *M. tuberculo-*

sis based on genetic analysis may also indirectly help detect phenotypic differences. It is known that some strains of *M. tuberculosis* are more virulent than others[2]. Are some strains also more likely to cause meningitis than others? Until the possibility of distinguishing different isolates, the emphasis has been on differences in the host's susceptibility. However, fingerprinting does not examine genes that might code for phenotypic differences, except in as much as the function of a particular gene may be disrupted by the insertion of an extra length of DNA. Whether closely related strains that shared similar fingerprints might also share similar determinants of virulence would depend on the relative frequency of change of fingerprint pattern compared with changes in phenotype. Once a strain has developed a particular characteristic, for instance multiple drug resistance, the progeny of that strain, which are likely also to be multiply resistant, will have identical or closely related fingerprint patterns. Small-scale surveillance to detect resistant strains more quickly than routine techniques might then be possible.

It has been known for some time that a limited range of strains of *M. avium-intracellulare* are found in patients with AIDS [34]. In Africa, *M. avium-intracellulare* has rarely been cultured from patients with HIV infection although it is cultivable from environmental samples (R. Brindle, personal communication). One explanation is that patients die earlier in the course of their HIV infection in Africa, before *M. avium-intracellulare* becomes established. However, other opportunist infections, such as cryptococcal meningitis, which also flourish only in the severely immunocompromised host, are seen quite commonly. Another question therefore is whether patients infected with HIV are particularly susceptible to some strains of *M. tuberculosis* or whether particular strains are more likely to reactivate.

17c.7 LIMITATIONS OF THE TECHNIQUE

As discussed earlier, to maximize the potential of fingerprinting for epidemiological studies, large numbers of isolates from different geographic regions will need to be compared. Current methods are sufficient to test the probabilities that a group of isolates of *M. tuberculosis* represent a cluster of infection. However, the difficulties with computerization make it much less likely that routine fingerprinting of isolates will allow a cluster to be detected *de novo*. Indeed, forensic DNA fingerprinting has tended to move away from multiple banding patterns towards single allele tests, partly because of difficulties in obtaining reliable comparisons between many bands. Sophisticated image-analysis systems already exist and it should prove possible to move from retrospective to prospective studies in the near future.

Fingerprinting may represent relatedness but it does not equate with genetic identity. The proportion of the genome studied is relatively small; only those restriction fragments that include a copy of the insertion element are visualized. In order to change the fingerprint pattern of an isolate a mutation would have to introduce a new restriction site close to a copy of the insertion element. Similarly, it would be possible for a large insertion or deletion to occur between two restriction sites with no insertion element affected and consequently no change in the fingerprint.

Before a fingerprint can be produced, a culture of *M. tuberculosis* has to be available. In studies of transmission this is frequently not the case. Similarly for looking for potentially drug-resistant secondary cases from a source there is an important delay while the bacilli grow. A method that used the polymerase chain reaction, or some other molecular amplification system, to detect polymorphisms based on the variable positions of insertion elements would be a real advance[35].

In view of the alarm caused by multi-drug

resistance in the USA, rapid methods for the detection of resistance will be a focus of research in the coming years. Mutations leading to resistance occur more frequently than transpositions, and fingerprint patterns do not change with the development of rifampicin resistance[36]. As mentioned above, once an isolate is known to be drug-resistant, fingerprint surveillance may detect transmission to other susceptible individuals. The finding that deletion of the mycobacterial catalase gene results in isoniazid resistance is the first molecular mechanism of resistance to be described in mycobacteria[37]. As others are described it will be possible to design rapid tests for the detection of resistance in cultured samples (Chapter 9, p. 171).

Fingerprinting with IS6110 produces patterns that distinguish individual isolates within the *M. tuberculosis* complex. It does not, however, separate the various species within the complex. Although *M. bovis* BCG has only one or two bands at fixed positions, as discussed above, the finding of bands in those positions does not rule out the possibility that the isolate is *M. tuberculosis* or a virulent *M. bovis*. The recent discovery of another unrelated insertion sequence, IS1081[38], may help. This element is much less mobile than IS6110. Fingerprinting with identical methods revealed a single pattern among 26 strains of *M. bovis* BCG that was not shared by any of 41 strains of *M. tuberculosis* and 32 strains of virulent *M. bovis*[39]. As further elements are described the particular uses that each may serve will need to be clarified.

17c.8 CONCLUSIONS

DNA fingerprinting of *M. tuberculosis* has already shown itself to be a useful new tool in studies of transmission of tuberculosis. It has given authority to observations on the changes that HIV has brought to the spread of tuberculosis. With the application of advances in image-analysis software and database handling, it should now prove possible to define the molecular epidemiology of tuberculosis on a global scale. Fundamental questions about pathogenesis and more pragmatic ones about clusters of cases can now be approached. The impact of the technique will be felt both among those in clinical care and among those in public health. Would more aggressive therapy reduce the chance of relapse in HIV-infected patients? Is the drug-resistant isolate spreading through our community? Is chemoprophylaxis a rational approach to tuberculosis control? The recent advances in our understanding of the molecular genetics of mycobacteria must rapidly be translated into innovative approaches to reverse the rising tide of tuberculosis.

REFERENCES

1. McFadden, J.J. (ed.) (1990) *Molecular Biology of the Mycobacteria*, Academic Press, London.
2. Grange, J.M., Aber, V., Allen, B. *et al.* (1978). The correlation of bacteriophage types of *Mycobacterium tuberculosis* with guinea-pig virulence and *in-vitro* indicators of virulence. *J. Gen. Microbiol.*, **108**, 1–7.
3. Jones, W.D. Jr. (1990) Geographic distribution of phage types among cultures of *Mycobacterium tuberculosis*. *Am. Rev. Respir. Dis.*, **142**, 1000–3.
4. Good, R.C. and Beam, R.E. (1984) Seroagglutination, in *The Mycobacteria: a Sourcebook*, (eds G.P. Kubica and L.G. Wayne), Marcel Decker, New York.
5. Butler, W.R., Jost, K.C. and Kolburn, J.O. (1991) Identification of mycobacteria by high-performance liquid chromatography. *J. Clin. Microbiol.*, **29**, 2468–72.
6. Daley, C.L., Small, P., Schecter, G. *et al.* (1992) An outbreak of tuberculosis with accelerated progresson among persons infected with human immunodeficiency virus. *N. Engl. J. Med.*, **326**, 231–5.
7. Selwyn, P.A., Hartel, D., Lewis, V.A. *et al.* (1989) A prospective study of the risk of tuberculosis among intravenous drug users with HIV infection. *N. Engl. J. Med.*, **320**, 545–50.
8. Elliott, A.M., Hayes, R.J., Halwindii, B. *et al.* The impact of human immunodeficiency virus

on infectiousness of pulmonary tuberculosis: a community study in Zambia. (Manuscript submitted.)

9. Britten, R.J. and Kohne, D.E. (1968) Repeated sequences in DNA. *Science*, **161**, 529–40.

10. Ohtsubo, H. and Otshubo, E. (1976) Isolation of inverted repeat sequences including IS1, IS2 and IS3, in *Escherichia coli* plasmids. *Proc. Natl. Acad. Sci. USA*, **73**, 2316–20.

11. Kiss, A., Sain, B. and Venetianer, P. (1977) The number of rRNA genes in *Escherichia coli*. *FEBS Lett.*, **79**, 77–9.

12. Stern, M.J., Ferro-Luzzi Ames, G., Smith, N.H. *et al.* (1984). Repetitive extragenic palindromic sequences: a major component of the bacterial chromosome. *Cell*, **37**, 1015–26.

13. Clewell, D.B., Tomich, P.K., Gawron-Burke, M.C. *et al.* (1982) Mapping of *Streptococcus faecalis* plasmids pAD1 and pAD2 and studies relating to transpostion of Tn917. *J. Bacteriol.*, **152**, 1220–30.

14. Campbell, A. (1981) Evolutionary significance of accessory DNA elements in bacteria. *Ann. Rev. Microbiol.*, **35**, 55–83.

15. Gill, P., Jeffreys, A.J. and Werret, D.J. (1985) Forensic application of DNA 'fingerprints'. *Nature*, **318**, 577–9.

16. Barker, R.H., Suebsaeng, H.L., Rooney, W. *et al.* (1986) Specific DNA probe for the diagnosis of *Plasmodium falciparum* malaria. *Science*, **231**, 1434–6.

17. Soll, D.R., Galsak R., Isley, S. *et al.* (1989), Switching of *Candida albicans* during successive episodes of recurrent vaginitis. *J. Clin. Microbiol.*, **27**, 681–90.

18. Reddi, P.P., Talwar, G.P. and Khandekar, P.S. (1988) Repetitive DNA sequence of *Mycobacterium tuberculosis*: analysis of differential hybridization pattern with other mycobacteria. *Int. J. Lepr.*, **56**, 592–7.

19. Eisenach, K.D., Crawford, J.T. and Bates, J.H. (1988) Repetitive DNA sequences as probes for *Mycobacterium tuberculosis*. *J. Clin. Micro.*, **26**, 2240–45.

20. Zainuddin, Z.F. and Dale, J.W. (1989) Polymorphic repetitive DNA sequences in *Mycobacterium tuberculosis* detected with a gene probe from a *Mycobacterium fortuitum* plasmid. *J. Gen. Microbiol.*, **135**, 2347–55.

21. McAdam, R.A., Hermans, P.W.M., van Soolingen, D. *et al.* (1990) Characterization of a *Mycobacterium tuberculosis* insertion sequence belonging to the IS3 family. *Molec. Microbiol.*, **4**, 1607–13.

22. Thierry, D., Cave, M.D., Eisenach, K.D. *et al.* (1990) IS6110, an IS-like element of *Mycobacterium tuberculosis* complex. *Nucleic Acids Res.*, **18**, 188.

23. Fomukong, N.G., Dale, J.W., Osborn, T.W. and Grange, J.M. (1992) Use of gene probes based on the insertion sequence IS986 to differentiate between BCG vaccine strains. *J. Appl. Bacteriol.*, **72**, 126–33.

24. Hermans, P.W.M., van Soolingen, D., Bik, E.M. *et al.* (1991) Insertion element IS987 from *Mycobacterium bovis* BCG is located in a hot-spot integration region for insertion elements in *Mycobacterium tuberculosis* complex strains. *Infect. Immun.*, **59**, 2695–705.

25. Godfrey-Faussett, P. and Stoker, N.G. (1992) Genetic 'fingerprinting' for clues to the pathogenesis of tuberculosis. *Trans. Roy. Soc. Trop. Med. Hyg.*, 86, 472–5.

26. van Soolingen, D., Hermans, P.W.M., de Haas, P.E.W. *et al.* (1991) Occurrence and stability of insertion sequences in *Mycobacterium tuberculosis* complex strains: evaluation of an insertion sequence-dependent DNA polymorphism as a tool in the epidemiology of tuberculosis *J. Clin. Microb.*, **29**, 2578–86.

27. Cave, M.D., Eisenach, K.D., McDermott, P.F. (1991) IS6110: conservation of sequence in the *Mycobacterium tuberculosis* complex and its utilization in DNA fingerprinting. *Mol. Cell. Probes*, **5**, 73–80.

28. Hermans, P.W.M., van Soolingen, D., Dale, J.W. *et al.* (1990) Insertion element IS986 from *Mycobacterium tuberculosis*: a useful tool for diagnosis and epidemiology of tuberculosis. *J. Clin. Microb.*, **28**, 2051–8.

29. Godfrey-Fausset, P., Mortimer, P.P., Jenkins, P.A. *et al* (1992) Evidence of transmission of tuberculosis by DNA fingerprinting. *Br. Med. J.*, **305**, 221–223.

30. Otal, I., Martin C., Vincent-Levy-Frebault, V. *et al.* (1991) Restriction fragment length polymorphism analysis using IS6110 as an epidemiological marker in tuberculosis. *J. Clin. Microb.*, **29**, 1252–4.

31. Godfrey-Fausset, P., Githui, W., Batchelor, B. *et al.* (1993) Recurrence of HIV-related tuberculosis in an endemic area may be due to relapse or reinfection *Tuberc. Lung Dis.* (in press).

32. Das, S., Chan, S.L., Allen, B.W. *et al.* (1993)

Application of DNA fingerprinting with IS*986* to sequential mycobacterial isolates obtained from pulmonary tuberculosis patients in Hong Kong before, during and after short-course chemotherapy. *Tuberc. Lung Dis.*, **74**, 47–51.

33. Schmid, J., Voss, E. and Soll, D.R. (1990) Computer-assisted methods for assessing strain relatedness in *Candida albicans* by fingerprinting with moderately repetitive sequence Ca3. *J. Clin. Microb.*, **28**, 1236–43.

34. Hampson, S.J., Portaels, F., Thompson, J. *et al.* (1989) DNA probes demonstrate a single highly conserved strain of *Mycobacterium avium* infecting AIDS patients. *Lancet*, **i**, 65–8.

35. Wilson, S.M., McNerney, R., Nye, P.M. *et al.* (1993) Progress toward a simplified Polymerase Chain Reaction and its application to the diagnosis of tuberculosis. *J. Clin. Microbiol.*, **31**, 776–82.

36. Godfrey-Faussett, P., Stoker, N.G., Scott, J.A.G. *et al.* (1993) DNA fingerprints of *Mycobacterium tuberculosis* do not change during the development of rifampicin resistance. *Tuberc. Lung Dis.* (in press).

37. Zhang, Y., Heym, B., Allen, B. *et al.* (1992) The catalase-peroxidase gene and isoniazid resistance of *Mycobacterium tuberculosis*. *Nature*, **358**, 591–3.

38. Collins, D.M. and Stephens, D.M. (1991) Identification of the insertion seequence, IS*1081*, in *Mycobacterium bovis*. *FEMS Microbiol. Lett.*, **83**, 11–16.

39. van Soolingen, D., Hermans, P.W.M., de Haas, P.E.W. *et al.* (1992) Insertion element IS*1081*-associated restriction fragment length polymorphisms in *Mycobacterium tuberculosis* complex species: a reliable tool for recognizing *Mycobacterium bovis* BCG. *J. Clin. Microb.*, **30**, 1772–7.

CONCLUSIONS

18

P.D.O. Davies

18.1 INTRODUCTION

Mycobacterium tuberculosis remains the single most successful pathogen in causing morbidity and mortality of the human race. There can now be little doubt that tuberculosis cases are increasing in so many areas of the globe that an increase in total cases year by year is resulting. Yet it is the relatively small increase in some developed countries, such as the USA and the UK, that has focused the world's attention once more on the disease it thought was dead, and forced the developed world to look once again to the developing world, parts of which are experiencing a several-fold increase in tuberculosis case rates within a decade.

The most important reason for this global increase is the spread of HIV infection, which causes immunocompromization and resultant increased susceptibility to tuberculosis infection so that overt disease develops in dually infected individuals. It is also becoming increasingly apparent that other factors may be implicated in this increase of disease, such as longevity of the elderly and worsening social deprivation among some sections of society in the developed nations.

The globe is now so small, and readiness of access so easy from one part to another, particularly with the demise of the Iron Curtain, that one nation's tuberculosis problem is every nation's tuberculosis problem. The enormous increases in tuberculosis we are witnessing is sub-Saharan Africa (Chapter 12b) may be only a foretaste of what is to come over the next few decades as HIV infection takes a hold in Asia, where four-fifths of the world population infected with the tubercle bacillus resides.

There is a temptation to feel that nothing can be done; to accept with resignation that the white plague will have to fall across the globe for a second time in two centuries, taking its toll without worthwhile resistance from modern medical science. But this would be too gloomy an outlook on the likely course of events.

Enarson (Chapter 2, p. 30) has pointed out that even in countries where HIV-related tuberculosis is rampant, rates of disease are an order of magnitude less than they were in the now developed world a century and a half ago, or than they were among some populations such as the Iniut Indians of Northern Canada as recently as 40 years ago. Despite the apparent large-scale fatality in some populations owing to HIV-related tuberculosis, there may be evidence that the global population is more resistant to the bacillus than it was during its last passage across the face of the earth.

The upsurge of disease has reawakened the scientific world to the need to apply 1990s technology to a disease that has traditionally been the Cinderella of all diseases in terms of the provision of research and resources for the past two decades.

Clinical Tuberculosis. Edited by P.D.O. Davies. Published in 1994 by Chapman & Hall, London. ISBN 0 412 48630 X

18.2 MICROBIOLOGY AND DIAGNOSIS

Identifying acid- and alcohol-fast bacilli from specimens by staining methods is in practice the only sure means of establishing a diagnosis of tuberculosis, and culturing bacilli the only means of confirming the diagnosis, 110 years after *M. tuberculosis* was identified as the causative organism. Microbiology therefore remains the only sure method of diagnosis but is both too insensitive for smear-negative or extra-pulmonary disease, and too slow for confirmation of a great proportion of cases.

Serological methods of diagnosis have no more than 90% specificity and 90% sensitivity but even with improved techniques will never be cheap or robust enough to use in developing countries (Chapter 17a). The polymerase chain-reaction technique (PCR) (Chapter 17b) has lead to a huge spate of publications but doubts remain as to its specificity to distinguish between *M. tuberculosis* and other mycobacteria or between overt disease, healed disease or infection. Even with massive improvements in technique, cost is likely to preclude its use in developing countries.

18.3 IMMUNOPATHOLOGY

Much of the immunopathology of tuberculosis remains to be elucidated. The two-stage process of the disease, primary and post-primary, results from a very complex series of immune reactions, which depend on genetic and environmental factors. The application of modern techniques has shown a number of factors, such as interferon gamma, tumour necrosis factor and calcitriol, to be implicated in the immune process and resultant disease and tissue damage of post-primary tuberculosis (Chapter 5, p. 55).

HIV infection suppresses the immune responses responsible for both the protection and the necrosis in post-primary disease so that progressive disseminated disease may result. Tuberculosis also enhances HIV replication, resulting in a speeding of the onset of AIDS.

Some workers in tuberculosis see a hope for treatment in the immuno-modulation of disease by vaccination with *M. vaccae*. Reports of its success remain anecdotal but are strong enough to warrant a full clinical trial, which is currently being planned (Chapter 12b, p. 259).

18.4 CLINICAL DISEASE

Forty years ago a textbook on tuberculosis would have had a relatively small section on non-respiratory disease. It is no accident that the chapter on non-respiratory disease in this book (Chapter 7) is larger than that on respiratory disease (Chapter 6). The increasingly common presentation of non-respiratory disease in immigrants to developed countries, and in HIV-infected patients, has confirmed the clinical importance of non-respiratory disease. It should therefore be borne in mind that tuberculosis can present in any site or organ of the body.

Symptoms and signs may be absent or occur relatively late on in the disease process. Commonly, tuberculosis presents with a gradual onset of malaise, weight loss and pyrexia. If pulmonary disease is present, respiratory symptoms such as cough, with or without haemoptysis, breathlessness or rarely chest pain may be present. Physical signs are usually fewer than chest radiology would suggest. Tuberculosis at any site is usually slow in onset and can easily be missed if not considered.

As with any infection the golden rule must be to try to obtain specimens for diagnosis, for smear and culture, before treatment is commenced. This is frequently not carried out when biopsies are taken from a non-respiratory site. A specimen should always be sent in normal saline for culture as well as in formalin for histology.

18.5 TREATMENT

Standard treatment for most forms of tuberculosis should now be isoniazid, rifampicin and pyrazinamide for 2 months followed by isoniazid and rifampicin for 4 months (2HRZ/ 4HR). The substitution of these drugs with others will prolong therapy; the addition of other drugs is unnecessary except where drug resistance is suspected. Most authorities would consider 2 months of the three drugs followed by 10 months of the two drugs necessary for adequate treatment of tuberculous meningitis. Treatment of relapsed cases may require longer therapy and, if drug resistance is suspected, ethambutol or streptomycin should be included initially.

Unfortunately the expense of rifampicin has meant that many countries have been unable to afford its use, thus prolonging chemotherapy and increasing the likelihood of default and relapse. The present plight of Africa may have been considerably prevented if rifampicin-containing regimens had been used during the 1970s and 1980s when it became available rather than the considerably less-effective thiacetazone. Co-ordinated international co-operation to supply rifampicin free to areas with suitable programmes, which may offer some help in ameliorating the present increase in cases, should be considered. The use of rifampicin-containing regimens in Asia where tuberculosis-related HIV is very likely to accelerate should also be considered an international priority. As Harries points out in Chapter 12b (p. 244), rifampicin-containing regimens, are in fact more cost-effective than the longer non-rifampicin regimens.

The use of steroids in the treatment of tuberculosis has always been a subject of contention. Corticosteroids are of proven efficacy in the treatment of pleural and pericardial disease (Chapter 6, p. 87; Chapter 7, p. 113) and are of probable value in reducing ureteric strictures in genitourinary disease provided they are given early enough (Chapter 7, p. 114). They have also been shown to reduce mortality and morbidity in tuberculous meningitis (Chapter 7, p. 106). Their use in other forms of tuberculosis remains controversial but should be investigated further with clinical trials.

18.6 DRUG-RESISTANT TUBERCULOSIS

Some drug resistance, whether primary or secondary, has been a feature of treating tuberculosis since streptomycin was first introduced in 1944. The strains of bacteria resistant to first- and second-line drugs now isolated mainly in parts of the USA, present a new and worrying prospect to the future chemotherapy of the disease (Chapter 9).

It is likely that a combination of poor prescribing, inadequate compliance and increased susceptibility to infection with HIV have combined to produce multi-drug resistant (MDR) tuberculosis. Provided adequate precautions are taken, such as isolation of those individuals affected until rendered sputum smear-negative, and suitable therapy given, which may include surgical intervention (Chapter 8c), there is no reason why MDR tuberculosis should become a global problem. Improved combined prescribing and dispensing the combination product Rifater (isoniazid, rifampicin and pyrazinamide) and the product Rifamate, Rimactazid or Rifinah (isoniazid and rifampicin) will play a major part in preventing the re-emergence of new MDR strains. It is important that such measures are undertaken where MDR tuberculosis is a problem. It would be the greatest tragedy of modern medicine if tuberculosis was once again rendered untreatable by medical means owing to bad medical practice.

18.7 TUBERCULOSIS OF IMMIGRANTS AND ETHNIC MINORITIES

Tuberculosis among immigrants and ethnic minorities probably represents the largest single reason for the increase in disease in the developed world (Chapter 10), as it is these groups where the highest rates of tuberculosis infection and disease reside. Where HIV has reached these groups, such as in areas of New York, rates of disease have risen dramatically. Tuberculosis services therefore need to be targeted to areas where these individuals live and appropriate screening procedures carried out, at port of entry or in the community.

Restriction of immigration owing to fear of disease is unhelpful and likely to be counterproductive. There is no evidence that tuberculosis among ethnic minorities is spread to the indigenous population but new techniques such as DNA fingerprinting (Chapter 17c) may be useful in investigating this possibility.

The reader will notice a contradiction between Enarson, who does not believe rates of disease are highest in new immigrants (Chapter 2, p. 26) and myself (Chapter 10, p. 200) who does. Enarson believes that the high rates seen in immigrants within 5 years of arrival are due to the high numbers of visiting immigrants such as students, who are only resident for a short time. High rates soon after immigration are therefore factitious due to an under-estimate of total numbers resident for 0–5 years in the country of adoption. It must be conceded that Canada has accurate data available on immigrants by year of entry and length of stay and these have enabled Enarson to draw his conclusions. The less accurate statistics from the UK certainly give the impression of higher rates soon after immigration, reducing steadily thereafter (Chapter 10, p. 196, Table 10.1). Evidence of high rates after a visit to the country of origin by an immigrant would tend to support this theory (Chapter 10, p. 197). It may be that experience differs between Canada and other nations. Either hypothesis does not affect the practical implications that these groups deserve targeted tuberculosis screening and resources.

18.8 PREVENTION

There is interesting division of the globe into countries that believe BCG has a place in the role of preventing tuberculosis infection and those, notably the USA, that do not. The arguments against BCG are, briefly, that trials of its efficacy are conflicting (Chapter 14b, p. 299) and that its use renders an individual tuberculin test positive, therefore confusing the interpretation of skin testing when considering chemoprophylaxis.

In contrast, BCG is used widely in developed and developing countries, where it may be given at birth, such as in parts of Africa, at about the time of puberty, such as in the UK, or both, such as in Hong Kong. Its efficacy of 75% protection over 15 years when given to teenage children has been consistently shown by UK studies since its first use 40 years ago. Though BCG does convert a tuberculin test-negative individual to tuberculin-positive, the degree of positivity from BCG alone can usually be distinguished from the degree of positivity from infection by *M. tuberculosis* (Chapter 15d. p. 347). Now that disease rates have fallen in developed countries, the debate is whether and when to stop such a vaccination programme.

Chemoprophylaxis of infected individuals is of proven efficacy (Chapter 14a) but there is an age cut-off where the frequency of adverse effects outweighs the possible benefit. Isoniazid alone for 6–12 months is the one form of prophylaxis that is clinically proven. Recent concern over isoniazid-induced hepatitis suggests that prophylaxis should be targeted carefully. There is increasing concern over the use of a single drug as prophylaxis in the presence of HIV infection where host immunity is compromised. This may cause a single drug to be ineffective and, of even greater concern, drug-resistant disease may emerge. Studies are currently in progress to investigate this.

Combined isoniazid and rifampicin for prophylaxis is used in some developed nations as this reduces the length of prophylaxis to 3 or 4 months and drug resistance would be most unlikely even if active disease developed. This regimen would be beyond the financial reach of most developing nations.

18.9 DISEASE CONTROL

WHO guidelines aim to achieve 85% cure and 75% case-finding of smear-positive cases. It is in areas of the developed world, such as inner cities, that have failed to achieve these guidelines, where tuberculosis rates are increasing rapidly. A recent paper from New York showed that only 10% of patients were followed-up long enough to achieve cure.

The principles of disease control are simple and cheap. They are:

1. The provision of a service for the diagnosis of patients presenting with disease, to treat those patients and to ensure full compliance for a period long enough to effect cure. In most cases where short-course chematherapy is used this is 6 months.
2. The provision of a service to screen those at greatest risk of developing tuberculosis. In practice, a minimal service would screen close contacts of those with smear-positive pulmonary disease.

This service could also provide strongly tuberculin-positive close contacts with follow-up and/or prophylaxis as appropriate and provide vaccination for tuberculin-negative individuals at risk of incurring infection.

This has traditionally been achieved using a system of compulsory notification so that a clinician diagnosing a case of tuberculosis is legally required to inform by notification the proper officer responsible for disease control for the local authority area in which the patient resides. The local authority officer responsible for disease control can then co-ordinate contact tracing. In practice a specialist tuberculosis nurse can carry out home visiting to ensure that patients being treated for tuberculosis take their treatment at home and attend clinic as required. The same nurse can also undertake contact tracing to ensure that contacts at risk of developing disease are screened. This system requires at least one full-time equivalent specialist tuberculosis nurse for each area per 50 cases per year (Chapter 15c). The larger the area or the more difficult the access to homes, the fewer cases a single nurse will be able to manage adequately.

Facilities for management of patients, and screening of contacts can usually be provided at a local chest clinic, for each authority area, staffed by a physician trained and experienced in the management of tuberculosis.

Current mishandling of tuberculosis at local and national level has arisen because the reduction in the number of cases in many developed countries has lead to a dismantling of the national notification system in some countries, a loss of specialist tuberculosis nurses in many areas, and an atrophy of expertise and experience among clinicians responsible for managing the disease.

The upsurge in tuberculosis in the developed and developing world has taught us that these services must be maintained until the last case of tuberculosis is cured. Ideally, a similar system for control should be available in developing countries but difficulty in communications may preclude national statistical collecting. Nationally agreed programmes are available (Chapter 15b, p. 335) where, despite few resources, the WHO target of near to 85% cure and 70% case-finding can be achieved.

National government commitment is fundamental to a successful control programme, which should be permanent and organized throughout the nation. Only then can the necessary structures be set up and staff be made available. A clear protocol needs to be drawn up so that co-ordination can take place at central, regional, district and dispensary level. The first requirement is for accurate recording of cases to provide a district register (Chapter 15b, p. 330). This should include outcome of treatment. The effectiveness of the programme can then be evaluated.

Sufficient drug supplies must be available and the means to provide directly observed therapy, through visits to dispensary, in-patient beds or home visitors, made possible. Tuberculosis programmes in developing countries are the most cost-effective of all medical interventions because of the importance to the national economy of the majority of the patients, who are in early adult life.

18.10 THE FUTURE

As far as anything can be foreseen, tuberculosis is likely to increase globally for the next decade and further. This is primarily due to HIV impacting on tuberculosis-infected individuals in Asia. HIV is unlikely to cause a substantial increase in tuberculosis in developed countries except among minorities where a high incidence of infection resides, such as ethnic minorities, recent immigrants from the developing world and the homeless.

The cost of drugs in the treatment of tuberculosis should not be a problem provided there is broad enough international co-operation. To cure everyone in the world who has disease at this moment, in drug terms alone would cost less than one billion US dollars (Chapter 15b, Table 15b.5). It is the co-ordination at local level that is the difficult aspect of disease control and where resources, both in the developed and developing world, need to be targeted.

These control programmes will have to be maintained or strengthened, or implemented as required, in all countries. A new generation of tuberculosis workers, visitors, nurses and doctors will need to be trained. Research into new drugs or existing drugs that are known to kill *M. tuberculosis* will need to be increased. New diagnostic techniques, particularly to obtain quicker confirmation of disease and sensitivities to confirm disease are urgently needed. The recently described methods of detecting drug resistance by bioilluminescence may prove a major step forward. Of most use would be a new vaccine, providing much more protection than BCG. The future does not look good, but neither did it in 1880 nor in 1940 when the greatest advances in the means to combat tuberculosis were about to be made.

REFERENCE

1. Israel, H.L. (1993) Chemoprophylaxis for tuberculosis (Editorial). *Respir. Med.*, **87**, 81–3.
2. Jacobs, W., Barletta, R.G., Udani, R. *et al.* Rapid assessment of drug susceptibilities of *M. tuberculosis* by means of luciferase reporter phages. *Science*, **260**, 819–22.

INDEX

Page numbers in **bold** refer to figures, those in *italics* refer to tables.